# Innovation and Change in Professional Education

Volume 17

**Series editor**

Wim H. Gijselaers, School of Business and Economics, Maastricht University,
The Netherlands

**Associate editors**

L.A. Wilkerson, Dell Medical School at the University of Texas at Austin, TX, USA
H.P.A. Boshuizen, Center for Learning Sciences and Technologies,
Open Universiteit Nederland, Heerlen, The Netherlands

**Editorial Board**

Eugene L. Anderson, Anderson Policy Consulting & APLU, Washington, DC, USA
Hans Gruber, Institute of Educational Science, University of Regensburg,
Regensburg, Germany
Rick Milter, Carey Business School, Johns Hopkins University, Baltimore, MD, USA
Eun Mi Park, JH Swami Institute for International Medical Education,
Johns Hopkins University School of Medicine, Baltimore, MD, USA

**SCOPE OF THE SERIES**

The primary aim of this book series is to provide a platform for exchanging experiences and knowledge about educational innovation and change in professional education and post-secondary education (engineering, law, medicine, management, health sciences, etc.). The series provides an opportunity to publish reviews, issues of general significance to theory development and research in professional education, and critical analysis of professional practice to the enhancement of educational innovation in the professions.

The series promotes publications that deal with pedagogical issues that arise in the context of innovation and change of professional education. It publishes work from leading practitioners in the field, and cutting edge researchers. Each volume is dedicated to a specific theme in professional education, providing a convenient resource of publications dedicated to further development of professional education.

More information about this series at http://www.springer.com/series/6087

Debra Nestel • Kirsten Dalrymple • John T. Paige
Rajesh Aggarwal
Editors

# Advancing Surgical Education

Theory, Evidence and Practice

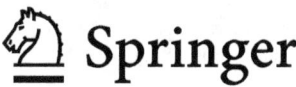

*Editors*
Debra Nestel
Faculty of Medicine, Nursing & Health
Sciences, Monash Institute for Health
and Clinical Education
Monash University
Clayton, VIC, Australia

Faculty of Medicine Dentistry & Health
Sciences, Department of Surgery,
Melbourne Medical School
University of Melbourne
Parkville, Australia

John T. Paige
Department of Surgery
Louisiana State University School
of Medicine
New Orleans, LA, USA

Kirsten Dalrymple
Faculty of Medicine
Imperial College London
London, UK

Rajesh Aggarwal
Department of Surgery, Sidney Kimmel
Medical College
Thomas Jefferson University
Philadelphia, PA, USA

Jefferson Strategic Ventures
Jefferson Health
Philadelphia, PA, USA

ISSN 1572-1957          ISSN 2542-9957    (electronic)
Innovation and Change in Professional Education
ISBN 978-981-13-3127-5     ISBN 978-981-13-3128-2   (eBook)
https://doi.org/10.1007/978-981-13-3128-2

© Springer Nature Singapore Pte Ltd. 2019
This work is subject to copyright. All rights are reserved by the Publisher, whether the whole or part of the material is concerned, specifically the rights of translation, reprinting, reuse of illustrations, recitation, broadcasting, reproduction on microfilms or in any other physical way, and transmission or information storage and retrieval, electronic adaptation, computer software, or by similar or dissimilar methodology now known or hereafter developed.
The use of general descriptive names, registered names, trademarks, service marks, etc. in this publication does not imply, even in the absence of a specific statement, that such names are exempt from the relevant protective laws and regulations and therefore free for general use.
The publisher, the authors, and the editors are safe to assume that the advice and information in this book are believed to be true and accurate at the date of publication. Neither the publisher nor the authors or the editors give a warranty, express or implied, with respect to the material contained herein or for any errors or omissions that may have been made. The publisher remains neutral with regard to jurisdictional claims in published maps and institutional affiliations.

This Springer imprint is published by the registered company Springer Nature Singapore Pte Ltd.
The registered company address is: 152 Beach Road, #21-01/04 Gateway East, Singapore 189721, Singapore

# Foreword by Richard Canter

This book is a timely and exciting addition to the surgical education literature. Let me explain why. The last 30 years or so has seen a transformation in surgical education with three distinct elements of change: organisational to university-based systems of quality, provider to demand-led delivery of service and surgeon to surgeon-educator. Arguably the most important of these has been surgeon to surgeon-educator because of the ability to scale up excellence. A highly skilled surgeon may, for example, complete 10,000 operations in a career and hopefully bring improvements to 10,000 patients. If at the same time they develop 20 surgical trainees to the same level of excellence, who themselves go onto complete 10,000 operations, then the spread of excellence is exponentially increased. The point is rapidly approaching when surgeons not only develop other surgeons to a standard of excellence but also pass on the educational skills for them to do the same. This means that there is the potential over a surgical generation or two for the excellent practice of a single surgeon to influence thousands or even millions of patients. So far, so good. Unfortunately, the same argument can be applied to the spread of poor practice and the capacity to do harm. This is the reason why research into surgical education, and how to develop excellence in yourself and others, is so important. This book is not only timely but also important for patient welfare.

The discipline of surgical education has spawned a real and increasing interest in education theory, practice and research with many choosing to adopt significant roles as educators in their institutions. The four editors have identified expertise from experienced researchers and brought together a set of fascinating chapters linking practice, theory, evidence and research methods. For anyone interested in surgical education, and in particular in education research, this has got to be a first choice book to read. Why? Because the breathtaking range of topics that now cover the field of surgical education will disturb some basic assumptions about relevant topic, what constitutes evidence, the choice of research paradigm, the selection of methodology and relevant literature so will encourage you to go on an intellectual journey of discovery. Don't be surprised if one evening you find yourself reading philosophers like Foucault and others and enjoying the challenge of new unexpected ideas that are relevant to surgery. Surgery, surgical education and surgeons have all changed so much in such a short time, and yet this is only the beginning.

Nuffield Department of Surgery  Richard Canter
University of Oxford
Oxford, UK

# Foreword by Christopher Christophi

The concept and the need of a textbook specifically on surgical education was envisaged and developed following the recognition of the global and broader need for professional development in health professions education.

The Royal Australasian College of Surgeons and the University of Melbourne's Department of Surgery have implemented the highly successful graduate programmes in surgical education, initiated by Prof. John Collins and implemented by one of the editors of this book – Prof. Debra Nestel. This book is a logical sequela to these programmes and makes compelling reading for any person committed to surgical education and aspires to leadership in this rapidly expanding field. The editors have brought together an outstanding group of contributors comprising experienced, internationally recognised authors and national contributors comprehensively addressing concepts and topics pertaining to surgical education.

Apart from being a knowledge and reference resource, this pioneering book is global in perspective, provocative and challenges established dogma. It is divided into five sections and follows a sequence initially addressing governance and theories of surgical education and the practical aspects faced by those at the coalface of this specialty. It concludes by addressing research aspects and the future directions.

This book will prove to be an indispensable armamentarium to those involved in this evolving field and reflects the expertise and enthusiasm of the editors and contributors.

Department of Surgery                                   Christopher Christophi
University of Melbourne
Parkville, VIC, Australia

# Foreword by Carlos Pellegrini

The focus of *Advancing Surgical Education: Theory, Evidence and Practice* is on residency and post-residency training. Recognizing that most of the training and education of surgeons is done by surgeons and that most surgeons are not necessarily equipped with the skills and knowledge needed to provide the most effective and efficient education and training to their trainees, the book is intended to fill this gap with a comprehensive description of the theories, the evidence and the practice of modern surgical education. Each of the five parts of the book provides unique insights into a different aspect related to education. The first part deals with a lot of the historical aspects, the role of leadership and governance in surgical education. The second part of the book delves deeply into the theories that underpin educational practices. It explores the science of learning and the science of teaching, and while this portion of the book will certainly appeal to those who are in charge of teaching programmes, I believe some of its chapters (like the role of power in surgical education, the construction of the surgeon identity, etc.,) will equally be of interest to those surgeons in the trenches – those that are involved in the daily teaching of residents and fellows. The third part of the book, dedicated to the practice of surgical education, is in itself a complete compendium dealing with the design and implementation of surgical education and training activities at the intersection of service and education. It provides advice on recruitment, on the role of feedback, on the role of assessment all the way to certification and revalidation, on the management of underperformance and on training and safety and is a "must" for everyone involved, including the trainees themselves. The fourth part of the book deals with research in surgical education, and this portion reflects the background and extraordinary expertise of the editors themselves, assembled from some of the best programmes around the world. This part of the book is recommended to young faculty members who wish to start their scholarly involvement in the field of education. The last part of the book describes the future state of surgical education and training and provides a "destination postcard" for 2030. All in all, this book provides a plethora of information and guidance that will serve surgeon-teachers around the world in the years to come.

Professor, Department of Surgery                                      Carlos Pellegrini
University of Washington
Seattle, WA, USA
Chief Medical Officer
UW Medicine
Seattle, WA, USA
Vice-President for Medical Affairs
University of Washington
Seattle, WA, USA

# Contents

1    **Celebrating Surgical Education**........................................................... 1
Debra Nestel, Kirsten Dalrymple, and John T. Paige

**Part I   Overview: Foundations of Surgical Education**

2    **Surgical Education: A Historical Perspective**....................................... 9
Roger Kneebone

3    **The Contemporary Context of Surgical Education**............................ 17
Adrian Anthony and Vijayaragavan Muralidharan

4    **Surgical Education Leadership and the Role of the Academy**........... 33
Peter Gogalniceanu, Margaret Hay, and Nizam Mamode

5    **The Governance of Surgical Education: The Role of the Colleges**..... 45
Ian Eardley

**Part II   Overview: Theories Informing Surgical Education**

6    **Cognitive Neuroscience and Design of Surgical Education**................ 57
David Bartle and Andrew Evans

7    **Expertise Theories and the Design of Surgical Education**................. 69
Alexander Harris

8    **Helping Learners Through Transitions: Threshold Concepts, Troublesome Knowledge and Threshold Capability Framework in Surgery** .......................................................................... 79
Simon Blackburn, Julian Smith, and Debra Nestel

9    **Communities of Practice and Surgical Training**................................. 95
Tasha A. K Gandamihardja and Debra Nestel

10   **Activity Theory and the Surgical Workplace**..................................... 105
Edward F. Ibrahim

| 11 | The Role of Power in Surgical Education: A Foucauldian Perspective | 115 |

Nancy McNaughton and Ryan Snelgrove

| 12 | Constructing Surgical Identities: Being and Becoming a Surgeon | 123 |

Roberto Di Napoli and Niall Sullivan

| 13 | Constructing Surgical Identities: Becoming a Surgeon Educator | 133 |

Tamzin Cuming and Jo Horsburgh

## Part III  Overview: The Practice of Surgical Education

| 14 | Designing Surgical Education Programs | 145 |

Jennifer Choi and Dimitrios Stefanidis

| 15 | Selection into Surgical Education and Training | 157 |

John P. Collins, Eva M. Doherty, and Oscar Traynor

| 16 | Models of Teaching and Learning in the Operating Theatre | 171 |

Alexandra Cope, Jeff Bezemer, and Gary Sutkin

| 17 | Supporting the Development of Psychomotor Skills | 183 |

Pamela Andreatta and Paul Dougherty

| 18 | Patients and Surgical Education: Rethinking Learning, Practice and Patient Engagement | 197 |

Rosamund Snow, Margaret Bearman, and Rick Iedema

| 19 | The Role of Verbal Feedback in Surgical Education | 209 |

Elizabeth Molloy and Charlotte Denniston

| 20 | The Role of Assessment in Surgical Education | 221 |

P. Szasz and T. P. Grantcharov

| 21 | Entrustable Professional Activities in Surgical Education | 229 |

Stephen Tobin

| 22 | Revalidation of Surgeons in Practice | 239 |

Ajit K. Sachdeva

| 23 | Demystifying Program Evaluation for Surgical Education | 255 |

Alexis Battista, Michelle Yoon, E. Matthew Ritter, and Debra Nestel

| 24 | Simulation in Surgical Education | 269 |

Rajesh Aggarwal

| 25 | Developing Surgical Teams: Theory | 279 |

John T. Paige

| 26 | Developing Surgical Teams: Application | 289 |

John T. Paige

| 27 | Supporting the Development of Professionalism in Surgeons in Practice: A Virtues-Based Approach to Exploring a Surgeon's Moral Agency | 303 |
|---|---|---|
| | Linda de Cossart CBE and Della Fish | |
| 28 | Managing Underperformance in Trainees | 313 |
| | Jonathan Beard and Hilary Sanfey | |
| 29 | Patient Safety and Surgical Education | 327 |
| | S. D. Marshall and R. M. Nataraja | |

## Part IV  Research in Surgical Education

| 30 | Researching in Surgical Education: An Orientation | 341 |
|---|---|---|
| | Rola Ajjawi and Craig McIlhenny | |
| 31 | Researching in Surgical Education: A Surgeon Perspective | 353 |
| | Rhea Liang | |
| 32 | From Dense Fog to Gentle Mist: Getting Started in Surgical Education Research | 363 |
| | Deb Colville and Catherine Green | |
| 33 | Reviewing Literature for and as Research | 377 |
| | Nigel D'Souza and Geoff Wong | |
| 34 | Measuring the Impact of Educational Interventions: A Quantitative Approach | 389 |
| | Jenepher A. Martin | |
| 35 | Understanding Learning: A Qualitative Approach | 405 |
| | Kirsten Dalrymple and Debra Nestel | |
| 36 | Ethical Issues in Surgical Education Research | 423 |
| | Martyn Kingsbury | |
| 37 | Remaining "Grounded" in a Laparoscopic Community of Practice: The Qualitative Paradigm | 439 |
| | Rory Kokelaar | |
| 38 | The Nature of Nurture in Surgery: A Drama in Four Acts (So Far) | 445 |
| | David Alderson | |
| 39 | Approaching Surgery Simulation Education from a Patient-Centered Pathway | 451 |
| | Kiyoyuki Miyasaka | |

**Part V  Future Directions in Surgical Education**

**40  Surgical Education in the Future** .......................................................... 459
Prem Rashid and Kurt McCammon

**41  Finally, the Future of Surgical Educators**............................................ 469
Debra Nestel, John T. Paige, and Kirsten Dalrymple

**Index**................................................................................................................. 483

# Chapter 1
# Celebrating Surgical Education

Debra Nestel, Kirsten Dalrymple, and John T. Paige

**Overview** The surgeon as educator faces the challenges of adequately preparing the next generation of surgeons while maintaining a busy practice and keeping up with the latest developments and innovations of the field through familiarity with best evidence in literature. This book helps with keeping up with the latest best evidence in education research and theory. As surgical care has a universal component related to the responsibility entrusted to the surgeon and the healing through combination of mind and hand, so too surgical education involves disseminating knowledge as well as skill. This book aims to address knowledge of surgical education. In this chapter, we share drivers for the book and personal perspectives that inform its shape. We also acknowledge the many influences on our own thinking and practices.

## 1.1 Introduction

Surgical education is in an exciting phase. This book celebrates some of its many achievements. In this chapter, we summarise key influencing factors in the development of this book, and we share personal perspectives and orientate readers to the content.

---

D. Nestel (✉)
Faculty of Medicine, Nursing & Health Sciences, Monash Institute for Health and Clinical Education, Monash University, Clayton, VIC, Australia

Faculty of Medicine Dentistry & Health Sciences, Department of Surgery, Melbourne Medical School, University of Melbourne, Parkville, Australia
e-mail: dnestel@unimelb.edu.au; debra.nestel@monash.edu

K. Dalrymple
Faculty of Medicine, Imperial College London, London, UK
e-mail: k.dalrymple@imperial.ac.uk

J. T. Paige
Department of Surgery, Louisiana State University School of Medicine, New Orleans, LA, USA
e-mail: jpaige@lsuhsc.edu

© Springer Nature Singapore Pte Ltd. 2019
D. Nestel et al. (eds.), *Advancing Surgical Education*, Innovation and Change in Professional Education 17, https://doi.org/10.1007/978-981-13-3128-2_1

Several factors influenced the initiation and development of this book. The shifting orientation of surgical education from an apprentice-based model to a competency-based one with interim variations has created an opportunity for the discipline to grow. This has occurred at a time with parallel development in theories that inform educational practice. These theories offer frameworks to make meaning of and guide educational program design, implementation and evaluation. During the last 30 years, there has been significant development in educational theories and practices, many of which have been 'overlooked' by surgical educators who have remained rooted solely in an apprenticeship model.

This book provides opportunities to access a broad range of theories – some theories enable us to take a *macro* view of practice (*social/cultural/political*), while others focus on the micro (*individual as learner and/or teacher*). We include offerings across this spectrum. These new opportunities to view surgical education as something amenable to structure, measurement, standardisation and examination through educational theory have moved the field forward. It has become fairer, safer and more knowledgeable of itself, in many regards, but these advances have sometimes come with costs and a realisation of the limitations of, for example, competency-based education. There is a growing recognition, and some might rightly call a reassertion of the importance of fostering meaningful, trusting, social relationships between learners and teachers as a basis for growing trainee surgeons' surgical judgement and skill and for considering their progress. Taking more holistic views of expertise, of what constitutes surgical 'community', and of surgery's end goal of improving the health and well-being of patients brings us back to considering the role of trust, not only as a facet of professional practice but of educational practice. If we subscribe to the argument that this is where significant development happens, for both educators and trainees, our efforts to understand and improve our practice as educators must also embrace the social, the cultural and the individual as a person. That this parallels arguments around the care of patients is not coincidental.

Being a surgical educator today affords new opportunities to develop an identity that goes beyond what it did in the past. It adds a knowledge-based, skill-based and the critical judgement of another professional practice to surgery's existing training traditions – it adds the field of education. Bringing the field of education to the surgical educator provides a wider repertoire of tools with which to examine difficult and complex educational problems.

With the professionalisation of surgical education comes greater acknowledgement and recognition of its expertise. This has become more evident through the development of standards for practice such as those published by the Faculty of Surgical Trainers in Edinburgh in 2014 [1]. In Australia, the Academy of Surgical Educators was launched in 2013 and seeks to 'foster excellence' [2]. In 2017, the American College of Surgeons established the Academy of Master Surgeon Educators which will function as a 'think tank' seeking to improve the quality of surgical education. Annual and biannual conferences in surgical education are focal events for surgical education scholars and educators – the International Conference on Surgical Education and Training (ICOSET) and the United States-based

> **Box 1.1 Examples of Journals Where Surgical Education Research May Be Published (Excluding Surgical Clinical Journals)**
> 1. Academic Medicine http://journals.lww.com/academicmedicine/pages/default.aspx
> 2. Advances in Health Sciences Education http://www.springer.com/education+&+language/journal/10459
> 3. BMC Medical Education http://www.biomedcentral.com/bmcmededuc
> 4. Journal of Surgical Education http://www.sciencedirect.com/science/journal/19317204
> 5. Medical Education http://www.mededuc.com/ or http://www.wiley.com/bw/journal.asp?ref=0308-0110
> 6. Medical Teacher http://www.medicalteacher.org/MEDTEACH_wip/pages/home.htm
> 7. Perspectives on Medical Education http://www.springer.com/education+%26+language/journal/40037
> 8. Teaching and Learning in Medicine http://www.siumed.edu/tlm/
> 9. The Clinical Teacher http://www.theclinicalteacher.com/

Association for Surgical Education (ASE) Conference. Although the landscape of surgical education differs internationally, this also provides opportunities to learn from each other. There is a growing body of specialist surgical education literature with edited books such as Fry and Kneebone [3], a collection of readings from theorists, researchers and practitioners (surgery and education), and, from Pugh and Sippel [4], a 'practical' guide to establishing a surgical education career in the United States. There are also several peer- reviewed health professions education journals that publish research from the surgical education research community (Box 1.1). These initiatives of communities of practice illustrate just how far surgical education has come in a relatively short time.

Graduate programs in health professions and clinical education are now quite common. Although surgical practice shares many features and concerns with other health professions, there is also a recognition of its highly specialised nature, and, hence, programmes designed for surgical educators have been offered, for example, at Imperial College London since 2005 [5] and through the University of Melbourne and the Royal Australasian College of Surgeons (RACS) since 2012 [6]. Like graduates with interests in surgical education from other programs, they usually undertake research that is adding to understanding ways in which surgical education is practised internationally. An important driver for this book is the provision of a reference book for students embarking on higher degrees where surgical education is a focus. We acknowledge that navigating this landscape can be challenging and thoughtfully described by Kneebone (2002) in his essay on internal reflection [7]. In this he describes the challenges of making meaning of the education literature after training in a biomedical positivist tradition.

This book sits in the Springer series: *Innovation and Change in Professional Education*. This is a logical home for several reasons. At its heart, the book is about innovation. Authors have been invited to contribute because of their innovative and often critical positioning and philosophising about ways to support the next generation of surgeons. The landscape of surgical practice and education is a dynamic one. This sort of change is inevitable and welcomed, as the community whose needs are to be met by the profession, and those who are to meet them also change. And, although surgery is a professional practice, the education of surgeons has often been of low value in departments of surgery. Surgical education has not been seen as requiring the development of educational expertise. This aligns with privileging the language of surgical training over surgical education in common parlance. Our position is that the responsibility of those charged with supporting the development of the next generation of surgeons needs more than a *training* focus. They also require a deep and deliberate consideration of *values* about teaching and learning. This book provides an opportunity to prompt critical reflection on the values and practices associated with surgical education.

In its very construction, the book attempts to model the bringing together of surgical education perspectives and the nurturing of a new generation of surgical education scholars. The authors are drawn from various parts of the globe and are comprised of teams of surgeons and academics from education, the social sciences and more. With their different backgrounds and perspectives come forms of writing and argument that may vary from those with which you are more familiar. We invite you to explore these varied ways of communicating knowledge and challenge you to make links with more familiar approaches. We believe that this book goes beyond those before it in its breadth, depth and examination of surgical education practices and the ways in which they are communicated.

## 1.2  Our Editorial Team

Our editorial team came together through our links with Imperial College London, three of us (DN, KD, RA) having worked at Imperial for extended periods, and JP has undertaken research with colleagues based at Imperial. Collectively, we have expertise in various facets of education and surgical knowledge and practice. During the development of this book, we have been living and working across four countries – Australia (DN), the United Kingdom (UK) (KD), Canada (RA) and the United States of America (USA) (JP and RA) – and we are all actively involved in surgical education.

Debra Nestel PhD FSSH has worked in surgical education for about 10 years and broader health professions education for over 30 years, in Hong Kong, London and Melbourne. Currently Professor of Surgical Education, Department of Surgery, University of Melbourne, and Professor of Simulation Education in Healthcare, Monash University, Australia, Debra spends her time approximately equally in education research and practice. She is Co-Director of the Graduate Programs in

Surgical Education and the Graduate Programs in Surgical Science. After Professor John Collins, then Dean of Education, RACS, had a proposal for post-graduate qualifications in surgical education approved, Debra was tasked with its implementation. A core reference book was an important driver for this project. Debra's first degree was in sociology, and this seeps through much of her current practice. She has a strong interest in simulation, especially simulated patient methodology and in faculty development. Debra mainly conducts qualitative research while appreciating the role of all research paradigms to address the broad range of questions relevant to surgical education. She has also edited books on simulated patient methodology and healthcare simulation and is editor-in-chief of the open access journal, Advances in Simulation, the journal of the Society in Europe for Simulation Applied to Medicine. She holds service roles in many professional organisations.

Kirsten Dalrymple, PhD, is Principal Teaching Fellow and Course Co-Director, Master's in Education in Surgical Education, Department of Surgery and Cancer, Faculty of Medicine, Imperial College London. She has worked in health professions education for over 15 years, having trained initially as a biomedical scientist. Before working in the United Kingdom, Kirsten played a lead role in major curricular changes and faculty development at the University of Southern California's School of Dentistry. She has been a key figure in the execution and ongoing development of Imperial's Master's in Surgical Education since 2008, having had the opportunity to work closely as tutor and research supervisor for surgeons from different countries, specialties and at different stages of their careers. Her work with clinical colleagues and her own scientific background have shaped her interest in how values and views of knowledge impact educational practice and have provided her with motivation to build links between education and surgery. She is currently working on a pedagogic project exploring how failure and mistakes are perceived by different disciplines, including surgery, and the impact this has on professional development. She serves on two of Imperial's educational research ethics committees.

John Paige MD, FACS, joined the Department of Surgery at Louisiana State University (LSU) School of Medicine in New Orleans in 2002 where he has practiced general and minimally invasive surgery. Currently, he is Professor of Clinical Surgery with additional appointments in the Departments of Anesthesiology and Radiology. He serves as both overall and surgical director of the American College of Surgeons Accredited Comprehensive Education Institute, the LSU Health New Orleans School of Medicine Learning Center. John has dedicated his academic career to surgical education and research. His published work in simulation and surgical education related to skills acquisition and interprofessional team training has led him to present nationally and internationally. He is an active member of several national surgical society simulation, education and faculty development committees, holding leadership positions. He is coeditor of a book on simulation in radiology. He has been a coinvestigator on federally funded grants exploring team training. John's areas of interest include simulation-based skills training, interprofessional education, team training, human factors, patient safety and debriefing.

Rajesh Aggarwal MD PhD FRCS FACS is a surgeon and educator. He trained as a surgeon in the United Kingdom and has held academic and clinical posts at Imperial College London, University of Pennsylvania and most recently at McGill University where he was also charged as director of the Steinberg Centre for Simulation and Interactive Learning. In 2002, he completed a PhD degree in virtual reality technologies for surgical education. In 2017, Rajesh has taken on his role in strategic business development at Thomas Jefferson University and Jefferson Health.

## 1.3 Conclusion

In closing this chapter, we acknowledge many of those who have influenced our thinking and practices, some of whom are contributors to this book. The five sections of the book commence with orientation notes offering linkages between the varied contributions. We hope you enjoy the contents of this book as much as we have in working with our colleagues from around the world in assembling examples of their scholarship. Time to celebrate.

## References

1. McIlhenny, C., & Pitts, D. (2014). *Standards for surgical trainers Edinburgh: Royal college of surgeons Edinburgh*. Available from: https://fst.rcsed.ac.uk/standards-for-surgical-trainers.aspx
2. Royal Australasian College of Surgeons. (2017). *Academy of surgical educators*. [Cited 2017 November 11]. Available from: https://www.surgeons.org/for-health-professionals/academy-of-surgical-educators/
3. Fry, H., & Kneebone, R. (2011). *Surgical education: Theorising an emerging domain*. London: Springer.
4. Pugh, C., & Sippel, R. (2013). *Success in academic surgery: Developing a career in surgical education*. London: Springer.
5. Imperial College London. *MEd surgical education*. [Cited 2017 November 11]. Available from: https://www.imperial.ac.uk/medicine/study/postgraduate/masters-programmes/med-surgical-education/
6. University of Melbourne and Royal Australasian College of Surgeons. *Master of surgical education*. [Cited 2017 November 11]. Available from: https://coursesearch.unimelb.edu.au/grad/1865-master-of-surgical-education
7. Kneebone, R. (2002). Total internal reflection: An essay on paradigms. *Medical Education, 36*(6), 514–518.

# Part I
# Overview: Foundations of Surgical Education

The first part of this book explores foundations of surgical education from its historical roots in apprenticeship to its transformation over time to address changes to medicine, surgery, and wider society. As noted in the introduction to the book, contemporary surgical practice and education are dynamic entities that interact with one another. In his historical perspective, Kneebone considers the relative certainties of surgical education over the last century and how recent practices have resulted in the current state of "fluidity and instability" (Chap. 2). He concludes this chapter "reflecting on the continual process by which innovation becomes established as a 'new normal,' only to be overtaken in its turn by continuing change." This offers further justification for this book to be located in the series: Innovation and Change in Professional Education.

Anthony and Muralidharan examine the shift to competency-based surgical education from the long history of apprenticeship (Chap. 3). Using the context of surgical training in Australia and New Zealand, they describe the Royal Australasian College of Surgeons (RACS) and other institutional approaches to developing an educationally aware community of surgical educators, essential to address contemporary drivers for surgical education. One important challenge is to balance the increasing demands on the surgical education workforce while delivering an expanded surgical curriculum that best serves the modern community. The authors acknowledge an orientation to actively develop *well-rounded* surgeons, where the "nontechnical" skills are valued alongside conventional and other characteristic skills of operating. For many issues, they consider its impact at macro-, meso-, and microlevels. Although their work has a regional context, many of the issues have relevance globally.

From Gogainaceu et al., we learn of the support of leadership development in surgical training (Chap. 4). This is an element of professional practice that has often not formed part of traditional curricula. The authors describe how leadership and education are similar transformative processes that "facilitate growth, foster collaborations and increase scientific knowledge, innovation and enterprise." They also explore the role of academy in the development of leaders and educators and, indeed, educational leaders.

Quality in surgical education must have a central role and one manifestation is governance. From a United Kingdom perspective, Eardley reviews the place of the Surgical Royal Colleges in the governance of surgical training – in curriculum development, assessment, selection, certification, quality assurance, and trainee support (Chap. 5). Additionally, the chapter describes the complex and changing relationship of the colleges with the regulator, the funder, and the education providers.

In summary, this part offers a status check on where we have been and where we are. Two focused topics that must be considered for developing excellence in surgical education – leadership and governance – illustrate essential foundations for change and quality.

# Chapter 2
# Surgical Education: A Historical Perspective

Roger Kneebone

**Overview** This chapter considers how the landscape of surgical education has changed over the past century and how the educational certainties of an earlier generation have been supplanted by fluidity and instability. After outlining the establishment of open surgery in the first half of the twentieth century, the chapter uses the introduction of minimally invasive (keyhole) surgery in the 1980s as a lens for examining the educational implications of surgical innovation and the processes by which such innovation can trigger educational change. At the same time, the discussion charts the emergence of professionalism of surgical education, shaped by expert perspectives from outside medicine. This has led to a broadening of methodological approaches to the investigation of educational questions and the establishment of surgical education as a scholarly field with its own identity. The chapter concludes by reflecting on the continual process by which innovation becomes established as a 'new normal', only to be overtaken in its turn by continuing change.

This chapter surveys how the landscape of surgical education has changed over the past century and how contemporary challenges have been shaped by the past. In that time, the surgical world – together with the sociopolitical world it responds to and reflects – has become increasingly fluid and unstable. Disciplinary boundaries are becoming blurred, and new technologies are overturning previously settled ways of knowing and of doing. The focus of surgical education has shifted from learning how to do things as they are already done to responding to (and moulding) a surgical world that is in continual flux. A professionalisation of education has taken place which has moved beyond the frame of surgical practice to include expert perspectives from outside medicine. This has profound implications for what it means to be a surgeon and a surgical educator.

R. Kneebone (✉)
Department of Surgery and Cancer, Imperial College London, London, UK
e-mail: r.kneebone@imperial.ac.uk

Two related developments – keyhole (minimally invasive) surgery and simulation-based training – provide the backdrop for a discussion about changes which have shaped the landscape of today. This account will inevitably oversimplify a complex picture. It presents the personal perspective of the author, a clinician who trained as a surgeon in the 1970s and 1980s, became a general practitioner in the 1990s, and has since specialised in surgical education at a large London university medical school.

Surgery in its current form is rooted in the upheavals and discoveries of eighteenth-century Europe [1, 2]. At that time, Paris emerged as a major centre of clinical innovation, while in Britain, the Hunter brothers (John and William) played a pivotal role in establishing surgery as a scholarly discipline underpinned by rigorous study. Wherever it was practised, a strong performative element to operative surgery was prompted by the need (before the discovery of anaesthesia) for surgeons to be rapid and decisive and influenced by a history of anatomical and surgical performance reaching back to earlier centuries.

The next hundred years saw the establishment of 'scientific' surgery, influenced by European (and especially German) practice. Advances in microbiology and biochemistry transformed clinical practice, framing surgery as the application of scientific knowledge and surgeons as applied scientists rather than performers. From the mid-nineteenth century onwards, developments such as anaesthesia, antisepsis and asepsis meant that previously inaccessible territories of the body could be safely operated upon – first the abdomen, then the brain, the heart and beyond. Approaches to investigation, diagnosis and treatment became increasingly influenced by the laboratory, and the body became seen as a mechanism which could be fixed by surgery.

At the same time, major changes were taking place in the landscape of clinical education. Concerns about standards in American medical schools led to Abraham Flexner's overhaul of undergraduate medical training and brought much-needed reforms. His report of 1910 sets standards for admission and graduation, highlighting the importance of science in the curriculum [3]. This led to the closure of many rural medical schools in America and laid the foundation for educational structures which persist to this day. Postgraduate education too was in flux. For example, in the late nineteenth century, the celebrated surgeon William Halsted introduced the concept of a formal surgical residency at Johns Hopkins Hospital in Baltimore [4–6]. In a model which became widely adopted and is still in place today, structured training combined clinical experience with graded supervision.

In the United Kingdom, the establishment of the National Health Service in 1948 marked a later watershed. For the first time, medical care became available to all, regardless of the ability to pay. In the decades that followed, surgical care was provided within a strong social professional framework. A clear hierarchical structure (established in the aftermath of World War II and reflecting the social structures of the time) was set in place. Education and training were central to this structure. Surgical 'firms', each led by a consultant, consisted of close-knit groups of surgeons in training who underwent an extended apprenticeship lasting many years. Almost all out-of-hours care was provided by those in training, and trainees gained extensive experience in operative surgery. The 'firm' system ensured continuity of care for patients and offered a supportive and collegial milieu for clinicians but required high levels of commitment and exceptionally long hours of work. An important effect of this demanding training was to develop a surgical identity amongst those who underwent it – a shared sense of what it meant to 'be' a surgeon as well as to do surgical work, as much about who a surgeon became as what he or she could do. In contrast to undergraduate medical education, with its focus on curriculum and formal learning, postgraduate surgical learning was assumed more than designed or prescribed. Assessment of fitness to progress within the system was unsystematic, opaque and based on the personal judgment of senior clinicians.

By the mid-twentieth century, surgery seemed to have reached a steady state. A stable social structure for interaction between patients and professionals was taken for granted, and – as with education in schools and universities more generally – what was to be learned appeared fixed and unchanging. This approach represented the wider sociopolitical context of the time, with its climate of deference and confidence in authority in general and in the medical profession in particular. Publics and politicians trusted clinicians to design and oversee their own educational as well as clinical practice, and post-war social assumptions were clearly visible.

By this time, surgical training had become well-established, with education accepted as a by-product of clinical care. The assumption was that by working within the healthcare system for long enough, a learner would eventually become expert. The extended apprenticeship system provided enormous experience in the skills of operating, while the 'firm' structure ensured that trainee surgeons became versed in all aspects of patient care (including continuity between ward and theatre) and became part of a close-knit (if closed and often inward-looking) professional community. For surgeons, therefore, education and clinical care were inseparable. There were few specific courses or programmes, and surgical learning took place from within, as part of being a practitioner. Senior surgeons were expected to teach in every aspect of their practice, from outpatient clinic and ward to operating theatre and emergency room, but there was no overt surgical curriculum. Learning took place by absorption, underpinned by an assumption that by the end of training, trainees would have been exposed to sufficient breadth and depth of experience to undertake full responsibility when they became consultants themselves. Professional examinations were more about factual knowledge than practical skill.

By the 1980s, all this began to change. Part of this disruption was technological. Discoveries and developments in areas such as imaging, energy sources, fibre optics and miniaturisation led to new opportunities within operative surgery and medicine as a whole. The power of surgery (until then confined to what could be done with relatively simple instruments) became enormously enlarged. At the same time, a shift from diagnosis to intervention meant that previously sharp distinctions between surgery, medicine, radiology and other disciplines started to become smudged. Intestinal endoscopy, for example, was developed by gastroenterologists and radiologists, and surgeons were no longer the only group who carried out delicate invasive procedures on patients.

Another aspect of this disruption was societal, reflecting equally profound political and social change at that time. Public faith in the skill and beneficence of doctors began to be questioned, challenging previously stable structures of authority and deference. A series of prominent cases in the UK included the Bristol heart surgeons (where it became clear that some paediatric cardiac surgeons continued to operate on small children while knowing that their results were worse than those of colleagues), the Alder Hey Children's Hospital scandal (where pathologists removed and retained body parts without parents' knowledge or consent) and the notorious Dr. Harold Shipman (who systematically murdered scores of patients). These and others started to erode the unquestioning trust of an earlier generation, reconfiguring relationships between clinicians, patients and society. Management structures within the health service were redesigned too, and clinical practice was no longer the exclusive province of clinicians. Clinical education too came under the microscope, and educational practice began to open up to specialist non-clinicians.

What became known as keyhole surgery provides a useful example of how technical innovation, public perception and a changing sociopolitical climate collectively precipitated educational change. This change was shockingly rapid. If it is difficult for trainees starting a surgical career today to envisage a world before minimally invasive surgery, it is perhaps even more difficult to imagine a world without the Internet, mobile phones or word processors. In the mid-1980s, none of these things were there. Yet within a single surgical generation, a radical new approach to operative surgery became embedded as the 'new normal'.

Keyhole surgery can be seen as a watershed in many ways. In surgical terms, it transformed perceptions of the need for surgery to be invasive, demonstrating that major interventions could be carried out through tiny incisions which dramatically reduced pain and shortened hospital stays. In social terms, it marked a shift in the balance of power between the profession and the public, showing how pressure from patients accelerated the adoption of a new approach [7]. In educational terms, it highlighted how a radical change in surgical practice (apparently a technical issue) continues to reverberate through surgical training.

The meteoric rise of keyhole surgery is instructive. In the 1980s, a number of clinicians were exploring how to minimise the trauma of open surgery, with its extensive incisions. Taking advantage of technical developments of the time (including advances in imaging, energy sources and fibre-optic technology), they developed innovative ways of collaborative working in order to solve technical challenges. The urologist John Wickham, for example, pioneered percutaneous nephrolithotomy for the removal of renal tract stones. Working closely with an interventional radiologist, instrument designer and other clinical colleagues, Wickham made a major contribution to what has now become a commonplace procedure. In the process, he modelled a new surgical approach, challenging the dominant role of the surgeon and suggesting instead that power be distributed within a surgical team to draw on multiple sources of expertise. The author has researched this process in detail, gathering first-hand accounts of a transformative time by using simulation-based re-enactment to document not only technical developments but relationships with patients and within clinical teams [8–10].

As surgery's power increased, so did its potential for causing harm. Once the benefits of minimally invasive therapy (as Wickham named it) started to become known, pressure from patients mounted for surgeons to perform procedures laparoscopically. A series of high-profile disasters raised public awareness of the dangers of the new surgery in inexpert hands. Iatrogenic damage during elective laparoscopic surgery showed that specific training was needed, even (perhaps especially) for experienced surgeons who had acquired great expertise in open surgery but struggled with making the transition to a different paradigm.

This posed an educational challenge. The manipulation of keyhole instruments required qualities which were not guaranteed by seniority and expertise in open surgery but required specific aptitudes, training and experience. The physical challenges of manipulating tissues and materials at a distance using unfamiliar instruments, viewed via screen-based images rather than direct vision, demanded unfamiliar perceptual and fine motor skills. The 'new surgery' was new for all surgeons and levelled the playing field. This triggered a systematic approach to learning these unfamiliar ways of seeing and doing. Because keyhole surgery was revolutionary rather than evolutionary, it became easier to make the case that all surgeons (not just beginners) needed formal training. There was no shame in a surgeon admitting that he or she was not an expert in this radically new approach (unlike admitting to uncertainty in a field in which they were already regarded as expert). The established approach of learning from seniors who had mastered what learners aspired to learn did not hold when the masters themselves were on uncertain ground. There was a need instead for education based on meeting the demands of the new rather than absorbing the ways of the old. Training courses multiplied and assessment took centre stage.

The requirement for specialised motor skills brought a new emphasis on technical aspects of surgery. A distinction between 'technical' and 'non-technical' skills arose, raising issues about how fine manipulative skills in particular might be taught, learned and assessed. 'Skills laboratories' were established, where surgeons could practise and perfect the manipulative skills which laparoscopic surgery required. The separation and privileging of technical skills over broader clinical expertise continue to reverberate today. In addition to its obvious benefits in ensuring high standards of manipulative skill, it has had the unintended effect within surgical education of displacing attention from other aspects of surgical practice, especially the holistic care of patients outside the operating theatre.

At the same time, a burgeoning patient safety movement was gathering momentum, and it became increasingly clear that clinical care in all specialties could inflict damage as well as conferring benefit. This contributed to the rise of simulation as a mainstay of education, arguing that many skills should be practised and perfected outside the operating theatre, where real patients would not be placed at risk of harm. Huge investment went into simulation facilities, with industries vying for position as suppliers of costly sophisticated simulators and related equipment. This focus on technical skills drew attention further away from the wider considerations of surgery as a holistic clinical practice (for its patients) and an educational community (for its practitioners).

At this point, assessment focused on details of technique, devising ways to measure what was measurable. Education became something to be measured, and assessment started to play a prominent role. Attention fixed upon what could be most easily captured and analysed. Metrics such as laparoscopic instrument 'path length, suture tension and time to completion of a procedure were used to assess progress and outcome. As outlined above, a growing sense of public unease and mistrust increased pressure to show that education was both formal and effective. One effect of a preoccupation with the technical aspects of keyhole surgery was to strive to show that training 'worked'. Here, the surgical community often framed its questions in a biomedical way, proposing and testing hypotheses and comparing groups of learners in the way that clinicians compare treatments or drugs. This quantitative approached dominated discourses of assessment and is still in evidence today.

The introduction of professional educators changed the way in which surgeons approached education. In the earlier part of the twentieth century, sociologists had observed surgeons but seldom worked directly with them as collaborators [11, 12]. Later on, educational expertise outside surgery began to make its way into the surgical world. The disciplinary traditions of education (rooted in the humanities and social sciences rather than the natural and physical sciences) brought a qualitative approach which in many ways was better suited to the questions which surgical education began to ask. A realisation grew that research into surgical practice and research into surgical education require different approaches.

As educationalists from outside medicine were brought in to provide specialist expertise, a tension between methodologies and philosophies of enquiry began to surface, with a growing sense that measuring what was easily measurable might not capture the complexities of clinical practice. Throughout these developments, there has been growing recognition that the educational side of surgical education resists 'simple' analysis of isolated skills and always plays out within a complex social context. Education in the current world shows a tendency for components of this whole to be hived off and separated. Many elements of current assessment are conducted outside the clinical setting and in assessment centres and simulation centres and performed by different kinds of expert. Although much has been gained – for example, in terms of demonstrating operative skill – other aspects (such as the expert but unquantifiable judgement of an experienced senior colleague) have been marginalised or devalued. Although formal curricula (such as the UK's Intercollegiate Surgical Curriculum Project) have articulated what is to be learned in terms of factual knowledge and technical skill, much remains implicit and eludes capture.

The unanticipated consequences of well-intentioned reform continue to defy prediction. For example, while mandatory reduction of duty hours has lessened the harmful impact of excessive working, the resulting fragmentation of clinical 'firms' has had serious repercussions on the development of surgical identity and a demoralising effect on social cohesion [13, 14]. Now surgical education is more nuanced, looking beyond isolated skills to seeing education as a process resulting in social and ontological change as well as the acquisition of knowledge and skill. There is great value in educationalists and clinicians working together, combining their perspectives and drawing on insights from other branches of medicine. In recent years, collaborative working between educationalists and surgeons has led to a growing body of surgeon educators, developing a distinct professionalism of their own. This has included insights into the pedagogical practices of the operating theatre [15–17].

Returning to keyhole surgery, the distinctiveness of the new (at that time) way of performing surgery took attention away from the need to embed it in the same values of care as applied to any other kind of surgery. Yet a technicist focus sometimes eclipsed humanist values, giving undue prominence to the technical. This led to a disconnection from relevant insights within education (both medical and beyond) such as the groundbreaking work within general practice around the teaching of consultation skills and the role of simulated patients in the teaching and learning of complex clinical issues.

Keyhole surgery is an example of a process which in retrospect seems smooth and unruffled but which in fact took place by a series of leaps. The author has worked extensively with teams of pioneering surgeons from that time, using simulation to re-enact and document surgical and educational practices. These personal accounts give a vivid sense of the uncertainties and difficulties of introducing change within a professional setting. Building on those insights, the challenge now is to integrate surgical and educational expertise in order to remain responsive to an increasingly unstable world. Part of this instability is a consequence of relentless technical innovation. New approaches are being developed all the time, and what has become the new 'normal' in many surgical specialties will presumably be superseded by a new 'new'. Already interventional radiology, robotics, personalised medicine, genomic and phenomic science and diagnosis based on big data are challenging traditional framings of surgical practice and what it is to be a surgeon. Previously secure disciplinary boundaries are dissolving as former certainties unravel.

Surgical education must concern itself as much with who surgeons are and what they will become as with the techniques and skills they master and develop. Flux gives rise to opportunity and innovation but can also create uncertainty and discomfort. Alongside continual technical change is a widespread social instability and a worrying decline in morale. Within the profession, surgical identity is having to be refashioned. Events such as the Mid Staffordshire hospital scandal (where appalling instances of neglect and lack of care came to light within an NHS Trust) and the subsequent Francis Report [18] have highlighted failings of humanity and professional practice. Relationships between clinicians, patients, publics and society are continually being reconfigured, and surgical education must take all this into account.

## 2.1 Conclusions

As a clinician entering surgery, it is easy to think that things have always been as they are now. It is salutary to reflect on how much has changed over a single professional lifetime. The constantly accelerating rate of change means that challenges will arise at ever-decreasing intervals. Surgical education is shaped and defined as much by its social setting as by its professional and technical context. Perhaps, instead of following clinical innovation, surgical education should accompany or lead it.

## References

1. Spary, E. C. (1999). The performance of surgery in enlightenment France. *Endeavour, 23*(4), 180–183.
2. Guerrini, A. (2006). Alexander Monro primus and the moral theatre of anatomy. *The Eighteenth Century, 47*(1), 1–18.
3. Flexner, A. (1910). *The Flexner report on medical education in the United States and Canada.* New York: Carnegie Foundation.
4. Imber, G. (2010). *Genius on the edge: The bizarre double life of Dr. William Stewart Halsted.* New York: Kaplan Publishers.
5. William, B. M. (1990). *Osler: A life in medicine.* Toronto: University of Toronto Press.
6. Harvey, B. M. (2005). *Cushing: A life in surgery.* Toronto: University of Toronto Press.
7. Schlich, T., & Tang, C. L. (2016). Patient choice and the history of minimally invasive surgery. *The Lancet, 388*(10052), 1369–1370.
8. Kneebone, R., & Woods, A. (2014). Recapturing the history of surgical practice through simulation- based re-enactment. *Medical History, 58*(1), 106–121.
9. Kneebone, R., & Woods, A. (2012). Bringing surgical history to life. *BMJ (Clinical Research Ed), 345*, e8135.
10. Frampton, S., & Kneebone, R. (2017). John Wickham's new surgery: 'Minimally invasive therapy', innovation, and approaches to medical practice in twentieth-century Britain. *Social History of Medicine, 30*(3), 544–566.
11. Becker, H., Geer, B., Hughes, E., & Strauss, A. (1961). *Boys in white.* New Brunswick: Transaction Books.
12. Bosk, C. (1979). *Forgive and remember: Managing medical failure.* Chicago: University of Chicago Press.
13. Brooks, J. V., & Bosk, C. L. (2012). Remaking surgical socialization: Work hour restrictions, rites of passage, and occupational identity. *Social Science & Medicine, 75*(9), 1625–1632.
14. Cope, A., Bezemer, J., Mavroveli, S., & Kneebone, R. (2017). What attitudes and values are incorporated into self as part of professional identity construction when becoming a surgeon? *Academic Medicine, 92*(4), 544–549.
15. Bezemer, J., Cope, A., Kress, G., & Kneebone, R. (2013). Holding the scalpel: Achieving surgical care in a learning environment. *Journal of Contemporary Ethnography, 43*(1), 38–63.
16. Bezemer, J., Cope, A., Kress, G., & Kneebone, R. (2011). 'Can I have a Johann, please?': Changing social and cultural contexts for professional communication. *Applied Linguistics Review., 2*, 313–334.
17. Bezemer, J., Kress, G., Cope, A., & Kneebone, R. (2011). Learning in the operating theatre: A social semiotic perspective. In V. Cook, C. Daly, & M. Newman (Eds.), *Innovative approaches to exploring learning in and through clinical practice* (pp. 125–141). Abingdon: Radcliffe.
18. Francis, R. (2013). *Report of the mid Staffordshire NHS Foundation Trust public inquiry.* London: The Stationery Office.

# Chapter 3
# The Contemporary Context of Surgical Education

**Adrian Anthony and Vijayaragavan Muralidharan**

**Overview** The development of a competent surgeon has evolved over centuries from a predominantly apprenticeship model to one that incorporates modern theories of learning accompanied by increasing awareness of the significant contribution from the hidden curriculum. Increasing public awareness and demands from educators and trainees have emphasised the importance of nontechnical competencies. The Royal Australasian College of Surgeons has determined nine core competencies as a basic requirement for surgical training. It has responded to emerging demands by the introduction of formal educational processes supporting the development of an educationally aware surgical teaching community. A challenge for surgical training is to balance the increasing demands on the surgical education workforce while delivering an expanded surgical curriculum that best serves the modern community. This chapter explores the changing field of surgical education and provides an overview of the future challenges.

---

A. Anthony (✉)
Upper Gastro-Intestinal Unit, The Queen Elizabeth Hospital, Department of Surgery, Discipline of Surgery, University of Adelaide, Adelaide, Australia

Board of Surgical Education & Training, Royal Australasian College of Surgeons, Melbourne, Australia
e-mail: adrian.anthony@adelaide.edu.au

V. Muralidharan
HPB & Transplant Unit, Austin Health, Melbourne, Australia

Department of Surgery, The University of Melbourne, Austin Health, Melbourne, Australia

Board in General Surgery, Royal Australasian College of Surgeons, Melbourne, Australia
e-mail: v.muralidharan@unimelb.edu.au

## 3.1 Introduction

In his report to the Carnegie Foundation in 1910, Abraham Flexner understood that failure to meet challenges in medical education would hinder advances in healthcare [1]. This sentiment is as relevant now as it was more than a hundred years ago. Challenges in surgical education inevitably arise from the ongoing interaction between the surgical profession and the society it serves. Society is better educated, better informed and more aware than ever about its own healthcare needs and rights. It has grown accustomed to and expects reliable access to high-quality and safe surgery. It is also acutely aware of the ever-increasing cost it is being asked to pay for surgical care. Consequently, society has become less passive in determining how it accesses surgical care and is seeking to have a greater say in how governments, the profession and surgeons service its needs. Surgical paternalism has had to make way for patient-centred models of care. The demand for greater accountability is not solely focused on maintaining standards of surgical care but also in reforming aspects of the system that society considers are wanting.

Expectations relating to healthcare reforms are no longer confined to its consumers. There is increasing awareness amongst doctors-in-training of the importance of educational quality as a means of shaping professional practice and improving patient care. Trainees recognise that if they are to be accountable for how they perform as future surgeons, they must share the ownership in ensuring their training needs are being met. Educational rigour is no longer determined only by assessment rigour as set by assessors although it continues to occupy a pre-eminent position. Trainees define educational rigour by the quality of the learning experience and the diligence and accountability in the teaching that supports their learning [2]. Surgical education is evolving towards learner-centred models of training just as surgical care is readjusting to patient-centred approaches. It appears that society and doctors-in-training have convergent expectations of the future direction of healthcare.

An understanding of the changing expectations of society, patients and trainees provides surgery with the opportunity to be responsive. Surgical education is the means by which the profession can strategically remain relevant in its relationship with its members, trainees and society. The dominant contemporary themes for surgical education revolve around a holistic approach to training across the breadth of surgical competencies, capacity and capability to train surgeons in an evolving landscape and preparing a workforce fit for servicing societal needs. How these themes contextualise the current state of play can be considered at the micro, meso and macro levels of surgical education.

## 3.2 Producing a Competent Surgeon

The intimate and invasive application of complex psychomotor skills to treat patients uniquely differentiates surgeons from the majority of medical disciplines. This characteristic of surgery has spurred a tailored approach to education and training when compared to other medical education programmes [3]. The focus on mastering "technical" skills in surgery has, however, not easily accommodated training in the so-called nontechnical competencies. Nontechnical competencies refer to a set of cognitive, social and personal resource skills [4]. They represent humanistic skills and professional behaviours, recognised in the social sciences as determinants of human factors [5]. The Royal Australasian College of Surgeons characterise a surgeon as being competent across nine domains that incorporate both technical and professional skills and which are comparable to domains articulated in the CanMEDS, GMC and ACGME frameworks. These are technical expertise, medical expertise, communication, judgement and decision-making, collaboration, management and leadership, professionalism, health advocacy and scholar and teacher [6].

### 3.2.1 The Importance of Professional Competence

From a patient's perspective, nothing less than a full complement of competencies is required in a competent surgeon [7]. This view is supported by evidence that illustrates how technical competence by itself is insufficient to guarantee optimal surgical outcomes [4, 8, 9]. The Bristol affair in the United Kingdom over a decade ago was a stark example of the consequences of individual surgeons failing in professional skills [10]. The Expert Advisory Group report on discrimination, bullying and harassment in surgery and surgical training [11] is another confronting example of the consequences of not adequately training surgeons in professional skills. The report identifies flaws in how surgeons behave and interact with trainees, international medical graduates, each other and those around them. The problem is not unique to the Australasian context or to surgery [12], but the report brings a sense of urgency to understand and act to redress the deficiencies in professional skills. There is ample evidence that lapses in professional behaviour are strong predictors of poor patient outcomes [9]. Therefore, the drive for change is not simply to ensure surgeons contribute to a respectful work and training environment but is necessarily aimed towards building a durable culture of patient safety.

Yet, it cannot be assumed that trainees and surgeons universally conceptualise surgical competence as an interdependent and inclusive set of technical and professional skills. Many regard competencies as something that can be ranked in order of importance, relevance and even choice [13]. This may be a product of how surgeons are trained and what they experience during training, perhaps reflected by the fact that most surgical curricula do not adequately articulate how the nontechnical competencies are to be learnt, measured or assessed. It is worthwhile considering why this may be so.

### 3.2.2 Nontechnical Skills and the Hidden Curriculum

Most surgeons are likely to have little understanding of how professional behaviours can be taught, nor have they been equipped to teach nontechnical skills (NTS). The dependence of patient safety on professional behaviour is not uniformly acknowledged by surgeons because this relationship has not been adequately explained. Furthermore, NTS are not regarded as skills that can be objectively defined, measured, practised and assessed. Such skills, often termed "soft skills", appear to be perceived as desirable without being essential. This may explain why there is a paucity of activities within surgical training and continuing professional development that focus on learning NTS. Much of what defines nontechnical competencies has typically resided in the hidden curriculum. Perhaps, too, the perception that medical and technical competencies are easily measurable, but not so the other competencies, reinforces the notion that measurable skills have greater relevance than skills that are seemingly intangible [13].

NTS are typically acquired through a process of socialisation, as trainees learn within a community of practice [14]. Although socialisation is an immensely effective process for instilling professional behaviours, it relies on acceptable role modelling on which to mould behaviours. It also remains the responsibility of trainees to calibrate observed behaviours in order to judge their appropriateness. This process is largely tacit without any scaffolding, monitoring, formal assessment or feedback. As such, the development of NTS occurs largely within the hidden curriculum. It is estimated that approximately 5% of surgical trainees struggle to progress due to deficiencies in NTS [15]. Without being defined in the curriculum, NTS are not easily opened to guided development, deliberate practice, feedback or remediation. Relying only on socialisation is neither adequate nor acceptable, and a more explicit approach is required.

Teaching NTS and behaviours is emerging globally as a new focus for medical education across the continuum [16]. Educational designs aimed at improving NTS, and behaviours need to be grounded in understanding related concepts, complexities of relationships (between surgeons, patients, the profession and society) and the roles of governments, regulators and colleges.

### 3.2.3 Teaching Nontechnical Skills

There is growing awareness and appreciation of the evidence that identifies what competencies are essential in surgical practice [17] and how deficiencies in nontechnical competencies are reliable predictors of adverse clinical outcomes [4, 9]. The literature attributes a number of competencies as fundamental elements of human factors: communication, decision-making, collaboration, leadership and professionalism [5]. The evidence that safe surgery is necessarily dependent on human factors is compelling and unsurprising [18]. The dependency of patient safety on human factors should prompt surgeons to conceptualise surgical care within a human factors framework. Such a framework brings the advantage of understanding how behaviours associated with nontechnical competencies have an immediate effect on patient safety. The revised CanMEDS competency framework eloquently constructs a patient safety framework that makes explicit how behavioural (nontechnical) competencies are inextricably linked to safe clinical practice [7].

The fact remains that many elements that define nontechnical competencies are learnt through tacit processes and therefore reside in the hidden curriculum [14]. The literature enlightens us that this need not be the case. Each of the surgical competencies refers to definable standards of behaviour where, for any given circumstance, requisite behaviours can be explicated [6]. In turn, professional behaviours can be deliberately taught, practised and learnt through reflection and simulation [14, 17–19]. Subsequently, behavioural skills can be measured and are therefore assessable [16, 20]. Contrary to the notion that only medical and technical expertise can be measured, all nine surgical competencies can indeed be taught, practised, learnt and assessed. Emerging evidence indicates that efficacy in nontechnical competencies correlates with improvement in technical competencies [4, 18], supporting the notion that technical and nontechnical competencies are in fact interdependent.

Teaching, learning and assessing NTS remain relatively unfamiliar to surgeons. This provides an opportunity for surgical education to promote technical and professional competencies in equal measure. At the macro level, regulators are beginning to explore the utility of revalidation of clinical practice. Here is an opportunity to incorporate behavioural and professional skills as core components of revalidation. Such a requirement would enable specialist colleges at the meso level to examine how nontechnical competencies can be strengthened through continuing professional development programmes. A greater emphasis on the importance of nontechnical competencies through CPD activities would prompt local clinical governance bodies to more critically measure surgical outcomes, not just through a biomedical lens, but according to humanistic criteria such as appropriateness of situational awareness, degree of collaboration, effectiveness of communication and strength of teamwork. At the micro level, individual surgeons and their peers can be expected to audit surgical practice against similar humanistic criteria. When reviewing an adverse outcome, factors relating to situational awareness, communication, teamwork, stress response and other professional behaviours can be explicitly considered in order to have a richer understanding of the influence of NTS on surgical outcome.

Educational processes to support trainees develop professional competencies would need to be incorporated into training programmes. While revalidation is one driver for reforming aspects of surgical training, the opportunity exists not to await "top-down" change to occur. A "bottom-up" approach can still proceed by those responsible for surgical training programmes; surgical colleges can show commitment to accept *all* competencies as mandatory and mutually dependent, to explicate nontechnical competencies in the surgical curriculum and to adopt evidence-based methods for practising and assessing professional behavioural skills.

## 3.3 Training Capacity and Capability

The derivative meaning of the word *Doctor* (*docere*) is to teach. The primary responsibility of surgical colleges globally is surgical education and training. There is an ingrained expectation that, as a self-regulating profession, surgeons will train surgeons. New fellows of the college accept the responsibility for teaching when they recite the RACS Fellowship Pledge. Teaching is regarded as a core surgical competency. However, despite embedded traditions of scholarship, surgical education faces threats to its capacity and capability to teach. The range of skills that surgical trainees need to learn and achieve competence has expanded leading to a change in the educational environment. There has been a distinct shift from a teacher-centred approach of surgical training to a learner-centred one. Consequently, the skills required for teaching are different and broader in repertoire and require time and effort to master. Surgeons appear less able to commit to teaching and to learn to teach effectively, despite being committed to teaching.

### *3.3.1 The Teaching "Supply"*

The demographic profile of surgeons in Australasia reveals an ageing surgical workforce [21, 22]. The current shortfall in surgical workforce is predicted to worsen. This will impact on training and education as surgeons experienced and skilled in teaching will be leaving the workplace over the next decade. As undergraduate and postgraduate surgical education moves into regional areas, the geographic mismatch in the distribution of surgeons will exacerbate any shortages in teaching capacity. In the past 7 years, the proportion of trainees who rotate through non-metropolitan hospitals has risen from 25% to 33%. The proportion of surgeons servicing these areas remained static at 30% [23]. As teaching occurs predominantly as pro bono work, the burden of teaching will gradually fall to a declining number of volunteers. It is estimated that less than 15% of surgeons commit to instructing on generic skills courses [24]. A more evenly distributed instructing load would require almost 25% of all surgeons to teach on skills courses.

While much of surgical learning occurs in the clinical workplace, surgeons often struggle to find opportunities for planned teaching. Day surgery, short-stay surgery, fast-track surgery, new models of acute surgical care, increasing subspecialisation, flexible training and safer working hours for surgeons and trainees have altered the training environment. These changes increase the throughput of work, necessitate greater expenditure of time and effort to ensure safe patient journeys and diminish opportunities for workplace teaching and learning. The changes have also eroded the time for surgeons and trainees to invest in a meaningful teacher-learner relationship. This may be compounded by a generational gap between senior surgeons and incoming trainees, real or perceived, particularly in terms of attitudes towards learning and expectations of behaviour. There is an increasing perception by surgeons of the multifactorial influences that lead to a potential reduction in the standards of entry to training, quality of training and attitudes exhibited by trainees. This combined with introspection of their own abilities to teach across all nine surgical competencies may well lead to disenfranchisement of a significant proportion of the surgical workforce. The increasing realisation that an expert surgeon has never really meant being an expert teacher needs to be addressed by investment in training the teachers.

### 3.3.2 The Learning "Demand"

The burden of teaching in the past decade has escalated as surgical training broadened its focus to include the nine competencies along with an increase in the intake of surgical trainees by 18.7% [25]. Surgeons are now expected to select, teach, feedback, assess and remediate on cognitive, behavioural and social competencies while having to assimilate the evidence base that underpins best educational practices. Surgeons are required to be proficient in using contemporary in-training and work-based assessment tools and develop performance improvement plans that engender different concepts to that of teacher-centred supervision and assessment, to which they are more accustomed. The responsibility to identify and manage the trainee in difficulty is important, requires due diligence and can be demanding. Contemporary methods of teaching using simulation and e-learning resources pose further challenges for surgeons to remain educationally engaged. While many surgeons bemoan the values associated with the current generation of trainees, many trainees become frustrated at the lack of adaptability of their trainers.

Another major challenge for future surgical education is the progressive reduction in clinical exposure which impacts on the development of both technical and NTS. Driven by occupational safety, financial and logistical concerns, the average hours worked by doctors-in-training continues to diminish. Shift work impacts on continuity of care and learning while increasing demands on teamwork and communications. Intelligent use of simulation training and judicious availability of e-learning resources will be required to offset the deficit in clinical exposure. The problems created by shift work may be creatively utilised to integrate formal teaching and training in nontechnical competencies such as communications and teamwork. The cost implications of utilising advanced technologies to compensate for educational time will need to be considered in the context that gathering clinical experience remains uncompressible in time. This along with the expanding knowledge base in medicine leads the training bodies to the politically vexing question of expanding the training time.

### 3.3.3 Accountability in Educational Practice

There is a risk that the growing sophistication of contemporary surgical education is outstripping the capacity and capability of surgeons to meet a range of educational requirements. As the rigour around surgical training increases, so too are the requisite skills for being a surgeon educator. In the present environment, surgeons need to be equipped with an evidence-based set of educational skills through formal training. Moves to formalise the educational practice of surgeons is, however, daunting and requires careful consideration through dialogue to ensure there is engagement and ownership of how this is achieved. Professionalism in the delivery of surgical education is inseparable from accountability in educational practice. The drivers for accountability originate from trainee expectations of meaningful learning experiences as well as fairness and transparency in educational processes [2]. These expectations are not unreasonable given surgical training is a high-stakes commitment. An equally important driver is the recognition that the quality of training influences the quality and safety of surgical care. As revalidation of surgeons becomes inevitable, educational practice can be expected to be part of the scope of revalidation. In the United Kingdom, surgical educators are already required to submit evidence of their educational practice and are one example of educational accountability [26]. The North American system that has traditionally incorporated faculty development with programme evaluation is another model of accountability, integrated into the practice of education.

In the Australasian context, amongst numerous other national contexts, professional development programmes exist to upskill surgeons in trainee selection, supervision, feedback, assessment and remediation (Table 3.1). More recently, the RACS has sought to equip surgeons with teaching skills via a raft of courses and programmes, some of which are mandatory and many of which are undertaken in significant partnerships with professional and educational bodies (Table 3.1).

These efforts may redress the shortfalls in capabilities, but capacity for teaching remains a major problem. Strategies to recruit more surgeons into active teaching roles must include measures to prioritise opportunities for training. The tension between service and training is inevitable but perhaps unnecessary. Viewing training and service provision as being interdependent rather than in conflict would allow management at the meso level to approve policies that enable surgeons at the micro level to balance training opportunities with service provision. Being accountable for education must be reciprocated with appropriate opportunities and conditions to educate and train. This could be strengthened by meso level jurisdictional and institutional policies that commit to valuing and prioritising surgical education in the workplace [27]. The degree of commitment can be measured against and mandated through macro level standards built into the accreditation process.

Adopting a peer-assisted programme to support surgeons in their educational practice has merit, based on the reported successes in undergraduate medical education [28]. It may also be appropriate to partner with experts who are not surgeons to teach selected nontechnical competencies to trainees. For some behavioural competencies such as teamwork, it may be feasible to collaborate with other colleges to share development and delivery of training modules and to use simulation-based methods to bring efficiency to skill acquisition.

An important feature of surgical education is the pro bono contribution of surgeons. Many surgeons view the ideal of teaching without extrinsic reward as an obligation of the social contract. To what extent this ideal undermines capacity

**Table 3.1** Examples of professional development of educational skills available for surgeons – short courses and degree programmes

| Course | Parent organisations and partnerships | Programme details |
|---|---|---|
| **NOTSS:** Nontechnical Skills for Surgeons | University of Aberdeen | NOTSS is a behaviour rating system based on a skills taxonomy that allows valid and reliable observation and assessment of four categories of surgeons' nontechnical skill: situation awareness, decision-making, communication and teamwork and leadership |
| | Royal Australasian College of Surgeons | |
| | Royal College of Surgeons of Edinburgh | |
| | Royal College of Surgeons of England | |
| **SATSET:** Supervisors as Trainers for Surgical Education and Training | Royal Australasian College of Surgeons | The Supervisors and Trainers for Surgical Education and Training (SAT SET) course enables supervisors and trainers to effectively fulfil the responsibilities |
| **KTOT:** Keeping Trainees on Track | Royal Australasian College of Surgeons | Aimed at early detection of trainee difficulty, performance management and holding difficult but necessary conversations |
| **FSSE:** Foundation Skills for Surgical Educators | Royal Australasian College of Surgeons | This is an introductory course to expand knowledge and skills in surgical teaching and education and establish a basic standard expected of RACS surgical educator |
| **EMST:** Instructor Course | American College of Surgeons | Aimed at developing the faculty for EMST courses |
| | Royal Australasian College of Surgeons | |
| Early Management of Severe Trauma | Academy of Medical Educators | |
| **CCrISP® Instructor Course:** Care of the Critically Ill Surgical Patient | Royal College of Surgeons of England | Aimed at developing the faculty for CCrISP® courses |
| | Royal Australasian College of Surgeons | The CCrISP® course aims to develop simple, useful skills for managing critically ill patients and coordination of multidisciplinary care |
| | Academy of Medical Educators | |

(continued)

**Table 3.1** (continued)

| Course | Parent organisations and partnerships | Programme details |
|---|---|---|
| **TIPS Instructor Course:** Training in Professional Skills | Royal Australasian College of Surgeons | Aimed at developing the faculty for TIPS courses. The TIPS course teaches junior doctors, surgical trainees and IMGs the importance of nontechnical skills |
| | Monash University | |
| | St Vincent's Medical Education Unit | |
| **Surgical Teachers Course** | Royal Australasian College of Surgeons | The Surgical Teachers Course builds upon the concepts and skills introduced in the SAT SET course |
| | St Vincent's Hospital Medical Education Unit | |
| **ELPS:** Educational Leadership Programme for Surgeons | Royal College of Surgeons of England | A highly interactive course for senior staff which considers different styles of leadership and the advanced skills and attitudes of an effective leader, manager and mentor |
| **TrACE:** Training and Assessment in the Clinical Environment | Royal College of Surgeons of England | A 1-day course that provides advanced training and assessment skills for clinical and educational supervisors |
| **Training the Trainers: Developing Teaching Skills** | Royal College of Surgeons of England | An interactive course to improve planning, developing, delivering and evaluating surgical training |
| **Surgeons as Educators** | American College of Surgeons | This 6-day intensive course is designed to provide surgeons with the knowledge and skills to enhance their abilities as teachers and administrators of surgical education programmes |
| **Graduate Programs in Surgical Education** | Royal Australasian College of Surgeons | This suite of programmes addresses the specialised needs of teaching and learning in a modern surgical environment. The programmes allow surgeons to gain formal skills in teaching and educational scholarship |
| Graduate certificate | The University of Melbourne | |
| Graduate diploma | RACS Academy of Surgical Educators (ASE) | |
| Masters | | |
| **Masters and Postgraduate Diploma in Education** | Imperial College London | An intensive face-to-face teaching, discussion and academic programme to challenge and develop the thinking and practice as a surgical educator |

building is difficult to know. It might be argued that those who align with the younger generations may feel less inclined to teach without extrinsic reward, but there is currently little evidence to substantiate this view. Appropriate recognition of teaching, whether or not it is pro bono, is important if education is to have perceived value. Negotiations with hospitals to prioritise time for teaching and learning are likely to be a key part of recognising and valuing teaching. It is time to rethink how teaching opportunities can be created to optimise learning in the changing environment. Accreditation standards pertaining to supervision and teaching may require strengthening and enforcement to support strategies in building teaching capacity.

## 3.4 Social Obligation

As a profession, surgery has a responsibility to not only serve the community but to do so in a way that best meets community needs. The laws of market economics dictate that a degree of equilibrium be reached between supply and demand. However, while the market is demanding that more surgeons reside and practice in non-metropolitan locations and have skill sets that are more generalist in scope, the reality is that these needs remain largely unmet. In the current climate, surgical education needs to determine and define its role in influencing a responsive supply of surgical services.

The literature provides some insight into how and why trainees choose a career in surgery [29]. What is poorly understood is how trainees gauge community needs and expectations in making career choices. It is also unclear to what extent trainees are guided to weighing up community needs to inform socially responsive career choices. Not everyone can become a superspecialist surgeon in a quaternary institution even if they aspire to this goal; it is neither realistic nor desirable for surgical training to accommodate such career preferences, particularly as surgical training relies on expensive, precious and finite public resources. Therefore, given the importance of making appropriately informed career choices, it seems prudent for surgical education to assume some stewardship in guiding socially responsive career choices. This requires an understanding of surgical workforce demographics, prevalence of surgical diseases within different population settings, foreseeable advances in surgical practice, resource allocation and evolving models of surgical care. It also requires an awareness of the imprecise nature of workforce predictions and planning. Simultaneously there must be awareness and transparency where training bodies become involved in future workforce planning and resource allocation as there is a significant potential for conflict of interest both real and perceived. Meaningful dialogue between training providers and government, who gatekeep resourcing of healthcare delivery, is necessary to demonstrate that surgical education is being socially accountable. The fact that surgical training occurs primarily within the public health system requires surgical education to be accountable for producing surgeons fit for servicing the needs of the public.

### 3.4.1 Supporting Socially Responsive Career Decisions

There are several indicators that surgical education should adopt a socially responsive approach to training surgeons. These include an ageing surgical workforce, disparity in access to surgical care between communities and within communities correlating with disparity in surgical outcomes, the evolution of different models of care such as acute surgical units to manage the burden of both emergency and elective surgery, the emergence of new technologies impacting on choice of treatment, the ever-rising cost of surgical care and rationalisation of surgical resources to achieve both efficacy and efficiency. Trainees require an appreciation of these complex factors in order to align career choices with sociopolitical imperatives. Ignoring these factors is contrary to the social contract that surgery has in acting in the best interest of patients and society. Surgical education has the potential to have an active role in advising career decisions that are socially responsive. Strengthening training capacity and capability in regional and rural settings and promoting the desirability of acquiring a generalist set of expert surgical skills are ways of supporting informed decisions. Specialty Training Boards also have a role in counselling trainees on specialty specific surgical services that are required to meet current and foreseeable community needs. Perhaps informing trainees on the future direction of surgery in terms of workforce requirements should be central to the career counselling offered through surgical education. Furthermore, highlighting the global responsibility of graduating surgeons to meet the needs of disadvantaged sectors of the community and of our Pacific Island nations is both socially responsible and an attraction to some trainees.

### 3.4.2 Social Accountability

A surgical education and training programme that is not seen to be socially responsible risks its autonomy in determining training priorities being supplanted by externally regulated requirements. It is therefore preferable that surgical education demonstrates initiative in producing surgeons with the skill set most appropriate to meet community needs. While surgical colleges, training boards and jurisdictions must maintain a dialogue around the surgical needs of the community, individual surgeons must also be prepared to counsel trainees on how to mould career aspirations with the realities of societal needs. Trainees can be encouraged to consider a range of surgical pathways that align with community needs while fulfilling personal preferences. It is also likely that surgical training programmes will be accredited taking into account how they manage the issue of providing education and training that is socially responsive. The question of awareness of social obligation in service provision is already being asked of prevocational doctors [30]. It is not unreasonable that surgery will be expected to articulate how its training programme seeks to prioritise community needs with the professional preferences of trainees.

## 3.4.3 Diversity and Inclusivity

There is growing awareness of the benefits of the surgical community being truly representative and reflective of the broader community [31]. Diversity and inclusion refers to gender, ethnicity, indigeneity, religion and minority groups, ultimately aimed at ensuring all surgeons are culturally competent. Cultural competence enables a more socially responsive model of surgical care with better patient outcomes, than would otherwise be possible [32]. Cultural safety and competence are clearly articulated standards for Australasian Specialist Training Programs [33]. There are several areas of surgical education where diversity and inclusion are yet to be fully achieved. These are evident by the disparity in gender and indigenous representation amongst trainees as well as on decision-making bodies, lower examination pass rates for international medical graduates (IMGs) and paucity of flexible (e.g. part-time) training opportunities. In turn, these factors discourage participation by women, IMGs and indigenous groups in surgical training. All policies relating to surgical education require scrutiny with the purpose of identifying those elements that impede diversity and inclusion. Educational processes and practices also require review to determine where inequitable training experiences exist. Those involved in surgical education must develop an awareness of how to adjust education practice in order to engender equity in surgical training. The notion that surgical education should assume social responsibility in administering training and formulating strategy needs to be accepted and realised by the surgical community if surgery is to continue to serve the community.

## 3.5 The Challenge Ahead

Surgeons are renowned for their adaptability and, paradoxically, their conservatism. The contextual elements outlined above represent challenges for surgical education, which require adaptability of educational design and processes and conservatism of ideals pertaining to what it means for surgery to be a profession. They affect all players across the spectrum, from trainees and surgeons to regulators and governments. There is little option but to engage with these challenges, as quality and safety of surgical care would be directly compromised by inaction. The college, as a sophisticated educational organisation, is well placed to lead in the necessary reforms, adaptations and innovations. The priority for the college is to develop strategic direction for sustainable surgical education through research, scholarship, innovation and collaboration. Collaboration and partnership will be necessary with governments, regulators, universities, professional educators, postgraduate medical councils, experts in professional skills and professionalism, surgical craft groups and other colleges. Change inevitably brings challenges, and challenges should be viewed as opportunities. Immense opportunities exist to position surgical education at the forefront of how best to train surgeons of the future.

# References

1. Flexner, A. (1910). *Medical education in the United States and Canada – A report to the Carnegie Foundation for the advancement of teaching.*
2. Scott, S. V. (2014). Practising what we preach: Towards a student-centred definition of feedback. *Teaching in Higher Education, 19*(January 2015), 49–57. https://doi.org/10.1080/13562 517.2013.827639.
3. Kneebone, R., & Fry, H. (2011). The environment of surgical training and education. In H. Fry & R. Kneebone (Eds.), *Surgical education – theorising and emerging domain* (Vol. 2, 1st ed., pp. 3–17). Dordrecht: Springer. https://doi.org/10.1007/978-94-007-1682-7.
4. Hull, L., Arora, S., Aggarwal, R., Darzi, A., Vincent, C., & Sevdalis, N. (2012). The impact of non-technical skills on technical performance in surgery: A systematic review data sources. *Journal of the American College of Surgeons, 214*(2), 214–230. https://doi.org/10.1016/j.jamcollsurg.2011.10.016.
5. Flin, R., O'Connor, P., & Crichton, M. (2008). *Safety at the sharp end: A guide to non-technical skills* (1st ed.). Hampshire: Ashgate Publishing Ltd..
6. RACS. (2012). *Becoming a competent and proficient surgeon: Training standards for the nine RACS competencies.*
7. Wong, B., Ackroyd-Stolarz, S., Bukowskyj, M., Calder, L., Ginzburg, A., Microys, S., … Wallace, G. (2014). *The CanMEDS 2015 patient safety and quality improvement expert working group report.*
8. Arora, S., Sevdalis, N., Nestel, D., Woloshynowych, M., Darzi, A., & Kneebone, R. (2010). The impact of stress on surgical performance: A systematic review of the literature. *Surgery, 147*(3), 318–330.e6. https://doi.org/10.1016/j.surg.2009.10.007.
9. Cooper, W. O., Guillamondegui, O., Hines, O. J., Hultman, C. S., Kelz, R. R., Shen, P., … Hickson, G. B. (2017). Use of unsolicited patient observations to identify surgeons with increased risk for postoperative complications. *JAMA Surgery, 37212*, E1–E8. https://doi.org/10.1001/jamasurg.2016.5703.
10. Kennedy, I. (2002). *Learning from Bristol.*
11. RACS. (2015). *Expert advisory group expert advisory group report to RACS on discrimination, bullying and sexual harassment expert advisory group expert advisory group report to RACS.* Retrieved from http://www.surgeons.org/about/building-respect,-improving-patient-safety/expert-advisory-group/
12. Fnais, N., Soobiah, C., Chen, M. H., Lillie, E., Perrier, L., Tashkhandi, M., … Tricco, A. C. (2014). Harassment and discrimination in medical training: A systematic review and meta-analysis. *Academic Medicine, 89*(5), 817–827. https://doi.org/10.1097/ACM.0000000000000200.
13. Arora, S., Sevdalis, N., Suliman, I., Athanasiou, T., Kneebone, R., & Darzi, A. (2009). What makes a competent surgeon?: Experts' and trainees' perceptions of the roles of a surgeon. *American Journal of Surgery, 198*(5), 726–732. https://doi.org/10.1016/j.amjsurg.2009.01.015.
14. Cruess, S. R., & Cruess, R. L. (2009). The cognitive base of professionalism. In *Teaching medical professionalism* (pp. 1–27).
15. Paice, E. (2009). Identification and management of the underperforming surgical trainee. *ANZ Journal of Surgery, 79*(3), 180–184.; ; discussion 185. https://doi.org/10.1111/j.1445-2197.2008.04837.x.
16. Hodges, B. D., Ginsburg, S., Cruess, R., Cruess, S., Delport, R., Hafferty, F., … Holtman, M. (2011). Assessment of professionalism: Recommendations from the Ottawa 2010 Conference. *Medical Teacher, 33*(5), 354–363. https://doi.org/10.3109/0142159X.2011.577300.
17. Bearman, M., O'Brien, R., Anthony, A., Civil, I., Flanagan, B., Jolly, B., … Nestel, D. (2012). Learning surgical communication, leadership and teamwork through simulation. *Journal of Surgical Education, 69*(2), 201–207. https://doi.org/10.1016/j.jsurg.2011.07.014.

18. Rao, R., Dumon, K. R., Neylan, C. J., Morris, J. B., Riddle, E. W., Sensenig, R., ... Brooks, A. D. (2016). Can simulated team tasks be used to improve nontechnical skills in the operating room? *Journal of Surgical Education, 73*(6), e42–e47. https://doi.org/10.1016/j.jsurg.2016.06.004.
19. Irby, D. M., & Hamstra, S. J. (2016). Parting the clouds: Three professionalism frameworks in medical education. *Academic Medicine, 91*(12), 1606–1611. https://doi.org/10.1097/ACM.0000000000001190.
20. Cruess, R., Mcilroy, J. H., Cruess, S., Ginsburg, S., & Steinert, Y. (2006). The professionalism mini-evaluation exercise: A preliminary investigation. *Academic Medicine, 81*(10), 574–578.
21. RACS. (2011b). *Surgical workforce projection to 2025: Volume 1 the Australian workforce* (Vol. 1).
22. HWA. (2012). *Health workforce 2025 doctors, nurses and midwives – volume 1* (Vol. 1).
23. Young, C. (2011). International medical graduate – can we do better? *General Surgeons Australia Newsletter, 12*(3), 2.
24. RACS. (2011a). *Surgical workforce 2011 census report*.
25. Commonwealth of Australia. (2012). *Medical training review panel fifteenth report*.
26. McIhenny, C., & Pitts, D. (2014). Royal College of Surgeons of Edinburgh, Faculty of Surgical Trainers: Standards for Surgical Trainers.
27. GMC. (2015). *Promoting excellence: Standards for medical education and training*.
28. Silbert, B. I., Lam, S. J. P., Henderson, R. D., & Lake, F. R. (2013). Students as teachers. *Medical Journal of Australia, 199*(3), 4–5. https://doi.org/10.5694/mja12.10970.
29. Sobral, D. T. (2006). Influences on choice of surgery as a career: A study of consecutive cohorts in a medical school. *Medical Education, 40*(6), 522–529. https://doi.org/10.1111/j.1365-2929.2006.02482.x.
30. Australian Health Ministers' Advisory Council. (2015). *Review of medical intern training*.
31. RACS. (2016). *Diversity & inclusion plan*.
32. Khoury, A., Mendoza, A., & Charles, A. (2012). Cultural competence: Why surgeons should care. *Bulletin of the American College of Surgeons, 97*, 13–18.
33. Australian Medical Council. (2015). *Standards for assessment and accreditation of specialist medical education programs and professional development programs*. Retrieved from https://amc-cms-prod.s3.amazonaws.com/files/fc6e591a9a87c6c2b45e1d744eafa41e5499717d_original.pdf

# Chapter 4
# Surgical Education Leadership and the Role of the Academy

**Peter Gogalniceanu, Margaret Hay, and Nizam Mamode**

**Overview** Leadership and education are similar in that they are both transformative processes that facilitate growth, foster collaborations and increase scientific knowledge, innovation and enterprise. Surgical academia poses increasingly greater challenges that are often outside the remit of regular professional training. Nevertheless, academy itself is a key modality of growth that informs the development of leaders and educators. This review highlights some key principles of effective surgical education and leadership and their relationship to academy.

## 4.1 Introduction

The exponential growth of academia driven by the digital revolution, globalisation and technological advances in the last 30 years has changed the way in which research is planned, conducted and disseminated. Consequently, a clinical research facility or laboratory is no longer a physical entity but a global virtual space in which individuals from a wide variety of cultural and professional backgrounds interact. Language barriers, time zone discrepancies, cultural differences, currency exchange rates and even political unrest have now become daily realities for academic surgical leaders. All too often surgeons in academia lack the leadership theoretical background taught in professional business administration degrees with unfavourable consequences for their research and clinical activity.

---

P. Gogalniceanu (✉) · N. Mamode
Department of Transplantation, Guy's Hospital, Guy's and St. Thomas'
NHS Foundation Trust, London, UK

King's College London, London, UK
e-mail: Nizam.Mamode@gstt.nhs.uk

M. Hay
Monash Institute for Health and Clinical Education, Monash University, Clayton, Australia
e-mail: margaret.hay@monash.edu

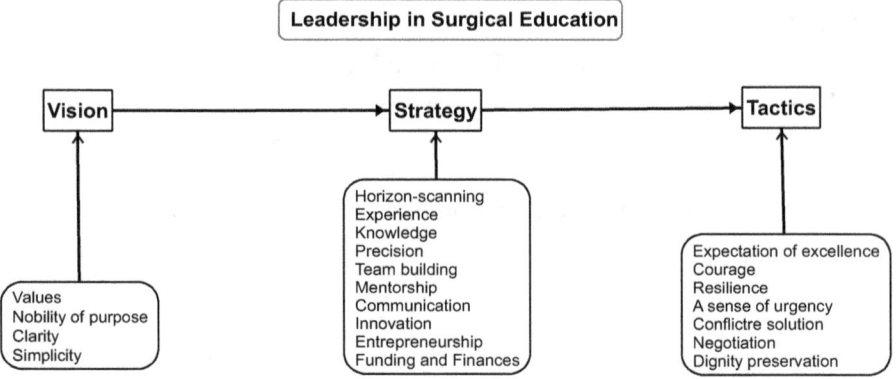

**Fig. 4.1** Summary model of leadership in surgical education

This chapter aims to subjectively define and review key leadership and educational processes that can help surgeons face the challenges of contemporary academic careers in the context of global surgical practice (Fig. 4.1).

## 4.2 What Is Leadership?

Effective leadership is a process responsible for the initiation and successful management of "change" [1]. As change is both inevitable and potentially attractive, it is not surprising that interest in leadership is both significant and sustained. However, the definition of leadership is vast, heterogeneous and context-dependent.

It can be more broadly defined as a process by which individuals in a position of authority use their power to influence a group in order to achieve a particular task [2]. Furthermore, we define it as a positive transformative process that shifts individuals or organisations from a lower to higher state of existence. In short, leadership adds value and safety. It is the positive and transformative nature of leadership that gives its true justification for authority, as it provides both a moral validation and a survival advantage for the community it represents. Consequently, true leaders are individuals who have the necessary creative, emotional, organisational and technical skills needed to become drivers for positive change.

Whilst leadership should always be representative and democratic, there are circumstances when leaders need to act on behalf of those they represent in the absence of consultation or group consensus. One such example was the landing of United Airlines Flight 1549 (in the Hudson River in January 2009). This demonstrates that it is the prerogative of those in command to make executive decisions in times of crisis, with the full knowledge that should failure occur (no matter how inevitable), they alone will be held responsible. As such, leadership requires an element of confidence (derived from competence), initiative and autonomy practised in exceptional circumstances and within the limits permitted by respect for each individual's rights. Nevertheless, this creates a central leadership dilemma, treading a fine line between courageous/moral statesmanship and irresponsible, unethical or dictatorial practices. In such cases, the suspension of individuals' freedoms for the "greater good" or their "best interests" represents an automatic disqualification from leadership for those in command. Respect for individuals' choices and rights should remain the moral compass needed to inform leaders regarding their commission to take unilateral action. In the context of surgery, clinicians are well aware of the importance of driving treatment and facilitating access to healthcare but also respecting patient choice in refusing it or withdrawing from it after due consideration has been given. Informed consent, multidisciplinary consultation and patient participation remain key clinical pillars of good surgical leadership.

Traditionally, effective leaders balance team- and task-related priorities. Authoritarian leaders focus on achieving their task at the cost of alienating their teams (or patients). In contrast, weak leaders constantly seek approval and lose the capacity of implementing their strategies. Current leadership theory has seen a shift away from the analysis of leadership "traits" or "styles" and a move towards a "contingency theory" [3], that is to say the selective application of different leadership approaches to match the task, team and environment in which the leader is performing.

## 4.3 What Are the Components of Leadership?

A simple theoretical model of leadership practice describes three processes needed to reach the desired outcome [4]:

1. Vision (objectives/goal): *why* is the task important?
2. Strategy (plan): *what* needs to be done for the task to be achieved?
3. Tactics (application): *how* will be the task achieved? By *who*? And *when*?

## 4.4 Education and Academy

Educators have a similar role to leaders, in that they guide moral and intellectual growth by creating opportunities and framing events in a way that allows their students not just to acquire knowledge but also to develop positive values and healthy attitudes.

Similarly, academy can be defined as the scientific pursuit of truth and morality though research, education and scholarship [5] leading to positive change. It is, in our view, a more fundamental process that can serve as an instrument for facilitating growth, including the development of other transformational activities such as leadership and education.

Consequently, this chapter defines education, leadership and academy not as separate entities but as identical transformative processes impacting on different scientific domains, namely:

- The acquisition of values and attitudes (education)
- The government of people (leadership)
- The discovery of new and truthful knowledge (research in all its forms)

As such, we will argue that surgical educational leadership is a complex process that can be developed through academic pursuits in order to improve clinical surgical practice. Consequently, academic leader-educators (ALE) are drivers of positive change within surgery education and practice. Their activity impacts not only on patient outcomes but also on the training of future surgeons and the development of the specialty as whole.

## 4.5 Vision Development

*Efforts and courage are not enough without purpose and direction* [6]
    JF Kennedy

**Defining the Vision** Leaders are individuals who are able to identify and differentiate what is essential and important from the mass of "white noise" of everyday activity [4]. In other words, they must find the "difference that makes the difference" and formulate it into a vision. *Constantin Brancusi* defines this "simplicity" as "complexity resolved" [7]. On the other hand, mediocre visions do not result from the distillation of complexity but are the outcome of a rushed and inconsistent analysis.

**Nobility of Purpose** The purpose of a vision is to "align, motivate and inspire" people about a specific task [1]. The concepts of goal identification and vision sharing have strong corporate roots and have often been imported in healthcare without careful discernment. In business environments, employees need to be aligned along a company's specific direction and commercial priorities. However, in healthcare academia, the ethical and professional values required are not only better defined but also legally enforced (e.g. the *Universal Declaration of Human Rights* [8] or the General Medical Council's Good Medical Practice guidance [9]). The *vision* must not only be clear but also address a worthy problem and carry moral weight in order to generate enthusiasm and legitimacy. As such, visions need to be value-based, representing the moral orientation of each team member, as well as the team's culture. This is crucial in establishing a *nobility of purpose* needed to generate intrinsic motivation, curiosity and dedication amongst the team. For example, a vision aiming to develop a cost-effective model of cataract surgery training in the third world as part of a global health programme is more likely to bring together a motivated team of surgeons compared to a project investigating mesh porosity in inguinal hernia repairs.

**Communication** It is also the ALE's duty to clearly outline and effectively communicate [10] visions so that they can be translated into behavioural changes. Leadership charisma, repetition and simplification are effective means of achieving this. Successful visions will therefore grow into the community's culture to create robust, autonomous and predictable team performance, as well as longer-lasting alignment with the original vision.

**Solutions** ALE need to offer a credible *solution* to the problem identified to create a sense of empowerment, focus, energy and enthusiasm. A lack of confidence in the capacity to resolve the task usually terminates any leadership capacity. The solution needs to be not just focussed and achievable but challenging enough to make it exciting and morally relevant enough to make it obligatory.

**Learning Points:**

- A vision is the outline of an important problem and its desired solution.
- Visions need to be values-based and problem-oriented. By combining values with strategy and tactics, effective ALE can find the balance of being both team- and task-oriented in reaching their goal.

## 4.6 Standard Setting

> *It must be done right* [11]
> R Linton, Massachusetts General Hospital

> *Inattention to detail is the hallmark of mediocrity* [12]
> M DeBakey, Houston Methodist Hospital

The ultimate responsibility of all leaders in science is discovery of *truth* ("veritas"). Interestingly, the same Latin term also translates as *correctness* or *rectitude*, which adequately describes the clinical principles of good surgical practice, that is to say to "do it right" [13] both from a technical, cognitive and ethical perspective.

First, it is essential for ALE to understand the meaning of quality, being aware that the search for "quality and excellence" in academia and in clinical practice has become a managerial cliché. In the context of surgical leadership, quality must be seen as a "capacity for excellence" [14], being interpreted in terms of precision, clarity, relevance as well as volume, efficiency and timeliness. Furthermore, it must be pragmatically assessed by insuring that all activity is outcome-oriented ("the end result") [15–17] but humane in its delivery. It remains the duty of surgical leaders therefore to educate their teams in the pursuit of quality.

Secondly, Kotter et al. have demonstrated that successful leaders are individuals who generate a *sense of urgency*, that is to say a rejection of complacent attitudes and an "alert and proactive" state which leads to a "determination to move, and win, now" [18].

Thirdly, ALE need to drive performance by creating a healthy sense of competition and "great expectations" [19]. Often this is done by contextualising the team's activity in relation to the practice of other successful competitors or elite institutions.

Fourthly, 360-degree feedback remains an important method for ALE to identify "quality blind spots" in their activity. However, caution must be exercised when engaging in unblinded peer-based feedback which remains largely inefficient due to collegial reluctance to offend. Leaders must instead be vigilant towards subtle or *occult negative feedback* manifested as poor staff retention, termination of collaborations or complaints from external teams or even the public.

Fifthly, ALE need to demonstrate the moral discipline and transparency needed not to rebrand failure or find justifications for mediocre outcomes. A capacity for critical analysis is essential, as well as the open-mindedness needed to modify both their activity and leadership style.

Finally, time-limited leadership appointments are necessary to ensure that institutional complacency, creativity decay and attrition of motivation do not develop amongst those established as leaders in surgical education.

**Learning Point** Quality can be defined as a sustained search for truth and excellence, driven by competition, precision, critical analysis and outcomes-oriented activity.

## 4.7 Courage

*In times of stress, be bold and valiant* [20]
   Horace

Academic pursuits are not without frequent and disheartening disappointments. ALE thus need to develop and demonstrate *courage* to thrive. Whilst the definition of courage in general is beyond the remit of this chapter, we would define it as the audacity to recover or progress against adversity through the suppression of fear [21, 22]. In the context of surgical academic practice, it should be seen as the ability to face personal, professional or financial risk for the benefit of patient care and the advancement of surgical science. This can be manifested either as resilience in the face of failure or as a determination to explore, innovate, build systems or change practice. Consequently, surgical leadership education must provide academics with the skills needed to negotiate institutional opposition, bureaucracy or the risk of losing professional or personal reputations. The historical case of Ignaz Semmelweis [23–25] and his research into the cause of puerperal fever is one of the many instances where academic courage has been met with personal and professional catastrophe. Semmelweis is considered a pioneer of antiseptic procedures today; however, his request to colleagues that they wash their hands between autopsy and patient examination work in an era prior to the acceptance of the germ theory of disease resulted in his professional ridicule and ostracisation. Nevertheless, the

ALE must assume this responsibility and be accountable for the team's failures on the road to success. Two characteristics have been identified that may aid the growth and application of courageous leadership. The first is the quality of self-awareness, which implies an understanding of one's values, motivations, strengths and weaknesses [26, 27]. The second is a strong belief in the essential moral worth of the objective pursued, which is essential in creating a higher sense of entitlement to succeed. Together, these create the ability to recover when suffering setbacks as well as to advance in the face of opposition. It is the duty of ALE therefore to educate and guide their teams into being realistically resilient [28], derive meaning out of hardship and become anti-fragile [29].

**Learning Point** Academic leaders must be strong, persistent and bold as well as motivated by a purpose that is perceived as being greater than themselves.

## 4.8 Conflict Resolution

*You have to get along to get ahead.*
    D.A. Cooley, Texas Heart Institute

Complexity generates discord, and this should be an expected daily reality for ALE. Hicks et al. identified "dignity violations" as an important source of human conflict. These can be defined as any conscious or subconscious threat to an individual's self-worth, giving rise to an instinctive emotional self-defence response [30]. *Dignity violations* may consist of erroneously perceived personal criticisms, failures to provide due care and recognition of an individual's values and identity or a more general lack of respect for one's intrinsic human worth (irrespective of their achievements or failures) [30]. *Dignity violations* therefore have toxic, catastrophic and even terminal consequences for teams and their collaborations. It is essential that ALE understand that the nature of conflict is primarily an emotional response to a social, intellectual or physical problem and that the solution offered must also be emotional rather than practical in nature. Often disproportionate reactions need to be contextualised in the plaintiff's own anxieties, expectations or personal circumstances. The concepts of honour, dignity and respect also display significant cultural variations, which are often muted in everyday social interactions and can consequently lead to unintentional violations. These may often continue to remain tacit but manifest through aggressive, irrational or inconsistent behaviours challenging a leader's authority.

If possible, ALE should aim to avoid conflict by transforming disagreements from a process of *debate* (one based on opposition, resulting in a loser and a winner) to one of *dialogue* (based on finding consensus). When conflict is inevitable, leaders should adopt collaborative and accommodative style, rather than being competitive, avoiding or abdicating their duty to resolve the crisis. Simple methods of conflict resolution involve active listening, expectation management as well as tactical compromises on behalf of ALE. Physical and mental health considerations must also be accounted for, and professional third-party mediation may be needed when these overwhelm a leader's management capacities. In addition, conflict resolutions must create a sense of mutual gain, rather than mutual loss, with a perceived sense of justice for both parties in order to facilitate permanent closure. ALE must also demonstrate neutral, consistent and unbiased behaviours when managing conflicts to maintain their authority as independent arbitrators. Furthermore, ALE must anticipate conflicts and consequently educate teams regarding the appropriate pathways and systems they must engage in should disagreement occur. These need to be clearly outlined in order to frame potential future actions taken by ALE and shape the team's understanding of expected behaviours. Furthermore, errors identified through such systems should be seen as learning lessons for the entire team rather than as occasions for allocating blame to individuals.

**Learning Point** ALE must concomitantly fulfil the roles of judges, advocates and negotiators to overcome conflicts. Their understanding of the concept of *dignity* is essential to this process.

## 4.9 Building Teams

Leaders are dependent on their collaborators, making successful team building an important factor in their success. Team members should share a common direction and enthusiasm, but not necessarily the same abilities, interests or personality profiles. Heterogeneity in skill set, experience and professional training are fundamental qualities that leaders need to consider when selecting and developing their team members. Polyvalent teams not only offer increased creativity but also anti-fragility [29] in the form of long-term stability against changing circumstances. An example of instability caused by inadequate multilateral team development was demonstrated by the introduction of laparoscopic, robotic-assisted and endovascular surgery in surgical communities of practice that were predominantly trained in open surgery. Institutions with progressive leadership were quick to train staff or employ new partners with the relevant skill set. In contrast, those that were slow or reluctant to adapt experienced a relative decline in their clinical and academic outcomes.

Secondly, leaders need to delegate specific roles to team members to foster personal development as well as to create time and opportunities for themselves. This highlights a second principle of leadership in team building, namely, that of "frontline leadership" (tactical command) versus "hilltop leadership" (strategic command), based on the degree to which leaders choose to be involved in the grassroot activities of their team [31]. Good academic leadership must allow a rapid interchange between tactical and strategic approaches in order to provide both action (e.g. writing a grant application) and direction (e.g. initiating collaborations with other centres), respectively.

Thirdly, effective leaders should pursue the development of sub-leaders that can incrementally take over limited and well-defined areas within the principal leaders' range of activity. This process not only consolidates growth but also allows principal leaders to expand their range of activities, increase volume and engage in alternative innovative or entrepreneurial pursuits. The process of allowing team members to gradually progress into sub-leaders provides both long-term professional satisfaction for those involved and diffusing any toxic leadership challenges that principal leaders may otherwise experience over a long duration of time.

**Learning Point** Academic surgeons should create polyvalent teams, foster growth, delegate responsibilities and raise a new generation of leaders.

## 4.10 Mentorship and Growth

The role of leadership has already been identified as a process of facilitating transformation both for the leader and individuals within a team. In pedagogical terms, a teacher is the active agent (or "scaffold") in the learner's zone of proximal development [32, 33] – meaning that they facilitate a progress that the learner would not have been able to achieve alone. In this way, the concept of leadership is analogous with that of education, in that they both act as a bridge between an inferior and a superior state of existence. In simple terms, the mentor (ALE) provides tuition and constructive feedback to allow learners to grow. However, true surgical leader-educators take a longer-term approach, creating experiential learning opportunities, as well as encouraging networking and collaborations to allow surgical pupils to develop as individuals. They realise that successful mentorship is about the transfer of generic skills, values and attitudes that students can apply to their own interests and careers. As such, a good academic leader is a catalyst and a creator of new leaders and researchers, often in unrelated fields of academia or clinical practice. *Bennis* and *Thomas* describe such individuals as creating "crucibles of leadership" whereby great expectations and demanding (often challenging) environments allow "opportunities for reinvention" [19]. Finally, ALE realise their own need to develop and engage in mentorship relationships with other experts. This not only facilitates their own process of continuing growth but also allows them to lead by example in teaching their own students the need to engage in a lifelong process of surgical learning.

**Learning Point** Academic surgeons should foster the growth of their team members by transferring their own values, skills and experience but allowing learners to develop according to their individual needs, talents and interests.

## 4.11 Finance and Entrepreneurship

*The entrepreneur shifts economic resources out of an area of lower and into an area of higher productivity and greater yield.* [34, 35]
　Jean-Baptiste Say

Increasingly, academia is being subjected to financial constraints. Public funding is both competitive, scarce and widely scrutinised, whilst private funding of research may be associated with restrictions. As such, ALE need to develop themselves and their students into successful fund-raisers and accountants, as well as scientists, researchers and clinicians. Surgical academic education must not ignore key human resources skills, such as staff recruitment and pension planning, the design of collaboration agreements and understanding of contract law. Surgical education needs to create academics which are able to create robust business plans and deliver results on time and on budget. Nevertheless, it is not sufficient for ALE to be merely financially competent and cost-neutral service providers. Instead, they should seek new opportunities of creating value, increasing productivity [36] and engaging in innovative activities in order to be true entrepreneurs. Risk and uncertainty [37] may often be the price of enterprise, reform and reorganisation, but ALE should help their students mitigate and control these. Whilst an entrepreneurial spirit is often found amongst surgical trainees, their leaders should provide the necessary training flexibility for them to seek development opportunities outside surgery and recognise these as a constructive way of employing their time.

**Learning Point** Leaders in surgical education need to both practice and teach cost-effective model of academic activity, innovation and entrepreneurship.

## 4.12 Conclusion

Leadership, education and academy are parallel but analogous processes seeking positive transformation. Change can be complex, unpleasant and costly. As such, those involved in its implementation require strong moral, emotional and intellectual attributes to negotiate this developmental ascent. Effective surgical leaders need to display a variety of characteristics, including a nobility of purpose, a commitment to the pursuit of truth and excellence, attention to detail as well as a sense of urgency and a respect for dignity. The role of academy is to provide the "crucible" in which surgical education leaders develop.

## References

1. Kotter, J. P. (1999). *John P. Kotter on what leaders really do*. Boston: Harvard Business Review Book: HBS Press.
2. Kotter, J. P. (1977). Power, dependence, and effective management. *Harvard Business Review, 55*, 125–136.
3. Goffee, R., & Jones, G. (2000). Why should anyone be led by you? *Harvard Business Review, 78*, 62–70.
4. Campbell, A. (2016). *Winners*. Random House.
5. Merriam-Webster, Inc. (1984). *Merriam-Webster's dictionary of synonyms*. Merriam-Webster.

6. Kennedy, J. F.. Speech of Senator John F. Kennedy, Raleigh, NC, Coliseum [Internet]. Available from: http://www.presidency.ucsb.edu/ws/?pid=74076
7. Gimenez, C., & Gale, M. (2004). *Constantin Brancusi*. London: Tate.
8. Assembly U. (1948). *Universal declaration of human rights*. UN General Assembly
9. Great Britain GMC. (2013). *Good medical practice*. Manchester: General Medical Council.
10. Kotter, J. P. (1977). Power, dependence, and effective management. In *Organizational influence processes* (pp. 128–143). Glenview.
11. Cutler, B. S.. Robert, R., & Linton, M. D. (1994). A legacy of "Doing it right": From the New England society for vascular surgery. *Journal of Vascular Surgery, 19*(6), 951–963.
12. Frazier, O. H. O.H. "Bud" Frazier interviewed by Donald A.B. Lindberg [Internet]. Available from: https://profiles.nlm.nih.gov/ps/access/FJBBWQ.pdf
13. Cutler, B. S., Robert, R., Linton, M. D. (1994). A legacy of "doing it right".
14. Eidt, J. F. (2012). The aviation model of vascular surgery education. *Journal of Vascular Surgery, 55*(6), 1801–1809.
15. Dervishaj, O., Wright, K. E., Saber, A. A., & Pappas, P. J. (2015). Ernest Amory Codman and the end-result system. *The American Surgeon, 81*(1), 12–15.
16. Kaska, S. C., & Weinstein, J. N. (1998). Ernest Amory Codman, 1869–1940: A pioneer of evidence-based medicine: The end result idea. *Spine, 23*(5), 629.
17. Brand, R. A. (2009). Ernest Amory Codman, MD, 1869–1940. *Clinical Orthopaedics and Related Research, 467*(11), 2763–2765.
18. Kotter, J. P.. (2008). *A sense of urgency*. Boston: Harvard Business School Publishing.
19. Bennis, W. G., & Thomas, R. J. (2002). Crucibles of leadership. *Harvard Business Review, 80*(9), 39–45 –124.
20. Cook, J. (1999). *The book of positive quotations*. New York: Gramercy.
21. Moran, L. (1987). *The anatomy of courage: The classic study of the soldier's struggle against fear*. Garden City Park: Avery.
22. Moran, C. (2007). *The anatomy of courage*. New York: Carroll & Graf.
23. Semmelweis, I. P. (1981). Childbed fever. *Clinical Infectious Diseases, 3*(4), 808–811.
24. Jay, V. (1999). Ignaz Semmelweis and the conquest of puerperal sepsis. *Archives of Pathology & Laboratory Medicine, 123*, 561–562.
25. Best, M., & Neuhauser, D. (2004). *Ignaz Semmelweis and the birth of infection control*. BMJ Publishing Group Ltd.
26. Goleman, D., & Boyatzis, R. (2001). *Primal leadership*. Harvard University Press.
27. Goleman, D., Boyatzis, R. E., & McKee, A. (2002). *The new leaders: Transforming the art of leadership into the science of results*. London: Little, Brown and Company.
28. Diane, L. C. (2002). How resilience works. *Harvard Business Review, 80*, 46–48.
29. Taleb, N. N. (2012). *Antifragile*. London: Penguin.
30. Hicks, D., & Tutu, D. (2011). *Dignity*. New Haven: Yale University Press.
31. Leonard, H., Cole C., Howitt, A., & Heymann, P. (2014). *Why was Boston strong? Lessons from the Boston marathon bombing*. Program on crisis leadership. President and Fellows of Harvard College.
32. Vygotsky, L. (1978). *Mind in society: The development of higher psychological processes*. Cambridge: Harvard University Press.
33. Vygotsky. (2013). *Philosophy and education*. Oxford: Wiley.
34. Hindle, T. (2009). *Entrepreneurship*. Available from: http://www.economist.com/node/13565718
35. Hindle, T. (2012). *The economist guide to management ideas and gurus*. London: Profile Books.
36. Hindle, T. (2008). *Guide to management ideas and gurus*. London: Profile Books.
37. Knight, F. H. (2012). *Risk, uncertainty and profit*. Wilmington: Vernon Press.

# Chapter 5
# The Governance of Surgical Education: The Role of the Colleges

Ian Eardley

**Overview** This chapter reviews the place of the Surgical Royal Colleges in the governance of surgical training in the UK. The College structures that oversee training include the Joint Committee for Surgical Training (JCST) and individual Specialty Accreditation Committees (SACs) and their roles in curriculum development, assessment, selection, certification, quality assurance and trainee support are described. The relationship of the Colleges with the regulator, the funder and the education providers is complex and has changed substantially from the time when the Colleges had a central responsibility for accrediting surgical training. The reasons for these changes are discussed. Although set in the UK, there are also commonalities for Colleges internationally.

## 5.1 Introduction

In the UK, the governance of surgical training rests between four organisations: the regulator (the General Medical Council or GMC); the arm of government that oversees and funds surgical training (currently Health Education England or HEE); the locations where surgical training actually happens, namely, the hospitals or Local Educating Providers (LEPs); and Surgical Royal Colleges. While the focus of this chapter is to discuss the role of the Colleges, it is not possible to do this without a description, where appropriate, of the roles of the other organisations and the consequences of these arrangements. Box 5.1 summarises the abbreviations of the organisations associated with governance of surgical training in the UK.

I. Eardley (✉)
Leeds Teaching Hospital Trust, Leeds, UK

> **Box 5.1: Abbreviations Relevant for Governance of Surgical Training in the UK**
> Certificate of Completion of Training (CCT)
> Certificate of Equivalence of Specialty Training (CESR)
> European Economic Community (EEC)
> Fellowship of the Royal College of Surgeons (FRCS)
> General Medical Council (GMC)
> Health Education England (HEE)
> Intercollegiate Committee for Basic Surgical Examinations (ICBSE)
> Joint Committee for Surgical Training (JCST)
> Local Education Providers (LEPs)
> Local Education and Training Boards (LETBs)
> Membership of the Royal College of Surgeons (MRCS)
> National Health Service (NHS)
> Objective Structured Clinical Examination (OSCE)
> Out of Program Research (OOPR)
> Out of Program Training (OOPT)
> Out of Programme Experience (OOPE)
> Postgraduate Medical Education and Training Board (PMETB)
> Quality Improvement Framework (QIF)
> Royal College of Physicians and Surgeons of Glasgow (RCPSGlas)
> Royal College of Surgeons of Edinburgh (RCSEdin)
> Royal College of Surgeons of England (RCSEng)
> Royal College of Surgeons of Ireland (RCSIre)
> Schools of Surgery (SoS)
> Specialty Accreditation Committees (SACs)
> Specialty Training Committees (STCs)

## 5.2 A Historical Perspective

The Barber Surgeons received their Royal Charter from King Henry VIII in 1540, but it was not until 1629 that King Charles I of England ordered the Barber Surgeons to establish a Court of Examiners that would certify ship's surgeons. The Surgeons separated from the Barbers in around 1745, and at that time, there were around 90 practicing surgeons within London. Training was by a process of apprenticeship, which at that time was set at 7 years, with an assessment at the end of that period by a Court of Examiners. In 1836, at an extraordinary General meeting of the Royal College of Surgeons of England, it was agreed that "no person would be recognised as a lecturer on anatomy, physiology, pathology or surgery in England until he shall have undergone an examination by the Council on two separate days, the first on anatomy and physiology and the second on pathology and the principles and practice of surgery". These examinations were embodied in the Royal Charter of 1843, which established the "Fellowship of the Royal College of Surgeons" (FRCS) as the indication that a surgeon had successfully completed their training.

In many ways, these structures and principles remained unchanged until the latter years of the twentieth century. This author trained when there was no written syllabus or curriculum, but simply a series of examinations with an assessment of "competency" at the end of training by the trainers who had overseen the training of that surgeon. The Colleges largely controlled surgical training, by setting the examinations and assessing the readiness of the trainees for certification while also overseeing the quality of the training posts themselves by means of regular visits to each training unit.

### 5.2.1 Drivers for Change

Much has changed in healthcare in the past 50 years. From the advent of the National Health Service (NHS) and the principle that treatment should be free at the point of delivery, there has been a progressive requirement by society that the outcomes of care are as good and reproducible as possible, with minimal harm to patients while they receive that care. In surgical education, this has resulted in a need for more standardised and objective outcomes of training, a greater emphasis upon patient safety with closer supervision of trainee surgeons and a need to demonstrate better value for money.

During the early years of the twenty-first century, these drivers resulted in a considerable change in the process of training and in the governance of surgical training and associated changes in the responsibilities and roles of the Colleges. There was a perception by the funders of medical training, the Government that the Colleges, being essentially membership organisations, were neither transparent nor democratic enough to be trusted to maintain their central position within medical training, despite their demonstrable expertise. Until that time, the Government had funded a considerable component of the training functions of the Colleges, but gradually this funding was withdrawn, while a new "regulator" of medical training was introduced, initially in the shape of the Postgraduate Medical Education and Training Board (PMETB) which began to function in 2005 and subsequently by the GMC which took over the functions of PMETB in 2010.

## 5.3 Current Architecture of UK Surgical Training

The GMC currently has a central position in UK medical and surgical training. It is the organisation that sets standards, approves curricula, certifies completion of training, approves equivalence of training for those who have trained outside the UK and quality assures medical training. However, it has neither the resources nor the expertise to actually do all those things themselves and has to delegate some of the day-to-day activities to others, including the Medical Royal Colleges.

HEE is currently the Governmental body that funds and manages medical training in the UK. It does this through a number of regional structures or Local Education and Training Boards (LETBs) most of which have a Postgraduate Dean to lead training in that locality. LETBs are often loosely referred to as "Deaneries". HEE has responsibility for managing the training not just of doctors but also of allied healthcare professionals including nurses, radiographers, physiotherapists and others. In medicine, they recruit the trainees, provide their salaries, arrange their clinical attachments, oversee the regular assessments of progression, manage trainees in difficulty and oversee the quality management of the clinical attachments. Inevitably, they have to work closely with the GMC, the local education providers and the Colleges. As the arm of government, they also have to deliver value for money and work within centrally determined budgets. The components that oversee surgical training within the LETB are the Schools of Surgery (SoS), with Heads of Schools who are employed by the Deaneries to manage surgical training in all specialties in that locality. Lying below the Schools are the individual Specialty Training Committees (STCs), which comprise a group of surgeons within that locality with a representative for each training unit. The Training Programme Director sits on that committee and has overall charge of the trainees in that specialty, in that locality.

The training units are located in hospitals and are termed the Local Education Providers (LEPs), and they actually deliver the educational attachments for trainees. They have a somewhat conflicted position because the UK NHS has largely been developed on the basis that trainees deliver much of the emergency care for patients, while the trainee salaries are largely paid for by the LETB with the intention that it pays for their training. This conflict between service and training is therefore complex. Many believe that service is essential in order to deliver experience, while others believe that this balance has veered too far in recent years towards service and to the detriment of training.

There are four Surgical Royal Colleges that oversee surgical training in the UK. The Royal College of Surgeons of England (RCSEng), Royal College of Surgeons of Edinburgh (RCSEdin), Royal College of Surgeons of Ireland (RCSIre) and the Royal College of Physicians and Surgeons of Glasgow (RCPSGlas) work together to oversee surgical training through a number of intercollegiate structures. The most senior structures are the Joint Committee for Surgical Training (JCST), the Joint Committee for Intercollegiate Examinations (JCIE) and the Intercollegiate Committee for Basic Surgical Examinations (ICBSE). Below JCST and JCIE, there are specialty-specific Specialty Accreditation Committees (SACs) and specialty-specific Intercollegiate Examination Boards. Currently, there are ten surgical specialties that sit within these structures, cardiothoracic, general, neurosurgery, oro-maxillo-facial, otolaryngology (ENT), paediatric, plastic, trauma and orthopaedic (T&O), urology and vascular, and the membership of each SAC is made up of specialty and College representatives.

## 5.4 Roles of the Surgical Royal Colleges in UK Surgical Education

### 5.4.1 Curriculum Development

In the early years of the twenty-first century, it became clear that there was a need for defined, written curricula to underpin postgraduate medical training. Currently, while the responsibility for curriculum approval of those curricula lies with the regulator, the responsibility for their actual development lies with the Colleges, and this responsibility is delegated to the individual SACs. Every 3 or 4 years, the SAC undertakes a review of the specialty curriculum and produces a document describing surgical training in that specialty. There is input from all relevant stakeholders including trainees, the lay public, the service (i.e. the NHS) and HEE, and when the final document is agreed, it is submitted for approval to the GMC. The curriculum must meet certain predefined standards that have been set by the GMC [1], and the GMC scrutinises the curriculum to ensure that those standards are met. There is often a formal panel review of the curriculum as part of this scrutinising process. When approved, it becomes the blueprint for training in that specialty until there is another review some time later.

Currently, the Colleges are the only organisations that have been given the responsibility to write curricula for medical and surgical training, and this ensures, perhaps more than any other single factor, that they remain central to the governance of surgical training in the UK.

Most curricula are now provided online for trainers and trainees in e-portfolios that describe the curriculum and provide real-time workplace-based assessment tools, logbooks for surgical procedures and systems that manage assessment and progression. The surgical curricula are housed in the Intercollegiate Surgical Curriculum Programme (ISCP) [2], and trainees currently pay an annual training fee that gives them access to the e-portfolio.

### 5.4.2 Assessment

The need to objectively assess trainees, and, in the case of surgery, to assess their ability to undertake technical tasks, has meant that there has been an increased emphasis upon assessment in the workplace. The development of workplace-based assessments as tools for providing formative and summative assessment of clinical, professional and technical skills has largely been led by clinical and surgical educators, sometimes in conjunction with the Colleges. However, while assessment in the workplace is undertaken by working surgeons, the annual review of the trainee progression lies with the SoS, and the determination of which assessments should be undertaken is still largely dictated by the Colleges, through the curricula.

Further, the College examinations first developed in the 1800s are still the basis for the summative assessment of knowledge in surgical training, although their structure and format have changed considerably over the years. Currently, there are two main sets of examinations: the Membership examinations that are taken after 1–2 years of surgical training, which deliver the post-nominal MRCS (Membership of the Royal College of Surgeons), and the Fellowship examinations that are taken towards the end of surgical training, which deliver the post-nominal FRCS (Fellowship of the Royal College of Surgeons). The examinations, being blueprinted to the curriculum, are an intrinsic part of the curriculum and accordingly are also regulated by the GMC, with an expectation that they adhere to the relevant standards [1].

The MRCS is an examination in two parts, a multiple-choice examination and an objective structured clinical examination (OSCE), and it covers the basic surgical sciences and the principles of surgery. It is written, marked and quality assured by the ICBSE and actually delivered as an examination by each of the Surgical Royal Colleges. Currently, all surgeons take this examination, although there is an equivalent alternative for trainees intending a career in ENT.

The FRCS is an examination in two or three parts, a multiple-choice examination, a clinical examination and/or a viva voce assessment, and there are ten specialty-specific versions. They are written, marked, delivered and quality assured by the JCIE and delivered by the specialty intercollegiate boards. Currently, all surgeons take an examination in their specialty FRCS examination. See Chap. 20 for further information on assessment.

### 5.4.3 Selection into Surgical Training

Surgery is traditionally a competitive specialty, certainly when compared to other medical specialties. Historically, when a vacancy arose, an individual hospital or Deanery advertised for a replacement trainee, and there was often stiff competition for training places. Such a process of local interview was both inefficient and not always transparent, and since 2007, national selection processes have been gradually introduced in every surgical specialty. There is also a further selection point into the early years of surgical training (core surgical training). See Chap. 15 for further information on selection.

Selection centre methodology has been incorporated with the intention of assessing all candidates equally and fairly. The principle is that this is an assessment, but for a different purpose (i.e. selection *into* a period of training). The format of the selection process is an OSCE-style assessment, with each candidate proceeding through a number of stations, where their skills and competencies are assessed. While the human resource components (advertising, contracts, logistics, contractual issues) of the selection process are undertaken by the Deaneries/LETBs, the design of the selection processes themselves (application criteria, standard setting, station design, marking, quality assurance) lies with the individual SACs, who now oversee selection into surgery on an annual basis.

## 5.4.4 Workforce Planning

The Colleges have no direct responsibility for workforce planning, but each College and each Specialty Association/SAC has a pretty good idea of current workforce numbers. The trainee numbers are supposed to reflect service needs, so that broadly speaking the number of trainees reflects the expected number of consultant jobs in the UK, but given the prolonged nature of the training process, workforce planning in surgical training sometimes gets it wrong! The most recent example of this was the period between 2005 and 2008 when the advent of drug-eluting coronary artery stents made it seem likely that the demand for cardiac surgeons would diminish over a very short time period. The Cardiothoracic SAC and the Colleges were at the centre of the response to that "crisis" including the year to year planning of recruitment numbers and the support for cardiac surgical trainees who might not have a consultant job at the end of their training. Happily for the cardiac surgeons, there still remains a need for their services, since the stents did not prove quite as effective as was once hoped!

## 5.4.5 Trainee Certification

The decision that a trainee has successfully completed surgical training and is now suitable to be certified is a decision for the regulator (i.e. the GMC), which in the UK holds the register of certified specialists for each specialty. There are currently three main routes to the register, via a UK-based training pathway that delivers a trainee with a Certificate of Completion of Training (CCT), via certification in another European country (at least until Brexit is complete) and via demonstration of equivalence for non-EEC nationals. This latter route requires the trainee to receive a Certificate of Equivalence of Specialty Training (CESR).

While the GMC actually delivers these certificates, it delegates much of the responsibility for determining whether a trainee has achieved the requisite standard to the Colleges, who in turn delegate that authority to the SACs. For the award of a CCT, the portfolio of the trainee is assessed firstly in the Deanery, by the annual review process. If approved, the SAC then reviews the whole portfolio, including examination results, logbooks and assessment portfolios. If approved, and the trainee is thought to be worthy of certification, this decision is passed to the GMC who then award the CCT. The GMC quality assures this process by independent review of a proportion of some of the applications (currently around 5–10%).

The SACs have developed a set of certification guidelines [3] that are intended to guide the trainee and which identify what a trainee will normally be expected to have achieved during their training programme. The guidelines cover such aspects of training as clinical and operative experience, operative competency, research, quality improvement and management and leadership.

For the award of a CESR, the applicant has to develop a portfolio of achievements that is mapped to the UK curricula and to the GMC's own Good Medical Practice [4], and when complete, the candidate submits that portfolio to the GMC for review. Again, the GMC delegates the review of that portfolio to the SACs who review the application before recommending an outcome back to the GMC, which may be to award a CESR, to reject the application or to ask for more evidence before making that award. Again, the GMC actually awards the certificate and quality assures a proportion of the SAC's decisions.

### 5.4.6 Quality Assurance

Historically, the sole responsibility for quality assurance of surgical training lay with the Colleges. Through the SACs, individual LEPs were regularly visited, with external assessments that were largely supportive, but in extreme cases resulted in immediate cessation of training in that unit. This in turn had the potential for enormous impact upon service provision and was in part why the UK government withdrew responsibility for quality assurance from the Colleges and delegated responsibility to an independent regulator. Although this was fought bitterly by the Colleges at the time, the subsequent years have gradually allowed the Colleges back into this essential area of surgical education.

The GMC currently has overall responsibility for setting and regulating standards for medical education and training in the UK. Its Quality Improvement Framework (QIF) sets out how it quality assures education and training and how it works with other organisations, for example, LETBs/Deaneries and Medical Royal Colleges, in this respect. There are three levels of quality activity: quality assurance, quality management and quality control. Quality assurance is the responsibility of the GMC and is the overarching activity under which both quality management and quality control sit. It includes all the policies, standards, systems and processes that are in place to maintain and improve the quality of training. Quality management is the responsibility of LETBs/Deaneries and refers to the processes through which they ensure that the training provided by the LEPs meets the GMC's standards. LEPs, for example, NHS hospitals, are responsible for the quality control of the training they provide by making sure it meets local and national standards.

The Colleges have developed a series of measures that sit alongside this quality framework, including a set of "quality indicators" that identify good training units, an annual survey of surgical trainees delivered to all surgical trainees [5], a process for externality which supports the annual review of trainee progression and a process of externality that supports Deanery visits to individual LEPs. They work closely with the SoS to quality assure surgical training, and while not in the position of central importance that they once held, they remain a crucial component of the system.

### 5.4.7 *Trainee Support*

When a surgical trainee is enrolled in surgical training, they are able to access support from a number of sources. At a local level, it will be from their trainer and mentor, while at a regional level, it will be from their programme director and Postgraduate Dean. At a national level, the JCST also supports trainees in a number of ways. They enrol trainees in the curriculum, they certify completion of training and they manage the duration of training, which may be affected by periods of time spent outside training for things such as research (Out of Program Research or OOPR), training (Out of Program Training or OOPT) or experience (Out of Programme Experience or OOPE). The rules for obtaining and accrediting these periods are often complex, and the JCST plays a central role in managing them. In addition, periods of time out of training for reasons of ill health or maternity need to be managed, while trainees who are less than full time also need support and clarity of when they can expect to be certified. JCST undertakes these processes and keeps a provisional CCT date for all trainees within the UK surgical training system.

## 5.5  An International Perspective

The governance of surgical training differs from country to country with a range of different bodies and roles existing in individual countries. No two systems are the same. However, the functions that need to be accomplished are broadly similar, and the differences are perhaps not as substantial as they might initially seem. Wherever surgical training is undertaken, there is the need to select trainees, to set standards, to write curricula, to assess trainees, to quality assure programmes and to certify the product of training. The strength of the College within an individual country varies enormously with government, funders, regulators, universities and hospitals all playing roles that vary from country to country.

## 5.6  Conclusion

The UK surgical training governance system is relatively centralised and reflects, in part, the existence of a centralised socialised healthcare system. The main players are the Colleges, the GMC, HEE and the NHS Hospital Trusts. Although the role of the Colleges is not as central as is once was, it remains a strong force in surgical education in the UK with its primacy in curriculum development (and all that goes with it) being perhaps the most important function that it currently undertakes.

## References

1. http://www.gmc-uk.org/education/postgraduate/standards_for_curricula_and_assessment_systems.asp
2. https://www.iscp.ac.uk
3. http://www.jcst.org/quality-assurance/certification-guidelines
4. http://www.gmc-uk.org/guidance/good_medical_practice.asp
5. http://www.jcst.org/quality-assurance/jcst-quality-indicators-and-trainee-survey

# Part II
# Overview: Theories Informing Surgical Education

This part orientates readers to the often *messy* world of theory. We use the term *theory* to describe *frameworks of ideas* that for some have become orthodoxy but for others may seem new and challenge ways of exploring the complex world of surgical education and practice. Although the theories inform *education*, they have disciplinary influences from, of course, education and also sociology, psychology, anthropology, politics and more. These disciplines also intersect, hence, the reference to *messy*. In selecting content, we could have chosen many other theories, but these are the ones that resonated for us and are often published as underpinning surgical education research, and we considered valuable for those engaging with surgical education in a scholarly way. In our individual practices, we have dominant influencing theories but also select from those listed here depending on the educational consideration at hand. We have aimed to demystify some of the language associated with these theories and offer simple orientations to their ontological (nature of reality) and epistemological (nature of knowledge) positions.

The first chapter from Bartle and Evans describes educational considerations from cognitive neuroscience (Chap. 6). They outline key concepts of information processing theory, cognitive load theory [1] and mastery learning. The latter popularised in simulation-based learning of procedural and operative skills [2]. Next, Harris offers insight to theories of expertise which have gained traction in surgical education literature through the notion of deliberate practice [3] (Chap. 7). This topic is usually of tremendous interest to surgical educators as it offers particular insights to the role of 'practice' in the development of excellence in operative (and other) skills. It seems to resonate/appeal for many reasons, including the analysis of 'elite' performance and of the need for sustained practice over many years (easily recognised) with goal setting and feedback/coaching.

Blackburn et al. introduce the theory of threshold concepts [4] and use their research with paediatric surgical trainees and *junior* cardiothoracic surgeons to identify threshold concepts and to share the value of applying the theory in these two contexts (Chap. 8). Gandamihardja and Nestel describe key concepts in a theoretical notion of communities of practice [5] and its value in using this lens to observe, design for and analyse workplace-based learning (Chap. 9). This chapter signals the role of communities of practice in the development of professional identity which is amplified in Chaps. 12 and 13.

Ibrahim offers an overview of activity theory and shifts learning to considerations of the entire surgical workplace – the environment, the history of the individuals, the culture, motivations and the complexity of real clinical activity – for educational design (Chap. 10). McNaughton and Selgrove focus our attention on the role of power in surgical education by viewing many aspects of practice from a Foucauldian perspective. This is an illuminating way to view common practices through what may be for many a different lens (Chap. 11).

The topic of identity development has seen recent scholarly interest in the health professions. Theories of identity have a long history in psychology and social psychology where there are literally scores of theories. Chapters 12 and 13 explore some that have been popularised in the health professions education literature and help us better understand the complex changes individuals undergo in becoming a surgeon. The first is from Di Napoli and Sullivan on the development of surgeon identities (Chap. 12). The second, from Cuming and Horsburgh (Chap. 13), a less studied focus, is on the development of the surgical educator identity. The authors' outline major approaches to developing surgical educators in ways that mirror the arguments made about developing surgeons in the previous chapter. This process is about much more than providing tips and tricks for educational practice. It requires a more fundamental engagement with surgical educators' beliefs about knowledge and identity and their agency as surgeons, on individual and institutional levels. Attending to these wider developmental concerns has implications for how we approach faculty and career development structures of those involved with surgical education and surgical education research.

In summary, this part offers a range of theories that reflect different worldviews. Variously, they are cited in health professions education literature, offer guidance for designing educational activities, make meaning of challenging educational experiences and likely broaden and deepen understanding of the many considerations in educational practice.

## References

1. van Merrienboer, J., & Sweller, J. (2010). Cognitive load theory in health professional education: Design principles and strategies. *Medical Education, 44*(1), 85–93.
2. McGaghie, W. C. (2015). When I say … mastery learning. *Medical Education, 49*(6), 558–559.
3. Ericsson, K. (2004). Deliberate practice and the acquisition and maintenance of expert performance in medicine and related domains. *Academic Medicine, 79*(10), S70.
4. Meyer, J., & Land, R. (2005). Threshold concepts and troublesome knowledge (2): Epistemological considerations and a conceptual framework for teaching and learning. *Higher Education, 49*(3), 373–388.
5. Wenger, E. (1998). *Communities of practice: Learning, meaning and identity*. Cambridge, UK: Cambridge University Press.

# Chapter 6
# Cognitive Neuroscience and Design of Surgical Education

**David Bartle and Andrew Evans**

**Overview** The surgical educator who understands human cognition is better able to design and implement educational activities. The cognitive neurosciences propose theories and models of learning which aid in this understanding. Information Processing Theory emphasises active thought processing whereby information is grouped and processed between the learner's working and long-term memory. As this information is synthesised, it develops into schema which can be more efficiently manipulated by the mind. Cognitive Load Theory draws on this theory and proposes that schema best develop when a learning activity is tailored to the audience. Mastery Learning contends that expertise occurs in stages and that it is best for a learner to master their current sphere of learning before progressing to the next. Optimal tuition recognises the learner's current sphere of learning and accelerates the attainment of mastery.

## 6.1 Introduction

Surgical education involves the synthesis of a great deal of knowledge, skill and attitude in what can be a fluid and at times chaotic learning environment. Cognitive neuroscience equips the surgical educator with tools to introduce purposeful design to the complex task of educating surgeons. Cognition is the mental action or process of acquiring knowledge and understanding through thought, experience and the senses. Cognitive processes are involved with simple processes such as learning a new scientific fact or developing a new procedural skill and are also involved with higher faculties such as reasoning and judgement. Cognitive processes are used in both concrete and abstract realms and span the continuum between conscious and unconscious thought [4, 6, 9, 11, 12].

D. Bartle (✉)
Tauranga Hospital, Tauranga, New Zealand

A. Evans
Townsville Hospital, Douglas, Australia

Using scientific process, the cognitive neurosciences investigate how we acquire knowledge and understanding and illustrate this through various models and theories. This brings coherent frameworks to the art and science of education and allows us to better understand how the human mind works and how it assimilates, processes, stores and retrieves information [2, 7, 8, 11].

This chapter presents key cognitive theories relevant to specialty level surgical education. These theories are Information Processing, Cognitive Load and Mastery Learning. Together these theories serve as a foundation upon which educational practice is based. With greater understanding of how the mind works, the surgical educator can design more effective learning activities (Box 6.1).

---

**Box 6.1 Key Cognitive Theories Relevant to Specialty Level Surgical Education Information Processing Theory**
*Key Concepts*:

*Cognitive processes may be likened to computer processes.*
*Working memory has limited capacity.*
*Grouping information together allows greater cognitive capacity.*
*Information Processing Theory is a foundational theory of cognitive neuroscience.*

*Key Theorist*:

*George Miller*

*Other Theorists*:

*Endel Tulving, Alan Baddeley, Graham Hitch, Henk Schimdt*

**Cognitive Load Theory**
*Key Concepts*:

*Schema is important for dealing with information.*
*We learn best under conditions aligned to our cognitive architecture.*
*Educational activities should reduce unnecessary cognitive load.*

*Key Theorist*:

*John Sweller*

*Other Theorists*:

*Fred Paas, Jeroen van Merrienboer*

---

(continued)

> **Box 6.1** (continued)
>
> **Mastery Learning**
> *Key Concepts*:
>
> *Explores methods of empowering students to achieve mastery.*
> *Students should achieve mastery in current activity before to moving to the next.*
> *Centres on the student rather than the educational system.*
> *Allows underperforming trainees to gain extra support.*
>
> *Key Theorist*:
>
> Benjamin Bloom
>
> *Other Theorists*:
>
> William McGaghie, Taylor Sawyer

## 6.2 Information Processing Theory

The Information Processing Theory recognises the active processes of learning and uses the model of a computer to illustrate aspects of human cognition. As with a computer, the brain receives information, processes and codes it in a meaningful way and then stores it for later use.

### *6.2.1 Active Thought Processes*

*Information Processing Theory emphasises active thought processes*

Information Processing Theory was introduced in the mid-twentieth century during an era in which behaviourism was the leading model for understanding human cognition [1, 2, 4, 6]. Behaviourism centred around a stimulus-response model in which a certain stimulus generated a certain response. The experiment with Pavlov's dogs illustrates this theory using what is termed classical conditioning. Behaviourism largely ignored the cognitive processes which mediated the relationship between stimulus and response. The underlying mechanisms involved with dealing with information in behaviourism are portrayed as being passive and dictated by the stimulus rather than our own mental capacity. Information Processing Theory emphasises active thought processing as central to how we deal with the received information and better illustrates the ability for higher-level cognitive function [1–3].

Input → Processing → Storage → Output

## 6.2.2 Types of Memory

*Working and long term memory work in tandem to permit cognitive function*

An understanding of memory is central to the Information Processing Theory and important to understanding educational processes.

Working memory is the function we use to hold small amounts of information in a readily available state for a short period of time. Working memory is characterised by those things of which we are presently conscious. The working memory has an extremely limited scope and can generally only hold a few elements for a short period of time [1–3].

In 1956, George Miller explored issues surrounding working memory, which at that time was referred to as short term memory [1–3]. He described how working memory is limited in its capacity and generally holds seven items with a range between five and nine. The theory became known as *seven plus or minus two* and has been demonstrated to be remarkably constant with some variation depending on the nature and familiarity of the presented information and the age of the subject [3].

In contrast to working memory, long-term memory has significant capacity and can hold information for an extended period of time. Long-term memory holds information out of conscious thought, and as we draw this into conscious thought, it starts functioning within working memory. Long-term memory is more than a repository of rote learnt facts but rather a complex system of organised structures that allow us to assimilate and process new information and to solve problems. Working memory and long-term memory work in tandem to permit efficient cognitive function [3, 4].

## 6.2.3 Chunks

*Grouping information together allows us to manipulate information more easily*

Miller also proposed that by organising information into chunks, we could expand the capacity of the working memory. This concept is very important as it provides insight as to how we manipulate information and is the basis for other cognitive theories [2, 4]. While it still holds true that the working memory can only function with a limited number of entities, if these entities themselves contain further information, the overall capacity of the working memory is significantly increased. By exploiting this phenomenon and organising information, people are able to hold a greater overall amount of information in their working memory. This concept is further explored under the Cognitive Load Theory [8].

## 6.2.4 Recency and Primacy

*We are more likely to remember the first and last items on a list*

The Information Processing Theory allows us to better understand certain observed phenomenon. Information presented to a person is not necessarily assimilated in a uniform fashion. The serial position effect is the tendency for an individual to be able to recall the first and last items with greater accuracy than the items in the middle [4]. The ability to recall early information is referred to as the primacy effect and is thought to take place because there is a greater amount of processing capacity available at that stage. The first item on a list can be rehearsed on its own, whereas the fourth item on a list has to be rehearsed with the first, second and third item. The ability to better recall the later information is termed a recency effect and is thought to take place because the information that remains in the working memory is easier to access without being crowded by yet further information. The serial position effect has important implications in education. When conducting a presentation, it is important to highlight key information at the beginning and end such as having clear objectives at the beginning and a clear summary at the end. Serial position effect is also likely to affect an examiner's recall of a student's performance. The first and last impressions are likely to be weighted greater in the examiner's mind than that from the middle of the assessment.

## 6.2.5 Information Processing Feedback Loop

*Cognitive processes contain inbuilt monitoring systems*

As part of the Information Processing Theory, Miller presented a model of how the human mind processes information. Whereas the prevailing belief from behaviourism was that of a simple stimulus-response reflex arc, Miller postulated a feedback loop much the same as is seen in physiological systems. This model is known as the Test-Observe-Test-Exit (TOTE) model [2]. In this model, a certain action is taken, and the response is monitored until the end result is achieved. A simple example is hammering a nail into wood. With each blow of the hammer, the position of the nail in the wood is monitored until such time that the nail is fully seated and the activity is complete.

When teaching a student how to incise skin, they will initially apply a certain amount of pressure to the scalpel and then observe for a result. If the pressure is not adequate, further pressure will be applied until the incision is made. Often a simple TOTE is embedded in a larger TOTE. A surgical operation can often be broken down into phases and each phase into smaller parts. As one part is completed, the surgeon moves to the next part until the phase is completed and so on until the operation itself is completed. This provides a hierarchical structure of how we carry out activities and how at each level a monitoring system is in place to ensure it is carried out satisfactorily.

### 6.2.6 Multicomponent Model

*Oral and visuospatial information interacts through information processing*

Building on the Information Processing Theory, Alan Baddeley and Graham Hitch recognised the complexity of working memory and developed a model of working memory in which they proposed two short-term storage mechanisms, one for dealing with language and the other for dealing with visuospatial information [4, 5]. The language component was termed the phonological loop and the other the visuospatial sketchpad. These components are controlled by the central executive which is responsible for directing relevant information to the appropriate area and suppressing irrelevant information. The phonological loop holds the sound of language and continually rehearses it in a loop, while concentration is directed towards that task, such as a phone number until the number is written down or dialled. The visuospatial sketchpad is used for constructing and manipulating images and mental maps. Visuospatial subsystems deal with the visual aspects such as shape and colour and spatial aspects such as location and relationship. A fourth component of the model is the episodic buffer which integrates information and aids in the storage of long-term memory. This multicomponent model emphasises the interaction between auditory and visuospatial learning and is especially relevant to surgical education which combines theoretical knowledge with visual and spatial awareness to carry out practical skills.

In summary, the Information Processing Theory provides a model for understanding human cognition. It emphasises the active processes of cognition and allows educationalists to further study and harness these processes to improve the delivery of effective education. The Information Processing Theory has served as the foundation upon which other theories are developed including the Cognitive Load Theory.

## 6.3 Cognitive Load Theory

Cognitive Load Theory suggests that we best learn under conditions which are aligned to our cognitive architecture. It is concerned with optimising educational activity so that the learner can retain as much of the content as possible. The theory, developed by John Sweller, is based on Information Processing Theory. Sweller's work focused on instructional design with cognitively complex and technically challenging material and is therefore appropriate for surgical education [8–12]. Sweller was particularly interested in the reasons why people may have difficulty learning complex material, and these insights can help us support underperforming trainees.

## 6.3.1 Schema

*Schema allow us to block information together which frees up cognitive resource*

Sweller uses the concept of a schema to illustrate how the mind can deal with large volumes of information. A schema is a cognitive construct stored in the long-term memory that permits us to treat multiple elements of information as a single element [8, 11]. As you read this text, your eye will be seeing individual letters; however your mind recognises certain groups of letters as specific words and treats the information as a word rather than a letter. The process of reading becomes much simpler as your mind has created a schema that allows you to treat multiple elements (letters) as a single element (word). Schemata are modular with smaller schema used to construct medium schema which can in turn construct larger schema. When manipulating information our mind is able to do this much more efficiently with discreet blocks than the thousands of smaller parts that make up those blocks.

As we develop schemata related to a particular problem, we are more likely to recognise the problem quickly and to apply the appropriate solution. A math student who has developed schemata for solving algebraic equations will be able to more easily recognise the problem and apply a solution than someone who is less familiar with this field. As the cognitive processes become more familiar, there is less load on the working memory, and the mind automates certain activities which previously required significant cognitive effort. The development of schemata is recognised as a defining feature of an expert in their field. With developed schema, the expert will be more fluent in their thought processes and when faced with a more challenging problem will have greater cognitive resource available to address the problem.

## 6.3.2 Cognitive Load

*Cognitive processes are loaded in different ways*

Cognitive Load Theory describes three types of load. These are (a) intrinsic, (b) germane and (c) extraneous [11].

Intrinsic load refers directly to the inherent difficulty of learning the subject matter. For a given subject matter, this load will depend on the learner's previous knowledge or experience in the domain. While the intrinsic load itself cannot be lowered, a learning task can be made more appropriate by aligning it to the learner's current level of experience. It is therefore important to know your audience and tailor educational activities appropriately.

Germane load refers to the cognitive load devoted to the construction of schema and is important for being able to retain information. This is the cognitive load involved with the various steps of processing and making sense of the intrinsic information and storing it in an appropriate schema.

Extraneous load refers to the cognitive load related to the presentation of information. Learning experiences which are confusing or difficult to follow have a high extraneous load, and this has the potential to saturate someone's cognitive capacity, meaning that they will be less able to assimilate the intrinsic load. Presenting educational activity appropriately will reduce the extraneous load. For example, when trying to convey the concept of a square shape, a simple diagram will achieve this much more efficiently than attempting to do so using a complex geometric definition.

Consider a builder working on a house. The intrinsic load refers to the essential work such as sawing and hammering. Germane load refers to activities such as erecting scaffolding which are not implicitly part of the building but necessary to complete the job. The extraneous load refers to unnecessary obstacles such as poorly drawn and confusing plans.

When designing educational activities, the intrinsic load will remain relatively constant but should be tailored to the audience. Germane load is important for retaining information. The challenge is to reduce the barriers to learning (extraneous cognitive load) and promote the tools for assisting learning (germane load). Understanding the processes involved with establishing schema allows for improved educational activities.

As students develop schema, they will become more agile with their thinking. Students who have developed appropriate schema and have begun to automate their cognitive activities will be at a stage where cognitive resource is available for new information to be assimilated. If a student has not yet mastered this initial information, they are unlikely to have adequate cognitive resource available to assimilate new information. This concept is key to understanding Mastery Learning.

## 6.4 Mastery Learning

*Mastery is achieved in stages*

Mastery Learning explores methods of empowering students to achieve mastery-level performance. Bloom contends that students should achieve a level of mastery in their current sphere of learning before progressing to the next [13]. By reaching this level of mastery, students will have developed appropriate schema and will be automating their cognitive activity. This allows students to free up cognitive resource and develop a robust foundation of knowledge upon which further knowledge can be built.

*Uniform tuition is not necessarily optimal tuition*

Mastery Learning confronts the reality that there is a normal range of aptitude among students and that people learn at different rates. Given this variation Bloom argued that a uniform system of tuition is unlikely to enable the majority of students to reach mastery within a similar time. Bloom contrasts uniform tuition in which each student receives the same tuition with optimal tuition where the student receives targeted tuition aligned with established educational strategies. Optimal tuition will positively skew the distribution curve towards mastery [13].

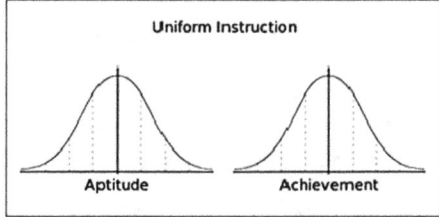
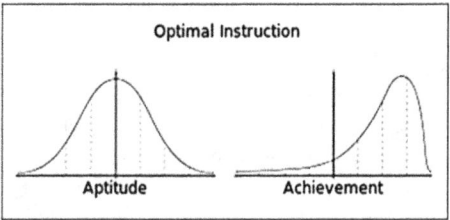

Mastery Learning shifts the focus of education from being an assessment activity (as might be the case for entry into a professional course) to being an equipping activity where the imparted knowledge and skill are essential parts of professional practice. Mastery Learning is especially relevant for vocational surgical training programs as the purpose of such programs is to ensure an appropriate level of mastery. This mastery is not just in technical areas but across a wide range of competencies.

### 6.4.1 Application

Teaching procedural skills is an important role of the surgical educator. Consider a student learning how to perform a new procedural skill. The session has been designed to involve theoretical learning and a demonstration of the procedure followed by a simulation activity in which the student will firstly practice the skill and then be formally assessed on the skill. Satisfactory performance during the simulation is a prerequisite before the student is able to perform this procedure on a person.

It is useful to consider the role of various cognitive models and how they affect the student's performance throughout this process. As a student faces the simulation activity, the newly presented information will be somewhat unfamiliar and not yet fully incorporated into cognitive schemata. The student's working memory will be loaded as it attempts to recall the theoretical information while concurrently executing the psychomotor skills of performing the simulated activity. It is possible that the student will struggle to achieve the necessary level of competency in such a task and until they do so it will be difficult for them to progress to the next level of learning.

In such a situation, the supervisor can help in a number of ways. They may be able to do this by drawing on the student's prior knowledge, explaining the rationale of the particular steps, breaking the procedure down into discrete phases each of which is easier to remember and encouraging mental rehearsal strategies or written plans which aid with committing the procedural steps to long-term memory. By providing these supportive educational strategies, the supervisor can accelerate the learning of the student and enable them to reach a level of mastery much sooner.

> **Box 6.2 Steps Associated with Mastery Learning (McGaghie)**
>
> 1. Baseline testing
> 2. Clear learning objectives
> 3. Educational activities focused on reaching the objectives
> 4. A set minimum passing standard for each educational unit
> 5. Formative testing to assess a minimum standard for mastery
> 6. Advancement to the next educational stage
> 7. Continued practice or study on an educational unit until the mastery standard is reached
>
> Source: McGaghie [15]

McGaghie has proposed certain steps associated with Mastery Learning (Box 6.2) which emphasise the need for the educator to understand baseline knowledge, establish clear objectives with focused educational activities and have a step-wise process for progression based on achieving certain minimum standards prior to moving to the next level [14].

## 6.5 Conclusion

The Information Processing Theory provides a foundational model of understanding cognition. The Cognitive Load Theory elaborates on this model and illustrates how cognitive processes come under load and how we use schema to better handle information processing. Mastery Learning recognises variation in individual aptitude and places importance on optimal tuition strategies to achieve mastery performance. Together these theories equip the surgical educator with scientific evidence to inform the design and implementation of educational activities.

## References

1. Miller, G. A. (1956). The magical number seven, plus or minus two: Some limits on our capacity for processing information. *Psychological Review, 63*, 81–97.
2. Miller, G. A., Galanter, E., & Pribram, K. H. (1960). *Plans and the structure of behavior.* New York: Holt, Rinehart & Winston.
3. Cowan, N. (2001). The magical number 4 in short-term memory: A reconsideration of mental storage capacity. *Behavioral and Brain Sciences, 24*(1), 87–114; discussion 114–85.
4. Baddeley, A. (1992). Working memory. *Science, 255*(5044), 556–559.
5. Baddeley, A. (2000). The episodic buffer: A new component of working memory? *Trends in Cognitive Sciences, 4*(11), 417–423.
6. Tulving, E., & Thomson, D. (1973). Encoding specificity and retrieval processes in episodic memory. *Psychological Review, 80*(5), 352–373.

7. Schmidt, H. G., Rotgans, J. I., & Yew, E. H. J. (2011). The process of problem-based learning: What works and why. *Medical Education, 45*(8), 792–806.
8. Sweller, J. (1988). Cognitive load during problem solving: Effects on learning. *Cognitive Science, 12*, 257–285.
9. Sweller, J. (1999). *Instructional design in technical areas*. Camberwell: Australian Council for Educational Research.
10. Paas, F. G. W. C., & Van Merriënboer, J. J. G. (1993). The efficiency of instructional conditions: An approach to combine mental effort and performance measures. *Human Factors: the Journal of the Human Factors and Ergonomics Society., 35*(4), 737–743.
11. Sweller, J., Van Merriënboer, J., & Paas, F. (1998). Cognitive architecture and instructional design. *Educational Psychology Review, 10*(3), 251–296.
12. Van Merriënboer, J. J. G., & Sweller, J. (2010). Cognitive load theory in health professional education: Design principles and strategies. *Medical Education, 44*, 85–93.
13. Bloom, B. S. (1968). *Learning for Mastery. Instruction and Curriculum*. Regional Education Laboratory for the Carolinas and Virginia, Topical Papers and Reprints, Number 1. Evaluation comment, 1(2), n2
14. McGaghie, W. C., & Fisichella, P. M. (2014). The science of learning and medical education. *Medical Education, 48*(2), 106–108.
15. McGaghie, W. C. (2015). Mastery learning: It is time for medical education to join the 21st century. *Academic Medicine, 90*(11), 1438–1441. https://doi.org/10.1097/ACM.0000000000000911.

# Chapter 7
# Expertise Theories and the Design of Surgical Education

**Alexander Harris**

**Overview** This chapter provides a critical analysis of key theories and models of expertise, in general and specific to surgery. The chapter will further consider the application of these theories to surgical education and skill acquisition, from a United Kingdom (UK) perspective, with a focus on simulation.

## 7.1 Introduction

Recent government white papers and surgical conferences [1–3] have used expertise as an underlying theme, without providing a structural framework for combining surgical expertise with surgical training and education. This chapter will summarily explore the concept of expertise and consider its potential application to the design of surgical education.

## 7.2 Theories on Expertise

The Oxford English Dictionary lists two definitions for expertise: (i) expert opinion or knowledge, often obtained through the action of submitting a matter to, and its consideration by, experts, an expert's appraisal, valuation, or report, and (ii) the quality or state of being expert, skill or expertness in a particular branch of study or sport [4]. These definitions, however, are vague and fail to provide any information on how expertise can be identified, achieved, or maintained.

---

*Please note that elements of this chapter have been submitted for consideration towards the fulfillment of the requirements for the degree Doctor of Philosophy at Imperial College London.*

---

A. Harris (✉)
Imperial College London, London, UK

NW London Deanery, London, UK
e-mail: alexander.harris00@imperial.ac.uk

Professor K. Anders Ericsson is a world authority on expertise. His edited tome, *The Cambridge Handbook of Expertise and Expert Performance* [5], provides a holistic examination of the research exploring expertise across numerous domains, with a particular spotlight on chess, music, and athletics.

Ericsson acknowledges the relevance of *historiometry*, defined as "…the statistical analysis of historical data in order to make a quantitative assessment or comparison of particular historical figures, events, or phenomena" [6], through his specific references to the work of Sir Francis Galton, a cousin of Charles Darwin. Galton, who researched the kinsfolk of eminent men, published his findings in the seminal book entitled *Hereditary Genius* in which he theorised that "a man's natural abilities are derived by inheritance" [7]. It was this controversial work that ultimately sparked the nature versus nurture debate that remains relevant to this day.

Ericsson's own theory of expertise is different to Galton's but also evidence-based. He broadly defines expertise as the consistent exhibition of superior performance for representative tasks within a specific domain and proposes that at least 10 years, or 10,000 hours, of sustained and deliberate goal-oriented practice is required to attain such expertise. An individual's motivation to improve, self and situational awareness, training environment, and coach are all identified as critically important concomitant factors. In addition, in a process akin to lifelong learning, experts continue to construct or seek out opportunities by which they may exceed their existing level of performance [5].

In forming his own definition of expertise, Ericsson has considered and extensively catalogued the work of others. He credits the concept of requiring 10 years of work to develop expertise in a subject to research on telegraphy that Bryan and Harter conducted in 1899 [8]. Their finding was subsequently confirmed by research in the domains of chess [9], as well as athletics, science, and the arts [10].

The theory of *deliberate practice* identifies how the maximum level of performance is not simply associated with time or experience but with deliberate efforts to improve. Deliberate practice is, therefore, defined by a highly structured set of activities with the explicit goal of improving performance [5]. This method has been employed with particular recent success in the domain of amateur and professional sports, where the aggregation of marginal gains in performing specific tasks has often been quoted as the perceived difference between success and failure [11].

Recent bestsellers [12, 13] and media outputs [14] have, however, tended to focus on the headline theory of 10,000 hours. This emphasis on time may represent a gross oversimplification of the subject. Furthermore, the generalisability of these theories to the medical and surgical fields is yet to be confirmed.

## 7.3 Models of Expertise

In addition to there being several theories on expertise – including (but not limited to) nature versus nurture, 10 years/10,000 hours of experience, and deliberate practice, as outlined above – various models of expertise have also been published. These have increased in complexity over time (Table 7.1). Fitts and Posner proposed a

Table 7.1 A timeline of the various models of expertise described

| Year | Author | Model |
|---|---|---|
| 1967 | Fitts and Posner | 3-stage model of skill acquisition |
| 1980 | Dreyfus and Dreyfus | 5-stage model of skill acquisition |
| 1996 | Hoffman | 7-point proficiency scale |
| 2007 | Collins | Periodic table of expertises |

three-stage model for learning a new skill [15]. The initial cognitive phase requires an intellectual approach that relies on both instruction and feedback. As the individual progresses in learning the skill, an associative stage is reached where co-ordination has developed. The final stage is reached when the individual becomes autonomous and is able to perform the task independently of cognitive control.

Dreyfus and Dreyfus subsequently proposed a five-stage model of the mental activities involved in directed skill acquisition [16]. The five stages described include novice, competence, proficiency, expertise, and mastery, which are attained through experience in a stepwise manner. Expertise is identified as the highest level of mental capacity and described as a non-analytical stage of performance where correct actions are intuitively made, in keeping with the Fitts and Posner model. Dreyfus and Dreyfus theorised that experts may, on occasion, transcend their usual high-performance levels to reach a stage of mastery.

Hoffman progressed to define expertise in terms of cognitive development, knowledge, and reasoning processes [17]. He described a seven-point proficiency scale with descriptions that appear readily transferable to the surgical domain: naivette, novice, initiate, apprentice, journeyman, expert, and master.

Collins, whose work is heavily influenced by that of Hubert Dreyfus, considered the processes involved with making tacit knowledge explicit [18]. He proposed a periodic table of expertises [19], which identifies the everyday knowledge required by members to live in society, e.g. speaking the same language. Collins states that such knowledge is located within society and that the individual merely draws upon it. However, like Ericsson, Collins identifies experience as an important marker of expertise.

## 7.4 Medical Expertise

Research into medical expertise has primarily focused on causal, analytical, and experiential knowledge. Elstein et al. began by considering the cognitive processes involved for peer-nominated expert diagnosticians in solving representative (simulated) hospital scenarios [20]. This reflected the manner in which de Groot had investigated the thought processes of world class chess players in an earlier seminal study on expertise. Whilst this line of research proved unsuccessful, what developed in time was an examination of the problem-solving process and how experts access memories of their past experiences in "chunks" such that a representative task would trigger an intuitive response based on extensive knowledge, pattern recognition, and non-analytical reasoning. These knowledge structures became termed *illness scripts* [21], which permitted the application of experiential knowledge to clinical reasoning using a forward thinking approach. This type of thinking is in contrast to the slower backward thinking, or analytical reasoning, approach that relies on the development and testing of hypotheses based on the information to hand.

More recently, it is the CanMEDS model that has attempted to provide a holistic framework for medical expertise. The CanMEDS framework is a consensus-based model of physician competencies that was adopted by the Royal College of Physicians and Surgeons of Canada in 1996. It was designed to ensure that postgraduate specialty training was fully responsive to societal needs [22]. It comprises seven roles, with the central role being that of medical expert. The role of medical expert also incorporates the knowledge, skills, and abilities of six other roles that are identified. These roles include communicator, collaborator, leader (manager), health advocate, scholar, and professional. Each role is clearly defined, described, and linked to key competencies on the college's website [23]. However, whilst some commentators view the CanMEDS framework positively with regard to surgical training [24, 25], others claim that the framework is too generic and must evolve to introduce "specialty specificity" [26].

## 7.5 Surgical Expertise

Sir John Tooke stated that "an aspiration to excellence must prevail in the interests of patients", in the findings and recommendations of an independent inquiry into Modernising Medical Careers [1]. Surgery is no exception to this aspiration. Nevertheless, in order to appreciate how surgical practice can move from its current focus on competence towards excellence, it is necessary to understand objectively what is meant by surgical expertise: how it is defined, identified, achieved, and maintained.

Whilst expertise and excellence have been extensively researched across multiple domains, expertise in surgery is under-researched. Publications associated with the field have largely focused on surgical heuristics, surgical competence, and countless novice-expert simulation studies (in which neither the novice, nor the expert, are generally accurately described). Although papers have been published that discuss the development of expertise in the surgical domain [27–31], they are largely anecdotal or merely relay the research so comprehensively compiled by Ericsson.

Ericsson has recently published his own commentary on surgical expertise with evidence-based insights into this emerging domain [32, 33]. At present, however, some of his original theories (founded upon expertise in other domains) lack evidence of transferability to the surgical domain. For example, one of the widest quoted theories concerning expertise is the 10,000 hours rule. Put simply (and placing the service provision versus training debate to one side), presuming that a UK-based higher surgical trainee works for 48 hours each week for 48 weeks of the year then, over a 6-year training period, he/she will have logged 13,824 hours of experience by the time that their training period is completed. Rather than being considered an expert by their peers, these graduating trainees are merely deemed *competent* for independent practice. Although Ericsson describes a number of factors, in addition to time, which can impact the development of expertise, this fact would suggest that surgery *might* be an exception to the established rules on expertise.

## 7.6 Stakeholder Opinion

Indeed, this argument raises another very important question: are all consultants experts? For example, if the clinical practice of the surgical consultant population were to follow a normal distribution, then it could be argued that the performance of half of the consultant population would be expected to fall below that of average. This statement, of course, presumes that a normal (rather than skewed) distribution is present. Either way, whether a skewed or normal distribution is present, it can be argued that consultants exhibiting superior performance to that of their peer group would be at the extreme end of the scale. In other words, surgical expertise, rather than being commonplace, could just as likely be rare.

It is therefore important to consider how expertise is viewed by key stakeholders – in particular, patients. As yet unpublished PhD research has revealed stakeholder (UK healthcare professionals and patients) consensus identifying operative skill as the key attribute of surgical expertise. The surgical community, however, has previously been divided over attempts to separate technical from non-technical skills [34]. It would therefore be naïve to suggest that operative skill encompasses mere technical ability alone. Instead, the previously divergent opinions expressed on surgical expertise in the published literature may imply that it represents a complex blend of multiple attributes, which are not easily distilled into separate entities.

## 7.7 Surgical Education

In recent years, the landscape of UK surgical education has been transformed. The introduction of working time restrictions [35], currently set at a maximum of 48 hours per week, has dramatically reduced opportunities for surgeons in training to gain operative experience [36], whilst traditional approaches to learning have also undergone radical revision. At the same time, a more structured approach to surgical training is moving towards detailed stipulation of specific competency outcomes [37].

Serious concerns have been raised about the impact of such changes on surgical training, with two potential solutions receiving particular attention. The first recommends making better use of existing clinical training opportunities within the 48 hours working week [2]; the second promotes supplementing clinical experience with simulation [38].

## 7.8 Skill Acquisition

Previous research into skill acquisition in non-surgical domains has demonstrated the conditions required for practice to consistently lead to improved performance [10]. These conditions included a defined goal, a motivated trainee, the provision of feedback, and the opportunity to refine performance with repetition of (similar) tasks. Deliberately identifying and addressing (i) areas of performance for improvement and (ii) better ways to perform tasks also helped to improve performance, although a daily limit may be required as such activities require full concentration [5].

## 7.9 Simulation

Simulation is one domain that seems to satisfy all of these conditions for improved performance, offering trainees the opportunity to advance their proficiency gain curve in a learner-centred environment away from the patient-centred operating theatre. Whilst simulation is now a mainstay of undergraduate medical education, its integration into mainstream postgraduate surgical training has proved more challenging.

Simulation-based training is widely established, especially within anaesthetic practice, and fully equipped simulated operating theatres are a key part of many dedicated simulation centres. Such centres, however, remain relatively scarce, are difficult to access, and are extremely costly to equip and run. Those instructors with access to simulation facilities must consider how best to implement simulation as a learning tool, tailoring programmes to trainees' specific learning needs [39]. Nevertheless, if utilised correctly, studies demonstrate that simulation training can improve operating room performance [40].

## 7.10 The Design of Surgical Education

A simulation-based curriculum has long been proposed for surgical training [41, 42]. Virtual reality programmes in particular permit trainees to log (virtual) operating experience in laparoscopic/robotic tasks, graded in difficulty, and with objective measures of performance that can be recorded to demonstrate an individual's learning curve but also to compare performance with that of his/her peer group. Whilst these are obvious benefits, the cost and limited access to such technology (especially in non-teaching hospitals) are well-recognised limitations. Furthermore, whilst computer graphics and haptic technology have greatly improved over the past 20 years, the perceived lack of realism, especially with regard to tissue handling, can restrict the usefulness of such programmes for more senior trainees.

Indeed, the London Postgraduate School of Surgery (the largest surgical training organisation in the UK) has a focused skills training programme integrated within a higher specialist clinical programme, which provides hands on training on anatomically realistic synthetic models and ex vivo porcine models with bench top simulators and box trainers. Training grade and specialty matched trainees are invited to attend distributed, structured, small group simulation sessions, overseen by teaching faculty with experience in both the clinical procedure being taught and the simulator being used. Both feasibility and acceptability of this programme have been demonstrated [43], but long-term outcome data are awaited.

## 7.11 Next Steps

The general conditions arising from expertise theories and suited to the design of surgical education appear well demarcated (e.g. deliberate practice), although progress with identifying which step of a task should be performed at what level of difficulty, at what frequency and interval, and in what environment, in order to achieve optimal performance improvement, remains unclear. Whilst various surgical training organisations and departments have developed their own curricula and adjuncts to surgical training, published outcomes and evidence of performance improvement from such programmes are still lacking, along with clinical correlation.

## 7.12 Conclusion

This chapter has summarily explored the evidence for expertise theories that can affect the design of surgical education programmes. Key concepts have been described and their application to the field of surgical expertise discussed, with a focus upon the role that simulation may have to play in augmenting surgical exposure and education training.

In conclusion, further research is required to demonstrate the generalisability of expertise theories to the surgical domain and the optimum schedule for performance improvement. However, certain key principles, such as deliberate practice, are already a feature of major surgical simulation programmes that are in various stages of development.

## References

1. Tooke, J. (2008). *Aspiring to excellence. Findings and final recommendations of the independent inquiry into modernising medical careers*. London: MMC Inquiry.
2. Temple, J. (2010). Time for training. A review of the impact of the European working time directive on the quality of training. [10th August 2013]; Available from: http://www.mee.nhs.uk/PDF/14274BookmarkWebVersion.pdf

3. ASGBI. (2012). *Expertise and excellence*.
4. OED. (2014). [14th September 2014]; Available from: http://www.oed.com
5. Ericsson, K., Charness, N., Feltovich, P., & Hoffman, R. (Eds.). (2006). *The Cambridge handbook of expertise and expert performance*. New York: Cambridge University Press.
6. OED. (2016). [19th June 2016]; Available from: http://www.oed.com
7. Galton, F. (1869). *Hereditary genius. An inquiry into its laws and consequences*. London: MacMillan and Co..
8. Bryan, W., & Harter, N. (1899). Studies on the telegraphic language: The acquisition of a hierarchy of habits. *Psychological Review, 6*, 345–375.
9. Simon, H., & Chase, W. (1973). Skill in chess. *American Scientist, 61*, 394–403.
10. Ericsson, K., Krampe, R., & Tesch-Romer, C. (1993). The role of deliberate practice in the acquisition of expert performance. *Psychological Review, 100*, 363–406.
11. Brailsford, D. (2014). [28th September 2014]. Available from: http://www.britishcycling.org.uk/gbcyclingteam/article/gbr20140411-British-Cycling%2D%2D-The-Brailsford-years-0
12. Gladwell, M. (2008). *Outliers. The story of success*. London: Penguin.
13. Syed, M. (2010). *Bounce*. London: Fourth Estate.
14. TV. Hidden Talent. 2012 [28th September 2014]; Available from: http://www.channel4.com/programmes/hidden-talent
15. Fitts, P., & Posner, M. (1967). *Human performance*. Belmont: Brooks/Cole.
16. Dreyfus, S., & Dreyfus, H. (1980). *A five-stage model of the mental activities involved in direct skill acquisition*.
17. Hoffman, R. (1996). How can expertise be defined? Implications of research from cognitive psychology. In R. Williams, W. Faulkner, & J. Fleck (Eds.), *Exploring expertise* (pp. 81–100). Edinburgh: University of Edinburgh Press.
18. Collins, H. (2010). *Tacit and explicit knowledge*. London: The University of Chicago Press.
19. Collins, H., & Evans, R. (2007). *Rethinking expertise*. London: The University of Chicago Press.
20. Elstein, A., Shulman, L., & Sprafka, S. (1978). *Medical problem solving: An analysis of clinical reasoning*. Cambridge, MA: Harvard University Press.
21. Schmidt, H., Norman, G., & Boshuizen, H. (1990). A cognitive perspective on medical expertise: Theory and implications. *Academic Medicine, 65*, 611–621.
22. CanMEDS. CanMEDS 2000. (2000). Extract from the CanMEDS 2000 project societal needs working group report. *Medical Teacher, 22*, 549–554.
23. CanMEDS. (2014). [20th August 2014]. Available from: http://www.royalcollege.ca/portal/page/portal/rc/canmeds/framework
24. Grantcharov, T., & Reznick, R. (2009). Training tomorrow's surgeons: What are we looking for and how can we achieve it? *ANZ Journal of Surgery, 79*, 104–107.
25. Arora, S., Sevdalis, N., Suliman, I., Athanasiou, T., Kneebone, R., & Darzi, A. (2009). What makes a competent surgeon?: Experts' and trainees' perceptions of the roles of a surgeon. *The American Journal of Surgery., 198*, 726–732.
26. Van der Lee, N., Fokkema, J., Westerman, M., Driessen, E., Van der Vleuten, C., Scherpbier, A., et al. (2013). The CanMEDS framework: Relevant but not quite the whole story. *Medical Teacher, 35*, 949–955.
27. Kirk, R. (1998). Surgical excellence – threats and opportunities. *Annals of the Royal College of Surgeons of England, 80*, 256–259.
28. Bulstrode, C. (2005). The essential attributes of a modern surgeon. *The Surgeon, 3*, 184–186.
29. Abernethy, B., Poolton, J., Masters, R., & Patil, N. (2008). Implications of an expertise model for surgical skills training. *ANZ Journal of Surgery, 78*, 1092–1095.
30. Alderson, D. (2010). Developing expertise in surgery. *Medical Teacher, 32*, 830–836.
31. Schaverien, M. (2010). Development of expertise in surgical training. *Journal of Surgical Education, 67*, 37–43.
32. Ericsson, K. (2011). The surgeon's expertise. In H. Fry & R. Kneebone (Eds.), *Surgical education: Theorising an emerging domain* (pp. 107–121). Netherlands: Springer.

33. Ericsson, K. (2015). Acquisition and maintenance of medical expertise: A perspective from the expert-performance approach with deliberate practice. *Academic Medicine, 90*, 1471–1486.
34. Ponton-Carss, A., Kortbeek, J., & Ma, I. (2016). Assessment of technical and non-technical skills in surgical residents. *The American Journal of Surgery., 212*, 1011–1019 In press.
35. EWTD. Directive 2003/88/EC of the European Parliament and of the Council of 4 November 2003 concerning certain aspects of the organisation of working time. [15th October 2012]. Available from: http://eur-lex.europa.eu/LexUriServ/LexUriServ.do?uri=CELEX:32003L0088:EN:NOT
36. Marron, C., Shah, J., Mole, D., Slade, D. (2006). European Working Time Directive, a position statement by the Association of Surgeons in Training. [15th October 2012]. Available from: http://www.asit.org/assets/documents/ASiT_EWTD_Final_310506.pdf
37. ISCP. Intercollegiate Surgical Curriculum Programme. [15th October 2012]; Available from: https://www.iscp.ac.uk
38. Donaldson, L. (2008). 150 years of the Annual Report of the Chief Medical Officer. [10th August 2013]. Available from: webarchive.nationalarchives.gov.uk/+/http://www.dh.gov.uk/en/publicationsandstatistics/publications/annualreports/dh_096206
39. Harris, A., Bello, F., & Kneebone, R. (2015). Simulation and training in minimal access surgery. In N. Francis, R. Bergamaschi, A. Fingerhut, & R. Motson (Eds.), *Training in minimal access surgery* (pp. 35–48). London: Springer.
40. Seymour, N., Gallagher, A., Roman, S., O'Brien, M., Bansal, V., Andersen, D., et al. (2002). Virtual reality training improves operating room performance. *Annals of Surgery, 236*, 458–464.
41. Aggarwal, R., Grantcharov, T., Eriksen, J., Blirup, D., Kristiansen, V., Funch-Jensen, P., et al. (2006). An evidence-based virtual reality training program for novice laparoscopic surgeons. *Annals of Surgery, 244*, 310–314.
42. McClusky, D., III, & Smith, C. (2008). Design and development of a surgical skills simulation curriculum. *World Journal of Surgery, 32*, 171–181.
43. Hanna, G., Mavroveli, S., Marchington, S., Allen-Mersh, T., Paice, E., & Standfield, N. (2012). The feasibility and acceptability of integrating regular centralised laboratory-based skills training into a surgical training programme. *Medical Teacher, 34*, e827–ee32.

# Chapter 8
# Helping Learners Through Transitions: Threshold Concepts, Troublesome Knowledge and Threshold Capability Framework in Surgery

**Simon Blackburn, Julian Smith, and Debra Nestel**

**Overview** This chapter explores a constructivist theory that can inform the design of surgical education and training programs, especially to address areas of particular challenge. Threshold concepts, troublesome knowledge and threshold capability are introduced and illustrated in paediatric surgical training and transition to cardiothoracic surgical practice. Like other theories in this section, threshold *concepts involve transformation of individuals' ways of thinking, movement through a* liminal state. This transformation is often associated with the development of a professional identity and represents an *ontological shift* in how the individual sees themselves and may reflect how others see them too. Learners can, however, sometimes find themselves in a *stuck* place where they can move neither forwards nor backwards. The ideas explored in this chapter may provide insights with which educators can help learners to move beyond their current state, to anticipate and plan for troublesome areas in learning, so that they can successfully navigate transitions.

---

S. Blackburn (✉)
Great Ormond Street Hospital for Children NHS Foundation Trust, London, UK
e-mail: sblackburn@doctors.org.uk

J. Smith
Department of Surgery (School of Clinical Sciences at Monash Health), Monash University, Clayton, Australia
e-mail: julian.smith@monash.edu

D. Nestel
Faculty of Medicine, Nursing & Health Sciences, Monash Institute for Health and Clinical Education, Monash University, Clayton, VIC, Australia

Faculty of Medicine Dentistry & Health Sciences, Department of Surgery, Melbourne Medical School, University of Melbourne, Parkville, Australia
e-mail: dnestel@unimelb.edu.au; debra.nestel@monash.edu

## 8.1 Introduction

The process of becoming a surgeon is a characterised by sustained study and practice over many years. Even after consultant surgeon status is conferred, professional development continues as surgeons adapt to changing technologies and processes of surgical practice. At any point in this development process, surgical trainees or consultants may get "stuck". That is, even with effortful practice they may be unable to advance to the next stage of development. Threshold concepts, troublesome knowledge and threshold capability offer surgical educators guidance in moving the trainee beyond the *stuck place*. This chapter explores these concepts in surgical education and training. We use italics to indicate features of the theoretical notion of threshold concepts.

## 8.2 Threshold Concepts

An Open University education report on education innovations identified ten new pedagogies and included threshold concepts [1]. In general terms, threshold concepts are "core" concepts/ideas/practices that must be understood (even embodied) before learners can progress. Sometimes these ideas (concepts) may seem counter-intuitive. They are characterised more precisely by the features listed in Box 8.1. For medical students, empathy has been identified as a threshold concept. Students may know what it is and do it (e.g. make empathic statements), but it may not be experienced as empathy by the intended recipient – patients. That is, the patient may experience the student's behaviour as going through the motions or mimicking

---

**Box 8.1 Threshold Concepts Have a Number of Common Defining Characteristics [2–4]**

1. *Transformative* – resulting in a sudden or lengthy shift in perception of a subject or discipline; once mastered the threshold concept alters the learner's view of the discipline; an epistemological shift.
2. *Integrative* – exposing and bringing together previously unappreciated interrelatedness within the discipline.
3. *Irreversible* – not being forgotten or unlearned without considerable effort.
4. *Bounded* – defining what is and what is not within a field or certain conceptual space, having a specific and limited purpose.
5. *Discursive* – using an enhanced and extended discipline-specific language in crossing a threshold.
6. *Reconstitutive* – altering a learner's subjectivity, sense of self or identity; an ontological shift.
7. *Troublesome* – see text.

empathy rather than being authentic. Unless the student realises that their empathic behaviour is not experienced by the recipient as such then they may be in a liminal state relative to the concept of empathic care. To illustrate, during a simulated patient-based consultation designed to support students in learning about empathic care, a simulated patient was able to share with a student that his empathic behaviour felt like "one of those drawings children do by joining the dots – it just felt like it was empathy by numbers, by joining the dots without any real commitment from you". This feedback had a profound impact on the student who was able to recognise that empathy in healthcare was much more than "joining the dots"; he had to personally feel committed to it. The student shared that he had experienced challenges in establishing rapport with patients and that he was somewhat *stuck* in developing productive student-patient relationships. This feedback had enabled him to move out of this *liminal* state.

Threshold concepts are described as being "akin to a portal, opening up a new and previously inaccessible way of thinking about something. They represent a transformed way of understanding, interpreting, or viewing something without which the learner cannot progress" [2]. Threshold concepts are, therefore, by their very nature *transformative*, in that they lead to a change in perception. It is argued that, in certain instances, this change may have an associated shift in identity. Neve et al. (2015) posit that threshold concepts "lead to a qualitatively different view of subject matter and are central to achieving mastery [sic] of a subject" [3]. Threshold concepts are further characterised as *irreversible*, in that, once acquired, the change in perspective or behaviour which has been produced by the threshold concept is unlikely to be unlearned. It may even be difficult to comprehend the state of those on the other side of the threshold who are unable to make meaning of what is happening because they do not understand it [2].

Another characteristic is that threshold concepts are *integrative*, "exposing the previously hidden interrelatedness of something" [2], but they are *bounded*, in that the understanding of one threshold concept is likely only to expose so much, before a new threshold is reached, and a further shift in perspective is required to make progress. See Box 8.1.

Threshold concepts can be challenging to identify [4, 5]. The importance of identification lies in their potential value as an aid to teaching and learning (as in the example above, to work with simulated patients to support the development of empathic care in healthcare students). Approaches to identifying threshold concepts include dialogue between teachers and learners and tools such as semi-structured interviews, questionnaires, surveys, short answer questions, review of old examination papers and observation of class room behaviours [4]. Controversy remains as to how many of the characteristics listed in Box 8.1 are required for a concept to be regarded as "threshold". Some characteristics might be more important than others. One of the theorists originally describing threshold concepts, Land, has stressed the importance of the *transformative* and *troublesome* elements in their definition [6], and these two elements have even been described as non-negotiable [4]. Authors have highlighted definitional problems [7] while others have questioned whether threshold concepts actually exist [5].

## 8.3 Troublesome Knowledge

*Troublesomeness* is perhaps the most interesting and relevant feature of threshold concepts. Troublesome knowledge may appear counterintuitive, alien or incoherent to the learner [8]. This feature of difficult learning has also been described as dissonance [9] or disorientating [10]. An important note on the characteristics of threshold concepts is that "all defining characteristics, except for troublesome [ones], describe the aftermath – not the experience – of student's successful acquisition of troublesome material" [11]. To identify threshold concepts in learners engaged in wrestling with them, it is troublesomeness that is likely to provide the clue to their recognition. Seeking areas of learning that are troublesome might point to threshold concepts – areas of learning which could benefit from educational intervention. The original notion of threshold concepts has its roots in university education, based on learning as intellectual understanding rather than learning in a professional, practical context. Meyer and Land (2003) have, however, drawn attention to the potential for the idea of threshold concepts to be applied to more practical disciplines [2]. Several authors have developed the idea in medical education [3, 12].

## 8.4 Liminal States

Transitional phases in training can be described in terms of *liminality* [13]. This term originates from ethnographic studies of tribal societies in which rituals associated with a transition from one state of being to another involve an *in between* period [14]. In some tribes, this liminal state involves being thrown out into the wild for a period, leaving the community a boy and returning a man. Meyer and Land (2005) argue that several characteristics of this liminal state are of use from an educational perspective. Liminality implies a transformative component; entering the liminal state describes a process of transition from one state of being to another. As a consequence, the individual acquires a new status but must also lose the old one:

> In order to do so, he or she must strip away, or have stripped from them, the old identity. The period in which the individual is naked of self – neither fully in one category or another – is the liminal state. [15]

This transformation may be protracted over time and involve oscillation between states. The other key characteristic of the liminal state is that once it is entered it is almost impossible to revert to the previous role, the old self has been lost but the new self has not been completely taken on. Linking these three ideas, troublesome knowledge may be reasons for a learner's liminality. Threshold concepts then represent changes that are substantive (*transformative* and *troublesome*) in knowledge or in practice that, once understood or achieved, will never be experienced from the same perspective.

## 8.5 Threshold Capability Framework

A further development in this field is the *threshold capability framework*. This framework provides an approach to dealing with previously unseen situations in professional, social and personal lives. Capability theory is concerned with the ability of learners to act effectively in future professional roles – of being able to deal with circumstances that cannot be specified in advance [16]. This theory, which has the potential to lead to the design of curricula to enhance a learner's transformative and capability building experiences, has had limited but promising applications [17]. It has particular appeal in surgery for its anticipatory nature, application to professional practice and the qualitative nature of *capability*.

## 8.6 Transitions in Surgery

We now shift our discussion to surgical education and practice. The personal development of surgeons traverses a number of important states: from medical student -> pre-vocational doctor -> surgical trainee -> consultant surgeon (Fig. 8.1). Through each state there will be an altered identity or sense of self where the individual feels that in some particular respect they are now thinking and practicing a little more like a surgeon [18]. Failing to address threshold concepts and troublesome knowledge encountered during each state may significantly impede learning and subsequent progression to the next state. There are particular challenges for newcomers to each state.

## 8.7 Threshold Concepts and Troublesome Knowledge in Surgery

Land and Meyer [18] explored ontological shifts across the careers of a small number of surgeons in London. They describe the threshold concept of *uncertainty* for surgical training – referring to the many surgical practices that are enacted to reduce, to manage and even to embrace uncertainty as part of the ontological shift in becoming a surgeon. They report surgeons' efforts during training of making sense of anatomy from a textbook relative to the patient on the operating theatre table. *Letting go* of learning anatomy from 2D textbooks requires an epistemological shift. The ability to deconstruct procedural practice was considered essential – this task analysis being key to error reduction. Surgical expertise is, of course, much more than the assemblage of the component parts; it requires integration, the achievement of which comprises an epistemological shift.

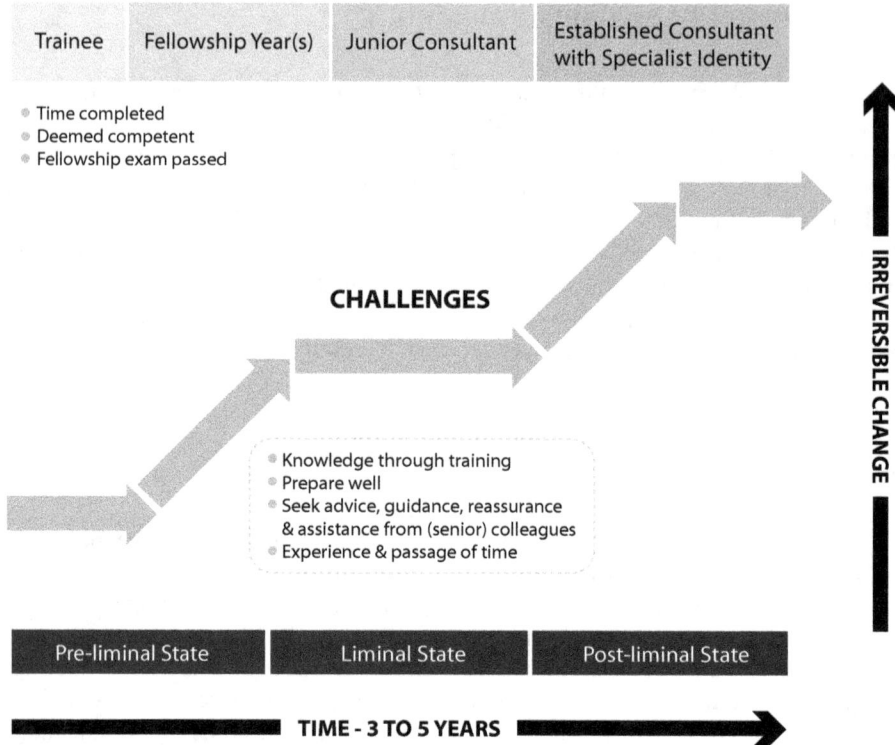

**Fig. 8.1** Transition from trainee to an established consultant with a specialist identity via a state of liminality

We now share two examples from our research with study features summarised in Box 8.2. Both studies involved individual interviews with learners – in the first example, paediatric surgical trainees in the United Kingdom and, in the second example, junior cardiothoracic surgeons establishing themselves in consultant practice in Australia.

### 8.7.1 Example 8.1 Exploring Threshold Concepts in Paediatric Surgical Training [19]

Troublesome areas of paediatric surgical training are listed in Box 8.2.

**Box 8.2 Summary of Our Studies Exploring Threshold Concepts**

| Paediatric surgery | Cardiothoracic surgery |
|---|---|
| Trainees in United Kingdom | Junior consultants in Australia |
| 8 individual semi-structured interviews | 13 individual semi-structured interviews |
| Purposively sampled surgical trainees across all years of the training programme | Purposively sampled cardiothoracic surgeons within 10 years of completing speciality training |
| Participants invited to consider technical skills, clinical judgement and knowledge derived from Intercollegiate Surgical Curriculum Project (ICSP, 2016) | Participants invited to consider theoretical and practical knowledge associated with cardiothoracic surgery including technical skill, clinical judgement, uncertainty, surgical complexity, etc. |
| Thematic analysis of transcribed interviews | Thematic analysis of transcribed interviews |
| Troublesome areas included: | Troublesome areas included: |
| 1. Knowledge | 1. Taking responsibility for patient care such as |
| 2. Clinical judgement | a. Clinical judgement |
| 3. Access opportunities for developing technical skills | b. Decision-making |
| 4. Transitions between roles (including validation as a paediatric surgeon) | c. Unsupervised operating |
| 5. Relationships with colleagues, especially consultant trainers | 2. Career design |
| 6. Impact of negative experiences | 3. New work environments |
| | 4. Relationships with colleagues, trainees and other team members |
| | 5. Technical challenges |
| | 6. Managing the previously unseen or unexpected |
| | 7. Coping with adverse events |
| | Uncertainty associated with handling each of these challenges was the most prominent threshold concept |

#### 8.7.1.1 Knowledge

The breadth of paediatric surgery as a specialty was identified as a source of difficulty. This was compounded by the rarity of some conditions encountered, particularly when neonatal surgery was considered. Specific topic areas were most notable by their absence from the discussion, although some areas of basic science were identified as difficult. Applied knowledge, the "know-how" of paediatric surgery, was perceived as being much more troublesome by participants:

> Well, there's what's written in the textbook and people know that there's an inner textbook. [Participant 3]

### 8.7.1.2 Access Opportunities for Technical Skills

There were few examples of technical operative skills that were identified as troublesome. Rather, accessing opportunities to operate sometimes proved troublesome.

### 8.7.1.3 Clinical Judgement

Developing clinical judgement, and recognising and reflecting on incorrect judgement, was a commonly occurring theme. Trainees often reflected on developing an ability to tolerate diagnostic doubt and the fact that their judgement had developed from experience. Clinical judgement was also an area in which the expectations of more junior trainees (of themselves) differed from those of more senior trainees. Paradoxically, junior trainees had an expectation that their own judgements should be independent, a different view from that expressed by more senior participants:

> I think, as a ST3 [Senior trainee] it's very difficult to make an independent decision about anything because everything is so overwhelming... [Participant 5]

Junior trainees moved from a position of expectation about their ability for independent clinical judgement to one expecting and accepting the shared nature of clinical judgement.

### 8.7.1.4 Transitions Between Roles

The transition to a higher surgical trainee was marked by an increased level of challenge; this was expressed in a perception of increased responsibility, increased expectations of technical skill and the demands placed by the fact that those being looked after are children. Associated with this increase in technical demand and responsibility, several trainees described difficulty with the sudden remoteness of support, with the consultant on call often at home and away from the hospital. Interestingly, this fear of seeking help seemed not to be recognised or recalled by the more senior trainees.

### 8.7.1.5 Validation as a Paediatric Surgeon

Alongside this transition in role, trainees described a desire to prove themselves, reflecting a lack of validation as a paediatric surgeon, one responded to a discussion about technical skills by saying:

> Yes, if you're a bit clumsy you'd be shown a better technique then that happens, but that's the default of the training pathway as opposed what is actually difficult for you as a trainee in those stages, the fact that you don't have any self-belief [Participant 1]

Some participants reflected on the importance of external support, particularly from their consultants, to their feelings of self-belief.

#### 8.7.1.6 Relationships with Trainers

All participants made reference to the importance of their relationship with their consultant trainer. The impact of this relationship was described across the domains of practice discussed and was seen to have an impact at all levels of training. Within this setting, trainees commonly remarked on the problems presented by frequently changing training consultants, who might have rather different views on the best way to perform a procedure.

#### 8.7.1.7 Impact of Negative Experiences

All participants described the impact on learning associated with *negative experiences*: situations where trainees had experienced an adverse outcome or had made a misjudgement. The emotional language associated with negative experiences was more marked in the interviews with junior trainees. The majority of the trainees were able to describe a specific instance in which a mistake or misjudgement on their part had led to a significant emotional response and also a process of reflection leading to a change in behaviour.

One participant summarised his understanding of this process in this way:

> I'd say it almost feels like the cerebral, cognitive part comes first…
> …then the emotional part helps to impress it on you. [Participant 2]

The emotional response to negative situations was quite marked, with trainees describing a profound impact on their sense of self as a consequence of negative experiences. The use of emotional language in the interviews was striking, with the term "cognitive scar" used by all trainees to describe their memory of such experiences.

Despite the profound emotional impact of these experiences, one interesting feature of the trainees' descriptions was that the eventual impact on learning was thought to be positive.

#### 8.7.1.8 Movement from Epistemological to Ontological Understanding

The impact of negative experiences on trainees was clear, and the descriptions obtained were very rich. There seemed to be a clear pattern of the response to these experiences having both emotional and cognitive components. The emotional aftermath and subsequent cognitive rationalisation were key points at which change occurred, with several trainees describing changes in their behaviour as a consequence of these experiences. This response could be viewed as a key event in development, analogous to a threshold.

The early stages of training in this study were characterised by a lack of self-belief and a feeling of a lack of validity as a paediatric surgeon, with some participants describing an abject fear of making mistakes. Some participants viewed the transition from their previous role into that of a higher surgical trainee as the greatest source of troublesomeness they had encountered. This moves the model of a threshold from an epistemological obstacle, where cognitive understanding is a key component, to a more complex process involving an ontological component, in which a change in identity is important. Emerging from this state, it might be argued that trainees acquire a "mature specialist identity" [20].

### 8.7.2 Example 8.2 Exploring Threshold Concepts in Cardiothoracic Surgeons (Junior Consultants)

Using similar methods to those in Example 8.1, threshold concepts and troublesome areas in the transition to consultant cardiothoracic practice were identified (Box 8.2). Knowledge acquired in preparing for the fellowship examination and the experience gained during local or international fellowships greatly assisted the transition from trainee to consultant. Successfully addressing some or all of the threshold concepts resulted in change as a person and as a surgeon that positively influenced each consultant's sense of worth and identity as a cardiothoracic surgeon:

> Well, I think I have moved on. I think I have an understanding now completely different from the beginning when I came out. I have matured. I have become more confident, comfortable dealing with a variety of routine or complex situations in cardiothoracic surgery. [Participant 1]

#### 8.7.2.1 Negotiating Threshold Concepts as a Junior Consultant Surgeon

In general, the threshold concepts and the associated challenges especially with respect to the actual conduct of cardiothoracic surgery were handled through having the requisite theoretical knowledge, preparing thoroughly for any challenging procedure and by seeking the advice, assistance or reassurance of experienced surgical colleagues. The accumulation of experience and reflection upon this experience over time resulted in a successful transformation in learning:

> I can actually do this job, you know, maybe I am actually all right, you know, as a surgeon; and I guess it gives you some confidence. [Participant 10]

#### 8.7.2.2 Uncertainty in the Operating Theatre

Faced with uncertainty in the operating theatre, the surgeons' response was to slow down, to move from a routine mode of practice to one that is more effortful and to recruit additional cognitive resources in a fashion previously described by

Moulton et al. [21]. On occasion, junior consultants would un-scrub, phone a colleague for advice or request a colleague come to the operating theatre to assist or take over. Factors influencing how they responded were both cognitive (e.g. heuristics, fatigue and distractions) and sociocultural (e.g. surgical culture, socialisation, hidden curriculum). How the junior surgeons sat within the social context of the cardiothoracic team had an impact on their clinical judgement and their intraoperative decision-making [22]. Positive relationships between junior consultants and their senior colleagues meant that there were few impediments in asking for help. Establishing trusting relationships with senior colleagues was important in managing uncertainty that cut across several of the troublesome areas. Effective socialisation within the cardiothoracic team combined with the successful completion of a demanding technical task, with a satisfactory patient outcome, provided the junior consultants with a huge boost in confidence. The self-belief to complete a task generated further successes in a positive feedback loop of self-efficacy. A balance was eventually reached between confidence, coping with uncertainty, personal image and technical performance [22]. It seemed apparent that this accumulated experience was a threshold through which the junior consultants passed and would never go back to seeing their work in the same way – an ontological shift.

### 8.7.2.3 The Previously Unseen or Unexpected

The junior cardiothoracic surgeon is constantly challenged by the uncertainty associated with previously unseen or unexpected situations:

> Certainly there are operations that you do when you're a consultant, but which you've never done as a registrar. [Participant 2]

Some of the strategies employed (and the influences underpinning them) to address these have been described above. The linking of threshold concepts with capability theory to create threshold capabilities [23] provides a framework for the design of a training programme aimed at preparing the surgeon to deal with previously unseen or unexpected circumstances. This theory recognises that in experiencing variation the surgeon develops the knowledge capability to deal with unexpected circumstances. Threshold capability theory has not, to our knowledge, been applied in surgery but the findings of this study suggest that such a theory would have significant appeal.

### 8.7.2.4 Coping with Adverse Events

Surgical complications and poor patient outcomes provoked a strong emotional response from the participants:

> ..... you see it all through your training, but it sort of just bounces off you emotionally until it happens to you, and you almost need grief counseling for the next few days. [Participant 4]

Sensations of being traumatised and strong grief reactions were common:

> The adverse outcomes traumatise you and they shake your confidence. [Participant 2]

They described to varying degrees the four phases identified by Luu et al. (fall, kick, recovery, long-term impact) following adverse events that relate to possible or actual surgeon error [24, 25]. There was also significant cognitive rationalisation especially when the adverse event was expected rather than unexpected. These experiences and responses to them were "troublesome" and were addressed through broad discourse with the cardiothoracic team and through being reflective (productive learning) and occasionally defensive (unproductive learning).

Schwartzman (2010), in proposing a theoretical foundation for threshold concepts, provides an explanation of these responses to adverse events as *rupture of the meaning frame* – "structures which embody the categories and rules that order new experience, shaping how we classify our encounters with the world: what we take in and how we act" [11]. Learning fills the meaning frame with content, whereas troublesome knowledge represented by the adverse event ruptures the meaning frame. A reflective response leads to reforming the meaning frame promoting transformative learning. A defensive response, however, preserves the existing meaning frame and limited if any learning occurs from the adverse event [11]. The attraction of this latter response could lie in the avoidance of cognitive dissonance [9]. Fortunately, the junior consultants saw adverse events as a positive learning experience, particularly in the context of discussions at morbidity and mortality meetings.

### 8.7.2.5 Liminality in the Transition to Consultant Cardiothoracic Surgical Practice

Each of the participants reported challenges in the transition from trainee to consultant.

> I don't think anything quite prepares you for consultant life. [Participant 5]

> The learning curve is so steep. [Participant 4]

> It's not a pleasant transition because there's always a degree of uncertainty. [Participant 9]

This transition commenced with the satisfactory completion of training (by achieving the requisite competencies) and with passing the Fellowship Examination. In preparing for consultant practice, the majority of consultants spent 1–3 years in a local or international Fellowship position to provide them with additional experience prior to commencing as a consultant. Time spent in this pre-liminal space [26] greatly assisted the participants in overcoming the uncertainty of responsibility (particularly in unsupervised operating) and of technical complexity. Upon appointment as a consultant the liminal space was entered and gradually traversed over several years. The anxiety and uncertainty of responsibility (particularly in decision-making), technical complexity (including the speed of operating), their place in a new institution and having adverse outcomes were overcome, and the consultants became confident, validated and more secure in their role. Successful patient outcomes from complex technical procedures were a major contributor to this ontological shift. Oscillations in and out of a liminal state, thereby creating a "provoked liminality", could occur even in the more experienced surgeons when previously unseen or unencountered technical complexities were faced. The overall process is shown in the Fig. 8.1.

#### 8.7.2.6 Implications for Surgical Education

Trainees or consultant surgeons seldom discuss, either formally or informally, the uncertainty and troublesomeness associated with the commencement of surgical practice. These troublesome areas need to be acknowledged and addressed by curriculum designers with respect to instruction and assessment. All participants stated that they were poorly prepared for consultant practice. The Royal Australasian College of Surgeons Preparation for Practice Course [27], which principally addressed the logistic aspects of career design (e.g. private practice), was attended by some but was deemed to be of limited overall value.

Each of the seven troublesome areas could serve as a curriculum target within surgical education. Workshops covering surgical decision-making, the various relationships in new work environments and handling the emotional impact of adverse events, for example, would be welcome. Robust discussion of these issues amongst senior trainees and junior consultants within cardiothoracic surgery and across other specialties would highlight many of the unseen or unspoken issues. Some of the transcripts analysed in this study could even form part of the educational materials for these workshops.

e-Learning [28] and simulation-based education [29] have been proposed as aids to the teaching and assessment of approaches to dealing with threshold concepts particularly uncertainty. Kneebone emphasised that the complexities of handling uncertainty must not be oversimplified during the simulated experience. In addition, it has been recognised that more senior surgeons soon forget the uncertainty and troublesomeness associated with commencing practice and simulated activities that have an "expert-centred focus with a learner-centred perspective" which could reconnect them with the transformative process being experienced by their junior colleagues [29].

Once in practice the junior cardiothoracic surgeons paid tribute to the advice, assistance and reassurance provided by their more senior colleagues. It is likely that a more formal mentoring programme might further enhance the interaction between junior and senior cardiothoracic surgeons.

## 8.8 Conclusions

Threshold concepts, troublesome knowledge and threshold capability all offer surgical educators a lens through which to view the complex pathways to becoming a surgeon. In our studies of paediatric surgical trainees and consultant cardiothoracic surgeons, the impact of negative experiences and coping with adverse effects had profound impact on the trainees and consultants, respectively. Learning to manage uncertainty usually resulted in some transformation of identity. Ensuring that negative experiences, coping with adverse events and managing uncertainty lead to learning is important so that trainees or consultants do not find themselves in a *stuck place*. Some suggestions have been proposed (e.g. e-learning, simulation, etc.), but these are unlikely to change individuals' ways of thinking as single events. Whole curriculum approaches that acknowledge threshold concepts that privilege their discussion between trainees, trainers and consultants, together with enactment of a range of strategies, are likely to support learners through these transitions.

**Resources**
The following website is an excellent resource for research and other resources associated with threshold concepts.

https://www.ee.ucl.ac.uk/~mflanaga/thresholds.html

## References

1. Sharples, M., et al. (2014). Innovating pedagogy 2014. In *Open University Innovation Report 3*. Milton Keynes: The Open University.
2. Meyer, R., & Land, R. (2003). Threshold concepts and troublesome knowledge: Linkages to ways of thinking and practising within the disciplines, In *ETL Project*. Coventry: Universities of Edinburgh.
3. Neve, H., Wearn, A., & Collett, T. (2015). What are threshold concepts and how can they inform medical education? *Medical Teacher,* 1–4.
4. Barradell, S. (2013). The identification of threshold concepts: A review of theoretical complexities and methodological challenges. *Higher Education, 65*, 265–276.
5. Rowbottom, D. P. (2007). Demystifying threshold concepts. *Journal of Philospophy of Education, 41*, 263–270.
6. Land, R. (2011). There could be trouble ahead: Using threshold concepts as a tool of analysis. *International Journal for Academic Development, 16*, 175–178.
7. O'Donnell, R. (2010). *A critique of the threshold concept hypothesis and an application in economics. Working paper 164*. [cited 2014 October 5th]. Available from: http://www.finance.uts.edu.au/research/wpapers/wp164.pdf
8. Perkins, D. (1999). The many faces of constructivism. *Educational Leadership, 57*, 6–11.
9. Festinger, L. (1957). *A theory of cognitive dissonance*. Stanford: Stanford University Press.
10. Mezirow, J. (2000). *Learning as transformation: Critical perspectives on a theory in Progress*. New York: Wiley.
11. Schwartzman, L. (2010). Transcending disciplinary boundaries. A proposed theoretical foundation for threshold concepts. In J. H. Meyer, R. Land, & C. Baillie (Eds.), *Threshold concepts and transformational learning* (pp. 21–44). Rotterdam: Sense Publishers.

12. Wearn, A., O'Callaghan, A., & Barrow, M. (2016). Becoming a different doctor: Identifying threshold concepts when doctors in training spend six months with a hospital palliative care team. In R. Land, J. Meyer, & M. Flanagan (Eds.), *Threshold concepts in practice*. Rotterdam: Sense Publishers.
13. Meyer, J., & Land, R. (2005). Threshold concepts and troublesome knowledge (2): Epistemological considerations and a conceptual framework for teaching and learning. *Higher Education, 49*(3), 373–388.
14. Gennep, A. V. (1960). *The rites of passage*. London: Routledge & Kegan Paul Ltd.
15. Goethe, R. (2003). *Ritual and liminality (NCSS theme: Culture) – purpose, background, and context*. Available from: http://www.uiowa.edu/~socialed/lessons/rituals.htm
16. Bowden, J. (2004). Capabilities driven curriculum design. In C. Baillie & I. Moore (Eds.), *Effective teaching and learning in engineering* (pp. 36–47). London: Kogan Page.
17. Male, S., et al. (2016). Students' experiences of threshold capability development with intensive mode teaching. In M. A. Davis & A. Goody (Eds.), *Research and development in higher education: The shape of higher education* (pp. 192–201). Hammondville: HERDSA.
18. Land, R., & Meyer, J. (2011). The scalpel and the 'Mask': Threshold concepts and surgical education. In H. Fry & R. Kneebone (Eds.), *Surgical education: Theorising an emerging domain* (pp. 91–106). London: Springer.
19. Blackburn, S., & Nestel, D. (2014). Troublesome knowledge in paediatric surgical trainees: A qualitative study. *Journal of Surgical Education, 71*(5), 756–761.
20. Rees-Lee, J., & O'Donoghue, J. (2009). Inspirational surgical education: The way to a mature specialist identity. *Journal of Plastic, Reconstructive & Aesthetic Surgery, 62*(5), 564–567.
21. Moulton, C. A., et al. (2007). Slowing down when you should: A new model of expert judgment. *Academic Medicine, 82*(10 Suppl), S109–S116.
22. Jin, C. J., et al. (2012). Pressures to "measure up" in surgery: Managing your image and managing your patient. *Annals of Surgery, 256*, 989–993.
23. Baillie, C., Bowden, J. A., & Meyer, J. H. (2013). Threshold capabilities: Threshold concepts and knowledge capability linked through variation theory. *Higher Education, 65*, 227–246.
24. Luu, S., Leung, S. O., & Moulton, C. A. (2012). When bad things happen to good surgeons: Reactions to adverse events. *The Surgical Clinics of North America, 92*(1), 153–161.
25. Luu, S., et al. (2012). Waking up the next morning: Surgeons' emotional reactions to adverse events. *Medical Education, 46*(12), 1179–1188.
26. Meyer, J. H., & Land, R. (2005). Threshold concepts and troublesome knowledge (2): Epistemological considerations and a conceptual framework for teaching and learning. *Higher Education, 49*, 373–388.
27. RACS. (2014). *Preparation for practice*. [cited 2014 October 5th]. Available from: http://www.surgeons.org/for-health-professionals/register-courses-events/professional-development/preparation-for-practice/
28. Evgeniou, E., & Loizou, P. (2012). The theoretical base of e-learning and its role in surgical education. *Journal of Surgical Education, 69*, 665–669.
29. Kneebone, R. (2009). Perspective: Simulation and transformational change: The paradox of expertise. *Academic Medicine, 84*, 954–957.

# Chapter 9
# Communities of Practice and Surgical Training

**Tasha A. K Gandamihardja and Debra Nestel**

**Overview** In this chapter, we share the theoretical notion of Community of Practice. We apply the theory to surgical training and use examples from Australia and the United Kingdom (UK). We summarize surgical training approaches then outline the theory and provide illustrations of how Community of Practice theory informs surgical training. By applying the theory to the surgical workplace, surgical trainers may improve the learning environment and thereby enhance learning experiences of medical students and junior doctors, attainment of competencies by surgical trainees and advance the production of surgical knowledge and practice.

## 9.1 Introduction

Changes in health services and surgical training have seen a shift from traditional apprenticeship-type learning to competency-based curricula with the workplace remaining the principal site for learning. Socio-cultural learning theories offer valuable lenses through which to observe, design for and analyse workplace learning. They acknowledge the importance of social relations for learning and the influences of cultural and historical factors in current practices. In this chapter, we consider the theoretical concept of Community of Practice described by Lave and Wenger [1] and later by Wenger [2] as a means to better understand surgical education and training within the workplace. We describe key elements – domain, community and practice and the valuable concept of legitimate peripheral

---

T. A. K. Gandamihardja (✉)
Chelmsford Breast Unit, Broomfield Hospital, Chelmsford, Essex, United Kingdom

D. Nestel
Faculty of Medicine, Nursing & Health Sciences, Monash Institute for Health and Clinical Education, Monash University, Clayton, VIC, Australia

Faculty of Medicine Dentistry & Health Sciences, Department of Surgery, Melbourne Medical School, University of Melbourne, Parkville, Australia
e-mail: dnestel@unimelb.edu.au; debra.nestel@monash.edu

participation. We use italics when introducing key terms in the theory. Community of Practice theory offers insights to the development of trainee, surgeon and surgeon educator identities which are further discussed in Chaps. 12, 13 and 37. We draw on our experiences of surgical training in Australia and the UK.

## 9.2 Contemporary Surgical Training

Over the past 30 years, surgical practice and training have changed in many ways. It has shifted from an apprenticeship model, where surgeons trained through long hours of learning on the job, a lack of a clear educational framework and an emphasis on opportunistic learning to the contemporary model – a consequence of surgical training being re-evaluated, restructured and re-modelled. Various factors have impacted this change, including the reduction of training hours, the challenges between training and service provision, 'on calls' with lack of continuity of patient care and the introduction of shift work (Chaps. 1 and 2). Unsurprisingly, these changes have had an impact on the way surgical trainees learn. In the UK, the quoted reduction in training from 30,000 to 6000 hours has meant that many trainees nearing completion of training would not have had as much clinical exposure compared to their predecessors [3]. However, the key goals of professional education remain – to steward knowledge, impart skills and instil the values of the surgical profession. This requires a balanced and integrated approach that orientates trainees to the cultural, social and humanistic aspects of surgery.

The contemporary surgical training model is now more structured. Continuous assessment and re-evaluation processes occur throughout training. Workplace assessments have been introduced, a minimum threshold of numbers required to be achieved of certain surgical procedures have been set, and logbook assessment and annual review of performances are now part of training. In addition, more emphasis has been placed on learning the importance of skills such as communication, teamwork, decision-making and professionalism.

Trainees have had to learn to adapt in order to navigate these changes successfully. They are aware that in order to succeed, they need to be able to target their learning, seek training opportunities and utilize any useful resource to achieve this goal. In addition to attending the formal structured educational days arranged by various training providers, trainees have had to explore additional avenues in order to enhance and facilitate their training. Increasingly, web-based learning resources have become available. Simulation-based learning and technical skills labs have also become a vital part of the educational process. However, while a structured educational framework is vital, a significant part of learning continues to take place while working in the day-to-day service of clinical care delivery. It is implicit, unintended, unstructured and opportunistic. Learning about how things are done by being exposed to a wide variety of different experiences is what makes surgery an exciting and rewarding specialty [4].

## 9.3 Situated Learning and Communities of Practice

Situated learning described by Lave and Wenger [1] views learning and development as occurring through participation in a community's activities. It is a type of learning that can only occur when an individual is immersed in a specific environment, with a specific group or type of people with a shared goal. Situated learning does not emphasize the role of a teacher or trainer, rather it argues that learning occurs through work (work-based learning) and that through engaging with other members within this environment, learners transform their understanding, roles and responsibilities as they participate [2]. Wenger describes a Community of Practice as 'groups of people who share a concern or passion for something they do and learn how to do it better through regular interaction' [2]. The Community of Practice theory posits the concept of social interaction as not only a way of learning but the vehicle of learning itself. In their ethnographic studies of craftspeople, Lave and Wenger coined the term – living curriculum – to describe this type of situated learning [1].

In a Community of Practice, there are key characteristics, namely, the domain, the community and the practice [5]. A shared domain of interest characterizes a Community of Practice. Being a member of this community implies commitment to the domain. Members interact, engage, learn from each other and share information thus creating a community. As a result, the members develop a practice where experiences, stories, problems and goals are shared as a community [5]. These concepts are summarized in Box 9.1.

**Box 9.1 Examples of the Structural Elements of Communities of Practice in a Surgical Training Environment (Surgical Unit)**

| Key concept | Description | Application in a surgical training environment |
|---|---|---|
| Domain | 'A community of practice … has an identity defined by a shared domain of interest. Membership therefore implies a commitment to the domain, and therefore a shared competence that distinguishes members from other people'<u>a</u> | The domain of a surgical Community of Practice is most likely to be the safe and effective delivery of surgical care, responsibility for evolution of surgical practice and development of surgical trainees. Depending on the boundary of the Community of Practice, the domain may be defined more specifically. Individuals may belong to many Communities of Practice at the same time, and some will fall within the overarching Community of Practice. For example, surgical trainees may have their own Community of Practice that involves them meeting informally to share experiences that advance their knowledge, practice and skills. Although their domain of interest includes safe and effective surgical care and so part of the broader surgical Community of Practice, passing the Fellowship Examinations will have prominence in their smaller community. They define themselves as others see them – as *surgical trainees* who are studying together to pass this specific exam. |

(continued)

**Box 9.1** (continued)

| Key concept | Description | Application in a surgical training environment |
|---|---|---|
| Community | 'In pursuing their interest in their domain, members engage in joint activities and discussions, help each other, and share information. They build relationships that enable them to learn from each other; they care about their standing with each other'[a] | The surgical Community of Practice in a hospital will have many opportunities for its members to interact. Formal interactions between members facilitate exchanges of experiences of the practice. For example, surgeons' (especially consultants and trainees) interactions in the ward, operating theatre, outpatient department and appraisal sessions, surgeons attending hospital level meetings and surgeons attending scientific conferences and surgical trainee special interest groups – all with the intent of developing and sustaining the practice. Informal interactions between members of the Community of Practice may include surgeons' opportunistic interactions in the tea room, surgeons attending hospital level meetings including corridor conversations and surgeons attending social events scientific conferences. |
| Practice | 'Members of a community of practice are practitioners. They develop a shared repertoire of resources: experiences, stories, tools, ways of addressing recurring problems – in short, a shared practice. This takes time and sustained interaction'[a] | This is how the community defines its activities, tools and products. This includes surgical knowledge and judgement, surgical techniques, surgical instruments, surgical practice documentation, operating theatre etiquette, surgical dress, surgical language, surgical journals and professional association websites. These are the elements of the community that help define it. |

[a]Wenger and Wenger-Trayner [5]. Retrieved from http://wenger-trayner.com/introduction-to-communities-of-practice/

Learning viewed as a situated activity has as its central defining characteristic a process known as *legitimate peripheral participation* (LPP) [1]. In order for *newcomers* to learn, they must be offered meaningful opportunities to contribute towards the common goal of that community. *Old timers* in the Community of Practice can facilitate or impede any participant's progression more centrally.

## 9.3.1 Communities of Practice and Surgical Training

In surgical training, there are many Communities of Practice (e.g. see Box 9.1). The community can be bounded by the physical environment (e.g. clinic, theatre, ward), the surgical specialty (e.g. general surgery, orthopaedics, neurosurgery) or the level of training (e.g. foundation trainee, higher surgical trainee) [6]. Some of these Communities of Practice will include members of different professional backgrounds such as nurses, pharmacists and occupational therapists to name a few, contributing to the social aspect of learning and giving the process a broader dimension.

The different work settings are potentially very rich communities in which to learn. A clinical ward offers different affordances for learning than an operating theatre, which in turn is different to an outpatient department, and these affordances will also vary by site. Yet, the surgical trainee will interact, engage and learn with and from other healthcare professionals within that Community of Practice. Learning therefore implies a relation to not only specific activities but also social communities. It is possible to belong to several Communities of Practice at any one time.

Surgical trainees usually enter a Community of Practice as a legitimate peripheral participant, requiring supervision and assistance, thus limiting potential risks and errors. Through participation, especially with old timers, the newcomers will learn how to practice and behave within the Community of Practice. Interactions enable sharing of the richness of the community. Trainees learn how old timers walk, talk and conduct their lives, observe what other trainees are doing and appreciate what is needed to become more central in that community. An important consideration is language and how trainees need to be able to talk the talk of the community. Surgical vocabulary is distinct from other disciplines and is an integral part of how surgeons communicate. The language of a surgical Community of Practice is an important factor in helping construct an identity within that community (see Chap. 12). Fluency with the language is used is an important indicator of belonging to the community [7]. Through shared experiences, the learning curve for surgical trainees should be improved, communication skills enhanced and collaborative work encouraged. Learning in the workplace not only fosters the development of surgical knowledge and skills but also the values central to the profession [8]. Areas considered tacit in surgical education such as the importance of teamwork, professionalism and communication skills are learnt and adopted while working and engaging with these role models [9]. This whole process of learning is cyclical and eventually the newcomers (medical students, junior doctors, surgical trainees) will replace the old timers, (the registrars and consultants). Each Community of Practice has their own rules and traditions which can create difficulties for trainees as they rotate through different units having to recognize, acknowledge and negotiate this variance. Not all learning that is situated functions productively. It is not uncommon for medical students and surgical trainees to report experiences of exclusion and intimidation. The legitimacy of their participation must be created by those within the community.

## 9.4 How Can Knowledge of This Theory Help a Surgical Educator?

Knowledge of Community of Practice theory can enable the surgical educator to appreciate learning opportunities and challenges and the multiple influences on students and trainees in the surgical workplace. They can help newcomers to the community through orientation of people, tasks, equipment and language. They can actively facilitate opportunities for participation in meaningful activities – learning from their peers, more advanced trainees, their consultants and other healthcare professionals around them. Box 9.2 provides three vignettes illustrating ways in which Community of Practice theory can be used to view learning. Awareness of the theory will not necessarily lead to learning per se but help the surgical educator to create a more suitable context in which learning can occur.

---

**Box 9.2 Vignettes of How Community of Practice Theory May Be Used to View Learning in Surgical Units for a Medical Student, a New Doctor and a Surgical Trainee**

**Medical student**

Steven McFee is nervous about his surgical rotation. He is quite certain that he wants to be a rural general practitioner but appreciates the value of the opportunity to experience a regional surgical practice as part of his medical degree. There has been no orientation to the surgical rotation, and he is not really sure where he has to go on his first day. Steven ended up missing much of his rotation through failure to engage. When he did attend, he was not made to feel welcome. He was not given anything meaningful to do. When he was scheduled to go to theatre, there was no one available to show him where to change. He found his way into the right theatre but felt unwelcome. He just stood against a wall planning his exit as soon as possible. He decided that he would just learn what he could from books to pass his exams. He figured he might get a surgical rotation during internship when he hoped the experience would be improved and he would gain knowledge to inform his planned general practice career.

*Community of Practice theory perspective: This is a lost opportunity to support Steven's learning even though he did not want to pursue a career in surgery. The experience has probably confirmed that surgery is not for him. Without knowing how to navigate even simple elements of surgical work – like getting changed and finding the right theatre, Steven has not even achieved legitimate peripheral participation. Even though Steven's goal for the rotation might have aligned with those of the surgical Community of Practice, he prioritized his curriculum requirements because of the absence of any meaningful engagement.*

(continued)

**Box 9.2** (continued)

**Junior doctor**

As a new graduate, Dr. Louise Peng is on a surgical rotation. She spends most of her time on the wards but has some opportunity to go into theatre. Dr. Peng is excited to be on the surgical rotation since she thinks she would like to pursue a career in surgery. She has been reading about general surgical conditions and surgical techniques. At the hospital, she has volunteered to participate in a surgical simulation research project as a subject! It has something to do with laparoscopy skills and stress. She can't wait. She hopes she will have some meaningful work in theatre. It was only a couple of weeks into the rotation when she was given the chance to go to theatre, but it was for relatively short periods. Most of her working day was on the wards. However, when she was in theatre, she was given the chance to assist. While assisting, Dr. Peng observed surgical trainees, registrars and consultants at work. She learned their language, noted their ways of interacting with each other and listened to discussions of intraoperative decision-making and of verbal and non-verbal instructional approaches at the operative site and how all members of the theatre communicated with each other. She was taught some basic operative techniques by one of the registrars. By the end of the attachment, she was managing her ward work effectively, and she was being supervised closing surgical wounds working with the registrar.

*Community of Practice theory perspective: As a gradual process, Dr. Peng moved from the position of a newcomer and legitimate peripheral participant to membership of the broader surgical Community of Practice associated with her rotation. The length of the attachment prevented more central movement, but the experience seemed invaluable in helping her acquire more than basic surgical knowledge and skills but also some of the language and professional values of other members.*

**Surgical trainee**

Dr. Wendy Black is a second-year general surgical trainee in a university teaching hospital. She participates in ward, outpatient and operating theatre activities. As part of her working day, she undertakes many tasks; some are shared with other trainees in the unit. To assist her integration into the surgical team, the lead consultant ensures that she has meaningful activities that contribute to the productivity of the surgical unit. These include the following activities:

Preoperative
  Conducting preoperative patient examination
  Selecting appropriate diagnostic and imaging tests
  Communicating operative plans to patient and relatives
  Participating in interdisciplinary surgical team meetings
  Presenting a coherent clinical assessment to colleagues
Intraoperative
  Positioning the patient for safe surgical access
  Performing common procedures under supervision
  Performing basic surgical skills (e.g. incision, diathermy, suction, retraction, suturing, etc.)
  Handling soft tissue appropriately
Post-operative
  Writing operative notes
  Conducting post-operative patient examinations
  Discharging surgical patients

(continued)

> **Box 9.2** (continued)
>
> These tasks are also expected competencies for her level of surgical training. The lead consultant seeks to align needs of the surgical service with training requirements by the provision of opportunities to undertake meaningful activities.
>
> *Community of Practice theory perspective: Again, as a gradual process, Dr. Black is moving more centrally to the surgical Community of Practice than Dr. Peng who had a more transitory engagement with the community. As a surgical trainee, it is essential that Dr. Black participates fully, and the nature of the activities she is performing (all meaningful) suggests that she is becoming a key member of the team. Dr. Black is perceived by patients and other members of the healthcare team as a surgeon/trainee which affirms Dr. Black's emerging identity as a surgeon. The lead consultant has made an effort to enable Dr. Black to participate in tasks that reflect her level of ability and has encouraged the registrars to work with Dr. Black in the pre- and post-operative tasks*

A second major thread with which Community of Practice theory may assist surgical educators is as an underpinning theoretical framework in educational research. It is beyond the scope of this chapter to demonstrate such applications. Box 9.3 shows an example from Quinn et al. (2014) in their study that used Community of Practice theory as an analytical lens to make meaning of a surgical journal club [10]. Additional examples are shared in Part IV of this book and specifically in Chap. 37 where Kokelaar shares his experiences of using this theory to explore the development of trainees' identities as members of a surgical laparoscopic community.

## 9.5 Conclusion

Socio-cultural learning theories can inform surgical training. Community of Practice theory is just one example. These theories acknowledge the importance of the workplace as a site of learning the practice of a community, where the practice is developed over time and where the culture of the social group is privileged over individual learning. Although it is not possible to design learning per se, it is possible to design for learning by considering ways in which the features of Community of Practice theory and legitimate peripheral participation occur. Although we have shared some key concepts of Community of Practice theory, it offers so much more, especially with respect to the development of professional identity. Chapters 12 and 13 develop further the ideas of Communities of Practice and the development of professional identity – of surgeons and of surgeon educators.

**Box 9.3 An Example of How the Community of Practice Theory Is Used as an Analytic Framework to Make Meaning of a Surgical Journal Club**
Quinn et al. (2014) used Community of Practice theory to better understand how surgical journal clubs support learning. The journal club comprised members of a surgical department (consultants, surgical trainees and students). The trainees were given a journal article to summarize and review through an oral presentation with the event occurring in a classroom arranged with rows of seats facing the presenter. Using case study method, two journal club events were observed and then purposively sampled participants interviewed individually about their experiences. The transcribed interview data was then mapped to key elements of Community of Practice. The authors reported the presence of four components of Community of Practice: *community* (learning as belonging), *meaning* (learning as experience), *identity* (learning as becoming) and *practice* (learning as doing). Although the joint enterprise and shared purpose were evident, the sense of community depended on the seniority of the participants. The most senior felt they belonged, while juniors who were on surgical rotations and could likely pursue non-surgical specialties were not engaged. Wenger describes these orientations as *peripheral* or even *outbound* trajectories. *Legitimate peripheral participation* was evidenced by the request that trainees present – a meaningful task. Ideally, the presentations would enable journal club members to discuss their relevant experiences. However, only the senior trainees' experiences and consultants' reactions seemed valued and respected. Some *newcomers* to the community deemed consultants to be the most important members to lead the journal club. Their low attendance threatened the perceived value of the activity and changed interactions between participants – less feedback was shared in their absence. Some participants clearly had expectations of *old timers* sharing their stories about practice in response to articles presented and their feedback helping to develop knowledge, skills and behaviours of the participants in the journal club. Opportunities for learning were lost for junior trainees, interns and students. Given trainees were on an inbound trajectory to the surgical Community of Practice, this seems less than optimal. By using a Community of Practice lens to view the journal club activity, the authors were able to identify elements to maintain and others to change within the journal club

# References

1. Lave, J., & Wenger, E. (1991). *Situated learning: Legitimate peripheral participation*. Cambridge, UK: Cambridge University Press.
2. Wenger, E. (1998). *Communities of practice: Learning, meaning and identity*. Cambridge, UK: Cambridge University Press.
3. Chikwe, J., de Souza, A. C., & Pepper, J. R. (2004). No time to train the surgeons. *BMJ, 328*(7437), 418–419.

4. Cox, A. (2005). What are communities of practice? A comparative review of four seminal works. *Journal of Information Science, 31*, 527–540.
5. Wenger, E., & Wenger-Trayner, B. (2015). *Introduction to communities of practice*. [Cited 2017 July 4]. Available from: http://wenger-trayner.com/introduction-to-communities-of-practice/.
6. Gandamihardja, T. A. (2014). The role of communities of practice in surgical education. *Journal of Surgical Education, 71*(4), 645–649.
7. Rogoff, B. (1990). *Apprenticeship in thinking. Cognitive development in social context*. New York: Oxford University Press.
8. Nestel, D., & Burgess, A. (2014). Surgical education and the theoretical concept of communities of practice. *Journal of Health Specialties, 2*, 49–53.
9. Dimitriadis, P., Iyer, S., & Evgeniou, E. (2014). Learning in the surgical community of practice. *Medical Science Educator, 24*(2), 211–214.
10. Quinn, E. M., et al. (2014). Surgical journal club as a community of practice: A case study. *Journal of Surgical Education, 71*(4), 606–612.

# Chapter 10
# Activity Theory and the Surgical Workplace

**Edward F. Ibrahim**

**Overview** This chapter explores the importance of the surgical workplace as a centre of learning. A sociocultural learning theory known as activity theory will be described and related to the field of surgery to help illuminate this multifaceted and complicated environment. Comparisons will be made with the theory of situated learning and communities of practice. Newer developments on activity theory such as knot-working and actor-network theory will be discussed. As a defining feature of activity theory, the prominent position of culturally mediated artefacts will be argued as both promoter and hinderer of expansive learning. Two published case studies of the surgical workplace will be critically considered to illustrate the strengths and weaknesses of an activity theory-based approach. Case study one examines the reality of collaborative multidisciplinary learning in practice, specifically the relationship across different specialities involved in the treatment of patients with suspected breast cancer. Case study two concerns what we can learn from how expert surgeons go about preparing to lead a theatre team towards excellent performance and how this knowledge is passed on to trainees.

## 10.1 The Surgical Workplace

The principal site of postgraduate surgical learning is in a hospital. In recent decades, the restriction in trainee surgeons' working hours has resulted in greater opportunity for personal study, structured course attendance and engagement with simulation technology. However, the vast majority of education is likely to occur in the workplace. The pivotal role of the workplace in the development of medical practitioners and the need to understand the process of 'informal learning' are now well recognised [1].

E. F. Ibrahim (✉)
Department of Trauma and Orthopaedic Surgery, West Middlesex University Hospital, Isleworth, UK

Chelsea and Westminster Hospital NHS Foundation Trust, London, UK
e-mail: edward.ibrahim@uclmail.net

In most countries, surgical training is hierarchical. The 'team' or 'firm' is led by one or more senior surgeons (attending or consultant). Accordingly, an apprenticeship model of learning has been popular [2]. This is predominantly a cognitive approach in which the learner makes sense of the surgical world by reconstitution and retention of the sensory input provided by his or her senior [1]. However, only a minority of the working day is spent with a more senior surgeon, and it is possible for learning to occur outside of this apprenticeship context [3].

The trainee surgeon's learning is situated in the hospital, but it will be imperative for them to transition between different environments such as the ward, the emergency department, the operating theatre and the outpatient clinic. Within each environment, they must engage with the typical type of patient encountered, the staff who work there on a more regular basis and, importantly, the objects and tools used as adjuncts to patient care in each geographical area.

## 10.2 An Introduction to Activity Theory

Sfard has made a distinction between two methods of learning [4]. *Acquisition* refers to the actions of an individual in seeking and gathering information, making cognitive sense of this information and being able to reproduce the information at an opportune time. *Participation* relates to the advancement of knowledge through the process of active collaboration with a group of colleagues or co-workers. These simple metaphors risk eliminating much of the complexity that might inform how surgical teams work [5]. However, they do provide a basis for understanding the progression from the previously dominant cognitive theories of learning to more sophisticated sociocultural learning theories of the twentieth century and beyond.

Activity theory is a significant and powerful theory that has advanced and expanded the participation metaphor [6], though interestingly its emergence began with a focus on the individual. In the 1920s Lev Vygotsky recognised the response of an individual to a stimulus for activity was mediated by a complex act [7]. It was Vygotsky's colleague Alexei Leont'ev who observed the limitations of individually focussed theory and expounded the difference between individual action and collective activity, thereby overlaying a social dimension [8]. Yrjo Engeström popularised activity theory by proposing that intricate social encounters should be interpreted in the context of an activity system [9]. The activity system accounts for the interaction of social, physical and organisational structure in the workplace. Analysis describes how a person negotiates a path within the system to achieve an objective. The organisation, structure and culture of the environment, community rules and norms and the perception of appropriate division of labour influence the individual's ability to reach their goal. Hence an activity system consists of six primary elements: individuals, objectives, tools, communities, rules and division of labour [9–12].

An activity has been described by Leont'ev as comprising subjects (e.g. healthcare workers engaged in the activity), an object (e.g. the goal of delivering patient care stimulates the activity), actions (goal-directed processes to accomplish the object, e.g. patient assessment and initial management followed by definite surgical management and subsequent rehabilitation) and operations (the way in which the action is carried out, e.g. the technique of surgical procedure). Operations themselves may become routine with practice. Activity theory recognises that conditions and personnel may change but the object remains central [8].

One of the central tenets of activity theory is the concept of mediation by artefacts [13]. Artefacts are created by people to govern their own activity. They include instruments, labels and technologies which persist through time and embody the history of previous objectives. They may be unique to one particular environment or pervade through many. Thus, the context of an activity system is the activity itself, stimulated by an objective and constituted through the actions of its people and artefacts. The *participation* of subjects is transformed by the *acquisition* of knowledge and the ability to use these tools in everyday practice.

## 10.3 Alternative and Complementary Sociocultural Education Theories in the Surgical Workplace

Given its components, one can imagine the community of surgical education being easily seduced by activity theory. The object is always to deliver high-quality patient care. The subjects (doctors, nurses, allied health professionals, managers) are employed by the hospital in defined roles. Stepwise actions are negotiated for the patient from their entry point into the system to discharge from hospital. The term 'operation' could not be more apt! The myriad of surgical equipment available makes the acknowledgement of the importance of artefacts particularly appealing. The surgical activity system is usually well governed by a series of historical protocols coded as artefact on paper or online. Division of labour is directed along well-established hierarchical lines. It is, however, important to recognise that other sociocultural learning theories do exist and have their place in the surgical workplace. At present, no solitary learning theory can fully explain or predict medical practice. A conglomerate of complementary theories is currently required to inform how old knowledge can be passed on and new knowledge produced [6]. Predominant and relevant examples include Lave and Wenger's theory of situated learning [3], which focuses on collaborative learning in a bounded hierarchal group and latterly Latour's actor-network theory [14], which locates learning in a web of human and non-human artefacts.

In many countries, doctors in training rotate through multiple hospitals and then through multiple medical teams within a hospital. Activity theory does not adequately explain how these newcomers will gain legitimate access to appropriate activity systems and, further, does not explain in detail what factors will be necessary for him or her to enhance their role in future systems in order to gain the necessary access to knowledge for further learning. These points are better addressed by the theory of situated learning [3] and the subsequent description of communities of practice [15]. Though described more fully in Chap. 9, it is important to note here that situated learning theory stresses responsiveness to a situation or environment. Activity grows out of the immediacy of the situation, and objectives follow. Activity theory differs by placing the object of activity at the starting point and, in this respect, may be more applicable to the vast majority of pre-planned surgical care.

Although situated learning enthusiasts do not deny that artefacts are important, they argue that the true focus should be the 'everyday activity of persons' [16]. As a craft specialist, a surgeon must recognise the need for mastery of the tools he or she uses. Building on the centrality of artefacts in activity theory, related sociomaterial approaches have been developed in order to further reclaim material and materiality in social life and rethink their relations with education [17]. These approaches argue for a more symmetrical approach to the study of workplace learning, claiming that educational analyses too often deny material things their vitality [18–20]. Surgeons will identify with the comments of Bleakley when he suggested that patient safety is frequently put at risk through lack of attention to the use and upkeep of materials [21].

Of the currently available sociomaterial-oriented learning theories, Latour's actor-network theory (ANT) perhaps shows the greatest explanatory power [21]. The term *actor* is used to describe any person *or* object involved in forming a network. *Network* refers to the way in which actors communicate, such that stronger and more numerous associations are formed with a view to promoting learning and excellent performance [14]. ANT therefore empowers objects with agency, in the sense that the functioning of an artefact can instigate the formation and development of a network [21]. ANT is not meant as an analytical apparatus but as a 'practice', a luminary source to visualise a phenomena more clearly [20]. The aim is not prescription or redefinition of protocols of action for network function but to identify and expand upon themes and possibilities emerging from the interaction of human and non-human elements. The following sections discuss learning points identified from two published examples of common surgical activity systems as examined through the lens of sociocultural theory.

## 10.4 Case Study 1: The Breast Multidisciplinary Team

An elegant example of an inter-professional activity system involving surgeons was described by Heldal. She followed a breast cancer unit in a Norwegian hospital for 18 months to qualitatively investigate how health professionals cross professional boundaries [22]. Particular emphasis was placed on the observation of the activity system during multidisciplinary team meetings. Here, the object was to create treatment pathways for a list of patients, and the subjects were surgeons, oncologists, radiologists, histopathologists and specialist breast cancer nurses. She found that subjects' professional relationships could be described as 'loosely coupled'. Connections occurred occasionally rather than constantly, and, although the collection of roles was always the same, the personnel differed from meeting to meeting. Surgeons would attend depending on availability, meaning connections were unstable and constructed on a sudden basis. Within this loosely coupled system, she also found evidence to support the notion that doctors' loyalties are sometimes more attributable to their speciality than the hospital and that professionals often fight to preserve their speciality boundaries. Activity theory would predict that these behaviours will be unhelpful in achieving the system objective.

The use of artefacts was found to have a profound effect on the apparently haphazard social system. The most important mediating object was the patient list, detailed with clinical information and constantly updated. This provided a constant reminder of the goals of the meeting and enabled integration among professionals. Heldal describes this as a *boundary object*, which has been previously described by Star and Griesemer as being 'plastic enough to fit into different contexts, but stable enough to establish a common identity across these contexts' [23]. However, some objects had the power to sever connections between subjects and made tighter coupling impossible. One example was radiological imaging. Even though pictures are intended to inform patient management, they were, in fact, fiercely guarded as the preserve of the radiologist who told the other professionals not to try to comprehend the imaging but simply trust the report.

Heldal's study highlights some of the problems often encountered within an activity system, in particular hindrances to learning across the boundaries marked by different specialists. It also provides emphasis for further research into a more recent development in activity theory known as *knot-working* [24]. The concept of knot-working acknowledges that each professional arrives at an inter-professional collaboration via his or her own activity system but has the ability to provide a 'different string in the knot' [25]. The centre of the knot is not fixed and shifts from moment to moment. Different professionals move the knot in different directions at different times, but the overall movement is towards co-configuration, 'often resulting in the creation of new tools for negotiated care' [24]. In this way boundary crossing has the potential to pave the way for *expansive learning*, i.e. something which has not been previously defined or understood is collectively learned at the point of creation by the group [5].

## 10.5 Case Study 2: Orthopaedic Trauma Surgery

Broadly speaking, understanding an inter-professional network requires examination of each member's activity system as viewed through their eyes. More specifically, to understand the participatory actions of a surgeon and potential for resultant learning, the activity system must be examined from his or her standpoint. Our group interviewed nine expert orthopaedic trauma surgeons in the UK to understand the process of planning for particularly challenging or unfamiliar complex surgical procedures [26]. The engagement process was found to be a classic example of *double stimulation*, previously described by Vygotsky [7]. The subject is provided with a demanding task (first stimulus – to cure a patient with a complex injury) and an external artefact (second stimulus – a radiograph or scan of the injury). Of course, the concept of an unfamiliar procedure or complex injury is relative to the experience of the surgeon. This method of double stimulation is commonly seen in the field of surgical education when a surgeon in training is encouraged to engage in an iterative process of problem-solving after being given a clinical vignette accompanied by a radiographic and/or surgical image.

Once engaged, the surgeons followed a typical sequence of learning actions that has been recognised in activity theory following the work of Davydov [27]. First, the conditions of the task are rationalised in order to make sense of the injury and impact on this particular patient. Second, the injury is modelled in artefactual form (usually through cross-sectional imaging). Third, the model is transformed to make it bespoke to the object in hand (not always possible with current technology but always played out in the mind's eye). Fourth, a sequence of actions is constructed that can be resolved following known or routine operations (a sequence of events is listed to allow the surgical procedure to take place). Fifth, the performance of these actions is monitored (the availability of the necessary equipment is checked, and the procedure is mentally rehearsed by the surgeon and often discussed with other surgeons). Finally, an evaluation of and reflection on the procedure is undertaken with a view to learning for next time. An example of a surgeon's activity system is shown in Fig. 10.1.

Rich descriptions of expansive learning by engagement in an activity system consisting of the surgeon's colleagues, company representatives and radiologists were generated. Artefacts were of central importance: computerised tomography scans of fractures, textbooks and online banks of knowledge, bone models with drawn-on fracture patterns and methods of fixation. Through collaboration with all the relevant actors a network was created with the sole aim of negotiating a path to the most successful outcome possible. The gap between the outcome that would have been produced at the moment of problem engagement and that which was eventually produced following the formation of a network could be conceived as a bespoke episode of learning for the surgeon. Vygotsky has previously recognised this distance as the *zone of proximal development* [7].

The surgeons could not have successfully treated their patients by engaging with a socially mediated activity system alone. This principle may hold greater relevance to the craft specialities such as surgery where perhaps the most vital aspect of the patient's care is for a solitary healthcare professional to produce a one-off 'performance' in a 'theatre'. There can be no doubt that a team is required to manage the patient from admission to discharge, but where the object is focussed on a complex operative procedure, the senior surgeon must take the great burden of responsibility. Our group found that surgeons engaged heavily with their previous memories and experience to produce the mental imagery required to prepare well. In many cases the balance of learning tipped from social to cognitive in nature [26]. In this particular scenario, the greater flexibility of actor-network theory may be a more appropriate descriptor than activity theory where the 'lead actor' can be afforded more importance than the system as a whole.

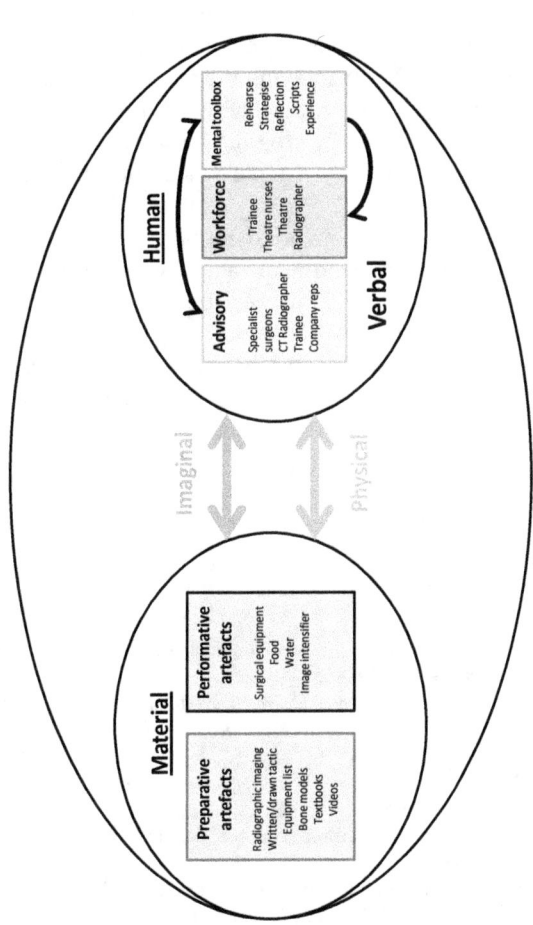

**Fig. 10.1** Diagrammatic representation of the interaction between human and material 'actors' in the preoperative preparatory network for a trauma procedure, as viewed from a surgeon's perspective. (Reproduced with permission from Ibrahim et al. [26]). Sociomaterial interactions are two-way and may be physical (e.g. manipulation of an object) or imaginal (e.g. the object stimulates the surgeon's thought processes). Materials are listed as those that aid preparation and those that are required to be in place at the time of procedure (performative). The people involved in the network may advise during preparation and be briefed to assist the surgeon on the day of the operation or both. The surgeon's own cognitive processes are included as a human actor and are heavily influenced by prior experience

## 10.6 Conclusions and Future Direction

Not all learning in surgery can be acquired through individualistic cognitive-based approaches. The surgical workplace is a complex, dynamic environment that cannot be ignored as a significant contributor to the education and training of medical professionals. Currently no one theory can simplify the situation so much as to be an all-encompassing guide to learning. However, learning theory rooted in sociocultural values such as activity theory may be more relevant, especially as they privilege the vitality of the artefacts that are so integral to the practice of surgery.

There is a paucity of published research studying the surgical workplace exclusively, but, from the literature available, it is clear that much more must be done to promote expansive learning such as boundary crossing between inter-professional disciplines. The concept of knot-working may provide a theoretical basis for further work.

Sociomaterial ontologies such as actor-network theory appear highly applicable to the objectives of an operating theatre. The role of each human and material component of a network is vital for patient care. However, it must not be forgotten that it is the cognitive processes of the surgeon who is taking overall responsibility for patient care that drives forwards the network. Whilst the surgeon's *acquisition* of knowledge and skill is paramount, *participation* within multiple activity systems throughout a career is essential not only for excellent performance but also for lifelong learning.

## References

1. Swanwick, T. (2005). Informal learning in postgraduate medical education: From cognitivism to 'culturism'. *Medical Education, 39*(8), 859–865.
2. Wright, S. M., Kern, D. E., Kolodner, K., Howard, D. M., & Brancati, F. L. (1998). Attributes of excellent attending-physician role models. *New England Journal of Medicine, 339*(27), 1986–1993.
3. Lave, J., & Wenger, E. (1991). *Situated learning: Legitimate peripheral participation*. Cambridge, UK: Cambridge university press.
4. Sfard, A. (1998). On two metaphors for learning and the dangers of choosing just one. *Educational Researcher, 27*(2), 4–13.
5. Engeström, Y. (2010). Activity theory and learning at work. In M. Malloch, L. Cairns, K. Evans, & B. N. O'Connor (Eds.), *The SAGE handbook of workplace learning* (p. 86). Los Angeles: Sage.
6. Bleakley, A. (2006). Broadening conceptions of learning in medical education: The message from teamworking. *Medical Education, 40*(2), 150–157.
7. Vygotsky, L. S. (1980). *Mind in society: The development of higher psychological processes*. Cambridge, MA: Harvard University Press.
8. Leont'ev, A. N. (1974). The problem of activity in psychology. *Soviet Psychology, 13*(2), 4–33.
9. Engestrom, Y. (1987). *Learning by expanding*. Helsinki: Orienta-Konsultit Oy.
10. Engeström, Y., & Blackler, F. (2005). On the life of the object. *Organization, 12*(3), 307–330.
11. Engeström, Y. (1999). Expansive visibilization of work: An activity-theoretical perspective. *Computer Supported Cooperative Work (CSCW), 8*(1–2), 63–93.

12. Cole, M., & Engeström, Y. (1993). A cultural-historical approach to distributed cognition. Distributed cognitions: Psychological and educational considerations (pp. 1–46).
13. Kuutti, K. (1991). Activity theory and its applications to information systems research and development. Information systems research: Contemporary approaches and emergent traditions (pp. 529–549).
14. Latour, B. (2005). Foreword by Bruno Latour. In B. Latour (Ed.), *Reassembling the social-an introduction to actor-network-theory* (p. 316). Oxford: Oxford University Press Sep 2005 ISBN-10: 0199256047 ISBN-13: 9780199256044. 2005; 1.
15. Wenger, E. (1998). *Communities of practice: Learning, meaning, and identity*. New York: Cambridge university press.
16. Lave, J. (1988). *Cognition in practice: Mind, mathematics and culture in everyday life*. New York: Cambridge University Press.
17. Fenwick, T., & Edwards, R. (2013). Performative ontologies. Sociomaterial approaches to researching adult education and lifelong learning. *European Journal for Research on the Education and Learning of Adults, 4*(1), 49–63.
18. Sørensen, E. (2009). *The materiality of learning: Technology and knowledge in educational practice*. New York: Cambridge University Press.
19. Waltz, S. B. (2006). Nonhumans unbound: Actor-network theory and the reconsideration of "Things" in educational foundations. *Educational Foundations, 20*(3), 51–68.
20. Fenwick, T., & Edwards, R. (2010). *Actor-network theory in education*. London: Routledge.
21. Bleakley, A. (2012). The proof is in the pudding: Putting actor-network-theory to work in medical education. *Medical Teacher, 34*(6), 462–467.
22. Heldal, F. (2010). Multidisciplinary collaboration as a loosely coupled system: Integrating and blocking professional boundaries with objects. *Journal of Interprofessional Care, 24*(1), 19–30.
23. Star, S. L., & Griesemer, J. R. (1989). Institutional ecology, translations' and boundary objects: Amateurs and professionals in Berkeley's Museum of Vertebrate Zoology, 1907–39. *Social Studies of Science, 19*(3), 387–420.
24. Engeström, Y., Engeström, R., & Vähäaho, T. (1999). When the center does not hold: The importance of knotworking. In S. Chaiklin, M. Hedegaard, & U. Jensen (Eds.), *Activity theory and social practice* (pp. 345–374). Aarhus: Aarhus University Press.
25. Varpio, L., Hall, P., Lingard, L., & Schryer, C. F. (2008). Interprofessional communication and medical error: A reframing of research questions and approaches. *Academic Medicine, 83*(10), S76–S81.
26. Ibrahim, E. F., Richardson, M. D., & Nestel, D. (2015). Mental imagery and learning: A qualitative study in orthopaedic trauma surgery. *Medical Education, 49*(9), 888–900.
27. Davydov, V. V. (1988). Problems of developmental teaching: The experience of theoretical and experimental psychological research. *Soviet Education, 30*(8), 6–97.

# Chapter 11
# The Role of Power in Surgical Education: A Foucauldian Perspective

**Nancy McNaughton and Ryan Snelgrove**

**Overview** A Foucauldian approach to the topic of power in surgical education engages constructivist and critical perspectives that consider social and clinical dimensions of training. A description of a Morbidity & Mortality (M&M) round is analysed using a Foucauldian concept of discourse to illustrate the different ways in which power is embedded in everyday practices. The authors focus on two discourses that discipline trainees beyond the scope of their knowledge and skill acquisition in order to make visible how implicit professional ideas influence surgical training.

## 11.1 Introduction

"[Michel] Foucault is a theorist who dealt directly with medical education. He wrote about the birth of clinical medicine and medical education, public health, psychiatry, schools and examinations, the body, physical and laboratory examination, sexuality and ethics" [1]. Foucault wrote during the mid-twentieth century in France at a time of political upheaval when traditional ways of doing things and looking at the world were being challenged by a critical school of scholars. Today there is growing interest in applying a Foucauldian lens to medical education. For example, Hodges et al. (2014) wrote about Foucauldian approaches in medical education research [1], and Bleakley and Bligh (2009) took up ideas related to his notion of the birth of the *clinical gaze* to raise questions about medicine's current drifts into simulation as a form of education [2]. Papadimos and Murray (2008) used Foucault's notion of *fearless speech* to examine the responsibility of medical schools to create

N. McNaughton (✉)
Centre for Learning Innovation and Simulation, Michener Institute for Education at UHN, Toronto, ON, Canada
e-mail: n.mcnaughton565@gmail.com

R. Snelgrove
Faculty of Medicine & Dentistry – Surgery Department, University of Alberta, Edmonton, AB, Canada
e-mail: rsnelgro@ualberta.ca

physicians as "able citizens who practice a fearless freedom of expression on behalf of their patients, the public, the medical profession, and themselves in the public and political arena" [3]. For our purposes we are interested in looking through a Foucauldian lens at power in surgical education.

This chapter examines the role of power in surgical education using a Foucauldian theoretical approach. Power within surgical education is often conceived as hierarchical, unilateral and uncontestable. In contrast, Foucault's philosophy defines power as relational and productive. It can have both positive and negative effects, with individuals at the same time being both recipients and wielders of power. It designates relationships between partners [4]. Power is not unidirectional but depends on the behaviour of all parties. Further, it is not held by a single agent. Instead, power is created and maintained by an entire system of practices and rules.

Traditionally, surgical education and clinical research are located within a positivist paradigm. Within this paradigm, a single truth exists and can be revealed through structured, empirical approaches such as randomized controlled trials and statistical analysis.

While this approach works well for hard sciences such as anatomy or biochemistry, when we widen our lens to consider the social world in which surgical training and practice take place, things become more complex. Reason cannot be isolated from the effects of power on what we come to believe is true. The form and use of empirical research are determined by people. In this way, values and interests may shape what comes to be considered knowledge and truth. A constructivist paradigm considers how these influences shape the social world around us. A Foucauldian approach falls within this paradigm and focuses on the ways in which truths that we take for granted are constructed in our daily practices through what Foucault calls "discourses".

According to Foucault, a discourse is an organized system of thought made up of "practices that systematically form the objects of which they speak" [5]. For example, ideas about clinical competence have changed over the years shifting from a focus on what people "know", as measured on written examinations, to what they can "do", as measured on performance-based assessments such as Objective Structured Clinical Examinations (OSCEs) [6]. This has led not only to new methods of teaching and assessing knowledge and skills but also to new accepted truths from one of rote, knowledge-based competence to one that can be recognized as a "performance discourse" of competence. Many different discourses are embedded both formally and informally in curricular structures, as well as in rules about what it is possible to say and do. Over time they become taken for granted and invisible – "It is just the way things work". Multiple discourses co-exist in the same place and time and intersect with each other creating tensions that need to be negotiated [5]. A discursive approach to the subject of surgical education brings to light the ways in which practices, ways of speaking, rules, and roles of authority engage pedagogically to construct systems of power that can reproduce 'truths' or knowledge about professionalism in the surgical field.

In the following section, we tell a story of a weekly Morbidity & Mortality (M&M) round in order to reflect on the effects of two discourses of power that are simultaneously active in surgical education practice and the potential effects on trainees and staff.

## 11.2 Discourses of Power Within M&M Rounds

A surgical resident approaches the podium at the weekly M&M rounds. The resident is presenting a common bile duct transection during a laparoscopic cholecystectomy. As he presents the case, the surgical faculty begin to grill him about the details: Did you obtain the critical view of safety before you clipped and cut? Why didn't you convert to an open cholecystectomy?

As he sweats at the podium, the resident pauses to think about his response. He was present during the operation with Dr. Gordon. The resident began the operation, and Dr. Gordon assisted. While dissecting the cystic duct of the gallbladder (the desired structure to transect), the resident believed that he was too medial and was at risk of damaging the common bile duct. He told Dr. Gordon this, but Dr. Gordon disagreed with his suggestion to move higher up on the gallbladder. The resident was uncomfortable proceeding and traded positions with Dr. Gordon. Dr. Gordon continued the dissection and asked the nurse for clips to place prior to transection. The resident protested again, suggesting a second opinion, and told Dr. Gordon that he believed the structure was tunneling back towards the liver and perhaps the common bile duct. Once again, Dr. Gordon ignored the resident's concerns and cut the structure. It became clear as Dr. Gordon began to dissect the gallbladder off the liver that they had indeed transected the common bile duct. At this point, Dr. Gordon did call for another opinion from a liver surgeon, and they spent the next 4 hours reconstructing the patient's biliary tree.

At the M&M round, the resident reviews these events in his head, but when he answers the questions from faculty, he accepts responsibility for the injury: "We thought we had a critical view before cutting…." The resident takes the blame for the injury, sensing that making a technical error was more acceptable to the audience than shirking responsibility and blaming the staff surgeon.

Dr. Gordon listens in the audience and remains silent. This is his second bile duct injury over the last few months. His practice is primarily breast surgery, and the only gallbladders he operates on are the difficult ones which come in overnight. He wished he could ask his colleagues for some mentorship and to come in to help him during these operations until he gets more comfortable, but he is worried that his colleagues would judge him for lacking confidence and skill. While the M&M is being presented, he is thinking about ways to get out of doing on-call gallbladders in the future.

## 11.3 Two Discourses

### 11.3.1 Biopower: A Disciplinary Discourse

Foucault was concerned with how knowledge was put to work through practices within institutional settings in order to regulate the conduct of others [7]. He coined the term biopower to describe the processes by which populations are regulated and bodies disciplined [8]. According to Jaye [9], sets of tacit and context-specific rules about how doctors should behave, think and feel are embedded within the institutional settings of the medical school and teaching hospital. "These rules are socially constructed and modelled in everyday clinical, teaching and learning settings by various practitioners, professionals, patients and students inhabiting this institutional space" [9]. The focus is on the relationships between the knowledge, the power, the body and the regulation of conduct according to a set of implicit truths. Disciplinary processes at an institutional level are most efficient and effective when, "individuals take up the task of self-regulation and self-disciplining, something that occurs as persons take up identities offered them through the discursive practices of social institutions and professions" [9]. The effect of these relationships is to produce a normalized set of practices that become invisible: the norm or "the way things are done" (i.e. the organizational culture). Examining surgical education through a lens of disciplinary power allows us to pull back a curtain and examine how particular practices get activated within professional settings and their effect on various players. Foucault's notion of biopower and in particular how it applies to the regulation and self-regulation of professional behaviours offers us insight into the role of power within a surgical training process.

The resident's actions during the surgery demonstrate knowledge of the biliary anatomy and an understanding of the consequences for complications arising from misidentification of its structures (i.e. mistaking the common bile duct for the cystic duct). His resulting actions during the case – to move aside and further to suggest a second opinion before having his staff proceed – may be judged as competent at the level of a resident. During M&M rounds, however, a discourse not directly related to anatomic knowledge is being invoked.

Examining the trainee's experience of the M&M rounds from the disciplinary perspective of biopower, we can see that this event is a specific regulating practice. This trainee's developing identity within the profession is tied to the manner in which he "performs" his understanding about his own skill and knowledge as well as his place in the professional hierarchy. It is a subjecting practice, that is, the resident is shaped into a particular kind of subject by the expectations of his professional community. By the resident's accepting blame for committing a technical error rather than "shirking responsibility" and blaming the staff surgeon for the complication, we see the resident's internalization of the values of the profession and the tension it causes with respect to the clinical facts as he represents the case. A disciplinary discourse then becomes visible during the resident's M&M presentation in his decision to defer to a norm of taking responsibility for a surgical procedure outcome and not shifting blame by recounting the actual sequence of events as they transpired (i.e. that the staff surgeon committed an error in identification of the biliary anatomy). It is a process of self-regulation that is a hallmark of professional training.

Another intersecting and overlapping discourse visible in the description of the M&M rounds is what Foucault referred to as "docile bodies" [10]. Foucault theorized the docile body as a malleable object on which disciplinary force is acted. Training is an important mechanism through which power creates docile bodies which are coaxed to respond to signals that are implicit and yet tightly organized through the networks of relations that maintain order. Surgical training is a discipline that is organized in such a way as to shape residents into surgeons who behave as professionals partly through respecting authority and following orders. Such discipline does not, however, necessarily teach residents how to become the person who is able to give the orders or direct their own behaviour.

One of the goals of practices such as M&M rounds is to create opportunities for trainees to internalize professional knowledge and skills as well as behavioural and attitudinal norms and values [11]. From a Foucauldian perspective, the weekly M&M round is a mechanism for reproducing a set of normalizing disciplinary techniques [12]. Social and professional mores are powerful shapers of professional conduct and are an influence on what we now identify as a "hidden curriculum". The hidden curriculum was first described in the medical education literature by Hafferty (1998) as "cultural mores that are transmitted, but not openly acknowledged, through formal and informal educational endeavours" [13]. The disciplinary discourses working within surgical training can be seen as one of the influences in creating a hidden curriculum or the understanding that there is a set of implicit social norms within the group that have to be obeyed in order to be successful.

M&M rounds then exist as an important disciplining medium that have high stakes for the trainee who is required to perform a professional identity as clinical role. There is much more going on in the resident's presentation than the facts of the case. This is social, professional and cultural territory with specific rules about taking responsibility, respecting authority and taking the blame even when the event may not be represented accurately. A disciplinary power of biomedicine can be seen in this example to operate through subjects internalizing how they should know and experience, behave, monitor and regulate themselves.

The tensions being negotiated by both the resident and the staff person indicate another powerful and overlapping discourse at play in our story.

### *11.3.2 Surgical Education as Pastoral Training*

*This form of power is linked with a production of truth—the truth of the individual himself.*
[14]

According to Foucault, over the course of modernity, pastoral power "spread and multiplied outside the ecclesiastical institution", and one of the most fertile areas for this development has been the realm of health and medicine [14].

With respect to surgical education, a pastoral discourse is relevant as another regulatory process in the socialization of surgical trainees. There is a complex reciprocity between a trainee and surgical attending who like Foucault's pastor is characterized by "the principle of analytical responsibility", according to which the pastor must account for "every act of each of his sheep, for everything that may have happened between them, and everything good and evil they may have done at any time" [15]. As Foucault observes, "[t]he pastor must really take charge of and observe daily life in order to form a never-ending knowledge of the behaviour and conduct of the members of the flock he supervises" [16]. The pastor's concern is with the daily workings and thoughts of the members of his flock – a procedure which involves the production and extraction of "a truth which binds one to the person who directs one's conscience" [15].

Within this discourse, the M&M round itself can be seen as a confessional performance during which the trainee is expected to outline all aspects of his decision-making and actions and confess his shortcomings before the pastorate. The expectation has been internalized and has become a form of self-regulation invisible to both trainee and staff alike. From a lens of pastoral power, we can see there is a complex tie between the pastor who exercises a minute and careful jurisdiction over the bodily actions and the souls of his flock in order to assure their salvation and the members of the flock who each owe him "a kind of exhaustive, total, and permanent relationship of individual obedience" [15].

A pastoral discourse captures the tension between discipline and protection that occurs during training processes. Being a good resident is very different from being a good surgeon. Training does not necessarily lead to the independent thinking required in practice. Training takes candidates who have shown independence, initiative and skill in order to gain entrance to the surgical discipline and trains them into compliance – "do as I say, not as I do" [9, 11]. On graduating these professionals are now expected to function independently and with confidence. The daily supervisory gaze to which a resident becomes so accustomed as a part of training is gone, replaced by an internalized disciplining gaze of the profession.

We can understand the surgical procedure described in the M&M round as a ritualized performance guided by the surgical attendings. The patient, although largely absent from the story, is here the ritual object upon which the two surgeons are ministering. In the M&M rounds, the tension between the trainee and the experienced surgeons about observations and decisions to act are resolved through the deference of the junior to the senior staff member who is ultimately responsible for the behaviour of his trainee/postulate as well as the outcome of the surgery (i.e. it is the name of the attending on the patient's wrist band not the resident's) which in turn is a salvation of sorts for the unconscious patient. This deference of the resident/postulate to the senior member/pastor may be so exacting that residents may actually begin to question their own memory, experience and ability to interpret reality. The constant reminders of position and/or rank can lead a resident to assume that their inexperience is the problem, that they are wrong and that the staff physician is right even in circumstances when they were not present during the event. It can be disconcerting at M&M rounds to see resident's question their first-hand experience of reality when a staff member who was never present starts authoritatively telling the room what happened and the room agrees with them. As identified in an article on M&M rounds by Kuper et al. [17], "Bosk, delineated the function of surgical M&M [round]s as moments when senior attending surgeons could claim and consolidate authority by taking public responsibility for the actions of their trainees, and from which their trainees and more junior colleagues could learn the moral qualities of senior clinicians" [11].

The resident's reflections during the M&M rounds about what to reveal during his presentation are a form of internalization and self-regulation. He recognizes the greater value of confessing to a wrong decision during the procedure than shaming his "pastor/teacher" to whom he is beholden. Reflected also in the M&M story is the staff surgeon's desire to receive mentorship himself regarding his gallbladder surgeries, as he is not confident in his own skills, but fears the effect of such an admission on his reputation and professional relationships. In this way, the individualizing nature of the pastoral discourse can be seen to act in both directions having a constraining effect on the trainee while also effectively isolating the staff surgeon from his profession and colleagues.

## 11.4 Conclusion

We have examined the role of power in surgical education using Foucault's concept of discourse to demonstrate the various ways in which taken-for-granted rules about professional conduct get built into daily processes and practices. There are implications for surgical trainees who internalize disciplinary and self-regulating practices. Surgical training environments are not static and undergo ongoing cultural shifts from multiple influences such as reduced resident work hours or increasing fragmentation in team and rotation assignment. Attention to power relations offers opportunities to examine the ways in which discourses may set up tensions for all players by implicitly creating unrealistic expectations about supervisory relationships and deference to authority.

Transition into practice after residency is one of the most difficult phases in a surgeon's career. Some of the reasons for this may be due to the systems of power within surgery. While these systems exist for a reason – responsibility for patient care is paramount in surgery – they are also not innocent. A resident who accepts blame without due process and follows orders without question may be seen as desirable during training. A staff physician who cannot make an independent decision, is afraid to call for help or ask for collegial advice can be dangerous.

The act of turning a familiar object like surgical training around and looking at it from a new vantage allows us to discover information that otherwise may remain hidden. Considering the effect of power as a daily set of practices potentially increases recognition that surgeons are created by a training system, encouraging surgical educators to step back and look at resident behaviour and the cultural values that fashion surgeons in a new light. The possible consequences of not looking anew at our professional practices are the reproduction of knowledge claims that may be less than effective and in some instances damaging for professional practice and health-care outcomes.

# References

1. Hodges, B. D., Martimianakis, M. A., McNaughton, N., & Whitehead, C. (2014). Medical education...meet Michel Foucault. *Medical Education, 48*, 563–571. https://doi.org/10.1111/medu.12411.
2. Bleakley, A., & Bligh, J. (2009). Who can resist Foucault? *The Journal of Medicine and Philosophy, 34*, 368–383.
3. Papadimos, T. J., & Murray, S. J. (2008). Foucault's "fearless speech" and the transformation and mentoring of medical students. *Philosophy, Ethics, and Humanities in Medicine, 17*, 3–12.
4. Foucault, M. (2006). In J. Khalfa (Ed.), *History of madness. Introduction* (pp. xiii–xxvii) (trans: Murphy, J.). London: Routledge.
5. Foucault, M. (1972). *The archaeology of knowledge: & the discourse on language* (trans: Sheridan Smith, A. M.). New York: Pantheon Books.
6. Hodges, B. (2012). The shifting discourses of competence. In B. Hodges & L. Lingard (Eds.), *The question of competence: Reconsidering medical education in the twenty-first century* (pp. 14–41). New York: Cornell University Press.
7. Foucault, H. S. (2001). Knowledge, power, and discourse. In M. Wetherall, S. Taylor, & S. J. Yates (Eds.), *Discourse theory and practice: A reader* (pp. 72–81). London: Sage Publications.
8. Foucault, M. (2004). *The birth of bio-politics. Lectures at the college de France 1978–1979*. New York: Palgrave Macmillan.
9. Jaye, C., Egan, T., & Parker, S. (2006). 'Do as I say, not as I do': Medical education and Foucault's normalizing technologies of self. *Anthropology & Medicine, 13*(2), 141–155. https://doi.org/10.1080/13648470600738450.
10. Foucault, M. (1995). *Discipline and punish. The birth of the prison*. New York: Vintage Books.
11. Bosk, C. L. (1979). *Forgive and remember: Managing medical failure*. Chicago: University of Chicago Press.
12. Nicoll, K. (1997). "Flexible learning"—unsettling practices'. *Studies in Continuing Education, 19*(2), 100–111.
13. Hafferty, F. (1998). Beyond curriculum reform: Confronting medicine's hidden curriculum. *Academic Medicine, 73*(4), 403–407.
14. Foucault, M. (1983). The subject and power. In H. Dreyfus & P. Rabinow (Eds.), *Michel Foucault: Beyond structuralism and hermeneutics* (pp. 208–226). Chicago: University of Chicago Press.
15. Foucault, M. (2007). *Security, territory, population: Lectures at the Collège de France, 1977–1978* (trans: Burchell, G.). New York: Palgrave Macmillan.
16. Golder, B. (2007). Foucault and the genealogy of pastoral power. *Radical Philosophy Revolution, 10*(2), 157–176.
17. Kuper, A., Nedden, N. Z., Etchells, E., Shadowitz, S., & Reeves, S. (2010). Teaching and learning in morbidity and mortality rounds: An ethnographic study. *Medical Education, 44*, 559.569. https://doi.org/10.1111/j.1365-2923.2010.03622.x.

# Chapter 12
# Constructing Surgical Identities: Being and Becoming a Surgeon

**Roberto Di Napoli and Niall Sullivan**

**Overview** This chapter focuses on the question of what surgical identities are and how they are constructed. It opens with clarification of the concept of professional identities before it considers, more specifically, surgical identities. Some possible meanings of surgical identities are subsequently unpacked from different theoretical angles (communities of practice, interprofessionalism and surgical identity construction). The resulting picture is one of the complexities, which depicts the surgical profession as being well beyond the acquisition of technical capabilities and scientific knowledge, highlighting its evolving nature in terms of what its members make of it over time and space. The chapter ends with a number of reflections on the importance of discussing surgical identities for the profession and for surgical education.

## 12.1 Introduction: The Rise of Professional Identities

Over the last few years, there has been an exponential increase in the discourse of professional identities [1–5]. Arguably, this is the result of wider, rapid changes in our societies, which have unsettled the traditional ways of looking at professions as rigid models around which people build their own professional roles and practice [6, 7]. Questions have emerged about the nature, scope, aims and ownership of different professions: Who is an academic today? Who is a lawyer? Who is a medic or, indeed, a surgeon?

R. Di Napoli (✉)
St. George's University of London, London, UK
e-mail: rdinapol@sgul.ac.uk

N. Sullivan
North Shore Hospital, Auckland, New Zealand
e-mail: niall.sullivan@uhbristol.nhs.uk

This chapter explores the question by juxtaposing theoretical constructs with examples taken from a case study in orthopaedic surgery [8]. This is an important exercise on two accounts: first, it helps with understanding the complexities of the surgical profession today; and second, it assists with the development of a type of surgical education that is related to a profession in evolution. We will explore moving from a static view of surgical education based on a toolbox of practical skills, knowledge and competencies to one that is mindful of how individuals make sense of their own role and practice in evolving professional and sociocultural contexts. Through an emphasis on the notion of surgical identities, at the end of this chapter, we argue for a type of surgical education that is dynamic, reflective and more aligned with the realities of our changing world, within and outside the surgical domain.

## 12.2 Conceptualising Professional Identities

The notion of 'professional identity' sits at the cusp between two important concepts: 'profession' and 'identity'.

Traditionally, a profession has been conceived of as a disciplined group of people who possess specialised knowledge and skills and abide by a given code of conduct. A profession has also been defined as an entity that is socially recognised and defends the needs and status of those who are part of it [9]. This view of a profession is arguably rather static in that it ignores the socialisation process into a profession and the identity issues this engenders; it says little about what it means to become part of a profession and the difficult identity work that is required to enter membership of this group and maintain a position in it. Being a professional is the result of a process of alignment with a profession and, to a lesser extent, alignment of the profession with its members, as their views of and vision for the profession evolve over time.

Although the concept of identity has, in the Western world, a long history going back as far as ancient Greece, it is the twentieth century that has seen a burgeoning of thinking and literature on the topic. Philosophers and social thinkers such as Mead, Bauman, Giddens and Foucault have been central in theorising the notion of identities as social constructs that are continuously being created and re-created at the interface between wider social forces and an individual's positioning and sense-making of those very forces. Seen from this angle, the notion of identity acquires both complexity and flexibility: individuals do not simply have fixed identities throughout their lives but negotiate these in relation to both changing circumstances and according to what they value and believe in at different points in their lives. Identities mix continuity and flexibility in complex ways [10].

The notion of 'professional identities' is predicated on both theories about 'profession' and 'identity'. As a starting point and in line with the work by Jarvis-Selinger et al. [11], we define these as points of integration between professionals' various statuses and roles and diverse professional and personal experiences, beliefs, values and worldviews that individuals bring into their work and that impact on the way they conceive of it. Professional identities are constructs through which professionals attempt to make sense of their profession (as a set of rules, expectations in terms of their own values and beliefs) [12].

In the next sections, we unpack the concept of surgical identities by making reference to a number of theoretical frameworks that are exemplified through a case study in orthopaedic surgery. The case study is taken from a master's degree research project studying the development of surgical identity and professionalism in Orthopaedic Registrars in UK training. The area explored related to the impact that attendance and participation at a regular morning meeting (trauma meeting) had on the registrars' identity development. The registrars' interactions within their communities of practice and the interplay between different communities were at the forefront of factors influencing the development of their surgical identities and professionalism.

## 12.3 Surgical Identities in Communities of Practice

The advent of the theoretical work going under the name of 'communities of practice' (COP) (Wenger) has played an important part in addressing the issue of professional identities [13]. It has highlighted the importance of identity work in the construction of professions. In line with this thinking, we conceive of professions as specific COPs. These are spaces that are defined by the shared rules, role expectations, interests, knowledge, values and practices held by a professional community. Within this identity field, professionals build, over time, their own sense of what it means to be and to become a lawyer, a teacher, a nurse or, indeed, a surgeon. This is what we call the process of professional identity formation.

In the case of surgical identities, these are progressively constructed, as individual surgeons increasingly embed themselves within the surgical COP and its specialising subcommunities (heart surgery, orthopaedic surgery, etc.). This community is the professional space within which individual surgeons navigate, as they shape and reshape their own surgical identities during their careers. This process happens through interactions with colleagues, exploring explicit or tacit rules and understandings of the surgical profession. In this process, surgeons expand on and deepen their understanding of surgery, both from its purely technical and more social aspects.

Surgical identities are formed within COPs and the professional space in which different COPs interact. In the case study about orthopaedic surgeons, for example, the orthopaedic registrar (like most surgical trainees) moves through varying COPs over the course of their training, from job to job and even from morning to evening. Their legitimacy and centrality are dictated by a number of factors: seniority, role, familiarity with other members, time in the community, makeup of the community, personality, values and beliefs about the profession. For example, a senior registrar who has worked in a department for a year who is on call and presenting in a trauma meeting would be seen as central. However, the same registrar in a new hospital, attending a trauma call on their first day, may be seen as less legitimate than the junior registrar who has previously worked in that department. This brings to mind the saying that 'respect must be earned'. In some ways, grade and experience allow for a transferrable legitimacy, yet there is more to attaining a position in a COP than simply the role one holds.

It is important to appreciate that within the surgical community, there are a multitude of COPs. These can be specialty and sub-specialty based such as orthopaedic surgeons, hospital based and grade based such as a junior doctor COP, task based such as a multidisciplinary team for cancer treatment and so on. Surgical trainees must interact with many of these COPs playing varying roles. As they do this, they inject their own practice into the profession, thus contributing to its evolution. Without having an explicit, formal knowledge about COP, the registrars in our case study were very clear in their understanding of their varying roles and centrality within the multitude of settings and teams they were involved in each day. Their COPs had indeed made the rules, expectations and forms of communication known to its participants. Professional communities play an important role in the formation of professional identities; they influence every aspect of a surgeon's working life.

## 12.4 Surgical Identities and Interprofessionalism

However, in line with the most recent work by Wenger-Trayner et al., our view is that surgical identities cannot be conceived as belonging to discreet, self-contained COPs [14]. We maintain that professional identities are built at the points of interaction between a specific COP and other communities. It is out of this dynamic that a professional identity is formed and evolves. Wenger-Trainer et al. encourage an ecological view of professional identities, as constructs that nurture and are nurtured by a variety of professional practices, behaviours and value systems, in an interprofessional fashion [15]. This means that one becomes a professional not just within a single-specific COP but in the interprofessional spaces between different COPs. Thus, being a surgeon means, first and foremost, interfacing with colleagues of one's specific specialism. This also implies being part of a wider community of surgeons, which is in turn nested within the wider medical profession. The medical profession interfaces with other COPs, such as those of nurses and social workers, for example. Seen through this lens, a surgical identity is a complex construct of roles in interrelated COPs.

This complexity was evident in our case study where at a trauma meeting a number of different professions and specialties would be in attendance. The presence of an anaesthetist, a nurse, a physiotherapist, etc. would alter the dynamic and thus how each member of the community interacts with those around them. Interprofessionalism relates to the ability of any member in a specific COP to communicate purposefully with members of other communities (surgical or otherwise) and learn from them in the liminal spaces in between these. Wenger-Trayner calls this ability to work across professional boundaries' 'knowledgeability', an important aspect of a surgeon's professional makeup.

## 12.5 Constructing Surgical Identities Through Reflections

Whilst the notion of COP is a powerful theoretical construct for understanding surgical identities, it does not tell us the whole story. To widen and complement our understanding, we make use of the work of theoreticians such as Archer [16] and Giddens [17]. These authors conceive of 'identity' as a complex and fluid entity that, within specific COPs, lies at the interface between structural factors (such as statutory definitions of surgery, its standards, desired behaviours and values, roles and role models) and the actualisation of these at the individual level, in relation to personal beliefs, values, perceptions and behaviours. We call this personal dimension the 'self'.

For people, building and maintaining their surgical identities mean enacting a constant work of sense-making between the structures within which they work and their own selves [18]. This is a true endeavour of socialisation, which goes well beyond the process of identification [6]. In terms of surgical identities this means that as individuals enter this particular COP, they bring into it their own views of and vision for the profession. This is nurtured by their own set of personal values and beliefs about what it is to be a surgeon in today's world.

Surgical identities are not simply models or sets of rules and expectations with which people align themselves a-critically and without reflection; rather, they are the result of ongoing sense-making and compromises between official definitions, stereotypes, real-time iterations and expectations of what it is to be a surgeon. Reflection is paramount in this process. Rhodes et al. [19] propose that there cannot be identity formation without reflection, and this idea is almost a constant in terms of identity formation [5, 20–24]. Reflection allows for understanding of the contexts which individual professionals inhabit whilst guiding practice.

Our orthopaedic registrars emphasised that they did not join their surgical and orthopaedic COPs as a blank canvas. Rather, they brought with them multiple identities upon which to construct their orthopaedic surgical identities. These pre-existing identities were built from their experiences as doctors, brothers, mothers, sports team members and so on. This was particularly important when they were exposed to unprofessional behaviour from central members of their COP. Using their pre-existing values and beliefs, they regularly chose not to align themselves with these unprofessional behaviours. By reflecting on behaviours they witness, through their own value system and beliefs about surgery, surgeons make conscious and unconscious decisions about who they want to be and, importantly, who they do not want to be. As they become more central themselves, they are progressively able to exert greater influence on their community so that it may align more to their own sense of the profession.

## 12.6 Being and Becoming a Surgeon

The formation of surgical identities is never a once-and-for-all accomplishment. As surgeons navigate in and through their COP and other professional communities throughout their career, they acquire a growing sense of the complexities of being a surgeon and becoming a more competent and sophisticated one. Importantly, they also increasingly contribute to their community/ies as they progress in their careers in different and more complex contexts. This progressive accumulation of experience and expertise adds an element of individual control to the notion of surgical identities. The extent to which an individual may influence the COP depends on how facilitative these different professional contexts are. All things being equal, surgeons are arguably shaped by their profession as much as shaping it. Surgical identities are not simply mirrors of the profession; they potentially have the power to help individuals and the whole profession to evolve.

The process of becoming a surgeon can begin even before medical school admission, as individuals make sense of their understanding of the perceived qualities and attributes of surgeons. In this sense, Burford talks of *anticipatory socialisation* [23]. This is where a person attempts to adopt an identity that they believe will be congruent with that of a desired community/profession to gain legitimacy, whether or not this identity is congruent with their own. Stereotypical traits of specialties may be perpetuated in this way with the medical student aspiring to be an orthopaedic surgeon taking up rugby, drinking beer and even playing down their intelligence! However, over time, as they embed themselves within a surgical community, individuals start building a more complex sense of themselves within it and, given the right circumstances, are able to influence it.

Kegan suggested five stages of identity formation or 'orders of mind': incorporative, impulsive, imperial, interpersonal and institutional [25]. Of these, two, three and four loosely correlate with acting, becoming and being, respectively. These stages were discussed by Jarvis-Selinger et al. in relation to 'crises' which challenge medics and bring about changes in their identity [11]. These crises relate to significant events during a doctor's training and working life that trigger reflection and re-evaluation. These events can be small such as placing one's first suture or large such as a traumatic cardiac arrest and patient death. Pratt et al. referred to 'integrity violations' that brought about similar identity evolution. An example from this work noted US surgical residents making sense of doing paperwork and menial tasks during their early working years rather than effecting dramatic changes in patient outcomes through operating [26].

From our orthopaedic case study, we identified 'challenges' to legitimacy which had a similar impact to crises or identity violations. Such episodes included trainees being criticised for lack of knowledge or trainees witnessing unprofessional behaviour of central members of their COP. These events made the trainees question themselves, their roles and their career desires both consciously and subconsciously. They reflected on these events, and this reflection shaped their ideas, values, beliefs and, ultimately, their surgical identities.

## 12.7 Alignment: The Tensions Between Individuality and Uniformity

Finally, there is a dichotomy in surgical training with the desire for diversity in the profession to meet the evolving demands of the job all whilst expecting standardisation of surgeons through rigid competency-based assessment. Frost and Regehr [27] discuss how diversity can 'engender more culturally competent, empathic, and service-oriented graduates who are better prepared to care for society's increasingly heterogeneous patient population' [27]. It is concerning that many in healthcare and education policy-making roles consider there to be a singular, standardised way of being a competent surgeon. Wald (2015) contemplated how we may support and enhance identity formation 'without homogenizing the distinctiveness of healthcare professional team members' [24]. As we have discussed, this alignment of personal surgical identity/identities with that of our COPs is not unilateral. This idea is supported by Ibarra (1999) who counters that there is *a negotiated adaptation by which people strive to improve the fit between themselves and their work environment* [28].

Our orthopaedic registrars had a strong sense of what was required to gain legitimacy in their chosen COP, with a goal of obtaining consultant posts at the end of training. They generally displayed views on communication, interpersonal relationships, personal appearance, work ethic and knowledge that aligned well with that of the wider orthopaedic community. They acknowledged that there was a need to 'fit in' to gain and maintain legitimacy within their COPs, even if that meant stifling aspects of their personality and demeanour. However, the most senior trainees were more bullish in their assertion that when they became consultants, they would stay true to their values and beliefs and their identities, even when moving to new units. The extent to which these trainees have already been homogenised is difficult to ascertain. However, that these senior trainees still consider there to be aspects where they are resisting aligning with their COPs is both relevant and important.

## 12.8 Conclusion: Surgical Identities and Surgical Education

In this chapter, we have theorised a complex view of surgical identities. These are constructs that are:

- Social in character, as they are embedded within specific COPs which, in turn, are part of wider social settings.
- Built at the cusp between structural forces and personal factors.
- Fairly stable yet moving in relation to how individuals make sense of themselves and their work within the profession over time.
- Evolving not just in relation to one single COP but along the intersections of many others, in an interprofessional fashion. This means that surgical identities are to be understood in an ecological way rather than being conceived as discrete constructs linked to one single, specialised COP.

- Intimately connected to reflectivity, which allows for sense-making and professional evolution.
- Subjected to temporal change, as individuals evolve in their career.

We deem that an emphasis on surgical identities in surgical education is paramount for a number of reasons:

- First of all, it widens the idea of surgery beyond the acquisition of purely technical competencies and the appropriation of scientific knowledge. Whilst the latter is obviously paramount, it is arguable that surgeons need to learn to be and become professionals within complex professional and interprofessional contexts. An understanding of these and of one's professional standing, along with an ability to comprehend others' professional identities and work, is key for a successful surgical career and the benefit of the surgical profession as a whole.
- Second, through reflection, it encourages consideration of the ethical dimension of surgery, thus generating important debates about issues such as caring and compassion, respect for/dignity of the patient and openness to dialogue within surgical and medical contexts.
- Third, as a corollary, it opens spaces for debating issues of autonomy, self-regulation and responsibility for and agency towards society. This is much needed at times when professional autonomy is being put into question worldwide by forms of rational managerialism that emphasise efficiency over effectiveness [16].
- Fourth, through ideas of 'being' and 'becoming', it explicitly encourages surgeons to think of surgery as a continuous professional and personal journey, during which, along with increasing technical knowledge and skills, they need to learn how to position and reposition themselves in wider sociocultural contexts. This is important to remember, as surgery is of this world and contributes to its well-being.

Of course, emphasising the need to give space to surgical identities in the surgical curriculum is a complex curriculum design endeavour, which goes well beyond the addition of communication or reflective skills. It calls for a rethinking of the way in which surgical education is conceived, as one which is capable of integrating with 'knowing' and 'acting', the dimension of 'being' [29]. This requires time and effort by versatile surgical educators who can stand up to the challenge.

# References

1. Cruess, R., Cruess, S., & Steinert, Y. (Eds.). (2016). *Teaching medical professionalism: Supporting the development of a professional identity* (2nd ed.). Cambridge, UK: Cambridge University Press.
2. Kinsella, A., & Pitman, A. (2012). *Phronesis as professional knowledge: Practical wisdom and the professions.* Rotterdam: Sense Publishers.
3. Barnett, R., & Di Napoli, R. (Eds.). (2008). *Changing identities in higher education: Voicing perspectives.* London: Routledge.

4. Berry, A., Clemans, A., & Kostogriz, A. (2007). *Dimensions of professional knowledge: Professionalism, practice and identity*. Rotterdam: Sense Publishers.
5. Barbour, J., & Lammers, J. (2015). Measuring professional identity: A review of the literature and a multilevel confirmatory factor analysis of professional identity constructs. *Journal of Professions and Organization, 2*(1), 38–60.
6. Halpern, C. (2016). *L'identité(s): l'individu, le groupe, la société*. Sciences HumainesÉditions.
7. Alasuutari, P. (2004). *Social theory and human reality*. London: Sage.
8. Sullivan, N. P. T. (2015). The trauma meeting: An opportunity for the development of professionalism and the enrichment of professional identities. (unpublished).
9. Freidson, E. (2001). *Professionalism: The third logic*. Cambridge, UK: Polity Press.
10. Jenkins, R. (2014). *Social identity* (4th ed.). London: Routledge.
11. Jarvis-Selinger, S., Pratt, D., & Regehr, G. (2012). Competency is not enough: Integrating identity formation into the medical education discourse. *Academic Medicine, 87*(9), 1185–1190.
12. Kreber, C. (2016). *Educating for civic-mindness: Nurturing authentic professional identities through transformative higher education*. London: Routlledge.
13. Wenger, E. (1998). *Communities of practice: Learning, meaning, and identity*. Cambridge, UK: Cambridge Univ. Press.
14. Wenger-Trayner, E., Fenton-O'Creeve, M., Hutchinson, S., Kubiak, C., & Wenger-Trayner, B. (2015). *Learning in landscapes of practice: Boundaries, identity, and knowledgeability in practice-based learning*. London: Routledge.
15. Crawford, K. (2012). *Interprofessional collaboration and social work*. London: Sage.
16. Archer, M. S. (2008). *Structure, agency and the internal conversation*. Cambridge, UK: Cambridge University Press.
17. Giddens, A. (1986). *The constitution of society: Outline of the theory of structuration*. Cambridge, UK: Polity Press.
18. Weick, K. E. (1995). *Sense making in organizations*. London: Sage.
19. Rhodes, R., & Smith, L. G. (2006). *Molding professional character. Lost virtue: Professional character development and medical education*. Oxford: Elsevier.
20. Ashforth, B., & Mael, F. (1989). Social identity theory and the organization. *Academy of Management Review, 14*(1), 20–39.
21. Stets, J. E., & Burke, P. J. (2000). Identity theory and social identity theory. *Social Psychology Quarterly, 63*, 224–237.
22. Owens, T., Robinson, D., & Smith-Lovin, L. (2010). Three faces of identity. *Sociology, 36*(1), 477.
23. Burford, B. (2012). Group processes in medical education: Learning from social identity theory. *Medical Education, 46*(2), 143–152.
24. Wald, H. (2015). Professional identity (trans) formation in medical education: Reflection, relationship, resilience. *Academic Medicine, 90*(6), 701–706.
25. Kegan, R. (1994). *In over our heads: The mental demands of modern life*. Cambridge, MA: Harvard University Press.
26. Pratt, M., Rockmann, K., & Kaufmann, J. (2006). Constructing professional identity: The role of work and identity learning cycles in the customization of identity among medical residents. *Academy of Management Journal, 49*(2), 235–262.
27. Frost, H., & Regehr, G. (2013). "I am a doctor": Negotiating the discourses of standardization and diversity in professional identity construction. *Academic Medicine, 88*(10), 1570–1577.
28. Ibarra, H. (1999). Provisional selves: Experimenting with image and identity in professional adaptation. *Administrative Science Quarterly, 44*(4), 764–791.
29. Barnett, R., & Coate, K. (Eds.). (2005). *Engaging the curriculum in higher education*. Maidenhead: SRHE and Open University Press.

# Chapter 13
# Constructing Surgical Identities: Becoming a Surgeon Educator

**Tamzin Cuming and Jo Horsburgh**

**Overview** The challenge of developing an identity as a surgeon educator stems from the widely differing standpoints of surgery, with its biomedical view of the world, and education in its context as a social science. We argue that a social science lens is necessary for exploring the complex educational problems that surgeons face. Various forms of faculty development exist to unite the disparate traditions of education and surgery, yet the transformation from surgeon to surgeon educator is likely to be fostered best from within a community of surgeons who also identify as educators. A surgeon educator is presented as one who is able to integrate the two world views of surgery and education, which will prove of benefit not only to those they educate but also to surgery as a whole.

## 13.1 Introduction

This chapter sets out ways in which the burgeoning area of surgical education represents a cross-fertilisation of two different areas of expertise: that of surgery and that of education. We examine how for many surgeons it is fundamental to their professional identity to be involved in educating the next generation, yet the process of forming an identity as an educator is beset by difficulties. We consider these difficulties and how they may be addressed.

Education has always been a vital and central part of surgery. Surgical tradition has a surgeon handing on their insight and skills from a proud inheritance rooted in the very history of the craft. In this model, operative secrets are 'golden nuggets' at the heart of surgical education, with the surgical expert, the possessor of them, sought out by aspiring surgeons.

---

T. Cuming (✉)
Homerton University Hospital NHS Foundation Trust, London, UK

J. Horsburgh
Educational Development Unit, Imperial College, London, UK
e-mail: j.horsburgh@imperial.ac.uk

Changes in society and in medicine have had an impact on the process of learning surgery across the world. Consequently some of the surgical expertise we value risks being lost in subsequent generations. Developing expert professional judgement and decision-making in young surgeons, a process that had been implicit within the traditional time-serving method of training, is particularly vulnerable as hours and continuity of training have dropped. Surgical postgraduate education has expanded in response to such a perceived gap, with courses and training programmes finding their place. There is resistance, however, from both surgeons and their trainees to changes that appear to have been imposed from an educational establishment outside of surgery, one that seems to have insufficient awareness of the differing nuances in culture between medical specialties and does not speak sufficiently to the needs of surgeons or surgeons in training.

Education as a field incorporates the social sciences, humanities and philosophy, amongst other traditions, and has the potential to influence the surgical profession profoundly and positively. We argue that education may steer surgery through a period in which there is increasing reliance on numeric data as the main representation of complex educational outcomes, a phenomena criticised as superficial by Biesta [1], who terms it 'the age of measurement'. As Carr suggests, we are put in a position of valuing what we can measure, over measuring what we value [2]. Given the vast and qualitatively-oriented traditions on which education draws, it is ironic that a reliance on data-related outcomes has given educational changes in surgery a bad name: instead of encouraging feedback on performance, the number of workplace-based assessments done is simply counted, and trainees are rated on how many they have persuaded a trainer to fill out, not their content, or the process of discussion that is the educational idea at their heart.

We also argue that although there are a variety of ways that a surgeon may develop him/herself as an educator, this professional identity development is best done over time, in a local community of practice where educational issues and problems are situated.

A word on terms: 'training' is used as a term familiar to surgeons progressing along a highly prescribed path to independent operating. 'Education' is used to distinguish between this and a more holistic, wider view of enabling someone to become a surgeon. 'Trainee' is used indiscriminately, for simplicity.

## 13.2 Motivation to Engage with Surgical Education and the Challenges of Doing So

There is motivation for surgeons to become good trainers and to be known as such. Being a good trainer confers status and recognition in the wider surgical world. It is also a practical validation of one's worth as a surgeon. Trainees gravitate towards famed surgical trainers because excellent surgical skills are highly prized, and these will be assumed in the trainee who has spent time with such a trainer. Another advantage is that trainees will help manage a trainer's patient workload efficiently and are likely in future years to become trusted consultant colleagues. There are in addition accolades such as the UK annual 'Silver Scalpel' which is awarded by the Association of Surgeons in Training (ASiT) to an elected top trainer [3].

However, there are several challenges to engaging with education in a surgical context that are distinguished by surgeons themselves from the process of training. Practices within surgical training are often mandated and are increasingly regulated. The current accumulation of multiple tick-box assessment forms within this system is a much-maligned aspect of what is considered by most trainers to be coming from the world of 'education'. Many trainers do become involved in managing the trainees' progress through this system without the benefit of sufficient insight into the social science context of education to influence it. Lack of control over the curriculum is an additional cause of disengagement with education by surgeons [4, 5] and can lead to frustration with the education system they are working within. The frustrations are not limited to established surgeons but are shared by their trainees [6].

In the UK, the recent introduction of regulation for trainers, whilst laudable, risks driving an additional wedge between a trainer and his or her interest in being 'involved in education' [7]. Combined with the perception by some that education has lower status than research and clinical expertise itself, the motivation to engage with new approaches may be further diminished.

In order to develop as an educator, a surgeon needs to look beyond the way such concepts have currently been incompletely applied and seek to resist the reductionism that has been a divisive development in the field of surgical education.

## 13.3 Crossing Paradigms

One of the key challenges of engaging with educational ideas and practices is that they are largely unfamiliar to those who have been raised in a biomedical paradigm. For surgeons in the UK, there has often been no education past age 16 other than in mathematics and science-based subjects. These subjects, along with much of surgical teaching, assume a positivist viewpoint that knowledge is a certain entity existing outside of any individual in an external reality. It is, in this sense, objective. This is appropriate for the anatomical path of the abdominal aorta through the body but is a more contestable approach to thinking about knowledge around breaking bad news to a patient.

Becher and Trowler refer to academic disciplines as 'tribes and territories', distinguished from each other in differing views about the nature and purpose of knowledge [8]. They describe a contrast between 'hard' sciences – and surgery could be considered as such – and 'soft' sciences such as education [9]. The disciplinary traditions in which academics develop professionally exert an influence on their outlook towards knowledge and what makes it valid. How teaching and learning are approached by each 'tribe' is often related to this attitude. For example, teaching styles typical of education include facilitating discussions about an idea rather than pursuing didactic transmission of content, and this reflects the constructivist ethos of the discipline. Tension between what constitutes knowledge within education and surgery can manifest as scepticism in accepting alternative approaches to teaching (e.g. reflective practice, problem-based learning) and to educational research, particularly qualitative research. Those raised in a scientific tradition find educational literature 'foreign, expressed in a language that is both woolly and obscure', writes Kneebone [10].

Crossing to another paradigm is difficult because surgeons are asked to engage in the concept that previously-assumed certainties are ambiguous and questionable. Of course surgeons do routinely employ differing perspectives in their clinical lives in many ways, for example, in considering how patients interpret medical explanations of disease and the need for a particular operation. It is the failure to acknowledge that there can be multiple perspectives, or multiple views of truth that Kneebone suggests is an 'uncritical adherence to an overly "scientific" mode of thinking' and acts as a limitation to the development of insight and understanding in the training of surgeons.

By negotiating the differing perspectives of surgery and education, a surgeon educator can develop their identity as such, discovering advantages and the potential for personal development by being rooted in both disciplines.

## 13.4 What Are the Benefits of Engaging with Education?

Given the challenges of engaging with the field of education as a discipline and developing a professional identity as an educator, it is worth considering what education brings to the training and development of surgeons. Education brings to surgery an entirely different standpoint on the production of knowledge and results in an alternative approach for both teachers and learners. In recent years there have been widespread changes in the working hours and the curricula at both undergraduate and postgraduate levels that have limited the hours available for training. This has impacted upon surgical training in particular. Temple's 'Time for Training' report [11] in the UK summarised the difficulties, mentioning reduced time to absorb and develop complex aspects of professional practice compared to apprenticeship-type models of learning. A wider repertoire of educational strategies and insight, Temple argued, may make the most of the time available.

In the digital age, knowledge is less exclusive to professionals than in previous eras. What remains theirs is the interpretation and application of knowledge. This brings surgery closer to the field of education, in that they are both, in essence, professional practices that require their proponents, both surgeons and teachers, to interpret complex and variable systems and individuals.

Attempts to impose educational concepts on surgical education, for example, with mandatory reflective pieces using workplace-based assessments, have suffered due to a lack of understanding of the genuine benefits, in this case, of a purposive reflection that draws on multiple perspectives. It has also failed to produce an attitude towards workplace-based assessments that is formative [12]. Concepts such as reflection in action map well to the surgeon's ongoing decision-making within a challenging operation; however, most surgeons do not use this concept in their operative teaching although it may benefit their trainees' learning about such decisions [13]. Hence for both surgeons and their trainees, the encouragement to use reflection has not resulted in widespread acceptance of it as a concept. Barriers to adopting an alien concept such as that of reflection are still present, due to its origins in the educational field.

Many opportunities for learning in surgery are ad hoc and unwittingly exclude some learners, for example, by taking place in a changing room or in a social setting like a pub. When these elements of the hidden curriculum are made explicit, with the exposure of complex arenas of practice to debate and analysis by the learning surgeon, the trainer behaves more like an educator. This process is one in which barriers to educational concepts are being broken down by understanding. They may usefully extend to self-awareness, dealing with complexity, and theories around expertise. A surgeon who is making use of an active interest in these concepts starts going beyond their role as a trainer and moving closer to becoming a surgeon educator. Implementing educational concepts will allow the surgeon educator a broader view of difficulties that trainees have and provide a wider range of responses to offer.

## 13.5 Developing as a Surgical Educator

There are many ways to gain experience and greater understanding in the field of education. Like acquiring a surgical identity, becoming an educator is a long-term process. In this section we consider various routes including educational workshops, postgraduate studies in education and engagement with local communities of practice. In all of these methods, the surgeon is required to assimilate educational theory to underpin the process of integrating educational ideas into surgery.

Faculty development can range from attendance at teaching and learning workshops and completion of online courses to integrated, longitudinal, postgraduate programmes lasting a number of years [14]. Faculty development at an organisational level is becoming increasingly common in line with requirements of professional bodies, such as the UK's General Medical Council's accreditation requirements for postgraduate supervisors [15].

Whilst it may be easy to dismiss short educational courses and workshops for surgeons that provide 'tips and tricks' as lacking in depth, such courses, under the banner of 'training', are normally underpinned by educational theory (albeit not always explicitly referred to) and by certain educational values such as adopting a constructivist approach to learning and being learner-centred. Most courses will also help participants to reflect on, challenge and shape their beliefs about education [16]. Furthermore, they can help pique an individual's interest in education that may lead them to engage more deeply with education in the future.

A Best Evidence Medical Education (BEME) review evaluated the effectiveness of faculty development programmes, recognising that such evidence can be difficult to establish [17]. Elements considered included the development of curriculum, changes in practice at organisational levels and dissemination of learning to colleagues. Most interventions reported and included in the review had had a self-reported or observed positive effect on teaching effectiveness. However, few studies had established long-term impact, with those programmes of a longer duration, spanning several months or more, showing more profound effects than shorter ones.

In a study by one author (TC) of a 2-day surgical Training the Trainers course [18], the quantitative assessment of the course was able to demonstrate Kirkpatrick Level 4 [19], in that surgeons being trained in a procedure had a shorter learning curve after their trainers had taken the course. The course incorporated a number of key educational concepts around operative learning including feedback, establishing rapport, reflection and modelling a non-judgemental attitude. Six months after taking the course, however, qualitative interviews with course participants demonstrated some dissatisfaction and a resistant attitude, suggesting that such a course could not change anything significant in their teaching. It was interesting that their trainees had nonetheless benefitted. Whilst teaching behaviour can be modified, in the short term, by a course, long-term change may be lacking without engagement of the participant around their beliefs as educators. What the short course lacked was enough transformative power to convince surgeons that these educational concepts had improved their teaching, despite objective evidence that they in fact had.

With rapid changes in surgical education, both at undergraduate and postgraduate level, there has been increased demand for surgeons involved in education to study the discipline at a higher level [20]. The number of Master's- and doctoral-level programmes in medical, clinical or surgical education has increased dramatically worldwide [21]. In their review of graduates of such programmes, Sethi et al. [22] found a self-reported increase in participation in educational research and scholarship, which was underpinned by an enhanced understanding of educational theory. These authors argue that a key feature of a Master's in education is the role that professional identity formation plays in the programme. Many programmes specifically set out to facilitate a shift in identity that reflects the values and goals of the interpretivist, constructivist field of education.

The benefits to undertaking postgraduate study in education are at risk however without a wider community for their graduates to return to. Unpublished research by one of the authors (JH) [23] found that graduates of a Master's in Surgical Education programme valued local education communities to help further develop their professional identity. Where these local networks were not evident, it was more difficult to engage in educational practice. There is a contrast between the process of forming an identity as a surgeon, where socialisation, seen by Biesta [1] as the first step in 'becoming', is provided by surgical peers and colleagues at work and that of becoming a surgeon educator, where the natural community of 'educational' peers in an average working hospital is provided mainly by non-surgical physician colleagues.

Wenger's concept of communities of practice is a useful lens through which to consider this longitudinal development as a surgeon educator. Wenger defines communities of practice as 'groups of people who share a concern or passion for something they do and learn how to do it better as they interact regularly' [24]. They deal with common issues of concern and share practices, language and common goals. The motivation to engage with professional development as an educator is participation in such a community. The network of formal surgical training programmes and the training programme directors could be this community of practice. However, the integration of educational attitudes and theory is not yet universal within such structures. Alternative networks of surgeon educators outwith this regional structure are in their infancy. The surgical Royal Colleges in the UK are promoting education with day conferences and networks of College representatives. More may be needed however to bring together surgeons and educationalists to carry out research, particularly qualitative research, as well as ongoing cross-disciplinary learning.

We are not advocating that all surgeons need to complete a Master's or doctorate in education in order to become educators, but it may be helpful if such degrees become more widespread within communities of surgeon educators. Leaders and researchers amongst surgeon educators, perhaps with such a degree, need to encourage others into this community, acting as broker between the disciplines of surgery and education. Furthermore, collaboration with education experts has the potential to develop surgical education as a discipline that genuinely blends the expertise of both fields. There may also be engagement with the wider medical and surgical education community such as through the Academy of Medical Educators (AoME).

As educational ideas gain currency with individual surgeons through their experience of them, the boundaries between the worlds of surgery and education are likely to become ever less distinct.

## 13.6 Conclusion

Combating an over-reliance on educational frameworks that privilege numbers and measurement requires a transformative inclusion of education within surgery. To become a surgeon educator is to be at the forefront of such a revolutionary progression within the discipline of surgery.

In a world in which successful surgical outcomes are so highly prized, the role of teamwork, the subtleties of interactions around operative decisions and the importance of another world view besides the operative surgeon's – be it patient, trainee or allied professional – are being appreciated as the next major stepwise improvement that is possible in developed healthcare systems. Assimilation of the social sciences holds out this possibility for surgery.

Respect for educational expertise and the fostering of a community of surgeon educators within and beyond the settings where they educate may once again make education at the centre of surgical practice and a matter of pride for good surgeons everywhere.

## References

1. Biesta, G. J. J. (2010). *Good education in an age of measurement*. London: Paradigm.
2. Carr, D. (1999). Is teaching a skill? Philosophy Ed, pp. 204–211.
3. Association of Surgeons in Training. The Silver Scalpel Award. https://www.asit.org/silver-scalpel-award. Accessed 15th Sept 2017.

4. Beard, J. D., Marriott, J., et al. (2011). Assessing the surgical skills of trainees in the operating theatre: A prospective observational study of the methodology. *Health Technology Assessment, 15*(1), i–xxi 1–162.
5. Pereira, E. A., & Dean, B. J. (2013). British surgeons' experiences of a mandatory online workplace based assessment portfolio resurveyed three years on. *Journal of Surgical Education, 70*(1), 59–67.
6. Shalhoub, J., Marshal, D. C., & Ippolito, K. (2017). Perspectives on procedure-based assessments: A thematic analysis of semi-structured interviews with 10 UK surgical trainees. *BMJ Open, 7*, e013417. https://doi.org/10.1136/bmjopen-2016-013417.
7. GMC's promoting excellence: Standards for medical education and training. www.gmc-uk.org/education/standards.asp. Accessed 15 Sept 2017.
8. Becher, T., & Trowler, P. (2001). *Academic tribes and territories. Intellectual enquiry and the cultures of disciplines* (2nd ed.). Buckingham: Open University Press/SRHE.
9. Neumann, R. (2001). Disciplinary differences and university teaching. *Studies in Higher Education., 26*(2), 135–146.
10. Kneebone, R. (2002). Total internal reflection: An essay on paradigms. *Medical Education, 36*, 514–518.
11. Temple, J. (2010). Time for training. A review of the impact of the European Working Time Directive on the quality of training. Medical Education England.
12. Miller, A., & Archer, J. (2010). Impact of workplace based assessment on doctors' education and performance: A systematic review. *BMJ, 341*, c5064.
13. Schön, D. (1983). *The reflective practitioner: How professionals think in action.* London: Temple Smith.
14. Steinert, Y. (2014). Developing medical educators. A journey not a destination. In T. Swanick (Ed.), *Understanding medical education: Evidence, theory and practice.* London: Wiley.
15. General Medical Council. (2012). *Recognising and approving trainers: A consultation document.* London: GMC.
16. Steinert, Y. (2014). *Faculty development in the health professions.* Dordrecht: Springer.
17. Steinert, Y., Mann, K., Centeno, A., Dolmans, D., Spencer, J., Gelula, M., Prideaux, D. (2006) A systematic review of faculty development initiatives designed to improve teaching effectiveness in medical education: BEME Guide No 8. *Medical Teacher, 28*(6), 497–526 updated in: Steinert Y, Mann K et al. A systematic review of faculty development initiatives designed to enhance teaching effectiveness: A 10-year update: BEME Guide No. 40. Med Teach. 2016 Aug;38(8):769–86.
18. Mackenzie, H., Cuming, T., et al. (2015). Design, delivery and validation of a trainer curriculum for the national laparoscopic colorectal training program in England. *Annals of Surgery, 261*(1), 149–156.
19. Kirkpatrick, D. L., & Kirkpatrick, J. D. (1994). Evaluating training programs. Berrett-Koehler Publishers 1994.
20. Tekian, A., & Harris, I. (2012). Preparing health professions education leaders worldwide: A description of masters-level programs. *Medical Teacher, 34*(1), 52–58.
21. Tekian, A., Roberts, T., et al. (2014). Preparing leaders in health professions education. *Medical Teacher, 36*(3), 269–271.
22. Sethi, A., Schofield, S., et al. (2015). How do postgraduate qualifications in medical education impact on health professionals. *Medical Teacher, 38*(2), 162–167.
23. Horsburgh, J. (2015). Surgeons as brokers? Exploring the professional identity development of surgical educators. (Unpublished thesis) King's College London.
24. Wenger-Trayner, E. (2017). Introduction to communities of practice. http://wenger-trayner.com/introduction-to-communities-of-practice/. Accessed 25 Sept 2017.

# Part III
# Overview: The Practice of Surgical Education

This part orientates the reader to different philosophical positions in designing educational activities. It raises the concept of the locus of control in educational processes and the tensions of the provision of service and education in the same setting. The chapter foci address conventional elements of educational design and target surgical education specifically and troublesome and/or complex educational activities. The aspiration for quality in surgical education links all chapters.

Stefanidis and Choi offer fundamentals for designing surgical education programmes while also addressing higher conceptual issues associated with learners being socialised in multiple work places over prolonged periods of time (Chap. 14). They consider the role of stakeholders, availability of resources and continued personal and professional development of teachers and learners in the design and implementation of curricula. The chapter includes the fundamental components of a curriculum (e.g. recruitment and selection, curriculum design, educational modalities, objectives, competencies, outcomes, assessment approaches and evaluation). It raises questions about the philosophy of education and how what we consider valuable in a surgeon should be articulated and integrated into all aspects of curriculum design and embodied by those who have the responsibility to implement it.

Collins et al. introduce concepts, approaches and current challenges of selection into surgical education programmes (Chap. 15). Entry to surgical practice is highly competitive. The profession has a responsibility to ensure that those who enter surgical training are those who are best suited to its technically, emotionally and ethically demanding work. Starting with a clear and well-justified view of what constitutes a good 'surgical trainee' for a particular context, the authors argue that selection should feature a range of complementary and rigorously implemented methods that together paint a clear and more reliable picture of the candidate. Past, current and emerging approaches to recruitment and selection are explored and challenged.

From Cope et al., we glean insights into contemporary and emerging models of teaching and learning in the operating theatre (Chap. 16). Their chapter explores the challenges and opportunities of learning in this experientially rich environment where teachers must balance the needs of patient and learner. Through a survey of theoretical ideas, pedagogic practices and empirical research (often observational, naturalistic enquiry), the authors argue that learning in theatre is complex and negotiated through the senses, particularly through sight, touch, movement and dialogue shared by teacher and learner. More deliberative orienting to and reflection on operative experience are advocated as a means to gain more from this environment in terms of elaborating knowledge, psychomotor skills and professional values.

Andreatta and Dougherty take Cope et al.'s ideas further by drilling down into two specific frameworks for developing psychomotor skills within the contextualised operative setting (Chap. 17). By embedding Dave's psychomotor taxonomy into the BID teaching and learning model [1], the authors provide a concrete illustration for how trainee progression can be structured and fostered to manage challenges and maximise opportunities to learn in theatre. Together, Chaps. 16 and 17 provide complementary perspectives, one mapping out the complex territory and the other providing a theoretically informed route through it.

Stepping away from the operating theatre, Snow et al. craft a compelling case for expanding and enhancing the role of patients in surgical education (Chap. 18). Policy makers, regulators, educators, patient groups and funding agencies have been driving an agenda to improve healthcare worldwide through developing the role of the patient. Through a series of worked examples, the authors provide us with an expanded view of what these roles in surgical education might look like and why they might help the surgical community reimagine surgical education and surgical practice itself.

Molloy and Dennison share insight into the role of verbal feedback in surgical education (Chap. 19). Feedback and debriefing are considered essential for learning and though it may emerge from many sources (visual, tactile, written), the authors focus on the prevalent and essential verbal feedback that transpires in the social clinical environment. Although the concepts are considered in other chapters, here they are the central focus. The authors draw from literature in higher education and medical education and acknowledge the shifting discourse in feedback from expert-led to trainee-seeking. They consider ways in which conventional workplace-based learning facilitates feedback and other types of *reflective conversations* that promote learning and emphasise the importance of trusting relationships in facilitating the acceptance of feedback.

Assessment is a critical element of educational design in any programme. Szasz and Grantcharov explore current approaches, their limitations and future directions in the context of surgical education (Chap. 20). Assessment is a highly specialised area of any educational practice and more so when professional licencing is associated with the outcomes. The authors focus on the design of summative assessments or high-stakes assessments, that is, those with consequences for the trainee and the training programme. An evidence-centred assessment design framework, drawn from general education, is used to guide this process and enhance the rigour and defensibility of high-stakes assessment.

Focusing on a specific assessment strategy, entrustable professional activities (EPAs) are described in the context of surgical education by Tobin (Chap. 21). These assessments reflect the work-based nature of surgical education and are thought to represent emerging surgical competence in more holistic ways. Trainees are observed directly undertaking complex, integrated activities that their supervisor would *entrust* them to perform. Feedback is guided by activity-specific rating forms intended to provide the opportunity for conversations about facets of professional practice. Suitable levels of supervision can be matched to the level of performance, so that patient care remains safe and quality outcomes are obtained.

With links to several chapters, Sachdeva offers deep insights to certification and revalidation for surgical practice (Chap. 22). The drivers are shared with a reminder that high-quality surgical care is the ultimate goal of these processes. We have a responsibility to identify surgeons who do not meet performance standards. These processes must be continuous, rigorous, transparent and meaningful. Battista et al. take a different look at quality. This is from the perspective of programme evaluation (Chap. 23). Programme evaluation has a strong theoretical foundation and is often neglected in surgical (and other professional) curricula. Rather than being an afterthought, programme evaluation strategies can be incorporated at the programme development stage. This chapter describes traditions in programme evaluation and then provides illustrations relevant to different types of surgical curricula. The chapter is intended for those who are engaging or considering engaging in programme evaluation for the first time or are doing so with limited support from a formal programme evaluator.

Simulation has emerged as a critical educational method for surgery with an exponential increase in peer-reviewed publications alongside the development of increasingly sophisticated and diverse simulators. Aggarwal reports current evidence for simulation in supporting trainees in the development and maintenance of technical surgical skills, team work and professional skills associated with sequential simulations (Chap. 24). While showing incredible advances, he highlights the need for simulation-based approaches to be framed around more complex clinical activity and to be more programmatic in their outlook, drawing not only on multiple simulation formats but on patient-centred models of care.

Paige offers two chapters on developing surgical teams (Chaps. 25 and 26). The first chapter orients readers to human factors and theories associated with team training while the second shifts to applications in surgical practice. In the latter, Paige builds on ideas from the chapter on simulation emphasising the role of interprofessional education and uses his own experiences of implementing team-based simulations. Together Paige's chapters serve as an illustration of how conceptual frameworks (e.g. human factors, interprofessional education) alongside educational theory (e.g. experiential learning and reflection) can be operationalised in educational practice.

de Cossart and Fish remind us that professionalism is not static (Chap. 27). While acknowledging surgical history and tradition, the authors take a *fresh* look at professionalism. They draw on their experiences to share ways in which surgical educators can facilitate raising awareness of the sensitive considerations about the person the trainee (or surgeon) brings to their work. They also remind us that professionalism is responsive to society and culture. They suggest that today's surgeons must see beyond overly technical and regulatory-driven views of professionalism and recentre themselves and their teaching on a moral mode of practice, one that acknowledges the complexity and ethical nature of the surgeon's work both with patients and their trainees. They draw on their experiences to share ways in which surgical educators can engage with trainees to develop their professional judgement through overt and supportive critical reflection on professional dilemmas in practice.

Managing underperformance in trainees can be emotional and time-consuming. Beard and Sanfey offer salutary words of the profound impact that underperformance can have on all those involved – individual, patients, other surgeons and colleagues and the health service (Chap. 28). They give insight to the level and possible sources of underperformance and strategies to identify, analyse and manage individuals who are underperforming.

The last chapter intersects with several earlier chapters while deserving its own headline. Patient safety is a powerful and contemporary driver for surgical education. From Marshall and Nataraja, we learn of safety science, its relationship to human factors and its application in healthcare, specifically surgical practice and implications for surgical education. Again, simulation plays an important role and the content builds on work in earlier chapters.

Collectively, these chapters offer readers insights to conventional approaches to surgical education. While the chapters are all theory-informed, readers may find themselves referring back to Part II recognising content from the theory-focused chapters.

# Reference

1. Roberts, N., et al. (2009). The briefing, intraoperative teaching, debriefing model for teaching in the operating room. *Journal of the American College of Surgeons, 208*(2), 288.

# Chapter 14
# Designing Surgical Education Programs

**Jennifer Choi and Dimitrios Stefanidis**

**Overview** Designing new residencies, fellowships, CME programs, or reentry programs can initially appear an overwhelming task, but identifying its major points makes this a manageable and worthwhile endeavor. In this chapter we explore surgical program design from the perspective of the ACGME General Surgery Residency Program. This framework can then be applied broadly to any surgical education program. Aspects considered in this chapter include choosing and developing faculty and administration; choosing the trainees; developing curriculum that is comprehensive in its approach to technical skills, medical knowledge, and nontechnical skills; and finally program evaluation and improvement.

## 14.1 Introduction

In 2015 the AAMC reported that the US surgical workforce will have a shortage of 17,000–25,000 surgeons by 2025 [1]. The underlying reasons include a growing and aging general population in need of surgical services and expanded healthcare coverage due to government-initiated healthcare reform efforts. Given this anticipated shortage, the development of new training positions in surgery appears to be urgently needed. This need may be accomplished by expanding current training programs but also by starting surgical training programs de novo. Further, the rapid evolution of surgical techniques and technology frequently necessitates new educational program development to address training needs.

Building new surgical training programs from the ground up is an exciting opportunity for those fortunate to experience it but can also be overwhelming given the magnitude of the task at hand. Balancing clinical requirements with educational needs of the trainees, weaving educational best practices in rotation design, securing funding and institutional support, designing effective curricula, incorporating

J. Choi (✉) · D. Stefanidis
Department of Surgery, Indiana University School of Medicine, Indianapolis, IN, USA
e-mail: jenchoi@iu.edu; dimstefa@iu.edu

meaningful assessments, choosing the right faculty, and offering research and other experiences to learners are some of the factors that need to be considered.

In this chapter, therefore, the authors will provide recommendations on the important steps that should be considered when designing new surgical programs. While many of our recommendations are based on developing residency programs, the provided suggestions can be easily applied to any surgical training program such as subspecialty surgical residencies, surgical fellowships, surgeon reentry, or continuing education programs. We will specifically address the institutional and human resources needed but also introduce the topics of effective curriculum development and program evaluation. Each of these topics will be considered in depth by other chapters in this text.

## 14.2 Required Resources

Multiple resources are required for the development of a strong and successful surgical education program. After an initial needs assessment, resources such as material support and funding will need to be provided by the institution; a shift in the institutional culture to accommodate learners may also be necessary. Further, to ensure its success, it is critically important to select the appropriate human capital that will be involved in training [2].

### 14.2.1 Institutional Resources

The first step for new program development starts with a comprehensive needs assessment. Besides having a strong rationale for the development of a new program, several other factors need to be considered. Does the institution have the case volume and diversity appropriate to train surgical residents? For training programs that have formal case number requirements by their accrediting bodies, this information is paramount for the viability of the program. For example, US surgical residents have defined case minimums (850 cases) that have to be distributed in defined case categories [3]. These cases represent the diversity and breadth of general surgery and specialty practice and are a surrogate for adequate training. The Surgical Council on Resident Education has defined the type of cases further, by breaking them down into those necessary to be mastered versus those where mere exposure is adequate [4]. Even if minimum case requirements do not exist, any new program should have a realistic assessment of what case volume would be required for its trainees to gain meaningful experience and graduate as competent surgeons.

Identifying funding support for trainees is another important early step. Depending on the type of program, funding sources may be institutional, departmental, or through other sources such as grant funding or industry. While industry used to support a number of training programs especially surgical fellowships, such support has waned dramatically in recent years. Funding has to be sustainable for the duration of the program and number of trainees as well as account for support staff required to run the program [2].

The institutional culture itself must be supportive of trainees. Does the institution see trainees in surgery as value-added? Is the institution willing to support the residency in a way that optimizes the clinical learning environment [2]? The institution should prepare its staff for working with trainees by setting expectations for both supervision and autonomy. Further, it should value patient safety and quality improvement and promote ongoing learning and professional development – all factors that create an ideal learning environment for trainees [2]. The development and ongoing support of dedicated skills labs and simulation centers that offer training opportunities to learners outside the operating room are essential elements today for the effective training of surgical trainees. Finally, the institution should ensure appropriate working conditions for trainees including adequate hospital staffing in all areas of the hospital (transportation, lab technicians, nurses, medical assistants, etc.), work spaces, conference spaces, call rooms, lockers, offices, break rooms, and any other resources needed by the program.

## 14.2.2 Human Capital: Program Directors, Coordinators, Faculty, and Learners

Once the institutional commitment to the training program has been established and its financial viability ensured, the next focus is that of human resources. This includes program leadership, faculty, and the actual trainees.

### 14.2.2.1 Program Leadership

Program leadership sets the tone for the program and will drive the remaining aspects of development. The ACGME Program Requirements for Surgery provide comprehensive guidelines for the qualifications and responsibilities of the surgery program director that are applicable to other programs as well [3]. Most importantly, the program director must have an adequate amount of protected time to design and effectively run the program. For a general surgery program director, this dedicated time should be at least 50% [3]; for smaller programs, the amount of protected time may vary but needs to be realistically aligned with the needs of the program and its trainees. Further, the PD must be able and willing to enter a longer-term commitment (the ACGME requires at least 6 years) as the learning curve of all the duties and responsibilities is long and shorter terms will likely limit the director's effectiveness. In addition, the PD should be board certified in the specialty and maintain appropriate hospital privileges as they, too, will be among the key teaching faculty, leading in both administration of the program but also in the role of key clinical educator setting the example for other faculty to follow. Further, trainees are more likely to look up to and relate to a program director who is clinically active rather than in a purely administrative role. Besides these basic requirements, however, the most important characteristic of PDs is their passion for education. They must fill the role of the leader, teacher, mentor, and parent to help trainees grow and achieve their full potential. They must be available, affable and capable, tenacious and durable, organized and flexible, fearless, and cautious to balance clinical and faculty needs and trainee education and well-being needs.

Program directors need orientation, development, and mentorship both as educators and leaders to fulfill their roles successfully. In the USA, specific resources include ACGME workshops, the New PD Workshop of the Association of Program Directors in Surgery and the Association for Surgical Education, and the Surgeons as Educators course through the American College of Surgeons. These resources will fully orient the individual to the PD role and the requirements of certifying and accrediting bodies such as the American Board of Surgery (ABS) and the Accreditation Council for Graduate Medical Education (ACGME). For other programs, PDs should review the requirements of their respective accrediting body and seek help from that body when needed. In addition, institutional resources may be available to help the new PD navigate their new responsibilities such as input from experienced PDs from other specialties.

Once the PD is chosen, assembling a team that includes associate PDs, program coordinator(s), and dedicated core teaching faculty is the next key step. All members of the education team must be wholly engaged in the process of developing the residency and must be fully aware of their responsibilities to the surgical trainee. Depending on the size of the program, identifying one to two capable associate PDs is extremely important as they can support and boost the effectiveness of the PD. Associate PDs further ensure the continuity and longevity of the program if and when the PD moves on as their accumulated experience will make any transition smoother.

### 14.2.2.2 Program Coordinator

The program coordinator is the heart and soul of any program and can keep it running smoothly and effectively or render it dysfunctional and inefficient. As such the person sought to occupy this role should bring a range of skills including a background in project management, medical education, accreditation, and exceptional organizational skills. The coordinator is a key mediator between the trainees and program leadership, may serve as liaison with the ACGME or other accrediting bodies, helps with elements of the curriculum, and addresses many trainee needs that arise. Further, the coordinator is the face of the program to prospective trainees and surgical faculty.

### 14.2.2.3 Faculty

Selecting and educating teaching faculty may take a substantial amount of time and effort on the part of both the PD and the faculty member, but the importance of this investment by both the PD and faculty cannot be overemphasized. The faculty recruited to participate in the training program should also be passionate about teaching trainees and should be willing to share their patients with the trainees. Initially, the faculty will need to recognize and plan for the typically longer operative case duration [5] and clinic appointments and to integrate the trainee in all aspects of patient care, including calls from nurses. Affording faculty the opportunity to work with trainees on a preliminary basis may allow them to experience surgery and patient care with a trainee, offering a first-hand look at how their practice may need to be changed to accommodate the learner.

Given that the majority of surgical faculty do not have formal training in education, the program should provide access to faculty development programs including workshops, mentorship, and seminars to support and optimally prepare them for their educational duties as well. Teaching, learning, and evaluation in clinical and nonclinical environments will be new skills to new faculty. The program leadership must set expectations that new teachers will develop their educational practice in addition to clinical practice. Just as one reflects on clinical outcomes as opportunities for improvement, new faculty will get feedback from learners and peers to inform this aspect of performance. Quality improvement drives surgical practice, and carrying this to educational practice will further enhance that ethos [6].

Finally, creating a sense of ownership and buy-in among teaching faculty will ensure the longevity and success of the program. Therefore, assigning and supporting specific faculty to lead various parts of the curriculum or to design some aspect of the program will allow the program to develop under the broad leadership of the faculty rather than relying solely on the named leader.

Once again, selecting and developing the appropriate teaching faculty are essential; faculty who are indifferent to the training process will have a significant negative impact on the program and may result in its failure. In contrast, faculty who are mentored and developed over time will undoubtedly shape the program positively. Chapter 13 in this textbook considers arguments around and suggestions for developing surgeon educators.

### 14.2.2.4 Trainees

Besides ensuring that the best possible leaders and teachers have been recruited to participate in the program, concerted efforts are also required for the selection of good trainees. Recruiting motivated trainees, eager to learn and determined to be successful are important determinants of the program's effectiveness. Poorly selected trainees may increase attrition rates that put extra strain on the program, poison collegiality among learners, and strain relationships with staff, lead to suboptimal skill acquisition at the end of training, and threaten the long-term viability of the program by damaging its reputation.

Approaches to recruitment and selection of trainees have been evolving, especially over the past decade, to increase their validity, reliability, and acceptability to stakeholders. Those involved in developing and implementing a new surgical training program should ensure they educate themselves in these approaches and their underpinnings so that they can make informed decisions about what methods to employ for their context and why. Chapter 15 discusses current thinking and evidence for recruitment and selection approaches in surgical training.

Finally, one may feel an obligation to maximally backfill a program upon its initiation (e.g., fill all available PGY 1–3 positions upon initiation of the program). The authors recommend, however, that the program consider adding each year in succession, e.g., PGY 1s only in year 1, as this will allow faculty to develop in parallel with the growth of the residents and residency program.

## 14.3 Curriculum

In education, a curriculum is broadly defined as the totality of student experiences that occur during the educational process [7]. The term typically refers to the knowledge and skills trainees are expected to learn, including the learning objectives they are expected to meet, the lectures that faculty teach, the educational material (books, materials, videos, presentations, readings, etc.) offered to the trainees, and the assessment methods to evaluate trainee learning and skill acquisition [8].

The curriculum drives educational effectiveness, and its quality likely represents the most important determinant of the eventual outcome of the learner. Surgical educators should, therefore, be familiar with key concepts of curriculum development so they can optimally incorporate sound teaching, learning, assessment, and evaluation methods in their training programs.

It should also be noted that the curriculum is typically divided into the explicit, implicit (including the hidden), excluded, and extracurricular categories [9]. In this section we will refer to the explicit and implicit components of the curriculum that are important to surgical programs. We will further break the explicit curriculum of surgical programs into the three learning domains of technical, nontechnical, and affective skills.

There are numerous theories and design approaches to curriculum development stemming from the educational philosophy, the values and beliefs of those who design it, and the institutions it originate from. While the description of all existing approaches is beyond the scope of this chapter, the authors recommend Kern's six-step approach to curriculum design that is specific to medical education [10]. Kern's approach includes entries found in Table 14.1.

Taking such a systematic and well-justified approach to curriculum design can greatly enhance surgical programs. For example, with respect to the medical knowledge underpinning the technical domain, the learners' needs are defined by the

**Table 14.1** Kern's six steps [10]

| | |
|---|---|
| Perform general needs assessment | Determine generally the content which needs to be taught |
| Perform targeted needs assessment | Identifies particular gaps requiring emphasis |
| Establish goals and objectives | Goals are broad and objectives are specific, measurable outcomes allowing for assessment |
| Choose educational strategies | How should the content be best delivered, with what resources, and in what environment |
| Implement the curriculum | Make it happen! |
| Evaluate the curriculum | Measure outcomes with assessment and with formal evaluation to determine curriculum efficacy. Make modifications |

specialty-specific knowledge required as defined by the specialty board. The goals and objectives for this curriculum can be defined by the program, the patient needs, and the specialty board to some extent. The content may come from a standardized curriculum, such as SCORE [11] in general surgery, but the optimal education strategy for the implementation and delivery of the curriculum (lecture, online, or discussion based) may have to be defined by the needs of the learners and the availability of local resources. Learner and teacher feedback on initially chosen content and delivery methods will help inform any needed modifications of the curriculum that will optimally address the needs of the learner.

A common pitfall for surgical educators not very familiar with the curriculum development process and the components of the curriculum is to focus their efforts on the clinical curriculum (direct patient care) of which they have better knowledge. While the clinical curriculum may represent ~80% of the learner's training experience by time spent, in the opinion of the authors, the remaining ~20% of the curriculum – medical knowledge, quality/safety, technical skills training, nontechnical team skills, and what is taken away by learners informally through extended socialization in the surgical community (namely, via what is referred to as the hidden curriculum) – determines the overall character and success of the training program. In the following paragraphs, we will provide recommendations for curriculum development broken down into the learning domains of technical, nontechnical, and affective skills as they often require different approaches and structure. Further details can be found in other chapters of this book.

The technical skills component of the curriculum is unique to surgery and other interventional disciplines and has traditionally been accomplished in the operating room under faculty supervision. Over the past couple decades and amidst the incorporation of increasingly complex techniques and procedures into surgical practice, ethical concerns about trainee learning on patients, trainee work hour restrictions, and mounting pressure for clinical productivity, surgical educators have recognized the importance of skills training outside the operating room. The development of dedicated skills labs and simulation centers and the introduction of numerous training models targeting acquisition of specific skills have led to a paradigm shift in the education of surgical trainees [12]. Basic surgical skills such as suturing and knot tying, electrosurgical techniques, use of various instruments and devices, and even complex surgical techniques and procedures can be effectively taught in a simulated setting that enables skill acquisition in a low-stress, low-risk practice environment (learning from errors) prior to entering the high-stakes operating room environment.

When designing the technical skills curriculum, a number of factors need to be taken into consideration [13]. The goal of such curricula should be to encourage deliberate practice of trainees as it is essential for the development of expertise [14]. This type of practice consists of a highly structured activity that individuals engage in with the specific goal of improving their performance. It is further characterized by expert feedback on performance that guides improvement efforts [14]. Proficiency-based curricula set expert-derived performance goals for trainees to achieve and promote deliberate practice [15]. They are tailored to the training needs of the individual and lead to uniform skill acquisition by not relying on a time or repetition-based training paradigm, which is associated with variable outcomes [13]. Besides setting performance goals, skills curricula need to incorporate an element of overtraining and maintenance training to maximize the robustness of acquired skill and minimize skill decay after initial proficiency is achieved, respectively [16]. Further, robust assessment metrics should be used, and the curriculum should be adjusted to the level of the trainee and incorporate increasing levels of task difficulty [17].

Training in the skills lab is not meant nor expected to replace clinical experience but rather to augment trainee skills so that they can benefit most from the actual clinical experience. An appropriately structured and implemented skills curriculum, besides supporting trainee clinical performance, can be informed and driven by training needs identified in the clinical environment by teaching faculty or the learners themselves. Today a number of skills curricula are available that address a variety of surgical skills and can be implemented into the program's curriculum off the shelf [18–21].

The nontechnical component of the curriculum should address ACGME competencies such as professionalism, communication, and systems-based practice and include interprofessional team training, leadership, and situational awareness among other taught skills. Such skills can be effectively taught using simulation by structuring scenario-based training sessions with targeted learning objectives and effective debriefs that leave lasting knowledge and impressions on the learners. Surgical educators may also want to pursue team training with other related disciplines to recreate clinical practice realities. A number of resources are available to support the development of such skills through the American College of Surgeons [21] and the AAMC and can be applied to a variety of training programs as they are not discipline-specific [22].

The affective component of the curriculum is often ignored but is equally important to the other components. This aspect of the curriculum focuses on self-management skills, well-being, stress management, and emotional reactions to significant events and may also include personal and professional growth and other aspects of performance and behavior. A commonly used example may include breaking bad news to patients and their families for which there are certainly training modules available for individual programs. On the other hand, stress management techniques and performance-enhancing strategies such as mental imagery, resilience training, mindfulness, performance routines, attention management, wellness programs, and other components have been shown in the literature to benefit trainees [23, 24]. While these types of skills have received little attention in the surgical curriculum, the authors of this chapter expect them to become a routine component of surgical curricula in the near future as the evidence of their effectiveness is mounting [23–25].

Finally, one cannot forget the so-called hidden curriculum. Hidden curriculum refers to "the unwritten, unofficial, and often unintended lessons, values, and perspectives" [26] that trainees learn during the practice of surgery. While the "formal" curriculum consists of the aforementioned components directed at the learner and other knowledge and skills intentionally taught to trainees by their faculty, the hidden curriculum consists of the "unspoken or implicit academic, social, and cultural messages that are communicated" to trainees, while they engage in clinical practice [26]. This curriculum is impossible to define and control but may be influenced by appropriate teaching faculty and environment selection given that trainee behaviors are often modeled after those of their faculty and the environment they practice in. Selecting the highest-quality faculty which embody desired competencies in all domains and choosing the appropriate educational environment may assist in the appropriate growth and personal and professional identity development of the trainees. Indeed, some authors have argued that today's focus on physician competencies may emphasize mainly questions of assessment (such as doing the work of a physician) rather than ensuring the development of professional identity by trainees (i.e., being a physician) [27]. This has led others to suggest that a more reliable indicator of professional behavior should be the incorporation of the values and attitudes of the trainee into the identity of the aspiring physician [28, 29].

It should also be noted that the administration of the curriculum can be a significant challenge to PDs and will require input and help from all involved in the program. For their clinical experience, a clear plan is needed for residents to rotate among surgical services, led by the chosen key core faculty. For a US general surgery program, these rotations typically include general surgery (both open and laparoscopic), endoscopy, vascular surgery, thoracic surgery, plastic surgery, trauma surgery, and surgical critical care [3]. Trainees must be facile in the perioperative care and the longitudinal care of the patients on all of those services. Both the technical and bedside experiences require appropriate supervision and graduated autonomy as the trainee moves through the program. Ideally, trainees should be placed on rotations with appropriate cases for their level of training as well as appropriate opportunities for growth in the nontechnical aspects as well. The block diagram represents a monthly schedule for the resident in the 60 months of surgical training; it consists of the type and order of the clinical rotation schedule the residents will follow during their training. This must be planned and prepared before a program can be accredited. For programs that do not have this requirement, a block diagram can still be extremely helpful in organizing and offering effectively the training experience [3].

Additionally, the current landscape of the US healthcare environment requires that trainees be instructed in monitoring of their own patient safety and quality of care outcomes, a service that should be provided by the program [3].

## 14.4 Evaluation: Trainees, Faculty, and Program

Evaluation should permeate all aspects of the training program. It is important to assess trainees, teaching faculty, and the training program itself to build up a full picture of the program's quality. Addressed briefly here, more extensive discussion of approaches to program evaluation and learner assessment (also referred to as learner evaluation in the US context) can be found in Chaps. 19, 20, 21, and 23. Learner assessments are important because they inform the PD and program faculty on learner progress and milestone achievement, help identify performance areas in need for improvement and targeted remediation, provide information on curriculum effectiveness, and represent an excellent source of performance feedback to the learners themselves. Such assessments need to be multimodal and address all learning domains (cognitive, technical, nontechnical, and affective) in order to be the most effective; in the absence of targeted assessments, learner performance improvement is very difficult as constructive performance feedback cannot be initiated without knowledge of what learners do well and what not. Programs should be aware which learning domains are being assessed by each evaluation as it is inappropriate to apply domain-specific assessments to other domains (i.e., surgery programs cannot use ABSITE scores that assess knowledge to extrapolate resident technical or nontechnical performance).

Further, combining end of rotation evaluations, immediate workplace-based evaluations, case-based evaluations, 360-degree evaluations, skills lab and simulation-based assessments, and other assessments will provide a more appropriate, accurate, and comprehensive assessment of trainee performance and identify specific areas of excellence or in need for improvement. Van der Vleuten et al. have proposed a model for programmatic assessment, which simultaneously optimizes assessment for learning and assessment for decision-making about learner progress. A key principle of this model is that individual (formative) assessments are used for learning and feedback value, whereas high-stake decisions are based on the aggregation of many data points (summative) [30]. They further emphasize the importance of bias reduction to deal with the inevitable subjectivity of human assessments and propose 12 simple tips to accomplish the incorporation of such programmatic assessment in training programs that the reader may find useful [30, 31].

Besides learner evaluations, teaching faculty evaluations are equally important as they can provide faculty with feedback on their teaching performance and identify areas for improvement. Such assessment can be obtained from the learners themselves, but third-party expert observers can provide additional perspectives that may be important for faculty coaching and growth.

Finally, program evaluation is invaluable for the long-term success and thriving of any educational program. Such program evaluation should be sought from multiple sources including trainees and faculty as well as a review of program goal and objective accomplishment. This information will help inform any needed changes to optimize curricula, instructional methods, and learner and teaching faculty performance. It will also allow for setting the bar higher the next time around which will promote program excellence over time. These topics are explored in greater depth in Chap. 23.

## 14.5 Final Thoughts

Designing surgical education programs is a challenging but also very rewarding task to those who undertake it. Ensuring that needed resources are available and maximizing the quality of human capital involved provides the foundation of a successful program. Designing a comprehensive curriculum that addresses and assesses all domains of surgical performance will enable effective skill acquisition and galvanize competent surgeons by the end of the training program. Implementing a robust program evaluation process will promote its optimization over time and support its growth and longevity.

## References

1. AAMC Physician Workforce Report 2015 2015 [cited 2017 June 16]. Available from: http://www.aamc.org.
2. Nuss, M. A., Robinson, B., & Buckley, P. F. A. (2015). Statewide strategy for expanding graduate medical education by establishing new teaching hospitals and residency programs. *Academic Medicine: Journal of the Association of American Medical Colleges, 90*(9), 1264–1268.
3. ACGME Program Requirements for Graduate Medical Education in General Surgery 2017–2018 2017 [cited 2017 June 16]. Available from: http://www.acgme.org/Portals/0/PFAssets/ProgramRequirements/440_general_surgery_2017-07-01.pdf?ver=2017-05-25-084853-043.
4. Curriculum outline for general surgery 2017–2018 2017 [cited 2017 June 16]. Available from: http://absurgery.org/xfer/curriculumoutline2017-18_book.pdf.
5. Allen, R. W., Pruitt, M., & Taaffe, K. M. (2016). Effect of resident involvement on operative time and operating room staffing costs. *Journal of Surgical Education, 73*(6), 979–985.
6. Steinert, Y., Mann, K., Anderson, B., Barnett, B. M., Centeno, A., Naismith, L., et al. (2016). A systematic review of faculty development initiatives designed to enhance teaching effectiveness: A 10-year update: BEME guide no. 40. *Medical Teacher, 38*(8), 769–786.
7. Kelly, A. V. (1977). *The curriculum: Theory and practice*. London: Harper and Row 202 p. p.
8. Adams, K. L., Adams, D. E., & NetLibrary Inc. (2003). *Urban education a reference handbook*. Santa Barbara:.ABC-CLIO Available from: http://www.netlibrary.com/urlapi.asp?action=summary&v=1&bookid=101147.
9. Smith, M. K. (2000). *Curriculum theory and practice' the encyclopedia of informal education 1996*. [Available from: www.infed.org/biblio/b-curric.htm.

10. Kern, D. E. T. P., Howard, D. M., & Bass, E. B. (1998). *Curriculum development for medical education: A six-step approach*. Baltimore: Johns Hopkins Press.
11. SCORE Portal 2017 [Available from: https://www.surgicalcore.org.
12. Reznick, R. K., & MacRae, H. (2006). Teaching surgical skills – changes in the wind. *The New England Journal of Medicine, 355*(25), 2664–2669.
13. Stefanidis, D., & Heniford, B. T. (2009). The formula for a successful laparoscopic skills curriculum. *Archives of Surgery, 144*(1), 77–82 discussion.
14. Ericsson, K. A., Krampe, R., & Tesch-Romer, C. (1993). The role of deliberate practice in the acquisition of expert performance. *Psychological Review, 100*(3), 363–406.
15. Stefanidis, D., Acker, C. E., & Greene, F. L. (2010). Performance goals on simulators boost resident motivation and skills laboratory attendance. *Journal of Surgical Education, 67*(2), 66–70.
16. Stefanidis, D., Scerbo, M. W., Montero, P. N., Acker, C. E., & Smith, W. D. (2012). Simulator training to automaticity leads to improved skill transfer compared with traditional proficiency-based training: A randomized controlled trial. *Annals of Surgery, 255*(1), 30–37.
17. Stefanidis, D. (2010). Optimal acquisition and assessment of proficiency on simulators in surgery. *The Surgical Clinics of North America, 90*(3), 475–489.
18. Fundamentals of laparoscopic surgery 2016 [cited 2017 June 16]. Available from: https://www.flsprogram.org.
19. Fundamentals of endoscopic surgery 2016 [cited 2017 June 16].
20. ACS/ASE medical student simulation-based surgical skills curriculum 2016 2016 [cited 2017 June 16]. Available from: https://www.facs.org/education/program/simulation-based.
21. ACS/APDS surgery resident skills curriculum 2017 [cited 2017 June 16]. Available from: https://www.facs.org/education/program/resident-skills.
22. VandeKieft, G. K. (2001). Breaking bad news. *American Family Physician, 64*(12), 1975–1978.
23. Stefanidis, D., Anton, N., Howley, L., Bean, E., Yurco, A., Pimentel, M., et al. (2017). Effectiveness of a comprehensive mental skills curriculum in enhancing surgical performance: Results of a randomized controlled trial. *American Journal of Surgery, 213*(2), 318–324.
24. Rao, A., Tait, I., & Alijani, A. (2015). Systematic review and meta-analysis of the role of mental training in the acquisition of technical skills in surgery. *American Journal of Surgery, 210*(3), 545–553.
25. Anton, N., Howley, L., Pimentel, M., Davis, C., Brown, C., & Stefanidis, D. (2016). Effectiveness of a mental skills curriculum to reduce novices' stress. *The Journal of Surgical Research, 206*(1), 199–205.
26. Hidden curriculum 2014 [cited 2017 June 16]. Available from: http://edglossary.org/hidden-curriculum/.
27. Jarvis-Selinger, S., Pra, D., & Regehr, G. (2012). From competencies to identities: Reconsidering the goals of medical education. *Academic Medicine, 87*(9), 1185–1190.
28. Cruess, R. L., Cruess, S. R., & Steinert, Y. (2016). Amending Miller's pyramid to include professional identity formation. *Academic Medicine: Journal of the Association of American Medical Colleges, 91*(2), 180–185.
29. Cruess, R. L., Cruess, S. R., Boudreau, J. D., Snell, L., & Steinert, Y. (2014). Reframing medical education to support professional identity formation. *Academic Medicine: Journal of the Association of American Medical Colleges, 89*(11), 1446–1451.
30. van der Vleuten, C. P., Schuwirth, L. W., Driessen, E. W., Dijkstra, J., Tigelaar, D., Baartman, L. K., et al. (2012). A model for programmatic assessment fit for purpose. *Medical Teacher, 34*(3), 205–214.
31. van der Vleuten, C. P., Schuwirth, L. W., Driessen, E. W., Govaerts, M. J., Heeneman, S. (2014). 12 tips for programmatic assessment. *Medical Teacher* 1–6.

# Chapter 15
# Selection into Surgical Education and Training

John P. Collins, Eva M. Doherty, and Oscar Traynor

**Overview** Recruitment and selection of appropriate medical graduates to join a surgical education and training programme is a complex, expensive and high-stakes process. Although there is general agreement on the goals of selection, debate continues on how this should be undertaken.

A number of selection methods are used which include the curriculum vitae, letters of recommendation and the interview. More recently, the addition of aptitude testing and personality assessment techniques has been proposed in an effort to recruit trainees with the highest aptitude for surgery and to avoid selecting those whose personality may be unsuitable for such a career.

A critical review of the processes, criteria and methods involved in selection has been undertaken. The key to effective selection is the identification of the person specification required through an analysis of the job of a surgeon and to then design selection criteria based on these requirements. Different and complimentary selection methods are used to provide the best measurements of each of these selection criteria in order to score each applicant. There is currently insufficient evidence of the value of aptitude tests and personality assessments for these to be included as a routine part of the selection of surgical trainees or residents.

## 15.1 Introduction

The education and training of tomorrow's surgeons is facing many challenges. Restricted work hours, demands for improved efficiency in the operating room and elsewhere in the health services and shorter and more streamlined educational

---

J. P. Collins (✉)
University of Melbourne, Melbourne, VIC, Australia

University of Oxford, Oxford, UK
e-mail: john.collins@hillviewlodge.co

E. M. Doherty · O. Traynor
Royal College of Surgeons in Ireland, Dublin, Ireland
e-mail: edoherty@rcsi.ie; otraynor@rcsi.ie

programmes are impacting on opportunities for teaching and learning. At the same time, the increasing complexity of surgical ailments and procedures, the inclusion of more difficult minimally invasive and other techniques into everyday surgical practice [1, 2] and the increasing demands of the public have placed greater expectations on the competence and performance of surgeons graduating from surgical programmes.

It is therefore more important than ever the right persons are selected and then appropriately educated and trained to cope with a career shown to have the highest levels of stress amongst medical specialists [3].

A common objective is to identify a cohort of professionals who can learn quickly, work effectively within an interdisciplinary and multifunctional healthcare team, make prudent clinical decisions and master the technical and other competencies necessary for safe independent surgical practice [1].

Recruitment and selection of such professionals involves an expensive, complex and high-stakes merit-based process that is subject to medical regulatory considerations and legal requirements, the outcome of which may be challenged by unsuccessful applicants. Traditional selection methods have focused on the applicant's record of academic and other achievements as recorded in their curriculum vitae, comments made in letters of recommendation by those with whom the applicant has worked, the impression given during interview and a combination of opportunity and luck [4]. The rationale for including some of these selection methods is based more on familiarity and ease of quantification than on evidence-based relevance to future surgical performance.

The aims of this chapter are to review the current processes and methods of selection and the more recent developments with a view to providing useful guidelines for best practice.

## 15.2 Melbourne International Consensus Statement on Selection

In an effort to define a set of principles for use as guidelines for selection, a group of international experts in surgical education from eight countries (Table 15.1) identified ten important principles. These were circulated to delegates from 17 countries who participated in the first International Conference on Surgical Education and Training (ICOSET) in Melbourne [5]. Following repeated discussion, the delegates agreed on a consensus statement on the principles of selection (Table 15.1). Reference will be made to these principles throughout this chapter.

**Table 15.1** Melbourne International Consensus Statement on Selection

| |
|---|
| 1. Responsibility for selection must involve trained members of the surgical profession and the agencies (including employers) responsible for the delivery of education and training |
| 2. Selection must aim to identify those doctors with the values, attitudes and aptitude required to become competent surgeons |
| 3. Eligibility criteria (long-listing) for application to specialist surgical education and training should include generic and specialty-specific components |
| 4. Selection methodology must be predetermined and transparent, include a broad range of approaches to maximise validity and reliability, involve multiple raters, contain clear criteria for marking and allocate weighting for each tool which permits ranking of applicants |
| 5. Potential for successful training in a speciality programme is the basis for selection and not the extent of prior knowledge, experience and skills in that specialty |
| 6. Structured curriculum vitae provide important verifiable biographical information on clinical experience and academic and other accomplishments |
| 7. Structured referees' reports can provide credible information from surgeons, colleagues, other healthcare professionals and employers based on their first-hand experience of a doctor's performance in the working and learning environment |
| 8. Structured interviews should use questions which target specific competencies identified through job analysis and yield important information not available from other selection tools |
| 9. Knowledge is an essential base for clinical reasoning and judgement. The extent of a candidate's knowledge at the extremes of performance is a good predictor of their future overall performance |
| 10. Early selection into a surgical education and training programme must be accompanied by clearly established grounds and methodology to ensure struggling or underperforming trainees do not progress unless competency deficiencies are rectified |

[Authors: John Collins, RACS Australasia; Richard Carter, RCSEng; Ian Civil RACS NZ; Timothy Flynn ACS; Richard Reznick RCPSC; David Rowley RCSEd; William Thomas RCSEng; Oscar Traynor RCSI]

## 15.3 Developing a "Person Specification" for Surgery

Selection aims to identify those doctors with the values, attitudes and aptitude required to become a competent surgeon. The process commences through the collection and analysis of job-related information [6]. For surgery, this involves identifying the common tasks, roles and responsibilities associated with effective performance in the job of a surgeon [7]. Based on this information, a set of competency domains are identified [8]. Although many of these competencies are common to all surgeons, individual specialties may prioritise some or identify others according to the perception of relevance to their specialty. These competency domains provide the knowledge, skills, attitudes and personal qualities or "person specification" required and are used when designing selection criteria. Example behavioural indicators are then developed and mapped to the relevant attributes within each competency domain for use in selection [9].

## 15.4 The Selection Process

Responsibility for selection must involve members of the surgical profession and representatives of the agencies (including employers) responsible for the delivery of education and training (Table 15.1). Each person taking part must be familiar with the selection process and appropriately trained in the use of the selection methods being used. Selection commences with recruitment through self-selection, followed by the completion of an application form, which is then used to clarify the applicant's eligibility for surgical training.

### 15.4.1 Recruitment and Career's Information

Cohort studies of graduating UK medical students have shown that around 20% [13–26] list surgery as their long-term career choice [10]. As the process begins through self-selection, career information should include the "person specification" being sought, data on competition ratios, workforce requirements and future employment prospects for each specialty. This may help to avoid the mismatch between expectations and reality which exists in the minds of some applicants and particularly so for oversubscribed specialties [11].

The application form seeks biographical information and relies on the principle of past behaviour being the best predictor of future behaviour [12]. This form must be in a standardised format to enable comparisons to be made between applicants and include generic and specialty-specific questions.

### 15.4.2 Eligibility Criteria

Eligibility criteria, or long-listing for entry to a surgical programme, are based on national regulatory and legal requirements and on generic and specialty-specific stipulations (Table 15.1), both of which must be educationally and clinically defensible. In addition, criteria may vary depending on whether an applicant is applying for seamless surgical training or to a programme with separate early (core) and advanced training components [13].

It is important that opportunities are widely available for all would-be applicants to obtain the necessary clinical experiences and other attainments listed as eligibility requirements, to avoid the possibility of discrimination. Although criminal records or enhanced disclosure checks may be carried out during the selection process, employers usually include these in their pre-employment checks.

## 15.5 Selection Methods

### 15.5.1 Curriculum Vitae

Structured curriculum vitae provide important verifiable biographical information on clinical experience and academic and other accomplishments (Table 15.1).

### 15.5.2 Clinical Experience

Although specific clinical experiences may be required as eligibility criteria, the hidden curriculum of some specialties may result in applicants being expected to demonstrate extensive surgical experience at the time of application. However, it is the potential for successful training in a specialty programme which should be the basis for selection and not the extent of prior knowledge, experience and skills in that specialty (Table 15.1).

## 15.6 Academic and Other Achievements

Academic performance in medical school has been a consistently used criterion in the selection for surgical training. There is good evidence that undergraduate academic achievement is a predictor of subsequent academic performance [14] but little to support its use as a predictor of the other elements of future surgical performance.

In the USA, the USMLE Step 1 results are increasingly used in selection. This examination is designed to facilitate decisions about medical licensure rather than later performance on a training programme. Nevertheless, it has been shown that performance in the USMLE Step 1 examination is a good predictor of subsequent performance in the American Board of Surgery qualifying examination [15].

Ranking in a medical school's graduating class is sometimes used as a selection criterion [16]. Class rank, rather than actual examination score, is a fairer index of academic performance, as it negates the impact of different marking thresholds in different medical schools. The use of centile scoring allows the top-performing students to be rewarded, irrespective of which medical school they attended or the actual marks awarded.

Research output is another element of academic performance frequently used in selection. It is relatively easy to assign a value or score to publications and presentations at scientific meetings, simply by counting numbers and factoring in the impact factor of journals or the prestige of national or international meetings. Published research or possessing a PhD is not a strong predictor of surgical performance although it does predict future research performance [17]. Nevertheless, it is important that selection makes provision for recruiting the next generation of academic surgeons.

Extracurricular activities are sometimes rated for selection. Whilst participation in activities outside medicine is clearly desirable for a balanced life, there is no evidence that mere participation predicts better surgical performance. On the other hand, there is good evidence that having an *exceptional* trait (e.g. in sports, the arts or literature) is strongly correlated with surgical performance [18]. This suggests that individuals who excel in one domain have the personal attributes to be high achievers in other domains (e.g. in surgery). However, deciding what level of weighting, if any, should be assigned to exceptional performance in extracurricular activities during the selection of surgical trainees remains controversial.

## 15.7 Letters of Recommendation and Personal Statements

Letters of recommendation or referees' reports can provide vital and essential information from surgeons, colleagues, other health professionals and employers, based on their first-hand experience of the applicant's performance in the workplace (Table 15.1). Although widely used in selection, potential defects have resulted in their true value being questioned [19].

Applicants inevitably nominate referees whom they believe will provide a supportive report. Free-text letters of recommendation can be highly subjective, often incomplete and contain language which may be evasive and difficult to interpret and evaluate. Reports rarely contain adverse comments, placing those who must score them in what has been termed "fantasy land" [20].

A number of steps have been proposed to improve the validity and reliability of letters of recommendation [21]. The selection panel may choose referees from amongst those nominated by the applicant. Structured pro forma letters completed on a standardised template provide greater objectivity but must avoid promoting a "tick the box" culture. Professional Performance Appraisals (PPAs) are somewhat like referee reports, except members of the selection panel speak directly to the referees in person or by phone and complete a structured form. Although PPAs may enable a more open and frank discussion about applicants, the process is time-consuming, subject to a halo effect and open to legal challenge, particularly if the conversation is not recorded electronically.

Applicants may be invited to submit a personal statement to support their application. The purpose is to evaluate the applicant's personal insight and ability to articulate the reasons why they should be selected. Unfortunately, exaggerated and sometimes false claims are occasionally made which are time-consuming or even impossible to confirm or deny. Furthermore, these statements are often professionally prepared or downloaded from the Internet. There is no evidence that personal statements predict future performance and sufficient evidence of their flawed nature is available for them to be omitted [22].

## 15.7.1 Aptitude Testing and Personality Assessment as Aids for Selection

Following a symposium on the role of aptitude testing and personality assessment in the selection of surgical trainees [4], great enthusiasm was generated for their addition to the selection process [23]. However, despite the eagerness, this did not eventuate and was largely due to the lack of agreed objective criteria of surgical ability in the different surgical specialties [24].

## 15.7.2 Aptitude Testing

Renewed interest in aptitude testing as a marker of innate technical skills at the time of selection has recently arisen for mainly two reasons. Because of the reduced opportunities for training and learning, it seems reasonable to try and select those with the optimum innate skills in the expectation they will reach the required level of technical and other competences in a shorter time. Secondly, complex technologies are increasingly involved in twenty-first-century surgical practice. Those who aspire to practice in high-tech areas, such as robotic surgery, catheter-based interventions, advanced endoscopic and minimally invasive surgery, microsurgery and computer- assisted surgery, require high levels of fundamental or innate abilities (e.g. psychomotor skills and visual spatial abilities) that may not be as critical for traditional open surgery [1, 25]. The successful experience with aptitude testing in other occupations, such as the aviation, military and aeronautical industry [26], has further encouraged the providers of surgical training to re-examine its place in selection.

Psychomotor ability refers to hand-eye coordination and fine motor dexterity, attributes which are particularly important in microsurgery, ophthalmic surgery, neurosurgery and vascular surgery. Visual spatial ability is the capability to mentally manipulate objects in three dimensions and is important in laparoscopic surgery, image-guided surgery and robotic surgery. Depth perception is the ability to mentally interpret 2-D images to produce a 3-D image in the observer's brain and is important in laparoscopic surgery, image-guided surgery and microsurgery.

Although a number of validated tests of these abilities are available [27–29], there is little evidence of their value in predicting surgical performance. This may be due to the difficulties in defining and measuring what constitutes good surgical performance. Further research is required before recommending the inclusion of such tests in selection.

### 15.7.3 Personality and Emotional Intelligence

Doctors with a history of behavioural issues during their medical school course have been shown to more likely to undergo disciplinary action following graduation [30]. In addition, there have been recent reports of "hazardous attitudes" (macho, impulsive, antiauthority, resignation, invulnerable and confident) amongst surgeons [31] and a reported association between these traits and preventable adverse events [32]. These studies have added to a growing recognition that certain individuals may possess personality traits that are long-standing and associated with an increased tendency to behave unprofessionally in the workplace.

Personality is a broad concept in psychology, and its assessment is complicated by the fact that it includes positive traits such as extraversion and openness and dysfunctional traits such as neuroticism and psychoticism. The decision facing surgical programme directors with respect to the assessment of personality is firstly whether they should be used at all, and if they are to be used, should this be to select individuals with the ideal traits or to screen out those with undesirable ones?

The relationship between scores on personality testing and academic and clinical performance is not straightforward, as traits such as conscientiousness may be advantageous for some aspects of medical performance but if combined with other traits such as neuroticism, for example, may be disadvantageous [33]. The current consensus is that the value of personality assessments in high-stakes selection is yet to be proven [34].

Managing one's emotions is a key skill necessary for the development of expertise. Emotional intelligence (EI) concerns the ability to carry out accurate reasoning about emotions and the ability to use emotions and emotional knowledge to enhance thought [35]. Emotional intelligence can be mapped to surgical competencies and predicts scores on tests of interpersonal skills [36]. The concept is relatively new to surgical education, and incorporating the assessment of EI into surgical selection is complicated by the number of different conceptual frameworks available, each with very different associated measures. There are essentially two different forms of measurement, one which relies on self-report and one which is based on the assessment of ability to choose the best options in response to a range of interpersonal scenarios. There is general agreement that measures which rely on self-report are not suitable due to the possibility for faking good and that the ability-based measures may in the future prove to be the more reliable and valid choice [34].

### 15.7.4 Interviews

Although there is a lack of evidence that the "interview" and in particular the "traditional" unstructured interview have substantial predictive validity of future surgical performance [34, 37], it has been an important and long-standing component of selection for surgical training. Concerns exist regarding its subjectivity and interviewer bias and the costs to training programmes and candidates [2, 38].

Notwithstanding these concerns, the interview is popular with applicants and selection committees and likely to remain an important component of selection. It is therefore important the following steps are taken to improve the reliability and validity of the interview process [39].

1. Shortlisting

It makes sense to restrict invitations for interview to those candidates who have a reasonable probability of being selected. This requires the construction of a shortlist based upon previously agreed minimum criteria or aggregate scores in letters of recommendation and the curriculum vitae.

2. Format

There is evidence that a multi mini-interview (MMI) format has better predictive validity than the traditional single-panel interview [40]. This is especially true if MMIs consist of objective structured interview stations, each addressing clearly defined subject areas. Multiple observers are preferred to a single interviewer. MMIs are however costlier and more resource-intensive than single-panel interviews [41].

3. Content

A clearly articulated definition of the purpose of the interview process must first be established as this will dictate its content, regardless of the format used. A written description of the desired traits being sought must be available to each member of the interview panel and accompanied by related standardised questions to be asked of every applicant. Provision of behaviour-specific anchors for rating scales should be provided for each interviewer and a scoring rubric used to improve interrater and intra-rater scoring.

If MMI stations are used, they should cover a range of both cognitive and non-cognitive areas [42]. Ideally, the MMI should be used to assess attributes that have not been assessed more objectively by other components of the selection process, e.g. personal attributes (motivation and drive, time management, professionalism and interpersonal skills). The inclusion of behavioural-based interviewing as part of the interview process has been suggested as a possible method for improving the likelihood of selecting candidates with the "right cultural fit" and to reduce attrition rates [43] although this has yet to be proven.

Situational judgement tests (SJTs) are useful for assessing professional and ethical skills, analytical and problem-solving skills and clinical reasoning [44]. These SJTs, combined with or incorporated into the MMI process, have shown positive results in terms of predictive validity [34].

4. Interviewer Bias

Interviewer bias is a significant issue in the interview process. It is part of human nature to favour individuals like ourselves [45]. This effect can be magnified if candidates have professional coaching in interview techniques [46]. Interviewers should not be aware of applicant's cognitive data to minimise bias, although this may be difficult to achieve for those specialties with fewer numbers. Each interviewer should mark each candidate independently and prior to inter-examiner discussion and before reaching a consensus score [47].

5. Interviewer Training

Training of interviewers in interview techniques, marking and scoring and the rules regarding the unacceptability of unethical and "illegal" questions is essential. Interviewers should learn to use the full range of the marking scores available to avoid "clustering" of candidates around the midpoint of the marking range. They must also be conversant with equality, diversity and aspects of employment law [39].

6. Documentation

Documentation of the performance of each applicant during the interview must be clear, concise and professional. These records must be legible or, preferably, be in an electronic format. They should be retained in a secure central place by the educational body as they will be required in the event of an appeal from an unsuccessful applicant.

## 15.8 Monitoring, Evaluation and Appeals

Agencies responsible for the independent external accreditation of training programmes require educational providers to undertake quality assurance of their selection practices through ongoing monitoring and evaluation. Although no single selection process or method is endorsed by such agencies, standards require those in use to be clearly documented, publicly available, feasible and sustainable in practice. They must also support merit-based selection, able to be consistently applied and prevent discrimination and bias [48]. In addition, selection criteria and the weightings allocated to them must be transparent, rigorous, fair and capable of withstanding external scrutiny.

The education body is required to monitor and evaluate its experience with, and the outcomes from, its selection processes including validity, reliability and feasibility against agreed standards. Feedback from surgical trainees, supervisors, employers and representatives of the community make an important contribution to the development, monitoring and evaluation of selection.

Unsuccessful applicants may choose to appeal the decision of the education body. An appeals process must therefore be in place to provide an impartial review of these decisions. Most appeals can be dealt with, by the organisation's internal appeals process, but some may need to be escalated to the organisation's independent appeal's committee. Elements of a strong and effective appeals process include procedural fairness, timeliness, transparency and clearly documented reasons for decisions [48].

## 15.9 Discussion

The hallmarks of a first-rate education and training programme include the recruitment and selection of the most appropriate trainees, the development and delivery of high-quality education and training programmes, an access to sufficient accredited training positions and an equipped, motivated and sustainable surgical education faculty.

The goal of selection is to choose a cohort of the best applicants to ensure a diverse workforce and avoid recruiting those who may turn out to be problematic trainees or surgeons. Despite years of discussion and debate, the best method for the selection of surgical trainees remains controversial. Although a number of approaches are in common use, there is a lack of properly conceived long-term studies comparing different methods or combinations of methods in terms of which will provide the most reliable predictive information of success in surgical practice.

In the meantime, selection of trainees must go on, and some might argue that the percentage who fails to succeed or become problematic is small. Nevertheless, the consequences of inappropriate trainee selection are considerable, in terms of the personal and financial costs to the individual, to the surgeon educators, to the health service and to the public. This is particularly relevant as surgeons have been shown to be the specialty most likely to exhibit disruptive behaviour [49]. Although the Melbourne International Consensus Statement was agreed some years ago [5], the principles espoused (Table 15.1) remain a useful guide for those charged with the important task of selecting tomorrow's surgeons.

Whilst it is important the selection process avoids as far as possible choosing those who might prove to be ill suited for a surgical career, multiple appraisals including workplace-based assessments take place throughout training and should ensure that those who exhibit ongoing disruptive behaviour or hazardous traits are identified and advised to seek an alternative career. Even if it was possible to exclude those with undesirable personality or other issues, this alone may be insufficient as trainees may observe and even learn to adopt unacceptable traits and behaviours from the presence of poor surgical role models during their training [50, 51]. Exemplary role modelling by surgeons is therefore necessary during undergraduate medical education and postgraduate surgical training programmes [52]. Recognition and rejection of unacceptable professional behaviour in the workplace is just as important as avoiding the selection of those with undesirable characteristics.

Identifying the person specification required is fundamental to selection and has greatly enhanced confidence in the development of appropriate criteria and methods. Each method has its own individual strengths and weaknesses, and provided selection committees are aware of these and follow the recommendations to achieve greater consistency, reliability and validity; they and the trainees should have confidence with their use. For example, despite the shortcomings of letters of recommendation, comments made by a referee who is recognised as one who takes this task very seriously and completes it well cannot be ignored. Similarly, it is unlikely that any training programme director would accept a trainee without the reassurance of some form of interview. Although behavioural-based interviewing has been suggested by some authors [43], vigilance is required to ensure that this method does not limit the diversity required in the modern workforce.

Consideration of the emotions and feelings of the surgeon, particularly in the face of adversity and human suffering, and their ability to manage these challenges, is important for the well-being of the surgeon and the surgeon-patient relationship. It is said that the "affective regimes typically involving self-control, emotional restraint and the tempering of passions" are connected to a skilful performance [53] and that "in the domain of emotional restraint, it is the surgeon who is said to be the master" [53]. The difficulties in predicting at the time of selection, how an applicant will deal with these emotions, must be compensated for during their training through ongoing workplace-based assessments.

There is little doubt that higher levels of fundamental ability are required for some of the more complex newer surgical technologies, and whilst aptitude testing may one day have a place, it is not yet sufficiently developed, validated and feasible for inclusion. It is much more likely that those selected for these more advanced programmes will be experienced surgeons who have already demonstrated higher levels of innate ability during their preceding specialist training.

## 15.10 Conclusion

Although no single test or combination of tests has been identified to validly and reliably predict performance in the workplace, educational institutions have extensive experience and confidence with the use of a broad combination of the methods. If the selection criteria and the methods used are based on the person specifications identified through job analysis and the process of selection follows strict guidelines, this confidence is justified. Even the best selection methods will not completely avoid the occasional problematic surgeon and must therefore be supplemented by ongoing workplace-based 360-degree appraisal of trainees. Further longitudinal research is required to identify the most appropriate predictive methods for selection.

## References

1. Louridas, M., Szasz, P., de Montbrun, S., et al. (2016). Can we predict technical aptitude? *Annals of Surgery, 263*, 673–691.
2. Schaverien, M. V. (2016). Selection for surgical training: An evidenced-based review. *Journal of Surgical Education, 73*, 723–729.
3. Nash, L. M., Daly, M. G., Kelly, P. J., et al. (2010). Factors associated with psychiatric morbidity and hazardous alcohol use in Australian doctors. *The Medical Journal of Australia, 193*, 161–166.
4. Gough, M. H., Holdsworth, R., Bell, J. A., et al. (1988). Personality assessment techniques and aptitude testing aids to the selection of surgical trainees. *Annals of the Royal College of Surgeons of England, 70*, 265–279.
5. Collins, J. P. (2009). Editorial overview of proceedings. *ANZ Journal of Surgery, 79*, 96–99.
6. Ash, R. A. (1998). Job analysis in the world of work. In S. Gael (Ed.), *The job analysis handbook* (pp. 3–13). New York: Wiley.
7. Stevenson, H., & Henley, S. (1989). *Job analysis report on the role of the surgeon*. Thames Ditton: Saville and Holdsworth Ltd.

8. Collins, J. P., Gough, I. R., Civil, I. D., & Stitz, R. W. (2007). A new surgical education and training programme. *ANZ Journal of Surgery, 77*, 497–501.
9. Patterson, F., Ferguson, E., & Thomas, S. (2008). Using job analysis to identify core and specific competencies: Implications for selection and recruitment. *Medical Education, 42*, 1195–1204.
10. Goldacre, M. J., Turner, G., & Lambert, T. W. (2004). Variation by medical school in career choices of UK graduates of 1999 and 2000. *Medical Education, 38*, 249–258.
11. Collins, J. P. (2010). Foundation for excellence – an evaluation of the foundation programme. www.agcas.org.uk/assets/download?file=2053&parent=793.
12. Barden, D. M. (2008). Chronical careers: The unreliability of references. The Chronicles of Higher Education. www.chronicle.com/article/the-unreliability-of/45931.
13. Selection requirements. (2017). www.surgeons.org/becoming-a-surgeon/surgery-as-a-career/selection-requirements/.
14. Kenny, S., McInnes, M., & Singh, V. (2013). Associations between residency selection strategies and doctor performance: A meta-analysis. *Medical Education, 47*(8), 790–800.
15. Maker, V. K., Zahedi, M. M., Villines, D., et al. (2012). Can we predict which residents are going to pass/fail the oral boards? *Journal of Surgical Education, 69*, 705–713.
16. Paolo, A. M., & Bonaminio, G. (2003). Measuring outcomes of undergraduate medical education: Residency directors' ratings of first-year residents. *Academic Medicine, 78*, 90–95.
17. Robertson, C. M., Klingensmith, M. E., & Coopersmith, C. M. (2007). Long-term outcomes of performing a postdoctoral research fellowship during general surgery residency. *Annals of Surgery, 245*, 516–523.
18. Daly, K. A., Levine, S. C., & Adams, G. L. (2006). Predictors for resident success in otolaryngology. *Journal of the American College of Surgeons, 202*, 649–654.
19. Dirschl, D. R., & Adams, G. L. (2000). Reliability in evaluating letters of recommendation. *Academic Medicine, 75*, 1029.
20. Friedman, R. B. (1983). Fantasy Land. *The New England Journal of Medicine, 308*, 651–653.
21. Oldfield, Z., Beasley, S. W., Smith, J., Anthony, A., et al. (2013). Correlation of selection scores with subsequent assessment scores during surgical training. *ANZ Journal of Surgery, 83*, 412–416.
22. White, J. S., Lemay, J. F., Brownell, K., et al. (2011). "A chance to show yourself" – how do applicants approach medical school admission essays? *Medical Teacher, 33*, e541–e548.
23. Gough, M., & Bell, J. (1989). Introducing aptitude testing into medicine – surgeons lead the way. *BMJ, 298*, 975–976.
24. Deary, I. J., Graham, K. S., & Maran, A. G. (1992). Relationships between surgical ability ratings and spatial abilities and personality. *Journal of the Royal College of Surgeons of Edinburgh, 37*, 74–79.
25. Gallagher, A. G., Cowie, R., Crothers, I., et al. (2003). PicSOr: An objective test of perceptual skill that predicts laparoscopic technical skill in three initial studies of laparoscopic performance. *Surgical Endoscopy, 17*, 1468–1471.
26. Carretta, T. R., & Ree, M. J. (1996). U.S. air force pilot selection tests: What is measured and what is predictive? *Aviation, Space, and Environmental Medicine, 67*, 279–283.
27. Buckley, C. E., Kavanagh, D. O., & Gallagher, T. K. (2013). Does aptitude influence the rate at which proficiency is achieved for laparoscopic appendectomy? *Journal of the American College of Surgeons, 217*, 1020–1027.
28. Buckley, C. E., Kavanagh, D. O., & Nugent, E. (2014). The impact of aptitude on the learning curve for laparoscopic suturing. *American Journal of Surgery, 207*, 263–270.
29. Gallagher, A. G., Leonard, G., & Traynor, O. J. (2009). Role and feasibility of psychomotor and dexterity testing in selection for surgical training. *ANZ Journal of Surgery, 79*, 108–113.
30. Papadakis, M. A., Teherani, A., Banach, M. A., et al. (2005). Disciplinary action by medical boards and prior behaviour in medical school. *The New England Journal of Medicine, 22*(353), 2673–2682.
31. Bruinsma, W. E., Becker, S. J., Guitton, T. G., et al. (2015). How prevalent are hazardous attitudes among orthopaedic surgeons? *Clinical Orthopaedics and Related Research, 473*, 1582–1589.

32. Kadzielski, J., McCormick, F., & Herndon, J. H. (2015). Surgeons' attitudes are associated with reoperation and readmission rates. *Clinical Orthopaedics and Related Research, 473*, 1544–1551.
33. Doherty, E. M., & Nugent, E. (2011). Personality factors and medical training: A review of the literature. *Medical Education, 45*, 132–140.
34. Patterson, F., Knight, A., Dowell, J., et al. (2015). How effective are selection methods in medical education? A systematic review. *Medical Education, 50*, 36–60.
35. Mayer, J. D., Roberts, R. D., & Barsade, S. G. (2008). Human abilities: Emotional intelligence. *Annual Review of Psychology, 59*, 507–536.
36. Cook, C. J., Cook, C. E., & Hilton, T. N. (2016). Does emotional intelligence influence success during medical school admissions and program matriculation? A systematic review. *Journal of Education Evaluation for Health Professions, 13*, 40.
37. Prideaux, D., Roberts, C., Eva, K., et al. (2011). Assessment for selection for the health care professions and specialty training: Consensus statement and recommendations from the Ottawa 2010 conference. *Medical Teacher, 33*, 215–223.
38. Rosenfeld, J. M., Reiter, H. I., Trinh, K., et al. (2008). A cost efficiency comparison between the multiple mini-interview and traditional admissions interviews. *Advances in Health Sciences Education: Theory and Practice, 13*, 43–58.
39. Stephenson-Famy, A., Houmard, B. S., Manyak, A., et al. (2015). Use of the interview in resident candidate selection: A review of the literature. *Journal of Graduate Medical Education, 7*, 539–548.
40. Eva, K. W., Rosenfeld, J., & Reiter, H. I. (2004). An admissions OSCE: The multiple mini-interview. *Medical Education, 38*, 314–326.
41. Knorr, M., & Hissbach, J. (2014). Multiple mini-interviews: Same concept, different approaches. *Medical Education, 48*, 1157–1175.
42. Reiter, H. I., Eva, K. W., & Rosenfeld, J. (2007). Multiple mini-interviews predict clerkship and licensing examination performance. *Medical Education, 41*, 378–384.
43. Smith, F. (2016). Will behavioural-based interviewing improve resident selection and decrease attrition? *Journal of Graduate Medical Education, 8*, 280.
44. Petty-Saphon, K., Walker, K. A., & Patterson, F. (2016). Situational judgment tests reliably measure professional attributes important for clinical practice. *Advances in Medical Education and Practice, 8*, 21–23.
45. Quintero, A. J., Segal, L. S., & King, T. S. (2009). The personal interview: Assessing the potential for personality similarity to bias the selection of orthopaedic residents. *Academic Medicine, 84*, 1364–1372.
46. Laurence, C. O., Zajac, I. T., Lorimer, M., et al. (2013). The impact of preparatory activities on medical school selection outcomes: A cross-sectional survey of applicants to the University of Adelaide Medical School in 2007. *BMC Medical Education, 13*, 159.
47. Roberts, C., Walton, M., & Rothnie, I. (2008). Factors affecting the utility of the multiple mini-interview in selecting candidates for graduate-entry medical school. *Medical Education, 42*, 396–404.
48. Standards for Assessment and Accreditation of Specialist Medical ... (Standards 6 &7). (2015). www.amc.org.au/files/2c1fb12996b0f6e6e5cb5478dde9d9e991409359_original.pdf.
49. Rosenstein, A. H., & O 'Danie, M. (2008). A survey of the impact of disruptive behaviour and communication defects on patient safety. *Joint Commission Journal on Quality and Patient Safety, 34*, 464–471.
50. Satin, B., & Kaups, K. (2015). The disruptive physician. *ACS Bull, 100*, 20–24.
51. Crebbin, W., Campbell, G., Hillis, D., et al. (2015). Prevalence of bullying, discrimination and sexual harassment in surgery in Australasia. *ANZ Journal of Surgery, 85*, 905–909.
52. Collins, J. P. (2011). International consensus statement on surgical education and training in an era of reduced working hours. *The Surgeon*, S2–S5.
53. Whitfield, N., & Schlich, T. (2015). Skills through history. *Medical History, 59*, 349–360.

# Chapter 16
# Models of Teaching and Learning in the Operating Theatre

**Alexandra Cope, Jeff Bezemer, and Gary Sutkin**

**Overview** This chapter presents an evidence-based overview of what is known about content and process of teaching and learning in the operating theatre. It starts out by identifying theoretical perspectives on learning and teaching and their methodological implications. Following that the possibilities and challenges of teaching and learning in the operating theatre are explored, highlighting its distinct features as an educational venue. In the following parts, various teaching methods and typologies of content domains of learning are discussed and illustrated. The remainder of the chapter is focused on the verbal, gestural and haptic features of interactions between surgical educator, trainees and other members of the team. The chapter ends with questions for further research and a summary.

## 16.1 Introduction

Surgery is a craft specialty, requiring integrated knowledge, skill and decision making. To allow for these components to come together, the operating theatre is a key venue for learning. There is a long history of education in the operating theatre as the early operating rooms of the 1800s were designed as amphitheatres with steeply

---

A. Cope (✉)
Department of General Surgery and University of Oxford: Department of Continuing Education, Frimley Health Foundation Trust, Frimley, UK
e-mail: alexandra.cope07@imperial.ac.uk; alexcope@doctors.org

J. Bezemer
UCL Institute of Education, University College London, London, UK
e-mail: j.bezemer@ucl.ac.uk

G. Sutkin
Female Pelvic Medicine and Reconstructive Surgery, Departments of Biomedical and Health Informatics and Obstetrics and Gynecology, University of Missouri-Kansas City School of Medicine, Kansas City, MO, USA
e-mail: sutking@umkc.edu

racked seating to afford a view to medical students and other surgeons. Yet, despite the long history of teaching and learning in the operating theatre, academic research into intraoperative teaching is a relatively young discipline.

## 16.2 Theoretical Perspectives

As surgical education researchers, we often get asked the big question: 'What is the best way to teach in the operating theatre?' There are two ways to go about answering this question:

1. Identifying which model works best. This is based on the idea of one-size-fits-all and caters for the 'average' learner. Methodologically this would be best studied using an experimental study design.
2. Abandoning the idea that there is a single best model of intraoperative teaching and instead assuming that there are a range of different ways of teaching and that the most apt approach will depend on the learner's prior knowledge and skill and the possibilities afforded by the case. This is more of a situated perspective, in which learning is individualised, opportunistic and unique for each case. Methodologically this would be best studied using naturalistic inquiry, a qualitative analysis of what occurs in practice.

Ultimately 'teaching models' differ in terms of the degree of agency – freedom to act – given to and taken by the learner. Indeed, surgical educators ask themselves: What do I let my trainee(s) do/how much control do I want? How much feedback do I give on what they do? What do I draw their attention to, and what do I let them notice themselves? What norms and strategies do I make explicit, and which ones do I let them discover themselves? Educators can only answer these questions with reference to a specific moment in a concrete case, with a known learner and team. So, a teaching model is not a static, stable configuration – it is likely to change in different cases and even as a single operation progresses.

Knowles' adult learning theory suggests that all educational efforts should be directed at and centred upon the learner, with past experience recognised and utilised [1]. However, wide differences have been found between surgical teachers and learners when reporting learner needs [2]. These differing perspectives may be as a result of threshold concepts [3], meaning that the surgical teacher cannot appreciate some of the challenges experienced by the learner.

Theory-based models of teaching in the operating theatre have foregrounded motor skills learning theory [4], with phases of learning marked as cognitive, integrative and autonomous [5, 6]. Other surgical educators have suggested that the postgraduate surgical trainee should be presented with a personalised and specific set of explicit objectives including a list of operations in which they should be competent at the end of the rotation [7].

Yet, despite its well-recognised importance as a venue for surgical learning, some have observed that there are long periods of time in the operating theatre where seemingly no form of education takes place [8–10]. Additionally, there are wide differences between faculty and student perceptions of the quality and frequency of teaching in the operating theatre [11–15]. These discrepancies suggest that some learning is not recognised unless it is a direct result of explicit teaching strategies. Indeed, tacit knowledge has been acknowledged as important in allied specialties such as anaesthesia [16, 17] and is acquired through participation in a community of practice [18].

This chapter presents an evidence-based overview of what is known about content and process of teaching and learning in the operating theatre.

## 16.3 The Affordances of the Operating Theatre as an Educational Venue

The operating theatre poses unique challenges to the surgical educator as learning is integrated within patient care episodes and cannot be separated from it [19]. In many ways, the operating theatre is an ideal venue for surgical learning as the learning opportunities presented may be highly relevant and interesting to the postgraduate surgical learner – especially if the cases will constitute part of their eventual practice. Compared with learning in a classroom or an online learning platform, there are multiple different sensory stimuli, the environment is 'real' and there are opportunities for interaction with senior surgeons.

For a medical student, the operating theatre 'presents an opportunity to observe real clinical problems and their surgical management [...] and to gain insight into the work of the surgeon as a member of a multi-professional team' [20]. Additionally, there are multiple different stimuli for the learner. Lyon writes of the 'sensual perceptual experience' that is afforded to medical students, enabling them to construct a 'clinical memory' by integrating tactile sensations of live pathology with visual images and verbal learning [20, 21]. Dunnington et al. write about the high regard that students place upon teachers that allow the student to 'feel' the pathology [22].

## 16.4 The Challenges of the Operating Theatre as an Educational Venue

For the teacher:

Because the operating theatre is a work environment, the educator has limited ability to design specific learning episodes; they are restricted to the cases on the list that particular day. This means that the cases may not be appropriate to the stage of learning of the student and it may be difficult to ensure curriculum coverage over the course of the placement.

The surgical teacher also needs to manage the social relations of work with a cross-disciplinary team who may be from differing professional backgrounds to create a positive learning environment [22, 23].

The teaching surgeon has competing priorities in keeping the patient safe whilst educating their trainees, and this is especially important in the most critical portions of a surgery. Moulton et al. elaborated on some strategies inherent to teaching whilst avoiding surgical complications [24]. The teaching surgeons in their study maintained constant control, both over the progress of the entire surgery as well as individual steps. This required conducting a needs assessment of the trainee, encouraging the trainee to slow down during critical steps and sometimes taking over the surgery from the trainee. Some surgeons espoused the ability to give the trainee the illusion of control, although it was actually just the opportunity to operate under the teaching surgeon's guidance. They described a 'bargaining' between teacher and trainee, in which trainees were rewarded for preparation for the case by getting to operate more and sometimes punished for showing up unprepared.

For the learner:

The operating theatre can be an unwelcoming and intimidating environment for the medical student who needs to learn the explicated (e.g. in protocols) and tacit, implicit behavioural expectations and norms (the (local) 'culture'), e.g. norms about where to position themselves without desterilising the operative field [20, 21]. The high-stakes nature of surgical work can also have an emotional impact upon medical students as they may witness complications and tensions between members of the surgical team [25].

For undergraduate and postgraduate trainees, the nature of the work itself, the type of operation and high-stakes nature of it, complexity and timing of the procedure all affect the ability of the surgeon to allow intraoperative hands-on involvement, for example, allowing the postgraduate surgical trainee to perform the case under supervision [9, 26, 27]. There therefore may be limited opportunities for hands-on practice.

## 16.5 Structuring Operating Theatre Teaching

In terms of improving surgical education, it is increasingly recognised that experience alone is insufficient. For example, operating on carefully selected cases without direct supervision may be ineffective and inefficient and does not guarantee that learning is optimal or that learning opportunities are maximised [28]. Roberts et al. argue that a more deliberate approach to operating room teaching is needed in which objectives are set for learners' performance and immediate and specific feedback is provided to guide further practice [29]. It is hoped that in this way every surgical case includes a deliberate effort to improve a trainee's knowledge and skills. Roberts et al. put forward the briefing, intraoperative teaching and debriefing model (BID model) in the context of a surgical case making use of two events that bracket any operation – scrubbing up and time spent closing – to discuss educational aims and objectives as well as an opportunity for reflection and reinforcement after the case [29].

Debriefing is a well-recognised strategy to facilitate learner reflection and to assist in 'making every moment count' [30] with regard to learning opportunities in the operating theatre. Debriefing strategies such as 'SHARP: 5-step feedback tool for surgery' provide a structured approach for the surgeon educator and has been shown to improve the quality of the educational feedback provided to the learner [31].

## 16.6 Content of Learning in the Operating Theatre

Whilst the theoretical perspectives in the introduction to this chapter foregrounded motor skills, we have also signposted that interpretations of tactile and visual cues are key aspects of learning to work with living tissues. Cope et al. describe learning in the operating theatre across six domains: 'factual knowledge', 'motor skills', 'sensory semiosis', 'adaptive strategies', 'team-working and management' and 'attitudes and behaviours' [32].

Some of these domains were thought to be prerequisites to being promoted to the role of primary surgeon. For example, postgraduate surgical learners were expected to know the anatomy, the steps of the operation and how to throw a surgical knot and take a clip on and off before they were invited to be the primary surgeon. In Lyon's study, surgeons suggested that they are more likely to provide learning opportunities to those medical students that give off strong signs of motivation and commitment [21].

Cope et al. describe the learning of sensory semiosis – the ability of the surgical learner to make meaning of what he or she was seeing or feeling. They describe learning to interpret visual and haptic cues as learning how to *translate* what they were seeing into the 'known' anatomy of the textbook [32]. In the words of one of the trainees interviewed in this study:

> [Y]ou need to be able to put your fingers into a small incision and know what you are feeling – like to be able to find the appendix through a tiny incision and more than that, you should be able to tell whether or not it is inflamed just by the feel. [32]

It is known that gaze patterns differ between novice and expert surgeons, in both simulated and real surgical environments, and theatre learning may involve learning to attend to and attribute meaning to specific aspects of the operative field [33, 34]. Ability to interpret visual and haptic cues within human tissues is not exclusive to surgery. In many clinical disciplines, making sense of information presented visually or by touch is an essential part of becoming a good diagnostician [35]. Clinicians examine patients looking for abnormal findings in the hands, face and skin that give pointers to the underlying diagnosis, the experienced clinician has learnt what 'normal' and 'abnormal' look and feel like.

## 16.6.1 Verbal Intraoperative Teaching

Intraoperative teaching requires verbal instruction and communication, and there is an increasing body of literature that has analysed verbal interactions between post graduate trainees and faculty in the operating theatre [36–39]. Verbal teaching has been parsed into multiple categorisations including 'informing', 'explaining', 'commanding', 'quizzing' and 'banter'. Roberts et al. simplify these descriptive categories to:

*Instrumental interaction* – utilised to instruct the resident what action will move the case forward [38]. They termed this instrumental as the surgeon uses the learner like an instrument, as a means to an end.

> [N]ow maybe if you grab right down… and pull that down and to the left there you go. Pull it up a little as well. [38]

*Pure teaching interaction* – intended primarily to benefit the learner through providing educational value. This usually necessitates a brief pause in the surgery.

> [W]hen people start getting disease in the anal canal and the rectum, the chance of curing them is essentially nil, and the other issue there is that when people start having disease in their anal canal that their immune systems have been compromised in some way so then you have to consider the possibility of immunocompromise [38]

*Instrumental and teaching interactions* – intended to achieve the pragmatic goal of moving the case forward while also conferring teaching.

> A little bit deeper. Get through, get through that, get that, see that? You see that white stuff there? That's still dermis. We want to see fat, Okay let's keep going up. [38]

*Banter* – conversation unrelated to the procedure.

Roberts et al. make a plea for noticing the 'teachable moment' intraoperatively. They describe this as an 'unplanned learning opportunity that arises during the course of teaching' in which the teacher has an opportunity to pair a teaching point with a current step of the surgery. This is especially powerful when an unexpected surgical event arises [38].

Quizzing was a specific teaching behaviour described by many authors in which the teaching surgeon uses Socratic style questioning to assess the surgical trainee's knowledge [39].

> Attending surgeon is discussing laparoscopic port placement while inserting a trocar through a lateral abdominal incision. As the port enters the abdominal wall, the attending asks the medical student, 'Which vessel am I avoiding?' Attending then proceeds to explain the relationship of the epigastric vessels to the port site. [39]

Quizzing is a well-recognised phenomenon in schools and colleges and will frequently follow the form of an Initiation, Response, Feedback/Evaluation (IRF/IRE) sequence [40, 41]. There is debate in the wider educational literature regarding the purpose and value of this type of teaching in which the questioner is already in possession of the answer but is using the opportunity to 'test' how closely the learner's answer matches their own version. Some would speculate that this form of teaching interaction may be primarily about exerting power and hierarchical relationships over the learner. Others argue that the tension experienced by the trainee during quizzing approximates the tension in a high-stakes surgery [42].

Verbal narratives are also used during intraoperative teaching to emphasise a variety of intraoperative teaching points [43]. Hu et al. relate that three types of story are told – practice changes from lessons learned, personal training stories and near misses and adverse events. The most commonly told types were practice changes from lessons learned, and these stories usually described parallel patients from which knowledge was gained and affected adjustments in the management of patients or personnel [43]. Personal training stories frequently communicated norms of surgical culture and professionalism.

### *16.6.2 Nonverbal Intraoperative Teaching*

We have already outlined that learning to 'feel the pathology' is an important content domain of learning in the operating theatre, but touch and gesture are used for educational direction too. Chen et al. include pointing with instruments, finger or even laparoscopic camera within their taxonomy of surgeons' guiding behaviours [44].

Sutkin et al. provide a fine-grained classification of physical actions and gestures used intraoperatively by surgeons to convey their meaning during teaching [45]. They categorise different forms of physical teaching guidance, such as 'figurative'. This category refers to instances where the attending surgeon moves hands in space to describe the anatomy, the instrument or the motions required to accomplish a surgical step. They provide the following example:

> Attending is directing resident how to use the LigaSure device to accomplish the next step. Attending gestures with his right hand in space towards Fellow "When you take the LigaSure, so you have the back side sealed". His right hand flexes into a position similar to the hand position used to operate the handle of the LigaSure device. He makes this gesture after "LigaSure". He beats with the back of his hand to the right, as if he is pushing something away, on "backside". [45]

Because faculty assistance in the form of retraction, repositioning and scaffolding is an embedded form of surgical instruction, it can become difficult to categorise residents' participation in operations as there are dynamic and fluid shifts of control throughout the operation [46]. It is often challenging to identify who is the primary operator. Because surgical trainees respond to the surgeon educator's body movements and changes in hand and instrument positions, the surgical operation is a much more collaborative venture than perhaps would be thought by looking solely at verbal transcripts [47].

Some content areas of learning within the operating theatre are best delivered by specific educational strategies – for example, factual knowledge transmission may be best delivered through quizzing trainees with regard to anatomy and steps of the procedure. However, learning to interpret the feel of the tissues or how to interpret visual cues in the tissue in order to find the correct plane for dissection may be best taught through collaborative strategies between the trainee and trainer [48].

Co-construction is a characteristic of teaching that has been observed in the operating theatre that can utilise both verbal and nonverbal instructional exchanges between trainer and trainee [47]. It is dialogic sequence between trainer and trainee as they 'figure out' the anatomy together. Whilst open surgery can afford access by pointing to structures to assist with meaning making, in laparoscopic surgery this can be difficult and there is on occasion an assumption that the intended audience knows what is referred to by 'this' or 'that' [45, 48]. In the following example, deictic words are underlined that correspond with the consultant pointing with the Maryland grasper and touching particular structures.

| | |
|---|---|
| *Consultant:* | *Look at that* |
| *Staff Grade:* | *It's it's weird. I would go into that space above* |
| *Consultant:* | *That might be the artery and that might be the duct* |
| | *Can you see this anatomy?* |
| *Staff Grade:* | *Yep, ustYep, Just twisted twisted* |
| *ST 7:* | *Yeah, it's really weird, it's twisting round each other* |
| *Consultant:* | *Yeah, and what that's doing is it's, torting the Hartmann's, and what that's doing is it's, torting the Hartmann's pouch over* |
| *Staff Grade:* | *Yeah, just move* |
| *ST 7:* | *And you think behind where you are now, back* |
| *Consultant:* | *This one?* |
| *ST 7:* | *No, no. Back, back, back* |
| *Consultant:* | *That?* |
| *ST 7:* | *No, next one. Back, that?* |
| *Staff Grade:* | *ThisThis is no, no maybe is no, no maybe* |
| *Consultant:* | *That could be accessory artery?* |
| *ST 7:* | *Do you think it's an accessory du* |
| *ST 7:* | *Could be* |
| *Consultant:* | *CouldCould be yeah be yeah* |

In this example, there is genuine co-construction of the anatomy at this part of the operation. The consultant, staff grade and trainee discuss this using verbal and nonverbal signs that stand for possible interpretations of what they are seeing and consider the different possibilities and hypotheses put forward. Co-construction sequences were found to end in 'resolution' when structures were assigned anatomical names or were discounted [48].

### 16.6.3 The Surgical Team

Of course, the operative team is much broader than just the teaching and training surgeons. Nurses, surgical technicians, anaesthesiologists and anaesthetists all interact with and have an impact on surgical learners. Team communication influences a learner's sense of professional identity and the role of the surgeon within the team. Although surgeons, trainees and nurses often interpret interprofessional communication differently, the trainee who recognises that a senior nurse can be a good teacher in the operating theatre will increase their sense of professional identity [49].

### 16.6.4 Questions for Future Research

These intraoperative teaching episodes involve interesting discussions, but how do they impact surgical learning? There are multiple interesting questions ripe for future surgical education research, including: How does the briefing, intraoperative teaching and debriefing model (BID model) impact retention of new knowledge? What content about the hidden curriculum are within an attending's verbal narratives? What are the ideal ways to use retraction to orient the training surgeon to the next step of the surgery? How does an attending assess a trainee's position on the learning curve and make the surgical lessons succinct and appropriate? Does banter contribute to a safe learning environment? When quizzing makes a trainee uncomfortable, does that impact their performance? How is learning impacted by the pace of surgery? These questions are rich start points when considering current knowledge about intraoperative surgical teaching, and they deserve dedicated academic study. What content about the hidden curriculum are within an attending's verbal narratives? What are the ideal ways to use retraction to orient the training surgeon to the next step of the surgery? How does an attending assess a trainee's position on the learning curve and make the surgical lessons succinct and appropriate? Does banter contribute to a safe learning environment? When quizzing makes a trainee uncomfortable, does that impact their performance? How is learning impacted by the pace of surgery? These questions are rich start points when considering current knowledge about intraoperative surgical teaching and they deserve dedicated academic study.

## 16.7 Conclusions

This chapter aims to serve as an introduction to the evidence base around teaching and learning in the operating theatre. Teaching has been found to be highly complex involving many different team members along with sophisticated social interactions that include verbal and nonverbal guidance. The surgeon educator has both clinician and educator roles which must be managed simultaneously, which in part is what makes this a challenging educational venue. It is worth considering that the learner surgeon also observes these role conflicts and learns professional attributes of being a surgeon through the modelling of these behaviours.

# References

1. Knowles, M. S. (1984). *Andragogy in action. Applying modern principles of adult education.* San Francisco: Jossey Bass.
2. Pugh, C. M., DaRosa, D. A., Glenn, D., & Bell, R. H., Jr. (2007). A comparison of faculty and resident perception of resident learning needs in the operating room. *Journal of Surgical Education, 64*(5), 250–255.
3. Land, R., Meyer, J., & Flanagan, M. (Eds.). (2016). *Threshold concepts in practice. Educational futures: Rethinking theory and practice.* Rotterdam: Sense Publishers.
4. Fitts, P., & Posner, M. (1967). *Human performance.* Co Belmont: Brooks/Cole Publishers.
5. Kopta, J. (1971). An approach to the evaluation of operative skills. *Surgery, 70*, 297–303.
6. DaRosa, D., Zwischenberger, J., Meyerson, S., George, B., Teitelbaum, E., Soper, N., & Fryer, J. (2013). A theory-based model for teaching and assessing residents in the operating room. *Journal of Surgical Education, 70*(1), 24–30.
7. Reznick, R. (1993). Teaching and testing technical skills. *American Journal of Surgery, 165*(3), 358–361.
8. Scallon, S. E., Fairholm, D. J., Cochrane, D. D., & Taylor, D. C. (1992). Evaluation of the operating room as a surgical teaching venue. *Canadian Journal of Surgery, 35*(2), 173–176.
9. Schwind, C. J., Boehler, M. L., Rogers, D. A., Williams, R. G., Dunnington, G., Folse, R., & Markwell, S. J. (2004). Variables influencing medical student learning in the operating room. *American Journal of Surgery, 187*(2), 198–200.
10. Fernando, N., McAdam, T., Youngson, G., McKenzie, H., Cleland, J., & Yule, S. (2007). Undergraduate medical students' perceptions and expectations of theatre-based learning: How can we improve the student learning experience? *Surgeon Journal of the Royal Colleges of Surgeons of Edinburgh & Ireland, 5*(5), 271–274.
11. Rose, J., Waibel, B., & Schenarts, P. (2011). Disparity between resident and faculty surgeons' perceptions of preoperative preparation, intraoperative teaching, and postoperative feedback. *Journal of Surgical Education, 68*(6), 459–464.
12. Vollmer, C., Newman, L., Huang, G., Irish, J., Hurst, J., & Horvath, K. (2011). Perspectives on intraoperative teaching: Divergence and convergence between learner and teacher. *Journal of Surgical Education, 68*(6), 485–494.
13. Butvidas, L., Anderson, C., Balogh, D., & Basson, M. (2011). Disparities between resident and attending surgeon perceptions of intraoperative teaching. *The American Journal of Surgery, 201*(3), 385–389.
14. Levinson, K., Barlin, J., Altman, K., & Satin, A. (2010). Disparity between resident and attending physician perceptions of intraoperative supervision and education. *Journal of Graduate Medical Education, 2*(1), 31–36.
15. Chen, X., Williams, R., & Smink, D. (2014). Do residents receive the same OR guidance as surgeons report? Difference between residents' and surgeons' perceptions of OR guidance. *Journal of Surgical Education, 71*(6), e79–e82.
16. Hindmarsh, J., & Pilnick, A. (2002). The tacit order of teamwork: Collaboration and embodied conduct in anaesthesia. *The Sociological Quarterly, 43*(2), 139–164.
17. Pope, C., Smith, A., Goodwin, D., & Mort, M. (2003). Passing on tacit knowledge in anaesthesia: A qualitative study. *Medical Education, 37*(7), 650–655.
18. Lave, J., & Wenger, E. (1991). *Situated learning: Legitimate peripheral participation.* Cambridge, UK: Press syndicate of University of Cambridge.
19. Aggarwal, R., & Darzi, A. (2006). Training in the operating theatre: Is it safe? *Thorax, 61*(4), 278–279.
20. Lyon, P. M. A. (2003). Making the most of learning in the operating theatre: Student strategies and curricular initiatives. *Medical Education, 37*(8), 680–688.
21. Lyon, P. (2004). A model of teaching and learning in the operating theatre. *Medical Education, 38*(12), 1278–1287.

22. Dunnington, G., DaRosa, D., & Kolm, P. (1993). Development of a model for evaluating teaching in the operating room. *Current Surgery, 50*(7), 523–527.
23. Cox, S., & Swanson, M. (2002). Identification of teaching excellence in operating room and clinic settings. *American Journal of Surgery, 183*(3), 251–255.
24. Moulton, C. (2010). Operating from the other side of the table: Control dynamics and the surgeon educator. *Journal of American College of Surgeons, 210*(1), 79–86.
25. Lingard, L. (2002). Team communications in the operating room: Talk patterns, sites of tension and implications for novices. *Academic Medicine, 77*(3), 232–237.
26. Crofts, T. J., Griffiths, J. M., Sharma, S., Wygrala, J., & Aitken, R. J. (1997). Surgical training: An objective assessment of recent changes for a single health board. *BMJ, 314*(7084), 891–895.
27. Raja, A. J., & Levin, A. V. (2003). Challenges of teaching surgery: Ethical framework. *World Journal of Surgery, 27*(8), 948–951.
28. Mayer, R. (2004). Should there be a three-strikes rule against pure discovery learning? The case for guided methods of instruction. *Am Psychology, 59*, 14–19.
29. Roberts, N., Williams, R., Kim, M., & Dunnington, G. (2009). The briefing, intraoperative teaching, debriefing model for teaching in the operating room. *Journal of the American College of Surgeons, 208*(2), 299–303.
30. Temple, J. (2010). Time for training: A review of the impact ofhte the European Working Time Directive on the quality of training.
31. Ahmed, M., Arora, S., Russ, S., Darzi, A., Vincent, C., & Sevdalis, N. (2013). Operation debrief – a SHARP improvement in performance feedback in the operating room. *Annals of Surgery, 258*(6), 958–963.
32. Cope, A., Mavroveli, S., Bezemer, J., Hanna, G., & Kneebone, R. (2015). Making meaning from sensory cues in the operating room – an important content area of post-graduate surgical learning. *Academic Medicine, 90*(8), 1125–1131.
33. Law, B., Atkins, M. S., Kirkpatrick, A. E., & Lomax, A. J. (2004). *Eye gaze patterns differentiate novice and experts in a virtual laparoscopic surgery training environment, Proceedings of the 2004 symposium on Eye tracking research & applications* (pp. 41–48). San Antonio: ACM.
34. Richstone, L., Schwartz, M., Seideman, C., Cadeddu, J., Marshall, S., & Kavoussi, L. (2010). Eye metrics as an objective assessment of surgical skill. *Annals of Surgery, 252*(1), 177–182.
35. Bleakley, A. (2006). *Towards an aesthetics of healthcare practice: Learning the art of clinical judgement*. Denmark: University of Aarhus.
36. Hauge, L. S., Wanzek, J. A., & Godellas, C. (2001). The reliability of an instrument for identifying and quantifying surgeons' teaching in the operating room. *American Journal of Surgery, 181*(4), 333–337.
37. Blom, E. M., Verdaasdonk, E. G. G., Stassen, L. P. S., Stassen, H. G., Wieringa, P. A., & Dankelman, J. (2007). Analysis of verbal communication during teaching in the operating room and the potentials for surgical training. *Surgical Endoscopy, 21*(9), 1560–1566.
38. Roberts, N., Brenner, M., Williams, R., Kim, M., & Dunnington, G. (2012). Capturing the teachable moment: A grounded theory study of verbal teaching interactions in the operating room. *Surgery, 151*(5), 643–650.
39. Sutkin, G., Littleton, E., & Kanter, S. (2015). How surgical mentors teach: A classification of in vivo teaching behaviors part 1: Verbal teaching guidance. *Journal of Surgical Education, 72*(2), 243–250.
40. Mehan, H. (1979). *Learning lessons: Social organisation in the classroom*. Cambridge, MA: Harvard Press.
41. Wells, G. (1993). Re-evaluating the IRF sequence: A proposal for the articulation of theories of activity and discourse for the analysis of teaching and learning in the classroom. *Linguistics and Education, 5*, 1–37.
42. Healy, J., & Yoo, P. In defense of "Pimping". *Journal of Surgical Education, 72*(1), 176–177.
43. Hu, Y., Peyre, S., Arriaga, A., Roth, E., Corso, K., & Greenberg, C. (2012). War stories: A qualitative analysis of narrative teaching strategies in the operating room. *The American Journal of Surgery, 203*(1), 63–68.

44. Chen, X., Williams, R., Sanfey, H., & Smink, D. (2015). A taxonomy of surgeons' guiding behaviors in the operating room. *The American Journal of Surgery, 209*(1), 15–20.
45. Sutkin, G., Littleton, E., & Kanter, S. (2015). How surgical mentors teach: A classification of in vivo teaching behaviors part 2: Physical teaching guidance. *Journal of Surgical Education, 72*(2), 251–257.
46. Bezemer, J., Cope, A., Faiz, O., & Kneebone, R. (2012). Participation of surgical residents in operations. *World Journal of Surgery, 36*(9), 2011–2014.
47. Bezemer, J., Cope, A., Kress, G., & Kneebone, R. (2013). Holding the scalpel: Achieving surgical care in a learning environment. *Journal of Contemporary Ethnography, 43*(1), 38–63.
48. Cope, A., Bezemer, J., Kneebone, R., & Lingard, L. (2015). 'You see?' Teaching and learning how to interpret visual cues during surgery. *Medical Education, 49*(11), 1103–1116.
49. Lingard, L., Reznick, R., DeVito, I., & Espin, S. (2002). Forming professional identities on the health care team: Discursive constructions of the 'other' in the operating room. *Medical Education, 36*, 728–734.

# Chapter 17
# Supporting the Development of Psychomotor Skills

**Pamela Andreatta and Paul Dougherty**

**Overview** Comprehensive acquisition and mastery of psychomotor skills for surgical procedures must eventually be facilitated in the context of applied surgery. Although simulation-supported instruction provides a benign environment for acquiring basic abilities such as suturing and knot tying, the application of those abilities within procedural contexts requires alignment of optimal techniques and integration of process sequences dictated by operative circumstances. Trainees acquire these abilities through direct guidance and supervision by operative faculty. The challenge for faculty and trainees is to align the abilities of trainees within a procedural context, so trainees are able to practice what they have learned, while safely acquiring new abilities. We introduce a framework based on the Dave taxonomy of the psychomotor domain and implemented through the briefing-intraoperative-debriefing (BID) model that allows faculty and trainees to deliberately and collaboratively plan and monitor the cycle of psychomotor acquisition and development of mastery in any surgical context.

## 17.1 Introduction

Discourses focused on the topic of surgical skills acquisition, mastery, and maintenance are frequently fluid, sometimes confounding, and rarely unified in their conceptualization of the challenges within the construct. Largely at the root of these disparate considerations is the idea that psychomotor skills can be developed without integration of the cognitive and affective components that significantly influence their execution in applied surgical practice. That is, the idea that mastering physical movements associated with instruments and techniques designed to effect a surgical task must be learned within the context of applied surgery, inclusive of the inherent

P. Andreatta (✉)
Metrics-Healthcare, LLC, FL, USA

P. Dougherty
University of Florida, Jacksonville, FL, USA
e-mail: Paul.Dougherty@jax.ufl.edu

cognitive and affective factors therein. Although it is certainly true that mastery in the applied surgical environment must eventually be demonstrated (inclusive of all performance dimensions), as long as deliberate strategies for sequenced integration are an essential component of instruction, it is reasonable to develop some elements of each performance dimension independent from the others. The uses of non-operative proxies for developing psychomotor skills, such as needlework, span the history of surgery. Modern simulators extend the reach of some of the traditional phantoms; however any reasonably considered facsimile of the performance construct may be effective for establishing foundational understanding of psychomotor abilities, inclusive of tool function and implementation, techniques, sequencing, precision, and criteria for acceptable performance.

For psychomotor skills in surgery, the point where integration becomes essential is the juncture where psychomotor proficiencies have been achieved in a non-operative performance context, such as simulation, and their application in an operative one. If it is not possible to master psychomotor abilities outside of the operative context, they must be mastered in any case within it. Therefore, we will focus on the acquisition of psychomotor abilities within operative contexts while at the same time emphasizing the value we believe deliberate practice outside of operative theater brings to the development and maintenance of mastery in the surgical psychomotor domain. We will begin with a discussion of the theoretical foundations of performance in the psychomotor domain.

## 17.2 Theoretical Foundations

There are several established and empirically supported taxonomies for the development of performance in the psychomotor domain [1–3]; however the Dave taxonomy includes a hierarchy of significant progressive mastery that aligns quite well with the development of surgical skills. The five-level taxonomy includes (1) Imitation, (2) Manipulation, (3) Precision, (4) Articulation, and (5) Naturalization. During the initial Imitation phase, individuals observe and pattern behavior after someone else, including performing while observing demonstration. This corresponds conceptually with the tradition of "see one, do one" (regardless of the other challenges associated with that concept). In the second Manipulation phase, individuals perform certain actions by memory or following guided instructions. In the third Precision phase, individuals refine their abilities to perform skills with a high degree of precision, efficiency, accuracy, proportion, and exactness without guided support. In the fourth Articulation phase, individuals coordinate and adapt action sequences to achieve synergy and internal consistency, including combining two or more skills or activities to meet a broader requirement or integrated objective. Finally, in the fifth Naturalization phase, individuals combine, sequence, and perform two or more skills with ease and consistency, with little physical or mental exertion. Individuals

**Table 17.1** The Dave taxonomy of psychomotor domain [3]

| Dave taxonomy of psychomotor domain | | |
|---|---|---|
| Level | Definition | Expected quality of performance |
| 1. Imitation | Being able to observe an expert surgeon and pattern behavior associated with surgical tasks and actions, including performing while observing expert demonstration | Low quality, inconsistent, inefficient, dependent execution, discrete tasks and actions, performance dependent on guidance/instruction |
| 2. Manipulation | Being able to perform certain surgical tasks and actions from memory, able to follow instructions and verbal guidance from expert to perform skills | Low-average quality, inconsistent, inefficient, dependent execution, discrete tasks and actions, performance dependent on facilitative verbal guidance |
| 3. Precision | Being able to perform certain surgical tasks and actions with a high degree of precision, efficiency, accuracy, exactness, and proportion without direction or guidance from expert. Expert provides facilitation and corrective feedback | Average-good quality, consistent, efficient, independent execution, discrete tasks and actions, performance dependent on facilitative corrective feedback |
| 4. Articulation | Being able to perform tasks and actions with consistently good quality, as well as coordinate and adapt a series or sequence of actions, including combining skills, tasks, or activities to meet a broader surgical requirement or integrated objective. Expert provides consultation and support | Good quality, consistent, efficient, independent execution, integrated action sequences, performance dependent on facilitative consultation |
| 5. Naturalization | Being able to perform sequences of actions or activities automatically without physical or mental exertion, performs with ease, control, and high quality. Expert provides progress strategy and consultation as needed | Very good quality, consistent, efficient, independent execution, integrated action sequences, performance independent of facilitative consultation |

performing at the Naturalization level will demonstrate a high level of performance mastery that is second nature or natural, without needing to think much about it, which allows them to perform well while thinking about other things.

We illustrate the conceptualization of surgical skills within the framework of the Dave psychomotor domain taxonomy in Table 17.1. By providing a definition of each taxonomy level using the context of surgical skills, we can also begin to define the expected quality of performance at each level. This is important for defining performance standards when designing instructional activities, especially associated with the development of mastery. We will expand on this table further to delineate strategies for teaching and performance assessment in the following sections.

## 17.3 Teaching Surgical Skills in Simulated Contexts

The applications of simulated environments to support the development and maintenance of surgical skills are as varied as they are indispensable in most modern surgical education programs. High-, medium-, low-, and mixed-technology solutions have demonstrated the potential to facilitate the development of abilities from level 1 (imitation) through level 4 (articulation) and are especially valuable for the types of repeated deliberate practice activities required at level 3 (precision) [4]. If only for the safety advantages gained for both patients and clinicians, the uses of surgical simulation will likely continue to advance with increasing breadth and depth of scope, precision, flexibility, and comprehensiveness. Aspects of simulation-supported surgical training are addressed elsewhere in this book, so we will focus our primary attentions on developing instructional activities within applied operative practice. However, we are strong advocates for trainees developing fundamental surgical skills to level 3 minimally before performing them in applied surgical contexts. Not only does this provide a safer, higher-quality experience for the patient, it provides a better operative learning experience for the trainee and faculty who are able to concentrate on higher-order procedural considerations, such as decision-making or cognitive and affective reflection, and not details associated with basic surgical skills.

## 17.4 Teaching Surgical Skills in Operative Theater

A clear-cut framework for organizing and overseeing the development of surgical skills in operative contexts is the BID model: Briefing (B), Intraoperative teaching (I), and Debriefing (D) [5]. The BID model encompasses three phases, each of which corresponds to a natural point of engagement between faculty and trainee during an operation.

### 17.4.1 Preoperative Briefing (B)

During the preoperative Briefing (B), the faculty and trainee review the skill requirements for the planned operation, evaluate the trainee's ability level (Dave taxonomy) for each of the skills, and determine performance expectations for the procedure. For example, if the procedure involves bowel anastomosis, the faculty can review the trainee's demonstrated performance capabilities in performing anastomoses in multiple contexts (simulated, animal, cadaver, operative) and determine the best course for developing his/her abilities further, as well as what level of supervision will be required. The faculty and trainee should identify and agree upon no more than two to three targeted performance areas to focus on in any procedure. Less experienced trainees who are performing at levels 1 and 2 of the psychomotor taxonomy will perform less of the procedure compared to senior trainees performing at levels 3 through 5. A mid-level trainee who has demonstrated abilities at level 3 for tasks associated with the procedure will more likely identify more advanced goals for the operative case. Likewise, a senior trainee with a record of demonstrable abilities at levels 4 or 5 may have the aim of performing the entire procedure with minimal or no direct assistance from faculty.

## *17.4.2 Intraoperative Teaching (I)*

At Intraoperative (I) points where the surgical tasks or action sequences align with the two to three predetermined focus areas, the trainee and faculty work together to facilitate the advancement of the trainee's abilities. For example, a trainee might be ready to work on efficient and precise placement of a guidewire for an intramedullary nail (level 3) in a fracture fixation case. The type of facilitation will depend upon the current level of trainee performance and may include direct step-by-step guidance with or without demonstration, through consultation as needed to help apply skills in particularly difficult contexts. Intraoperative teaching to predetermine focused areas provides the trainee with direction about how to advance their abilities beyond his or her current level while at the same time providing faculty with concise and deliberate expectations for the trainee's overall participation in the case itself.

Intraoperative facilitation by faculty should strive to identify the levels at which the trainee is performing discrete skills and action sequences, including those areas where level 5 automaticity has been achieved. Allowing trainees to perform those areas of a procedure not only encourages trainees to work at developing their abilities, it serves to reinforce and expand their foundational understanding of the relationship of those actions to the broader procedural context. It also serves to introduce the natural dynamic that occurs in all procedures, where some sequences require more effort than others either because of unanticipated challenges or the inherent complexity of the procedure itself [6, 7]. Other sequences become more automatic over time, either because of routine application of the required tasks or the straightforward consistency of the surgical context. Faculty can facilitate successful execution of those behaviors requiring more effort by helping the trainee slow down, focus, and concentrate on the critical performance points for the case. Similarly, those predetermined one to three target performance areas identified during the briefing will necessitate trainee effort, and faculty should facilitate the trainee successfully working through those challenges using the same processes of slowing down, focusing, and concentrating on critical performance parameters, with or without direct guidance.

### 17.4.3 Postoperative Debrief (D)

Postoperative debriefing (D) between faculty and trainee serves to facilitate a discussion about how well the targeted skills were performed relative to the expected standards, as well as to formulate strategic plans for further skill development efforts. The faculty should help the trainee self-assess his or her performance; provide insights, guidance, and correction as needed; and formulate a plan of action for next steps required to advance the trainee's skills. For example, the faculty might inform the trainee that although he or she successfully placed the guidewire for the intramedullary nail, it required more than the recommended number of attempts and greater than the recommended amount of fluoroscopy to accomplish it. The faculty and trainee would then determine how the trainee should proceed to work on placing the guidewire more efficiently. The discussion should involve all aspects of the trainee's targeted skills for the case, including feedback on how the performance was executed relative to the expected standards and recommendations for next steps that the trainee can use for self-study or development in another operative context with the same or different faculty. To the extent possible, the trainee should create a written summary of the discussion for his or her records. This will help with subsequent operative planning with the same faculty or another, as well as provide a record of achievement for faculty members to reference as needed. The postoperative debriefing thus serves as a mechanism for trainees to learn to identify performance gaps, elicit expert feedback, and develop an action plan for further improvement; all of which are foundational elements for self-assessment and the types of self-regulated learning associated with maintenance of competency over the duration of a surgical career.

## 17.5 An Integrated Approach to Developing Surgical Skills

Supporting the acquisition, development, and maintenance of surgical skills can be implemented through various methods and instructional contexts. Historically, these abilities were acquired, developed, and maintained in operative contexts, with independent practice using low-technology proxies for some routine skills such as suturing and knot tying (needlepoint, embroidery, chicken parts, etc.). Modern educational practices across all surgical specialties are largely adaptive responses to challenges imposed by socioeconomic and medicolegal drivers, which have shifted both the quality and quantity of teaching opportunities between faculty and trainees. Competency-based education is being considered as a potential solution for many of these challenges; however the expertise required to substantively reformulate training processes and practices without sacrificing quality of care and safety for both clinicians and patients is outside the bailiwick of most pundits in the surgical education domain [8, 9]. The taxonomy of the psychomotor domain provides a foundation for structuring the acquisition and development of surgical skills performance mastery without substantial changes to what is being informally implemented in most graduate medical education programs, globally.

Using the Dave taxonomy, we can consider each hierarchical level as a developmental step toward being able to perform in the psychomotor domain but also as a progressive generation of the conceptual and procedural foundations for specific procedures and surgical science in its broadest implementation. That is, psychomotor abilities are inextricably tied to cognitive processing and decision-making associated with the performance construct, and the extent to which surgical skills are acquired and mastered through multimodal facilitation, the greater the integration of capabilities will be sustained in applied practice [10, 11]. There are many ways to facilitate multimodal processing during learning; however we propose a solution designed to easily fit within most modern surgical training programs [12]. Using the Dave taxonomy, we illustrate a process model for deliberate facilitation of surgical skills that includes the generation of both psychomotor abilities and foundational understanding of associated surgical application, reasoning, and implementation in Table 17.2. Potential facilitative behaviors are provided for both faculty and trainee at each hierarchical level.

**Table 17.2** Facilitative behaviors for surgical skill development using the Dave psychomotor taxonomy

| Dave taxonomy of psychomotor domain | | |
|---|---|---|
| Level | Faculty facilitative behaviors | Trainee facilitative behaviors |
| 1. Imitation | Facilitate trainee observation of behaviors by performing skill, task, or action while providing step-by-step explanation of what is being done and why | Observe faculty perform skill, task, or action |
| | Provide direct guidance to trainee as he/she attempts the skill, task, or action | Perform skill, task, or action while observing faculty or with direct faculty guidance |
| | Provide corrective feedback | Patterns faculty behavior, while providing step-by-step explanation of what he/she is doing and why |
| | Ask/answer questions | Ask/answer questions |
| 2. Manipulation | Facilitate acquisition of sequencing behaviors by performing skill, task, or action while trainee provides step-by-step explanation of what is being done and why | Explains each step and why it is being done while faculty performs skill, task, or action |
| | Provide verbal guidance to trainee while he/she performs skill, task, or action | Demonstrate skill, task, or action while explaining each step and why it is done |
| | Direct trainee to perform skill, task, or action in appropriate context | Respond to facilitative verbal guidance from faculty during performance |
| | Provide corrective feedback | Adjust performance based on faculty corrective feedback |
| | Ask/answer questions | Ask/answer questions |

(continued)

**Table 17.2** (continued)

| Dave taxonomy of psychomotor domain | | |
|---|---|---|
| Level | Faculty facilitative behaviors | Trainee facilitative behaviors |
| 3. Precision | Provide trainee with expected performance standards | Perform skill using deliberate practice techniques |
| | Facilitate skill development activities with simulation or operative experiences | Focus on developing performance accuracy, precision, efficiency, and consistency |
| | Devise skill development strategies with trainee | Adjust performance based on faculty corrective feedback |
| | Provide corrective feedback | |
| 4. Articulation | Facilitate skill development activities through operative experiences | Perform skill, task, and action sequences automatically with mastery |
| | Devise integrated, procedural approach to development strategies with trainee | Adjust performance of skill, task, and action sequences to unanticipated surgical or contextual challenges |
| | Provide consultation and support | Determine and demonstrate alternate approaches to skill, task, and action sequences to adapt to surgical or contextual challenges |
| | | Consult with faculty |
| 5. Naturalization | Facilitate skill development activities through operative experiences | Perform skill, task, and action sequences while explaining what factors contribute to procedural pacing ebbs/flows |
| | Provide trainee with progress strategy for acquiring new performance abilities | Perform skill, task, and action sequences while planning to monitor for potential procedural complications |
| | Provide consultation and support | Devise alternate techniques/devices to improve procedural task performance |
| | | Demonstrate skill, task, and action sequence to another trainee, with step-by-step explanation |
| | | Consult with faculty |

The illustrated facilitative behaviors in Table 17.2 are by no means exclusive or even prescriptive, however they provide a conceptual framework for instructional strategies that may be useful for both faculty and trainees. In anchoring facilitative strategies to a strong theoretical framework, we are able to provide a standardized instructional approach to surgical skills development that is not overly prescriptive but includes the essential elements for successful acquisition of skills integrated with the cognitive components of surgical science. The proposed approach begins with the big picture in the context of applied surgery, including reasoning attributes to establish the contextual foundations for skills within the procedure specifically and surgery generally. This lays the foundational knowledge for the trainee without the trainee being distracted by his or her own hand movements. It also serves to help trainees develop operative reasoning, surgical judgment, and decision-making early in the process of acquisition, which establishes the value of quality and safety throughout the training process.

The delineation of facilitative behaviors for both faculty and trainee conveys to each that they are jointly responsible for the successful development of the trainee's abilities. It also describes the process by which this can be achieved through deliberate and routine exchanges of information, strategic planning, coordination, and effort by faculty and trainees. Additionally, the process integrates the language of surgery to describe all relevant facets of surgical skills and associated competency standards for performance. This, in turn, establishes the bases for deliberate practice toward mastery, including precision, accuracy, consistency, efficiency, and ultimately automaticity. Mastery of surgical skills reduces cognitive load associated with processing psychomotor actions, which releases processing resources for higher-level analyses and decision-making [13, 14]. The development of mastery also facilitates expansion of practice and synthesis cognition by developing alternate approaches, as described for trainee behaviors associated with levels 4 and 5.

To illustrate how the Dave psychomotor taxonomy with facilitative behaviors and BID model could be applied to a specific surgical skill set, we provide a relatively straightforward example for facilitating the application of an intramedullary nail for surgical management of a diaphyseal tibial fracture in Table 17.3.

Table 17.3 Example skills development: intramedullary (IM) nailing of diaphyseal tibial fracture

| BID Step | Level 1 Imitation | Level 2 Manipulation | Level 3 Precision | Level 4 Articulation | Level 5 Naturalization |
|---|---|---|---|---|---|
| Brief: faculty (F) and trainee (T) decide the itemized goals for procedure | Observe intramedullary nailing process | With direct faculty guidance: | Identify, mark entry site | Identify, mark entry site | Operative exposure |
| | Provide instruments to surgeon when requested by name | Identify, mark entry site | Make incision, entry site | Make incision, entry site | Internal fracture reduction |
| | Identify placed guidewire, reamer, nail with fluoroscopy | Make incision, entry site | Penetrate metaphyseal bone with guidewire or awl | Penetrate metaphyseal bone with guidewire | Place guidewire |
| | | Penetrate metaphyseal bone with guidewire or awl | | Insert guidewire, tibial shaft axis | Ream medullary canal |

(continued)

**Table 17.3** (continued)

| BID Step | Level 1 Imitation | Level 2 Manipulation | Level 3 Precision | Level 4 Articulation | Level 5 Naturalization |
|---|---|---|---|---|---|
| | | | | Incrementally advance guidewire to fracture site | Insert intramedullary nail |
| | | | | Coordinate assists, manipulate distal fragment | Complete intramedullary nail fixation |
| | | | | Pass guidewire past fracture | |
| | | | | Confirm guidewire with fluoroscopy | |
| Intraoperative: faculty (F) and trainee (T) collaborate to achieve the predetermined goals for the procedure | (F) Perform internal fixation with explanation | (F) Guide trainee to identify, mark entry site | (T) Identify, mark entry site | (T) Identify, mark entry site | (T) Operative exposure |
| | (T) Observe internal fixation process | (T) Identify, mark entry site | (F) Provide corrective feedback | (T) Make incision, entry site | (T) Internal fracture reduction |
| | (F) Request instruments by name | (F) Guide trainee to make incision, entry site | (T) Make incision, entry site | (T) Penetrate metaphyseal bone with guidewire | (T) Place guidewire |
| | (T) Provide instruments to surgeon | (T) Make incision, entry site | (F) Provide corrective feedback | (F) Facilitate integrated sequencing of additional steps | (T) Ream medullary canal |
| | (F) Capture images of placed guidewire, reamer, nail with fluoroscopy | (F) Guide trainee to penetrate metaphyseal bone with guidewire | (T) Penetrate metaphyseal bone with guidewire | (T) Insert guidewire, tibial shaft axis | (T) Insert intramedullary nail |

(continued)

**Table 17.3** (continued)

| BID Step | Level 1 Imitation | Level 2 Manipulation | Level 3 Precision | Level 4 Articulation | Level 5 Naturalization |
|---|---|---|---|---|---|
| | (T) Identify placed guidewire, reamer, nail with fluoroscopy | (T) Penetrate metaphyseal bone with guidewire | (F) Provide corrective feedback | (T) Incrementally advance guidewire to fracture site | (T) Complete intramedullary nail fixation |
| | | | | (T) Coordinate assists, manipulate distal fragment | (T) Confirm fixation with fluoroscopy |
| | | | | (T) Pass guidewire past fracture | (F) Provide consultation |
| | | | | Confirm guidewire with fluoroscopy | |
| | | | | (F) Provide feedback | |
| Debrief: faculty (F) and trainee (T) review performance against standards, discuss development strategies and next steps | (T) Self-assess performance for each goal | (T) Self-assess performance for each goal | (T) Self-assess performance for each goal | (T) Self-assess performance for each goal | (T) Self-assess performance for each goal |
| | (F) Assess trainee performance for each goal | (F) Assess trainee performance for each goal | (F) Assess trainee performance for each goal | (F) Assess trainee performance for each goal | (F) Assess trainee performance for each goal |
| | (F/T) Determine areas for further development | (F/T) Determine areas for further development | (F/T) Determine areas for further development | (F/T) Determine areas for further development | (F/T) Determine areas for further development |
| | (F/T) Create plan of action for development efforts | (F/T) Create plan of action for development efforts | (F/T) Create plan of action for development efforts | (F/T) Create plan of action for development efforts | (F/T) Create plan of action for development efforts |
| | (T) Document debriefing outcomes, progress strategy | (T) Document debriefing outcomes, progress strategy | (T) Document debriefing outcomes, progress strategy | (T) Document debriefing outcomes and progress strategy | (T) Document debriefing outcomes and progress strategy |

## 17.6 Benefits of the BID Model with the Dave Taxonomy

The simplicity of the BID model belies its effective power in maximizing training efficiencies, especially when combined with the Dave taxonomy of the psychomotor domain. The approach facilitates the development of surgical skills within the context of operative procedures by focusing the attention of faculty and trainees in a way that maximizes the benefits of the surgical context while safely aligning performance expectations within the trainee's zone of proximal development [15]. The benefits for trainees are that they have targeted performance goals aligned to advance their current abilities, which allows them to focus and process information without extending beyond what is possible to safely achieve. At the early stages of level 1 skills development, the targeted goals may be to attempt a few simple tasks and then to actively observe faculty throughout the procedure as a way of establishing a foundational frame of reference for the overall procedure, its complexities, and how the discrete skills, steps, and sequencing integrate together through its completion. A paced deliberate strategy that facilitates dynamic exchanges of information across multiple performance domains facilitates richer and more durable ability development [10]. Encouraging trainees to routinely perform the abilities they have mastered while focusing more effortful attention toward advancing their abilities in a few targeted areas of natural expansion will assure that trainees maintain what they have learned and successfully achieve new abilities they are ready for. Building upon simpler experiences to become increasingly competent and autonomous is the ultimate objective of teaching in operative theater. By identifying where each trainee is performing within the taxonomy, astute faculty and training program directors can design strategies for building and strengthening the surgical skills of all trainees through rotational sequences, as well as longitudinally across the duration of the training program.

For faculty, being able to predetermine which aspects of a case will be supported by a trainee and in what capacity allows them to plan more effectively, as well as reduce stressors associated with trainees performing unsafely. Faculty members will rightfully assert control of a case to ensure that the appropriate balance between safety and training is maintained. However, the dynamics of how control is established, relinquished, and re-established when difficulties arise during a case may lead to hard feelings between faculty and trainee if the trainee believes he or she is capable of performing safely [6, 7]. Faculty will often facilitate trainees performing more routine procedural steps and guide trainees through parts of a case they believe the trainee can safely manage. Over time, and with earned trust, faculty will facilitate increasing autonomy as the trainee gains expertise and demonstrates safe practice. Difficulties may arise when the faculty and trainee are not in synch with each other about which part of the case the trainee will perform. Agreement between trainees and faculty about which parts of a case they are ready to perform, based on their demonstrated abilities, can be an incentive for achieving performance standards through deliberate sustained efforts. Ideally, this discussion occurs during the debriefing time after a completed case, so that trainees are able to prepare well before the next procedural opportunity. However, it should minimally occur as part of the preoperative briefing of all procedures.

## 17.7 Conclusions

The model we outline in this chapter supports trainees working with a single faculty member for a rotation or with larger teams and multiple faculty members over the duration of a training program. The advantages of the BID technique, coupled with the Dave psychomotor taxonomy, are that it is straightforward and familiar in concept to many, especially those who have used both briefing and debriefing components as part of their operative team management strategies. Advantages also include the deliberate uses of real-time, corrective feedback and performance assessment against standards, which is one of the most important facets of teaching in the operating room. This becomes increasingly achievable through mobile performance assessment systems designed to create and archive records for both trainees and faculty. However, the value of the BID model is easily lost if faculty and trainees do not employ the technique each time they work together. Although relatively simple to enact, professional development of faculty educators to teach them how to facilitate the processes is merited, especially if it instills an understanding of the benefits realized by trainees, faculty, and patients. Faculty development requires some resources and time; however the expenditures required to introduce the proposed approach are modest when compared to the risks associated with trainees performing below or above their ability level.

## References

1. Simpson, E. J. (1972). *The classification of educational objectives in the psychomotor domain.* Washington, DC: Gryphon House.
2. Harrow, A. (1972). *A taxonomy of the psychomotor domain: A guide for developing behavioral objectives.* New York: David McKay.
3. Dave, R. H. (1970). Psychomotor levels. In R. J. Armstrong (Ed.), *Developing and writing behavioral objectives* (pp. 20–21). Tucson: Educational Innovators Press.
4. Ericsson, K. A., Krampe, R. T., & Tesch-Roemer, C. (1993). The role of deliberate practice in the acquisition of expert performance. *Psychological Review, 100,* 363–406.
5. Roberts, N. K., Williams, R. G., Kim, M. J., & Dunnington, G. L. (2009). The briefing, intraoperative teaching, debriefing model for teaching in the operating room. *Journal of the American College of Surgeons, 208*(2), 299–303.
6. Moulton, C. A., Regehr, G., Lingard, L., Merritt, C., & Macrae, H. (2010). Operating from the other side of the table: Control dynamics and the surgeon educator. *Journal of the American College of Surgeons, 210*(1), 79–86.
7. Moulton, C. A., Regehr, G., Lingard, L., Merritt, C., & Macrae, H. (2010). 'Slowing down when you should': Initiators and influences of the transition from the routine to the effortful. *Journal of Gastrointestinal Surgery, 14*(6), 1019–1026.
8. Hodges, B. D., & Kuper, A. (2012). Theory and practice in the design and conduct of graduate medical education. *Academic Medicine, 87*(1), 25–33.
9. Rieselbach, R., Sundwall, D., Shine, K. (2015). Graduate medical education: The need for new leadership in governance and financing. Health Affairs Blog. http://healthaffairs.org/blog/2015/01/14/graduate-medical-education-the-need-for-new-leadership-in-governance-and-financing/.

10. Anderson, O. R. (1997). A neurocognitive perspective on current learning theory and science instructional strategies. *Science Education, 81*, 67–89.
11. Clark, J. M., & Paivio, A. (1991). Dual coding theory and education. *Educational Psychology Review, 3*(3), 149–210.
12. Moreno, R., & Mayer, R. (2007). Interactive multimodal learning environments. *Educational Psychology Review, 19*(3), 309–326.
13. Van Merriënboer, J. J. G., & Sweller, J. (2005). Cognitive load theory and complex learning: Recent developments and future directions. *Educational Psychology Review, 17*(2), 147–177.
14. Pollock, E., Chandler, P., & Sweller, J. (2002). Assimilating complex information. *Learning and Instruction, 12*(1), 61–86.
15. Vygotsky, L. (1978). *Interaction between learning and development. Mind and society* (pp. 79–91). Cambridge, MA: Harvard University Press.

# Chapter 18
# Patients and Surgical Education: Rethinking Learning, Practice and Patient Engagement

**Rosamund Snow, Margaret Bearman, and Rick Iedema**

**Overview** Patient involvement offers many opportunities for surgical education. This chapter presents ideas and examples to stimulate new ways of designing educational experiences. Patient involvement in medical education is presented as more than storytelling; it is how patients can be active teachers, curriculum developers and assessors. Involving patients may change surgical education and even surgical practice. In particular, patient involvement may shift (1) where the lesson starts and ends, (2) who decides what 'good' looks like, (3) what skills need to be learnt, (4) the role of the patient and (5) how to provide a good surgical service.

*I learn so much from my patients* is a common aphorism in medical education. However, patients can contribute more to surgical education than an opportunity for practice and/or being a role model of fortitude. This potential for patient involvement is mostly unexplored. There is relatively little literature with respect to patient engagement in surgical *practice* and even less literature describing patient involvement in surgical *education*. This presents an opportunity as other areas such as interprofessional education or chronic care education have a longer history of patient involvement [1], and surgical education can build on this work. Moreover, by thinking about surgical education differently, surgical practice itself can be rethought.

---

Sadly, Dr Rosamund Snow passed away in early 2017. Please take a moment to read her obituary in the British Medical Journal (BMJ 2017;346:j850). Rosamund was a compelling thinker, a fierce advocate and a delightful colleague. We shall miss her.

---

R. Snow (Deceased)

M. Bearman (✉)
Centre for Research in Assessment and Digital Learning (CRADLE), Deakin University, Geelong, Australia
e-mail: margaret.bearman@monash.edu

R. Iedema
Centre for Team Based Practice & Learning in Health Care, King's College London, London, United Kingdom
e-mail: rick.iedema@kcl.ac.uk

The 2016 'Vancouver statement' regarding the 'patient's voice in health and social care professional education' outlines a consensus view of current endeavours in this field [2]. According to this statement, the value of the patient voice is seen as being on the 'fringes', and while studies are increasing, patient participation in health professional education has not been studied in a way which demonstrates the impact or lack thereof on longer-term patient outcomes. However, programmes that promote patient participation in education have shown positive benefits for undergraduate students. To give a specific example, Ruitenberg and Towle [3] describe, through detailed qualitative analysis, the value of an inter-professional student group being mentored by a person with a chronic health condition. Studies indicate benefits to patients, such as a more 'positive sense of self' [4] and the reward of making a valued contribution [5]. They also suggest potential harms that can come to patients, if the approaches taken are not carefully considered, such as the negative emotions associated with vulnerability [5]. Finally, there is a distinct deficit in literature regarding patient involvement in advanced training programmes, which is where much of surgical education takes place. Nestel and Bentley [6] describe the contribution of real patient input into designing hybrid simulated patient scenarios for surgical trainees, but there appear to be few other examples.

This chapter presents ideas and examples to stimulate change. We describe what we mean by 'patient involvement' and then suggest how patient partnerships in surgical education have the potential to transform learning. We provide concrete ways of thinking about how this might be done, drawing from practical examples from outside surgery. Finally, we suggest how patient collaboration in surgical education may change surgical practice itself.

## 18.1 Thinking About 'Patient Involvement'

The phrase 'patient involvement' can mean very different things to people, depending on their background, location, and the way they think about the role of patients and clinicians. There are often semantic issues, such as who is a 'patient' and what constitutes a 'lay' perspective [7]. In general, there are a number of frameworks based on the 1969 ladder of citizen participation [8]. These map to stages of patient involvement from none to collaboration arrangements where the power differential between clinician and patient are flattened or reversed. These frameworks are cited in the patient involvement medical education literature [7] and are increasingly part of health service delivery. For example, patient involvement in developing patient safety is noted as aspirational from a report in the National Health Service in England [9]. We present the following, more informal, spectrum of possible responses from healthcare professionals.

*Stage 1: I don't know what patient involvement is*

For some, patients are seen as either recipients of care or participants in research. In this case, 'involvement' or 'engagement' may be interpreted as 'patient understanding' where clinicians try to increase a population's health literacy.

In these cases, information tends to flow from clinician to patient as outlined in Mulsow et al.'s 2012 study of surgical patient consent [10]. This is not what we mean by involvement; when patients are fully involved in education, the patient actively teaches the clinician (as described in Stage 5).

*Stage 2: 'I don't see how patients would have anything to contribute'*

Healthcare professionals listen to patients' histories and symptoms with a view to making decisions (or shared decisions) about an individual's care. In this worldview, the clinician is the expert, and the patient only interprets this expertise in the light of his or her own preferences. The next step is for the clinician to appreciate how much they can learn from patient's practical insights about their own bodies and contexts as well as biomedical knowledge, which in some instances is considerable, for example, after years of disease self-management.

*Stage 3: 'I can see how patients might contribute to learning, but it wouldn't be appropriate to ask them – and who would I ask?'*

Ethical concerns and worries over 'representativeness' tend to dominate this stage of patient involvement, alongside fears that patients asked to teach have an 'axe to grind' and will damage the learning experience. Certainly, a patient in receipt of care should not be made to feel that that care is dependent on agreeing to teach or help with education; but in general, the ethics of working with patients (including issues of payment) is the same as the ethics of working with anyone else.

Representativeness is another thorny issue perhaps left over from thinking of patients as research participants. No patient can represent others, but nor do they need to, any more than any one medical educator is expected to represent all doctors. Similarly, any teacher can have an 'axe to grind'; teacher training can help turn that passion into useful learning outcomes to pass on to the next generation.

*Stage 4: 'Storytelling is a great way to learn. I can get patients to tell the story of their experience'*

Often, the first step in patient involvement is to get a layperson to describe their disease or offer the life context around a biomedical issue. Such patient stories can be very powerful and useful ways of providing information. However, the impact of patient stories can be limited if the rest of the curriculum, and crucially, assessment, do not offer other opportunities for patient involvement. Emotional resonance and patient perspectives are very valuable; however, patients can and do contribute significantly more to medical and surgical education.

*Stage 5: 'Patients can work alongside me to design, deliver and assess education'*

In this chapter, when we discuss patient involvement, we are referring to the idea that patients can be active teachers, curriculum setters and assessors. In this way, patients may actively contribute to, and possibly *change*, surgical education. In the next section, we outline some substantive ways by which patients can contribute to surgical education – and surgical practice. We offer examples, most drawn from outside of surgery, to provide concrete illustrations of the possibilities or issues at hand.

## 18.2 How Patients Can Change Education and Practice

The fundamental point about working with patients is that their contributions will necessarily be different from the clinicians. Patient involvement may alter the clinicians', educators' and organisation's concept of surgical education and surgical practice. In particular, patients may change thinking about:

1. Where the lesson starts and ends
2. Who decides what 'good' looks like
3. What skills need to be learnt
4. The role of the patient
5. How to provide a good surgical service

### 18.2.1 Where the Lesson Starts and Ends

Whenever a set of skills is taught or a particular scenario chosen as a teaching medium, a decision is made about where to start and end, and what counts as the point where learning begins. For example, in simulation environments, learners may enter a room where a mannikin is already prepped and 'unconscious' or where a part task trainer is laid out for a specific skill to be tested. When patients are asked to define the scope of learning, however, they may start earlier and end later; they may focus on how preparation for surgery can change their experience and recovery, and how surgical decisions can impact on their later quality of life. This also means that the life experience of the patient, prior to the treatment at hand, may be more salient in a particular lesson. For example, patients with co-morbidities are likely to provide valuable information on what they need to know to self-manage safely, and what they will need from healthcare professionals while in hospital [11].

We suggest that to concentrate on teaching one part of a surgical pathway is the equivalent of learning to fly a plane without knowing how take off or land; it will work in a simulator, but great damage can be done if the pilot isn't prepared for a real-life journey. For an example of how patient-led lessons can vary, see Box 18.1.

> **Box 18.1: Real-Life Skills: Surgery Derailed**
> People with insulin-dependent diabetes designed and implemented a simulation scenario based on their own experiences. In this scenario, a young man who had lived with type 1 diabetes for 20 years presents to an emergency department with a serious fracture requiring surgery. The actor was trained by patient tutors with type 1 diabetes, who also guided him via in-ear communication during the simulation.

(continued)

**Box 18.1** (continued)

During the scenario, the patient experiences hypoglycaemia and asks to have his bag passed to him so he can self-treat with lucozade. In repeated runs of the simulation, different groups of candidates (junior doctors or final year medical students), aware that he should ideally be kept nil by mouth, refuse to comply with the patient's request. Due to hypoglycaemia, the patient becomes angry and aggressive when asked to test his blood glucose or consider a glucose drip. The scenario usually ends with him untreated and unconscious.

Patients with type 1 diabetes helped debrief the candidates about the issues they had most struggled with. This included the fact that – however much they wished to manage this patient according to textbooks – the optimum solution was to respect the patient's own expertise and allow him to self-treat by simply handing him his bag.

Candidates were asked to consider the following: after 20 years with type 1 diabetes, the patient probably would have self-treated several thousand mild hypoglycaemic episodes already, with skills developed since childhood. He would be extremely familiar with his personal 'hypo' symptoms, so a blood test would be less crucial than it might seem to a clinician, and it would seem pointless to an already angry patient to have a test when symptoms were very clear to him. Hypoglycaemia reactions are enormously varied, and medical textbooks barely touch on the range of responses; those who respond to hypoglycaemia with aggression may actually do physical harm to those they feel threatened by, so pragmatism is vital. Finally, any patient who was left to slip into coma due to a delay in treatment is unlikely to be accepted for immediate surgery in any case – and far more likely to sue.

## 18.2.2 Who Decides What 'Good' Looks Like

Traditionally, senior doctors or medical practitioners who are academics decide what the next generation is assessed on and to what standards. This is based on their own experience, learning and observations. This gives only a partial picture. While an experienced doctor is well placed to check things like technical ability and biomedical knowledge, it is much harder to argue for a medical practitioner's ability to assess patient-centred care, appropriate communication skills or patient comfort. Increasingly, patients are voicing concerns about what 'good' looks like in these areas [12]. In medical schools where patients are involved in assessment, changes have been made to both communication and practical skills requirements for students. See Box 18.2 for an example.

> **Box 18.2: Assessment by Patients**
> At many medical schools in the UK and USA, undergraduate students are taught how to perform vaginal exam by laywomen who use their own bodies to teach [13]. At the University of Oxford, these women, known as Clinical Teaching Associates (CTAs), worked with gynaecological surgeons to co-produce the students' final exam; the CTAs themselves act as assessors. Students are required to insert a speculum into their examiner, who will give them a mark based not only on communication skills but also on the technical skills that make the experience comfortable and safe. In the process, CTAs have changed the standards for consent. Students must not only ensure that the woman is happy for them to begin, they are also required to tell her that they will stop at any time if she becomes uncomfortable or upset – thus empowering the patient and restoring agency and dignity during what can be a very difficult procedure for many women. Prior to the introduction of this exam, students were tested on a plastic pelvic model with no pubic hair or realistic vulva (consent presumed), and a clinical examiner decided from external observation whether the student had performed the task adequately. The patient-led exam is, obviously, a more appropriate test of the skills these young doctors will need in practice.

## 18.2.3 What Skills Need to Be Learnt

A patient does not necessarily distinguish between technical and so-called 'non-technical' skills; moreover, they may not actually be independent of each other in practice [14]. Although communication and 'soft' skills are taught more than they used to be, they are still often part of a separate curriculum, perhaps involving role-playing actors who have no experience of the conditions or situations they are simulating. Practising on a silent mannikin or part task trainer can reinforce this skill split. A student or trainee may be able to perform a technical task such as suturing perfectly as long as she or he doesn't have to talk. Managing this kind of situation takes practice, and yet traditional medical education rarely supports students to acquire these skills. In patient-led scenarios, candidates may be explicitly asked to work on this task-combining, and learn how to negotiate situations where it is more difficult to respond to patients [15]. We provide an example of such a scenario in Box 18.3.

> **Box 18.3: 'She Asked the Questions in the Wrong Order!'**
> In one patient-designed emergency room simulation, candidates were asked to manage a drip and ongoing treatment while the patient herself (a mannikin voiced by a woman who had experienced the situation in real life) regained consciousness and asked questions about what was going on. Students who were very good at explaining a diagnosis in lay language when that was all they were required to do struggled when the patient asked questions in what they felt was 'the wrong order', while they were also trying to monitor vital signs. In particular, they found it hard to answer the question the patient had herself asked at diagnosis: 'will I be normal?' The patients who helped to design these scenarios all reported the enormous impact of doctors' responses to them at diagnosis, including difficult silences or doctors avoiding questions (even if those silences were due to the doctor trying to do something else of practical value).

### *18.2.4 The Role of the Patient*

If asked, patients may choose learning outcomes that have a very practical emphasis and real impact on long-term health. Patients coming out of surgery and returning to self-management are part of the healthcare team and require a handover just as useful and practical as those clinicians are taught to make to their colleagues. Learning how to do such a handover can make the difference between a patient being able to care for themselves and a patient being readmitted or requiring out-of-hours advice in an already hard-pressed healthcare service. This is particularly pertinent to patients who are self-managing chronic conditions, an increasing part of all medical work as the population lives longer and acute diseases become more curable.

Again, using an undergraduate example, Box 18.4 illustrates how patient design of learning can fundamentally shift teaching.

> **Box 18.4: Miscarriage Management**
> In the University of Oxford, women who have experienced miscarriage have designed teaching and assessment alongside clinicians. While the doctors' version of assessment involved a role play with an actress and focussed on communication skills and 'breaking bad news', the patient tutors set a different range of learning outcomes. These included students' ability to give the miscarrying woman enough information and empowerment to handle the subsequent few days safely: discussion of home pain relief, advice on how to tell what was 'normal' in terms of bleeding and pain after natural and/or surgical miscarriage, when to call emergency services and whether the process meant that the woman would actually see her foetus.

## 18.2.5 How to Provide a Good Surgical Service

Patients' role in surgical education is not restricted to training junior surgeons. Patients have relevance for how surgeons understand their role in the overall surgical service. The effect of patient involvement may go beyond focusing on the surgeon's 'soft skills' critical to functional and safe relationship with patients. What matters to patients are not just the safety of the surgery, the quality of surgical treatment and surgical outcomes and the experience of their relationship with their surgeon. What matters also to patients is the impact of the surgical service as a whole on their bio-physiological, psychological and social well-being. To return to the metaphor of the surgeon as a pilot in charge of the entire surgical journey, the surgeon-pilot is skilled not just in flying the plane but also in taking off and landing. That is, a surgeon should ensure the patient is prepared for the surgery and equipped to manage its aftermath. But from a patient perspective 'taking off' and 'landing' refer not merely to ensuring the patient has the necessary information before and after the surgery. These metaphors also refer to the treating surgeon's awareness about what happens with the patient along the entire treatment journey.

Consider Box 18.5 for an insight into the kinds of things this patient (a nurse herself) would see as central to how surgeons are educated.

> **Box 18.5: A Patient's Experience of Fragmented and Inadequate Surgical Care**
> A 68-year-old patient with a background in nursing was admitted to the emergency department with severe abdominal pain. She had surgery and then spent 5 days in the intensive care unit before transferring to a ward. While on the ward, she developed a bedsore and an infection in the wound site. Then on discharge, her treatment plan did not include follow-up by a community nurse, and the patient had to look after this infection herself. She was given no information about how to dress the wound but managed to look after the wound herself, with difficulty. She was very angry about this and wrote a letter of complaint to the hospital. The hospital responded that she was not entitled to community nursing. At her follow-up appointment with the surgeon, medical students were present, and she explained that she felt that she did not have the opportunity to raise the concerns she had about her care. A few weeks later, she developed pain on her side which became severe and continued for 1 year undiagnosed until her GP discovered a hernia. The pain was so severe that the patient felt suicidal at times because she could not function in her everyday life. Her experience of her original surgeon was such that she refused to go back to him and so was referred to another surgeon who found an incisional hernia, a complication of the first surgery. The patient then

> **Box 18.5** (continued)
> underwent a second operation to repair the hernia. Judging from the attitude of her second surgeon, she believes that the first surgeon is still unaware of this complication. The patient feels very angry about both her surgical care and nursing care. She has been given no opportunity to provide any feedback to the hospital or clinicians. She knows there has been no incident report made about the complication of the first surgery. She has not had a meeting granted with the hospital, denying her an explanation about what happened and an apology for what happened. She still has some days when she suffers severe pain.

Were the first surgeon to have practised the 'soft skills' discussed above, some of the problems described in this example might have been avoided. However, what is at issue here too is how the surgeon relates to and identifies with the service she or he provides. In saying this, we do not underestimate the incentives and constraints that bear on how surgeons practise and that perversely tend to limit the control that surgeons have over how their service is run, such as throughput targets, long theatre hours, inter-professional competition for theatre access, specialty control over what happens to surgery patients in intensive care and so forth. These social and environmental factors are far from immaterial to patients, their surgical care and their experiences of this treatment and its outcomes. However, patients are not given the opportunity to engage with any of these aspects of their treatment. These matters may be of great interest to patients who are open to becoming involved in surgical education. Specifically, if were patients like the nurse in the example above were given the opportunity, they might educate surgeons about two overarching issues: surgical service design, and surgeon identity. These are discussed each in turn.

The patient's contribution to *surgical service design* may highlight the importance of balancing official targets and service-internal pressures against continuity and consistency of surgical care for the patient, patient safety, transparency about surgical outcomes (including complications and incidents, and national policy mandating incident disclosure and the 'duty of candour'). These issues pertain not just to how surgeons *and the surgical team* communicate with their patients; they pertain also to how clinical teams structure, coordinate and organise their care processes for individual patients from the moment they enter the service to when (and how) their care is transferred on to primary and/or community care. From the patient's perspective, surgery encompasses clinical, interpersonal *and* organisational skills.

It is important to acknowledge that these service issues bear significantly on *surgeons' identity*. The relevance for surgeons' identity becomes apparent when we acknowledge that, for patients, surgical authority must encompass a surgeon's *personal* sense of responsibility for the organisational, managerial and temporal dimensions of their service. As this entire chapter highlights, the notion of 'surgery' does not apply merely to what happens shortly before, during and shortly after the operating theatre. Critically, for patients, the concept of surgery applies to the entire care experience and ultimate outcomes of the patient's treatment. This in turn broadens 'being a surgeon' from the role of the technician who negotiates an incision on a patient to the role of the professional who has responsibility for how patients journey through the whole trajectory of surgical care. This includes tracking, investigating and learning about mishaps that occur during patients' care. This may require negotiating information provision and activities with the surgical team as well as previous and future care providers.

Put together, the educational contributions that the nurse patient in the example above might want to make foreground the surgeon's responsibility for ensuring their service is safe and for making the patient feel safe. This underlines the notion that the surgeon's overall role and attendant skills are far from mostly 'hard' complemented with some that are 'soft'. The contemporary surgeon's skills are *multivariate*. These multivariate skills correspond to *all* the surgery treatment values that matter to patients and that play a role in their healing. As noted above, these skills include informing patients about what will happen and what has happened, understanding and acting on patients' preferences, organising patients' care as it traverses surgery and any other domains such as intensive care and the hospital ward and taming the constraints and pressures that are inherent in day-to-day hospital work such that patients remain safe and their outcomes are optimal. Engaging with patients at every step of the educational journey, from university student to trainee to senior practice, is critical to shifting the notions of surgeon identity, surgery care and surgical professionalism.

## 18.3 Conclusions

Surgical education has, to date, not engaged with patient involvement in any significant sense. However, the world of education and practice is shifting. Patients are increasingly contributing to the shape of medical education as well as medical practice. This offers huge opportunities for surgical education and surgery as a craft group. If patients are involved, surgical education and practice will inevitably change. In this brave new world, there is a tremendous opportunity to work with patients in designing surgical education and by extension, surgical service. It may be that despite the fears, patients will have better outcomes and be more satisfied with their treatment, if they are included in shaping surgical training and service rather than being the grateful or long-suffering recipient of care.

# References

1. Jha, V., Quinton, N. D., Bekker, H. L., & Roberts, T. E. (2009). Strategies and interventions for the involvement of real patients in medical education: A systematic review. *Medical Education, 43*(1), 10–20.
2. Towle, A., Farrell, C., Gaines, M. E., Godolphin, W., John, G., Kline, C., et al. (2016). The patient's voice in health and social care professional education: The Vancouver statement. *International Journal of Health Governance, 21*(1), 18–25.
3. Ruitenberg, C. W., & Towle, A. (2015). "How to do things with words" in health professions education. *Advances in Health Sciences Education, 20*(4), 857–872.
4. McKeown, M., Malihi-Shoja, L., Hogarth, R., Jones, F., Holt, K., Sullivan, P., et al. (2012). The value of involvement from the perspective of service users and carers engaged in practitioner education: Not just a cash nexus. *Nurse Education Today, 32*(2), 178–184.
5. Lauckner, H., Doucet, S., & Wells, S. (2012). Patients as educators: The challenges and benefits of sharing experiences with students. *Medical Education, 46*(10), 992–1000.
6. Nestel, D., & Bentley, L. (2011). The role of patients in surgical education. In H. Fry & R. Kneebone (Eds.), *Surgical education: Theorising an emerging domain* (pp. 151–168). Dordrecht: Springer.
7. Towle, A., Bainbridge, L., Godolphin, W., Katz, A., Kline, C., Lown, B., et al. (2010). Active patient involvement in the education of health professionals. *Medical Education, 44*(1), 64–74.
8. Arnstein, S. R. (1969). A ladder of citizen participation. *Journal of the American Institute of Planners, 35*(4), 216–224.
9. *Patient engagement in patient safety: A framework for the NHS*. National Health Service England. 2016.
10. Mulsow, J. J. W., Feeley, T. M., & Tierney, S. (2012). Beyond consent—Improving understanding in surgical patients. *The American Journal of Surgery, 203*(1), 112–120.
11. Misra, S., & Oliver, N. S. (2015). Diabetic ketoacidosis in adults. *BMJ: British Medical Journal, 351*, 1.
12. *Patient and public involvement in undergraduate medical education*. UK: General Medical Council. 2009.
13. Jha, V., Setna, Z., Al-Hity, A., Quinton, N. D., & Roberts, T. E. (2010). Patient involvement in teaching and assessing intimate examination skills: A systematic review. *Medical Education, 44*(4), 347–357.
14. Riem, N., Boet, S., Bould, M. D., Tavares, W., & Naik, V. N. (2012). Do technical skills correlate with non-technical skills in crisis resource management: A simulation study. *British Journal of Anaesthesia, 109*, 723–728.
15. Kneebone, R., Nestel, D., Yadollahi, F., Brown, R., Nolan, C., Durack, J., et al. (2006). Assessing procedural skills in context: Exploring the feasibility of an integrated procedural performance instrument (IPPI). *Medical Education, 40*(11), 1105–1114.

# Chapter 19
# The Role of Verbal Feedback in Surgical Education

**Elizabeth Molloy and Charlotte Denniston**

**Overview** This chapter synthesises findings from observational studies of feedback in surgical education and the broader health workplace which illuminate the failure of feedback to do its job in improving trainee performance. Given this state of affairs, we argue for an alternative way of looking at feedback practices in surgical education. The recent frameworks proposed by Boud and Molloy (Assess Eval Higher Educ 38:698–712, 2013), Feedback Mark 1 and Mark 2, reconceptualise feedback as an activity driven by learners rather than an act of 'telling' imposed on learners. Through identifying their own needs, concerns and practice goals, learners are more likely to take on board the strategies raised for improvement. This dialogic form of feedback is more likely to develop self-regulatory capacities in the learner, but this requires displays of vulnerability and establishment of trust between parties. We argue that these dialogic communication strategies, centred around respect, trust and development of 'the other' in terms of reaching their goals, may transfer to surgeons' skills in patient-centred care.

## 19.1 Introduction

There are different forms of feedback in surgical education, all of which play important roles in improving learner performance. The learner uses haptic feedback to alter angles or force during procedures and responds to written comments on their observed performance such as checklists, scale ratings, or qualitative comments as part of workplace-based assessments. The learner also uses verbal, or oral, feedback from patients, peers and supervisors to help improve subsequent performance on tasks.

---

E. Molloy (✉)
The University of Melbourne, Parkville, VIC, Australia
e-mail: elizabeth.molloy@unimelb.edu.au

C. Denniston
The University of Melbourne, Parkville, VIC, Australia

Monash University, Clayton, VIC, Australia

Contemporary literature in surgical education, and broader medical education, points to the importance of the learner-teacher relationship in optimising feedback. The degree of personal trust established, the trust in the assessment/training process itself and the perceived credibility of the teacher all play a role in determining the weight of performance-based information and the likelihood of the learner incorporating changes into practice [2, 3]. The 'educational alliance' [4], building from the notion of therapeutic alliance in psychotherapy, has been described as a potential helpful frame from which to build conditions that support dialogic exchanges. Drawing on this educational alliance and learner-centred feedback literature, this chapter will identify key design features (macro level) that are likely to promote optimal feedback practices in contemporary surgical education. In addition, we will outline the skills (micro level), including prompts, questions and, most importantly, pauses, that may facilitate a learner-centred feedback approach. The following section will describe unique opportunities for feedback in the surgical education context, including advances in simulation and e-learning, as well as highlight problematic aspects of contemporary surgical training that may challenge the enactment of best-practice feedback principles.

## 19.2 What Does Feedback Look Like in Surgical Education?

### 19.2.1 Feedback on Performance in Surgical Training

Despite evidence that feedback is important for learning in surgical education [5], verbal (oral) feedback is seen as one of the most challenging aspects of the trainee experience [6, 7]. Learners across medical education complain that they do not receive enough feedback, and when they do, it is difficult to use [7]. Learners report they are exposed to destructive forms of verbal feedback that can have a negative bearing on immediate learning outcomes and have longer-lasting effects on career [8]. Likewise, educators often anticipate the emotional impact of their feedback on colleagues or trainees and can approach these encounters with trepidation [2]. The feedback 'conversation' often takes the form of a supervisor monologue, albeit a 'mealy mouthed' version of what they really wanted to say to improve trainee performance. Both parties report wearing their 'thickest skin' in the hope that they will get through the feedback encounter with minimal scarring [9]. More specifically, surgical education typically takes place in a complex and high stress context, relative to other settings in medical education [10]. In theatre, there are multiple team members negotiating multiple functions, there is often limited time, interruptions and distraction, and the consequences of making mistakes are high. Feedback may be provided 'on the run' while trainees are performing a procedure or may occur retrospectively, in an informal sense, in between cases or at the end of a day of operating.

Verbal feedback is an essential, but not always utilised component of work-based assessment in surgical training world-wide. Chapters 20 and 21 outline the key approaches of both formative and summative assessment in the workplace, and in both these high and low stakes assessment approaches, feedback is a fundamental ingredient designed to drive trainee improvement. Multisource, or 360 degree, feedback is an increasingly accepted and validated approach to feedback where information from external sources including supervisors, patients and peers is viewed as key to the development of learners [8, 11]. Feedback from multiple sources has been reported to provide learners with a more complete picture of their performance/behaviours, and this 'triangulated viewpoint' can be particularly important given the reported low reliability of self-assessment [12, 13].

Feedback is not limited to face-to-face human encounters. Technology, in the form of high-fidelity simulation, is commonly used in surgical education and may be used to provide performance information to learners. Innovative approaches to feedback have incorporated technology-mediated feedback *with* multisource feedback. For example, Nestel et al. [5] incorporate the Integrated Procedural Performance Instrument (IPPI) in patient-focussed simulations (a hybrid simulation including simulated patients and part-task trainers) with multiple sources of verbal and written feedback. Learners are videoed completing a scenario, and this audio-visual capture and the independent judgements from clinical assessor, learner and simulated patient are collated and provided to the learner to inform decisions about learning and future performance [5]. Audio-visual capture via Google Glass is another mechanism used to support learner self-evaluation and the feedback conversation between educator and learner by providing visual evidence of performance [14]. As these examples demonstrate, there are many ways in which feedback can be sought and used in surgical education to benefit the learner. Although trainees and surgeons are encouraged to seek feedback from multiple sources, including from video recordings, simulators, patients and peers, the 'weight' or credibility they ascribe to the 'source of the feedback' will affect how they hear and use the information [3, 15]. Technology might be seen as a means to gather information about performance, but conversations about performance, including strategies for improvement, are still crucial for consolidation and advancement of learning.

## *19.2.2 Problematic Aspects of Feedback in Surgical Education*

### 19.2.2.1 Changing Nature of Surgical Education: Knowing the Trainee

The stresses inherent in surgical education are well documented [16, 17], and the role of supervision can add to these demands in the workplace. With more trainees in the health care system, it is challenging for supervisors to make assumptions about learners' prior educational experiences and skill levels. This can make task selection more challenging, as well as decision-making relating to how much direct supervision is required [18]. Shorter rotations also make it harder for supervisors to get to know the trainee and therefore tailor feedback to their needs. A recent study by Ong, Dodds and Nestel [19] highlighted that surgical trainees are not only learning new technical skills but are navigating case variability, operating team interactions and environmental cues and case scheduling, all of which affect learning and performance.

### 19.2.2.2 Feedback Should Be Based on Observed Behaviours But Often It Comes Second Hand

The continuity of the supervisory relationship is being increasingly threatened in postgraduate medical education. Often a learner has multiple supervisors, and often the 'supervisor of training' responsible for feedback delivery or progress decisions has not had many occasions of direct observation of the trainee in practice [20]. This means in feedback conversations that it can be difficult for the supervisors to answer learner's questions relating to the feedback or to provide examples of behaviour.

### 19.2.2.3 Diagnostics Without Strategies

Studies in both surgical education and medical education reveal that feedback information is focused on learner deficits rather than on strategies to improve performance (supervisor derived or collaboratively derived) [6, 7, 21]. Although tools have been developed that encourage planning for improvement such as the SHARP tool 5-step feedback tool for surgery [22], many feedback conversations in practice involve the identification of problems, without strategies to address deficits. This is unlikely to result in positive changes in the learner's next attempt at a similar task [9]. In other words, the 'feedforward' is often lacking.

### 19.2.2.4 Feedback Is Taken Personally, Despite Best Intentions

Even if delivered skilfully with a behavioural focus, information that serves to highlight how performance can be improved (developmental aim) can still be interpreted as overly 'critical'. The feedback can be taken personally by the learner if they are highly invested in the work [2]. As reported by Boud and Molloy [21], 'learners care about their work and they care about how it will be judged' (p. 1).

### 19.2.2.5 Inherent Tension Between Learning and Assessment in Workplace Training

Feedback should be about learner improvement, and many models of feedback encourage learners to articulate their deficits in practice (e.g. questions such as what would you do differently next time? What didn't go well?). The tension for learners in surgical education is that their mentors/senior colleagues are often also responsible for summatively assessing their performance. That is, supervisors often have a gatekeeping as well as a mentoring/developmental role. Learners, when self-evaluating their performance, are much less likely to expose their deficits to an assessor compared with a feedback conversation with a peer or a mentor. Training in medical specialty colleges does not often inspire exposure of deficits, and learners and supervisors need to work together to establish a climate of trust to facilitate honest, helpful performance discussions [20].

#### 19.2.2.6 Intersection Between Bullying and Feedback

Unfortunately, poor interactions between trainees and supervisors of training have attracted widespread attention in recent years. The intersection between feedback and bullying in surgical education and the mistreatment of medical trainees is not a new phenomenon, with reported issues in medical education since the 1990s [23]. In Australia in 2015, the Royal Australasian College of Surgeons (RACS) established an Expert Advisory Group (EAG) to provide advice on strategies to prevent discrimination, bullying and sexual harassment in the practice of surgery in Australian and New Zealand hospitals and in the College [24]. The EAG produced three key areas for action to help change this culture, one of which focuses on surgical education. RACS set forth to improve the capability of all surgeons involved in education to provide effective surgical education based on the principles of respect, transparency and professionalism [25]. One specific goal is to 'equip all surgical educators and supervisors to teach and provide constructive clear and timely feedback' *(goal 2.4)*. The next two sections highlight concepts of feedback design and the educational alliance as a means of 'equipping' educators to move towards achieving this goal.

## 19.3 Emerging Models of Feedback

### *19.3.1 Feedback Mark 1 and 2*

Conceptions of feedback as a practice have started to broaden in higher and professional education. A more recent definition of feedback [18], built on constructivist principles, is:

> Feedback is a process whereby learners obtain information about their work in order to appreciate the similarities and differences between the appropriate standards for any given work, and the qualities of the work itself, in order to generate improved work

Some defining characteristics that emerge from this broader notion of feedback are that feedback is not a single act but rather a *process* that evolves over time and learners are positioned as *agents* who seek the information for their own purposes (rather than recipients of 'news') and that a necessary element of feedback is that the information is *used* to generate new work or behaviour. In essence, this definition of feedback reframes the notion of the practice of feedback (input) around the effects on learners (output). This notion, known as Feedback Mark 1, is not a new one but rather signals a return to the roots of feedback in engineering and biology where the input in the system results in an output [18]. Feedback based on this approach challenges workplace learning cultures where there are established patterns of 'learning as apprenticeship' with accompanying feedback rituals resembling experts telling apprentices what is going right and what is going wrong [7].

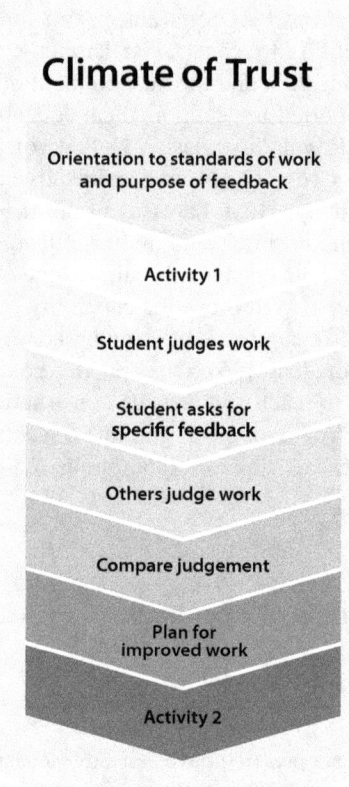

**Fig. 19.1** Feedback Mark 2 in the workplace context. (Based on Boud and Molloy [1] Fig. 2.4)

Feedback Mark 2 as represented in Fig. 19.1 acknowledges that humans have volition and that they may respond differently to the same stimulus (e.g. performance information) based on their circumstance, preferences, prior experience, values and knowledge. The model privileges (1) priming of both trainee and supervisor in terms of what occurs before the task and production of commentary on performance, (2) what occurs in the 'instance' of communication about performance and (3) what occurs subsequent to the exchange, the most important facet being an opportunity to put new behavioural strategies into practice.

Traditionally, the mechanism described as item 2 (the instance of communication post performance) is deemed to be feedback. Feedback Mark 2 acknowledges that the designing of tasks and cues before, during and after performance (or production of work) is integral to the feedback process.

## 19.3.2 Enacting Feedback Mark 1 and 2 in Surgical Education: What Does This Mean for Learners and Supervisors?

In order for learners and supervisors to take up more productive feedback practices, the following processes are recommended:

1. Orientating both parties to the purpose of feedback, this includes signposting that the 'traditional feedback ritual' is going to be challenged.
2. Purposeful design of tasks on placement, e.g. workplace-based assessments, cases with overlapping tasks, i.e. similar surgical techniques required so that strategies for change can be enacted and monitored for degree of success.
3. Supervisor probing learner for 'what should I look for in your performance?', i.e. during the scrubbing process, prior to a surgical procedure, the learner primes the supervisor for aspects of practice that they feel need improvement, similar to the first step in the SHARP tool, which explores learning objectives a priori [22].
4. Sending invitations for learner self-evaluation [6, 26]. This includes pausing for learner responses and potentially following up with more detailed probing for information if the learner deflects self-evaluation.
5. Following the learner self-evaluation with supervisor commentary to validate or challenge the learner's perspective (encouraging development of learner evaluative judgement [27]).

This form of feedback practice has two clear, and mutually informing, aims. The first is to improve performance on task at hand, and the second is to help generate a self-regulating practitioner who seeks information about their performance from the environment (instruments, video, patients, peers and teachers) in an effort to internalise standards for their future practice. These strategies can be enacted across the spectrum of surgical education contexts including the operating theatre, hospital ward and the outpatient setting.

## 19.4 Feedback for Learners and Feedback for Patients: What Are the Parallels?

### 19.4.1 Parallels in Surgical Education and Surgical Consultation

The parallel between educational and therapeutic practice has been drawn elsewhere in medical education literature with Molloy [6] drawing comparisons between patient-centred practice and learner-centred education in an observational study of verbal feedback in the workplace. Similarly, Sommer et al. [28] have used a familiar patient-centred communication skills teaching model (Calgary Cambridge Guides) to highlight the parallel between doctor-patient communication and educator-learner communication. Both these studies have suggested that clinicians' skills in patient-centred communication could be translated to learner-centred conversations on performance (feedback/teaching) and vice versa. We have considered these corresponding principles and present the parallel between Feedback Mark 2 with patient-centred consultation (see Table 19.1).

**Table 19.1** Distinguishing features of Feedback Mark 2 and patient-centred communication

| | Features of feedback mark 2 | What might this look like? | Corresponding feature in patient-centred consultation | What might this look like? |
|---|---|---|---|---|
| A | Orientation to standards of work and purpose of feedback | Explicitly outlining to a trainee the standards they are expected to perform to and that the purpose of feedback is improved performance | Orient the patient to the expectations and the purpose of the consultation interaction | Introduce self and other members of the health care team. Outline roles and the goal for the consultation |
| B | Learner judges their own work | Trainee evaluates own performance of work. Build trainee engagement in self-evaluation | Patient makes judgement on own situation | Invite the patient's perspective on situation |
| C | Learner asks for specific feedback on their work that matters to them most | Trainee seeks specific feedback about performance (e.g. a technical procedure or the flow of his/her history taking effort) | Patient asks surgeon for specific information on their situation that matters to them most | Patient enquires about surgical and non-surgical options based on their perspective or asks about time frames (e.g. 'Will I be walking in time for my son's wedding in June?') |
| D | Others judge work | Surgical educator judges the trainee's performance on the task | Surgeon judges the situation | Surgeon takes in all appropriate information and makes a judgement on the situation |
| E | Compare judgements | Creation of channels for dialogic discussion of judgements | Surgeon and patient compare judgements | Compare patient's perspective with surgeon's perspective |
| F | Generate plan for improved work | Collaborative development of a plan for improved work, clear strategies and time frames | Surgeon and patient make a plan to improve the situation including strategies and time frames | A shared decision is made for the next steps in the patient's journey (i.e. surgical pathway) |
| G | Implementation of strategies in subsequent tasks | Scheduling of future opportunities (e.g. additional case, simulation in clinical skills for the learner to improve work | Implement the plan and reassess situation | Plan is made to schedule future appointments, interventions or referrals to improve patient's health |

The Feedback Mark 2 model shares many similarities with key tenets of patient-centred care [29]: the exploration of the learner/patient goals and perspectives, the sharing of information with the learner/patient and collaboration to generate a plan for the future (e.g. improved performance, improved health). *Patient*-centredness is a requirement of registered doctors, proposed in many codes of practice. Developing these skills in *learner*-centred feedback conversations may facilitate educators' internalisation of this approach to feedback in the surgical setting. The benefits of learner-centred feedback are likely to be threefold. Firstly, by the learners identifying their own needs, concerns and practice goals, they are more likely to take on board the strategies raised for performance improvement. Secondly, the self-identification of deficits in performance has the potential to diffuse the emotional sting of educator-delivered feedback so commonly reported in the literature. Thirdly, this dialogical form of feedback puts the trainee in the position of self-regulator. By committing to self-evaluation, and then receiving comments that validate, challenge or build on their evaluation, trainees are given the opportunity to develop skills of professional judgement [27].

Challenges to this type of health care or education dialogue also exist. For example, when invited to share their own opinion, there are many contextual factors that impede patients from doing so. Likewise, in feedback conversations, it can be difficult for our learners to highlight their 'main concern' or aspect of their performance they would most like comment on. This phase requires both learner and patient to expose some vulnerability to the surgeon; the success of this phases hinges on overcoming this vulnerability. This may involve the educator/clinician taking time to pause and allowing the learner/patient to share their perspective [6]. This moment of space is often avoided with educators/clinicians jumping to Step D in Table 19.1 – offering judgement on the situation [7].

In an observational study of feedback [6], we found that educators often asked for the learners' perspective in a tokenistic manner, hoping they would 'be swift in their appraisal' so they educator could 'tell' the student their own thoughts on the situation. Similarly, communication skills teaching emphasises the seeking of the patient's perspective, because in practice this does not readily occur. Patients and clinicians may leave consultations with differing perceptions of the interaction, with clinicians thinking they have said things and their patients thinking differently. In a study that surveyed both surgical residents and faculty members, Jensen and colleagues [30] found a dissonance between perceptions of feedback provision with faculty members more likely to believe that they had delivered quality feedback than the residents in the study and mirrors findings published elsewhere [7]. This lack of opportunity to compare judgements and collaboratively plan for the 'where to next' impacts the quality of a feedback and patient care conversations [18, 31].

## 19.4.2 Educational Alliance and Empowering Trainees

Just as patients form a therapeutic alliance with their surgeon, trainees could be seen to form an 'educational alliance' with their supervisor [15]. Telio et al. [15] position feedback as a 'social negotiation enacted in the context of a relationship' (p. 934). The Educational Alliance as a framework for feedback relies on the quality of the relationship and the collaboration of both parties and is key to successful feedback interactions in surgical education [32]. The patient-centred care movement has pushed for the empowerment of care seekers. Within this relationship agency is shared, power is shared and the interaction represents a dialogue rather than a monologue. Telio et al. [4] emphasise the importance of a feedback *dialogue* involving two active parties. Active participation of the patient/learner is a key tenet of health care/education. Moving away from a feedback process based on telling, or transmitting information to the learner, Mark 2 and the Educational Alliance advocate for a collaborative discussion of learners' performance. Although this prospect may appear daunting to some, particularly given the current climate of short rotations and multiple supervisors working with trainees [33], evidence is building for a change in how feedback is viewed, and enacted [4]. Systems and processes will need to be adapted for this new conceptualisation of feedback to be adopted [34]. To challenge the historical methods of feedback in surgical education, not only do educators need to equip themselves with feedback skills but need to create an environment to empower trainees to be active in these conversations. Professional development of both parties (feedback theory and practice) and assessment structures that allow for iterative task attempts and formative feedback conversations will be important steps in this cultural change.

## 19.5 Conclusion (and Feedforward)

Feedback in surgical education is challenging for both learners and educators, and the time is ripe for a revolution in feedback practice. This chapter presents an alternative way of conceiving feedback where the learner actively seeks information about specific aspects of their performance and is encouraged to make sense of internal and external judgements, in order to plan for performance on future tasks. We propose that practices informed by the model of Feedback Mark 2 may have the potential to generate more productive outcomes for surgical trainees and colleagues and that these communication strategies may transfer into patient-centred care. Although perhaps a less familiar discourse in surgical education, the authors wish to reconceptualise feedback as a process that is mutually constructed rather than 'provided' and 'accepted'.

An important step in feedback research is to evaluate the effect of training of both learner and educator in 'collaborative feedback' on performance outcomes. The other key research direction is to investigate how the dedicated training in learner-centred feedback impacts on surgeons' mode of communication with other stakeholders-patients, peers and managers within the complex ecology that is the health care system.

## References

1. Boud, D., & Molloy, E. K. (2013). Rethinking models of feedback for learning: The challenge of design. *Assessment & Evaluation in Higher Education, 38*(6), 698–712.
2. Molloy, E., Borello, F., & Epstein, R. (2013). The impact of emotion in feedback. In D. Boud & E. Molloy (Eds.), *Feedback in higher and professional education* (pp. 50–72). London: Routledge.
3. Watling, C., Driessen, E., van der Vleuten, C. P., & Lingard, L. (2012). Learning from clinical work: The roles of learning cues and credibility judgements. *Medical Education, 46*(2), 192–200.
4. Telio, S., Ajjawi, R., & Regehr, G. (2015). The "educational alliance" as a framework for reconceptualizing feedback in medical education. *Academic Medicine: Journal of the Association of American Medical Colleges, 90*(5), 609–614.
5. Nestel, D., Bello, F., & Kneebone, R. (2013). Feedback in clinical procedural skills simulations. In D. Boud & E. Molloy (Eds.), *Feedback in higher and professional education* (pp. 140–157). London: Routledge.
6. Molloy, E. (2009). Time to pause: Feedback in clinical education. In C. Delany & E. Molloy (Eds.), *Clinical education in the health professions* (pp. 128–146). Sydney: Elsevier.
7. Sender Liberman, A., Liberman, M., Steinert, Y., McLeod, P., & Meterissian, S. (2005). Surgery residents and attending surgeons have different perceptions of feedback. *Medical Teacher, 27*(5), 470–472.
8. Archer, J. C. (2010). State of the science in health professional education: Effective feedback. *Medical Education, 44*(1), 101–108.
9. Molloy, E., & Boud, D. (2013). Changing conceptions of feedback. In D. Boud & E. Molloy (Eds.), *Feedback in higher and professional education* (pp. 11–33). London: Routledge.
10. Arora, S., Hull, L., Sevdalis, N., Tierney, T., Nestel, D., Woloshynowych, M., et al. (2010). Factors compromising safety in surgery: Stressful events in the operating room. *American Journal of Surgery, 199*(1), 60–65.
11. Sargeant, J., Armson, H., Chesluk, B., Dornan, T., Eva, K., Holmboe, E., et al. (2010). The processes and dimensions of informed self-assessment: A conceptual model. *Academic Medicine, 85*(7), 1212–1220.
12. Eva, K. W., & Regehr, G. (2005). Self-assessment in the health professions: A reformulation and research agenda. *Academic Medicine, 80*(10), S46–S54.
13. Kruger, J., & Dunning, D. (1999). Unskilled and unaware of it: How difficulties in recognizing one's own incompetence lead to inflated self-assessments. *Journal of Personality and Social Psychology, 77*(6), 1121–1134.
14. Tully, J., Dameff, C., Kaib, S., & Moffitt, M. (2015). Recording medical students' encounters with standardized patients using Google glass: Providing end-of-life clinical education. *Academic medicine: journal of the Association of American Medical Colleges., 90*(3), 314–316.
15. Telio, S., Regehr, G., & Ajjawi, R. (2016). Feedback and the educational alliance: Examining credibility judgements and their consequences. *Medical Education, 50*(9), 933–942.
16. Arora, S., Sevdalis, N., Nestel, D., Woloshynowych, M., Darzi, A., & Kneebone, R. (2010). The impact of stress on surgical performance: A systematic review of the literature. *Surgery, 147*(3), 318–330 30 e1–6.

17. Campbell, D. A. J., Sonnad, S. S., Eckhauser, F. E., Campbell, K. K., & Greenfield, L. J. (2001). Burnout among American surgeons. *Surgery, 130*, 695–702.
18. Boud, D., & Molloy, E. K. (Eds.). (2013). *Feedback in higher and professional education.* London: Routledge.
19. Ong, C. C., Dodds, A., & Nestel, D. (2016). Beliefs and values about intra-operative teaching and learning: A case study of surgical teachers and trainees. *Advances in Health Sciences Education: Theory and Practice, 21*(3), 587–607.
20. Castanelli, D. J., Jowsey, T., Chen, Y., & Weller, J. M. (2016). Perceptions of purpose, value, and process of the mini-clinical evaluation exercise in anesthesia training. *Canadian Journal of Anesthesia/Journal Canadien D'anesthésie, 63*(12), 1345–1356.
21. Molloy, E., & Boud, D. (2013). Seeking a different angle on feedback in clinical education: The learner as seeker, judge and user of performance information. *Medical Education, 47*(3), 227–229.
22. Ahmed, M., Arora, S., Russ, S., Darzi, A., Vincent, C., & Sevdalis, N. (2013). Operation debrief: A SHARP improvement in performance feedback in the operating room. *Annals of Surgery, 258*(6), 958–963.
23. Major, A. (2014). To bully and be bullied: Harassment and mistreatment in medical education. *The Virtual Mentor: VM, 16*(3), 155–160.
24. Expert Advisory Group. Advising the Royal Australasian College of Surgeons on discrimination, bullying and sexual harassment 2015. Available from: https://www.surgeons.org/media/22045685/EAG-Report-to-RACS-Draft-08-Sept-2015.pdf.
25. Royal Australasian College of Surgeons. Building respect, improving patient safety 2015. Available from: https://www.surgeons.org/media/22260415/RACS-Action-Plan_Bullying-Harassment_F-Low-Res_FINAL.pdf.
26. Johnson, C. E., Keating, J. L., Boud, D. J., Dalton, M., Kiegaldie, D., Hay, M., et al. (2016). Identifying educator behaviours for high quality verbal feedback in health professions education: Literature review and expert refinement. *BMC Medical Education, 16*(1), 96.
27. Tai, J., Canny, B., Haines, T., & Molloy, E. (2015). Building evaluative judgement through peer-assisted learning: Opportunities in clinical medical education. *Advances in Health Sciences Education, 21*, 659–676.
28. Sommer, J., Lanier, C., Perron, N. J., Nendaz, M., Clavet, D., & Audétat, M.-C. (2016). A teaching skills assessment tool inspired by the Calgary–Cambridge model and the patient-centered approach. *Patient Education and Counseling, 99*(4), 600–609.
29. Mead, N., & Bower, P. (2000). Patient-centredness: A conceptual framework and review of the empirical literature. *Social Science & Medicine, 51*(7), 1087–1110.
30. Jensen, A. R., Wright, A. S., Kim, S., Horvath, K. D., & Calhoun, K. E. (2012). Educational feedback in the operating room: A gap between resident and faculty perceptions. *American Journal of Surgery, 204*(2), 248–255.
31. Shay, L. A., & Lafata, J. E. (2014). Understanding patient perceptions of shared decision making. *Patient Education and Counseling, 96*(3), 295–301.
32. Ross, S., Dudek, N., Halman, S., & Humphrey-Murto, S. (2016). Context, time, and building relationships: Bringing in situ feedback into the conversation. *Medical Education, 50*(9), 893–895.
33. Pugh, D., & Hatala, R. (2016). Being a good supervisor: it's all about the relationship. *Medical Education, 50*(4), 395–397.
34. Wearne, S. (2016). Effective feedback and the educational alliance. *Medical Education, 50*(9), 891–892.

# Chapter 20
# The Role of Assessment in Surgical Education

P. Szasz and T. P. Grantcharov

**Overview** As competency-based medical education (CBME) continues to infiltrate postgraduate training, the focus among educators and researchers has shifted toward trainee assessment. Summative assessments are those from which consequences arise for both the trainee and training program. The main intent of summative assessments is to differentiate between different trainee states. Thus psychometric rigor must be at the center of such assessments to ensure defensible results. While no model has been created specifically to design such assessments, the evidence-centered assessment design (ECD) framework can be adapted to serve this purpose. Furthermore, there is published literature which outlines the criteria for "good" assessments – which taken together can serve a great starting point in the creation of summative assessments. Although progress has been made to date, the current summative assessments have limitations. As such more evidence is needed to support the interpretation of the results of such assessments.

## 20.1 Introduction

As competency-based medical education (CBME) continues to infiltrate postgraduate training, the focus among educators and researchers has shifted, albeit slowly, toward trainee assessment [1, 2]. Assessment can broadly take on two forms, formative and summative [3, 4]. Formative assessments, as discussed in Chap. 19, are used to improve trainee learning in various domains through appropriate feedback and the development of a student-teacher relationship [3–5]. Summative assessments on the other hand are used to evaluate and judge what trainees have learned to date [2, 3]. In this chapter, our focus will be on summative assessments. First, we will outline their purpose and compare/contrast them to their formative assessment counterparts. We will then discuss general design and evaluation strategies to ensure

P. Szasz (✉) · T. P. Grantcharov
University of Toronto, Toronto, ON, Canada
e-mail: peter.szasz@utoronto.ca; GrantcharovT@smh.ca

that appropriate results are obtained at the time of these summative assessments. Finally, we will examine how they are currently utilized in surgical education, with a conclusive focus on future directions to address some of the existing limitations.

## 20.2 Summative Assessments

Summative assessments, alternatively called high-stakes assessments, are those from which consequences arise for both the trainee and training program [1–3]. For the most part, summative assessments are carried out infrequently at the completion of a postgraduate year (PGY), at the transition in resident standing (i.e., from a junior to senior level trainee), or at the time of specialty/subspecialty certification [2]. These types of assessments can take on many forms, but they are usually formalized and standardized either written, oral, or based on clinical performance [3]. Examples of summative assessments during postgraduate training include part 3 of the United States Medical Licensing Examination (USMLE) and part 2 of the Medical Council of Canada Qualifying Examination (MCCQE) [6, 7], while examples of summative assessments at the completion of training include the American Board of Surgery (ABS) and the Royal College of Physicians and Surgeons of Canada (RCPSC) certification examinations [8, 9]. The main intent of summative assessments is to differentiate between different trainee states, be it pass/fail or competent/noncompetent [2, 3]. These assessments can then inform decisions about trainees' progression within a residency training program or trainee certification and matriculation into independent practice [2, 3].

Often discussed as two separate entities, formative and summative assessments share some fundamental similarities, are intertwined in practice, and are complex in their own right. One essential difference between them is their underlying purpose, a point that cannot be understated [10–13]. The psychometric rigor focusing on the outcome of formative assessments, which drive learning, is often downplayed with more importance placed on the educational process and effective trainee feedback [10–12, 14]. For summative assessments, however, which evaluate learning, psychometric rigor focusing on the outcome (i.e., competent/noncompetent) is paramount to ensure that assessment results are valid, reliable, and equivalent in order to make defensible decisions [10, 11]. As a result, summative assessments must be designed and implemented using a prescribed approach [10, 15].

## 20.3 Design Strategies for Summative Assessments

While no model has been created specifically to design summative assessments in medicine or surgery, the evidence-centered assessment design (ECD) framework can be adapted to serve this purpose with a particular focus on aspects surrounding the psychometric rigor required of such assessments [15]. This ECD framework has been used successfully to create summative assessments for high school students' course progression and for teacher certification [15–17]. The ECD framework is based on the concept that evaluations/assessments are evidentiary arguments, combining the purpose and content of an assessment into an operational process [15, 18]. It is composed of five domains: (1) *domain analysis*, (2) *domain modeling*, (3) *conceptual assessment framework (CAF)*, (4) *assessment implementation*, and (5) *assessment delivery*, which are built upon in an iterative manner [15].

In the setting of summative assessments, *domain analysis* precisely describes the content/tasks to be assessed, through a review of the available literature, guidelines, and educational standards, with a specific focus on the abilities (knowledge, skill, judgment, communication, etc.) that are required to accomplish this task [15, 18, 19]. The information that is gathered can also be compared to known exemplars of appropriate and exceptional task performance [18, 19]. As this domain requires a focus on an array of specific abilities, early and varied stakeholder buy-in from governing bodies, health-care providers, training programs, staff surgeons, trainees, and patients is crucial [15]. Domain analysis sets the foundation for the overall assessment and the domains to follow [15, 18, 19].

In *domain modeling*, the goal is to come up with an assessment schema (structure of an assessment argument) [15, 18, 19]. In this schema, the abilities described in *domain analysis* (referred to as warrants in ECD) for a particular task are compared to the data to be gathered about a trainee performing that task and data gathered about the assessment situation that together lend credibility to the claim that the trainee can complete the task (i.e., is competent) [15, 18, 19]. Furthermore in *domain modeling*, there should be a focus on alternative explanations that may lead to making a claim about a trainee that is inappropriate [15, 18]. This can be a result of either the assessment failing to induce the targeted abilities required of a particular task or the requirement to utilize abilities to complete the task, which are beyond the target level of the summative assessment [15, 20]. In *domain modeling*, stakeholders decide on what the assessment is to measure specifically [18].

The *CAF* uses the information from the previous two domains to create an outline for the summative assessment, centering on the assessment context, the instruments that will evaluate the task, and the way the data will be analyzed/utilized [15]. There are a variety of *CAF* models that together may be employed to design the specific task, and while beyond the scope of this chapter, we draw the reader's attention to reference numbers 18 and 19 for more information [18, 19]. Regardless of the models utilized, the results (scores) that arise from the chosen assessment instruments must have substantial evidence to support their interpretation and subsequent use for that particular task, befitting Messick's framework of validity [21–24]. This is also in keeping with the overall notion of the ECD framework, which again views assessment as an evidentiary argument, whereby evidence is collected to support the inferences that arise from the assessment [19]. Furthermore, for summative assessments, the results should be utilized to create criterion-referenced performance standards that provide defensible evidence to differentiate between trainees that are truly competent and those that are not [2, 25–27].

*Assessment implementation* focuses on operationalizing the assessment, with regard to the logistics of employing it into residency training, finalizing assessment techniques, and preparing evaluation materials and assessor training and calibration [15, 18]. Although seen as important, assessor training and calibration is infrequently completed, and this has been documented as a major unmet need in medical education [28, 29]. Downing et al. and Norcini et al. have suggested that such training is imperative and that prescribed formats should be utilized, the specifics of which depend on the type of summative assessment to be undertaken and the error which is most important to mitigate [28–30].

*Assessment delivery* focuses on trainees' completing the assessment, the actual procedures of carrying out assessment scoring, and result dissemination among stakeholders to determine and document whether trainees are deemed competent at the time of this summative assessment [15, 18].

In summary, although not specifically designed for the creation of summative assessments, the ECD framework with its five distinct and iterative domains can be adopted to serve this purpose and aid in creating such assessments within surgical education [15].

## 20.4 Criteria for "Good" Summative Assessments

Building on the design strategies discussed above, Norcini et al. published a consensus document outlining the required criteria for "good" assessments at the 2010 Ottawa Conference [10]. They outline seven such criteria including validity, reproducibility (reliability), feasibility, acceptability, educational effect, catalytic effect, and equivalence [10]. Although the first four of these criteria are well known and accepted in the education literature, as well as being integrated into the design strategies discussed above, the last three require some explanation [10, 15, 18, 19]. Educational effect refers to the assessment encouraging those who are to embark on it, to prepare in a manner that will benefit their education [10]. Catalytic effect refers to the results of the assessment producing feedback that will subsequently improve future performance (primarily relevant in the setting of formative assessments) [10]. Finally, equivalence refers to the need for the same assessment to produce comparable results when administered to trainees across various institutions and assessment cycles [10].

The degree to which each of these seven criteria is important is influenced by (1) the purpose of the assessment (formative or summative) and (2) the perceptions of involved stakeholders (governing bodies, training programs, staff surgeons, trainees) [10]. For summative assessments, the most important criteria are validity, reproducibility, and equivalence, given that defensible decisions will need to arise from such assessments [10]. Although important, feasibility, acceptability, and educational effect are seen as secondary, while catalytic effect is seen as unimportant for summative assessments, except for perhaps influencing a trainee's future educational endeavors [10]. In terms of stakeholder groups, differing criteria are seen as more/less important. For trainees, assessment objectivity is seen as essential, while for training programs and governing bodies, sound resident training and accountability for the performance of these residents as independent practitioners are seen as essential [10]. As such, the most important criteria in the setting of summative assessments are again validity, reproducibility, and equivalence, with specific criteria being more important to some stakeholders compared to others (i.e., acceptability for trainees, educational effect for training programs, and feasibility for governing bodies) [10]. Thusly, for summative assessments, the specific purpose of the assessment, how high stake it is (in-training promotion versus certification), and the interplay of stakeholders must all be taken into consideration when selecting specific criteria to determine whether it is a "good" assessment [10].

## 20.5 Current Summative Assessments in Surgery

Summative assessments in surgery are, for the most part, related to certification examinations taken by trainees at the end of training or in certain cases examinations taken for in-training promotion with a particular focus on knowledge and judgment [8, 9, 31]. More recently, summative assessments have been slowly making their way into performance aspects of surgical training as evidenced by the main panel discussion at the 2015 American College of Surgeons-Accredited Education Institutes (ACS-AEI) consortium and a recent systematic review [32, 33].

The ACS-AEI panel discussion outlined the rationale for summative assessments that are based in simulation and described examples currently used in surgery [32]. Exemplars in general surgery include the Fundamentals of Laparoscopic Surgery (FLS) examination, composed of both technical and cognitive portions, with a focus on basic laparoscopic knowledge and skills, as well as a multi-station summative technical skills examination based on the Objective Structured Assessment of Technical Skills (OSATS), completed by all postgraduate year (PGY) 1 surgical trainees at the University of Toronto [27, 32, 34, 35]. Exemplars in colon and rectal surgery include the Colorectal Objective Structured Assessment of Technical Skills (COSATS), composed of a multi-station technical skills examination taken by fellows concurrently completing the American Board of Colon and Rectal Surgery (ABCRS) written and oral certification examinations [32, 36]. Finally, exemplars in orthopedic surgery include a summative assessment evaluating an arthroscopic Bankart repair (ABR) on a cadaveric shoulder completed by senior level orthopedic trainees [32, 37].

In their systematic review, Goldenberg et al. evaluated absolute standard setting methodologies utilized for procedural assessments, with some discussion revolving around the implications of these findings for summative-type evaluations [33]. Broadly speaking, standard setting is a set of methodologies whereby cut scores on evaluations or examinations are created in a prescribed manner that then allow for the differentiation between those trainees that have met the appropriate standard and are deemed to have "passed" and those that have not (i.e., pass/fail, competent/ noncompetent, etc.) [26]. Several of the included studies' main objectives were to set performance standards for specific assessments that then may contribute to, or serve as, summative assessments themselves [27, 33, 36, 38–43]. The specialties/subspecialties included orthopedic surgery, urology, ophthalmology, general surgery, vascular surgery, and colon and rectal surgery [27, 33, 36, 38–43].

Although progress has been made compared to the paucity of performance-based summative assessments that were available even half a decade ago, the current summative assessments have limitations. These include an almost complete focus on technical performance, with no real assessments focusing on the other competencies within CBME in a summative manner. Additionally, although incorporating several of the criteria required for "good" assessments according to Norcini et al., very few document the design strategies used for their summative assessments [15, 18, 19]. However, this documentation is imperative, for both the psychometric rigor of the assessment and best practice sharing among different surgical specialties attempting to create summative assessments themselves [10, 15, 18, 19].

## 20.6 Conclusions

Based on the limitations identified above, the focus on moving forward should be to both utilize and document the strategies used to design and implement summative assessments into surgical training [15, 18, 19]. Furthermore, ongoing evidence should be sought to support the interpretation of the results of such assessments [10, 21–26]. Finally, with the implementation of CBME into surgical training, assessments need to be designed that can assess the various competencies that are required of trainees, not just medical knowledge/technical performance, the mainstay of "traditional" summative assessments. One possible way to do this is to incorporate narrative/qualitative comments into summative assessments, with strategies previously developed, to ensure these narrative comments also have acceptable psychometric rigor [1, 44–48]. This incorporation of qualitative comments also leads nicely into the work completed by Govaerts et al., who suggest that in complex environments such as surgical education, metrics in addition to quantitative measures for summative assessments should be sought, as learning is not necessarily linear and competence not necessarily fixed [49].

## References

1. Hawkins, R. E., Welcher, C. M., Holmboe, E. S., Kirk, L. M., Norcini, J. J., Simons, K. B., et al. (2015). Implementation of competency-based medical education: Are we addressing the concerns and challenges? *Medical Education, 49*(11), 1086–1102.
2. Holmboe, E. S., Sherbino, J., Long, D. M., Swing, S. R., & Frank, J. R. (2010). The role of assessment in competency-based medical education. *Medical Teacher, 32*(8), 676–682.
3. Epstein, R. M. (2007). Assessment in medical education. *The New England Journal of Medicine, 356*(4), 387–396.
4. Konopasek, L., Norcini, J., & Krupat, E. (2016). Focusing on the formative: Building an assessment system aimed at student growth and development. *Academic Medicine: Journal of the Association of American Medical Colleges, 91*, 1492–1497.
5. Ramani, S., & Krackov, S. K. (2012). Twelve tips for giving feedback effectively in the clinical environment. *Medical Teacher, 34*(10), 787–791.
6. Woloschuk, W., McLaughlin, K., & Wright, B. (2013). Predicting performance on the Medical Council of Canada qualifying exam part II. *Teaching and Learning in Medicine, 25*(3), 237–241.
7. (2014). *USMLE bulletin of information 2015*. Philadelphia: Federation of State Medical Boards of the United States, Inc., and the National Board of Medical Examiners.
8. (2015). *ABS booklet of information surgery*. Philadelphia: American Board of Surgery.
9. (2015). *RCPSC specialty training requirements in general surgery*. Ottawa: Royal College of Physicians and Surgeons of Canada.

10. Norcini, J., Anderson, B., Bollela, V., Burch, V., Costa, M. J., Duvivier, R., et al. (2011). Criteria for good assessment: Consensus statement and recommendations from the Ottawa 2010 conference. *Medical Teacher, 33*(3), 206–214.
11. Rolfe, I., & McPherson, J. (1995). Formative assessment: How am I doing? *Lancet, 345*(8953), 837–839.
12. Schuwirth, L. W., & Van der Vleuten, C. P. (2011). Programmatic assessment: From assessment of learning to assessment for learning. *Medical Teacher, 33*(6), 478–485.
13. Wass, V., Van der Vleuten, C., Shatzer, J., & Jones, R. (2001). Assessment of clinical competence. *Lancet, 357*(9260), 945–949.
14. Pereira, E. A., & Dean, B. J. (2013). British surgeons' experiences of a mandatory online workplace based assessment portfolio resurveyed three years on. *Journal of Surgical Education, 70*(1), 59–67.
15. Mislevy, R. J. (2011). *Evidence-centered design for simulation-based assessment – CRESST report 800*. Los Angeles: The National Center for Research on Evaluation, Standards, and Student Testing (CRESST).
16. Pearlman, M. (2008). The design architecture of NBPTS certification assessments. In R. E. Stake, S. Kushner, L. Ingvarson, & J. Hattie (Eds.), *Assessing teachers for professional certification: The first decade of the national board for professional teaching standards advances in program evaluation* (Vol. 11, pp. 55–91). Bingley: Emerald.
17. Huff, K., Steinberg, L., & Matts, T. (2010). The promises and challenges of implementing evidence-centered design in large-scale assessment. *Applied Measurement in Education, 23*, 310–324.
18. Mislevy, R. J., & Haertel, G. D. (2006). Implications of evidence-centered design for educational testing. *Educational Measurement: Issues and Practice, 25*(4), 6–20.
19. Mislevy, R. J., Steinberg, L. S., & Almond, R. G. (2003). On the structure of educational assessments. *Measurement: Interdisciplinary Research and Perspectives, 1*(1), 3–62.
20. Messick, S. (1994). The interplay of evidence and consequences in the validation of performance assessments. *Educational Researcher, 23*(2), 13–23.
21. Downing, S. M. (2003). Validity: On meaningful interpretation of assessment data. *Medical Education, 37*(9), 830–837.
22. Cook, D. A., & Beckman, T. J. (2006). Current concepts in validity and reliability for psychometric instruments: Theory and application. *The American Journal of Medicine, 119*(2), 166 e7–166 16.
23. Messick, S. (1989). Validity. In R. L. Linn (Ed.), *Educational measurement* (3rd ed.). New York: American Council on Education and Macmillan.
24. Ghaderi, I., Manji, F., Park, Y. S., Juul, D., Ott, M., Harris, I., et al. (2015). Technical skills assessment toolbox: A review using the unitary framework of validity. *Annals of Surgery, 261*(2), 251–262.
25. Schindler, N., Corcoran, J., & DaRosa, D. (2007). Description and impact of using a standard-setting method for determining pass/fail scores in a surgery clerkship. *American Journal of Surgery, 193*(2), 252–257.
26. Norcini, J. J. (2003). Setting standards on educational tests. *Medical Education, 37*(5), 464–469.
27. de Montbrun, S., Satterthwaite, L., & Grantcharov, T. P. (2016). Setting pass scores for assessment of technical performance by surgical trainees. *The British Journal of Surgery, 103*(3), 300–306.
28. Norcini JJ, Holmboe, E.S., Hawkins, R.E. Evaluation challenges in the era of outcomes-based education. Holmboe E.S., Hawkins, R.E. Practical guide to the evaluation of clinical competence. 1st Philadelphia: Mosby; 2008. 1–9.
29. McGaghie, W. C., Butter, J., & Kaye, M. (2009). Observational assessment. In S. M. Downing & R. Yudkowsky (Eds.), *Assessment in health professions education* (1st ed., pp. 185–215). New York: Taylor and Francis.
30. Feldman, M., Lazzara, E. H., Vanderbilt, A. A., & DiazGranados, D. (2012). Rater training to support high-stakes simulation-based assessments. *The Journal of Continuing Education in the Health Professions, 32*(4), 279–286.

31. (2014). *RCPSC objectives of surgical foundations training*. Ottawa: Royal College of Physicians and Surgeons of Canada.
32. Szasz, P., Grantcharov, T.P., Sweet, R.M., Korndorffer, J.R., Pedowitz, R.A., Roberts, P.L., Sachdeva, A.K. (2016). Simulation-based summative assessments in surgery. *Surgery* (in press).
33. Goldenberg, M., Garbesn, A., Szasz, P., Hauer, T., Grantcharov, T. P.(2016). Establishing absolute standards for technical performance in surgery: A systematic review. *British Journal of Surgery* (Submitted).
34. (2016). *Fundamentals of laparoscopic surgery (FLS)*. Los Angeles: Society of American Gastrointestinal and Endoscopic Surgeons (SAGES). Available from: http://www.flsprogram.org/about-fls/.
35. Peters, J. H., Fried, G. M., Swanstrom, L. L., Soper, N. J., Sillin, L. F., Schirmer, B., et al. (2004). Development and validation of a comprehensive program of education and assessment of the basic fundamentals of laparoscopic surgery. *Surgery, 135*(1), 21–27.
36. de Montbrun, S., Roberts, P. L., Satterthwaite, L., & MacRae, H. (2016). Implementing and evaluating a national certification technical skills examination: The colorectal objective structured assessment of technical skill. *Annals of Surgery, 264*, 1–6.
37. Angelo, R. L., Ryu, R. K., Pedowitz, R. A., Beach, W., Burns, J., Dodds, J., et al. (2015). A proficiency-based progression training curriculum coupled with a model simulator results in the acquisition of a superior arthroscopic Bankart skill set. *Arthroscopy: The Journal of Arthroscopic & Related Surgery: Official Publication of the Arthroscopy Association of North America and the International Arthroscopy Association, 31*(10), 1854–1871.
38. Pedersen, P., Palm, H., Ringsted, C., & Konge, L. (2014). Virtual-reality simulation to assess performance in hip fracture surgery. *Acta Orthopaedica, 85*(4), 403–407.
39. Thomsen, A. S., Kiilgaard, J. F., Kjaerbo, H., la Cour, M., & Konge, L. (2015). Simulation-based certification for cataract surgery. *Acta Ophthalmologica, 93*(5), 416–421.
40. Vassiliou, M. C., Dunkin, B. J., Fried, G. M., Mellinger, J. D., Trus, T., Kaneva, P., et al. (2014). Fundamentals of endoscopic surgery: Creation and validation of the hands-on test. *Surgical Endoscopy, 28*(3), 704–711.
41. Tjiam, I. M., Schout, B. M., Hendrikx, A. J., Muijtjens, A. M., Scherpbier, A. J., Witjes, J. A., et al. (2013). Program for laparoscopic urological skills assessment: Setting certification standards for residents. *Minimally Invasive Therapy & Allied Technologies: MITAT: Official Journal of the Society for Minimally Invasive Therapy, 22*(1), 26–32.
42. Beard, J. D. (2005). Education, training committee of the Vascular Society of Great B, Ireland. Setting standards for the assessment of operative competence. *European Journal of Vascular and Endovascular Surgery: The Official Journal of the European Society for Vascular Surgery, 30*(2), 215–218.
43. Teitelbaum, E. N., Soper, N. J., Santos, B. F., Rooney, D. M., Patel, P., Nagle, A. P., et al. (2014). A simulator-based resident curriculum for laparoscopic common bile duct exploration. *Surgery, 156*(4), 880–887 90–3.
44. Ginsburg, S., Eva, K., & Regehr, G. (2013). Do in-training evaluation reports deserve their bad reputations? A study of the reliability and predictive ability of ITER scores and narrative comments. *Academic Medicine: Journal of the Association of American Medical Colleges, 88*(10), 1539–1544.
45. Ginsburg, S., Gold, W., Cavalcanti, R. B., Kurabi, B., & McDonald-Blumer, H. (2011). Competencies "plus": The nature of written comments on internal medicine residents' evaluation forms. *Academic Medicine: Journal of the Association of American Medical Colleges, 86*(10 Suppl), S30–S34.
46. Driessen, E., van der Vleuten, C., Schuwirth, L., van Tartwijk, J., & Vermunt, J. (2005). The use of qualitative research criteria for portfolio assessment as an alternative to reliability evaluation: A case study. *Medical Education, 39*(2), 214–220.
47. van der Vleuten, C. P., & Schuwirth, L. W. (2005). Assessing professional competence: From methods to programmes. *Medical Education, 39*(3), 309–317.
48. Frohna, A., & Stern, D. (2005). The nature of qualitative comments in evaluating professionalism. *Medical Education, 39*(8), 763–768.
49. Govaerts, M., & van der Vleuten, C. P. (2013). Validity in work-based assessment: Expanding our horizons. *Medical Education, 47*(12), 1164–1174.

# Chapter 21
# Entrustable Professional Activities in Surgical Education

**Stephen Tobin**

**Overview** Surgical education and training has evolved considerably within the last 10 years. During this time, surgical colleges and many surgeons involved with postgraduate surgical education have recognized the need for direct observation, constructive feedback and linked summative assessments for residents and surgical trainees. There are many tasks that surgeons perform as part of their professional role. It cannot be simply about operative surgery. As trainees progress towards becoming surgeons, entrustable professional activities (EPAs) provide suitable constructs for trainees and their surgical teachers and supervisors. As the trainee employs their competencies within these clinical tasks, their progress can be observed, assessed and discussed. Suitable levels of supervision can be matched to the level of performance, so that patient care remains safe and quality outcomes are obtained. Feedback and assessment are supported by EPAs in the workplace.

## 21.1 Introduction

Entrustable professional activities (EPAs) were proposed in 2005 by Prof Olle ten Cate [1] in a perspective article and subsequently reported in 2007 [2]. The concept has shown itself to build well on competency-based medical education (CBME), linking the competencies to the trainee's performance at work. As introduced by ten Cate, EPAs also provide structure around the traditional apprenticeship model, where tasks are learned from experts or masters in their fields. These

---

S. Tobin (✉)
Royal Australasian College of Surgeons, Melbourne, VIC, Australia

University of Melbourne, Melbourne, VIC, Australia

Deakin University, Geelong, VIC, Australia

University of Notre Dame (Sydney), Sydney, NSW, Australia

Central Highlands Surgeons, Ballarat, VIC, Australia
e-mail: apstobin@icloud.com

apprenticeships required knowledge about the field, taught and learned in the field. There has often been a technical aspect to such workers, who in turn are defined by their jobs. This chapter is about use of EPAs in surgical education.

The structure of the EPA process, whatever is the clinical task, needs description. The activity should be able to be described within context, for example, the urgency. Performance requires certain knowledge, skills and attitudes, thus utilizing the competencies learned by the doctor. These components of the EPA may become criteria and methods to assess progress. Once the EPA is observed and performed competently on several (6–10) occasions, then independent performance can be entrusted.

EPAs are well suited to the postgraduate medical training environment, although some of the original work involved Dutch operating theatre technical assistants [3] for whom it was considered there were 5–7 essential tasks for their work role. For medicine with its many specialties, ten Cate has proposed that there are around 15–20 core EPAs for each medical specialty. Development has varied around the world, from the encyclopaedic lists defining paediatrics in the USA [4] to the 140 EPAs used in both training and formal summative assessment in psychiatry training in Australia and New Zealand [5].

EPAs can also be 'nested', meaning that within one major work, the task performed within a particular specialty can be subdivided into smaller EPAs at different levels. For example, the management of normal pregnancy could include competent performance of the antenatal care, as well as the common conditions that may develop during pregnancy, and the common problems related to delivery [6, 7].

Levels of supervision are described (Table 21.1), to match the observed level of trainee performance, with eventual independent safe practice and an ability to supervise the novice. They thus reflect true CBME, allowing safe development within the several major disciplines contained in one medical specialty. They allow consideration of competency utilization and demonstration, so that constructive feedback looks at these areas, as performance improves. EPAs also fit well with an observed global assessment, providing consideration of areas for improvement.

Within surgery, with its combination of principle-based practice and technical skills, it is proposed that most specialties could be described by 15–20 EPAs. RACS has taken this approach by defining 18 'key clinical tasks' to be achieved in the pre-vocational years (Table 21.2): these map to the performance necessary for the entry-level surgical trainee [8]. Early discussions have commenced within speciality training programs associated with RACS about use of EPAs within surgical training

**Table 21.1** Levels of supervision (From ten Cate [6])

| Level of supervision |
|---|
| 1. Observing the activity |
| 2. Acting with direct (proactive) supervision |
| 3. Acting with reactive supervision (within minutes) |
| 4. Acting unsupervised (under remote oversight) |
| 5. Providing supervision to juniors |

**Table 21.2** Key clinical tasks (JDocs) = EPAS for entry-level surgical trainees into RACS Surgical Education and Training (SET)

| | |
|---|---|
| 1 | Lead a ward round |
| 2 | Manage the acutely 'sick' patient |
| 3 | Consultation of the new patient |
| 4 | Organize the patient's operating room journey |
| 5 | Plan an operating list |
| 6 | Be a team member for CPR or trauma calls |
| 7 | Lead multidisciplinary team discussion |
| 8 | Present actively at morbidity and mortality meeting |
| 9 | Conduct empathic 'bad news' discussion |
| 10 | Provide perioperative medical management of the surgical patient |
| 11 | Demonstrate competence with an index procedure required for selection into SET |
| 12 | Supervise and delegate tasks to junior doctors and medical students |
| 13 | Regularly teach relevant surgery to the attached medical students |
| 14 | Develop a clinical research project suitable for major presentation or publication |
| 15 | Display appropriate professional behaviour and address poor behaviours |
| 16 | Participate in open disclosure process |
| 17 | Use ISBAR or other structured approach for handovers and clinical requests |
| 18 | Discharge the patient from in-patient care |

with pilots underway and planned. Proposed use towards the end of training and final fellowship eligibility will relate to the expected work performance of the newly graduated surgeon.

Comprehensive literature has been published since 2007 – notably this is rarely critical. The literature has considered EPAs favourably, with many reviewed articles considering and reporting implementation. As they have considerable face validity, EPAs have been used as alternatives to previous WBA approaches, to complement existing programs as well as for program renewal. The literature does not compare the impact of EPAs with other approaches. Limitations reported relate to the construct approach and the need for faculty and trainee engagement [9].

## 21.2 EPAs and Surgical Residencies

Selection into surgical training differs around the world, both in method and in timing in terms of postgraduate year at time of entry. The length of training programs varies as well – typically 4–8 years are involved. Most programs are still significantly time-framed; purely competency-based training programs have not commonly been sustainable except in Ontario [10].

During surgical residency, technical skill development – how to operate – has previously dominated traditional surgical thinking. Fortunately, CBME has influenced programs so becoming a surgeon involves far more than developing independence with operative surgery alone. EPAs can assist with work-based assessment prior to training, during training and at the completion of training.

## 21.3 EPAs for Readiness for Surgical Training

Selection into surgical training can occur within the completion of medical school year (USA, Canada), during the first one to two intern years or later than that. In Australia and New Zealand, selection typically occurs in PGY4-6, meaning commencement of training in PGY5-7. In Britain, selection often occurs in PGY4 (after the two foundation years there are two core years). The work performance of the just-graduated doctors will be less than that of the doctor with 4–6 years of clinical work behind them.

Graduation from medical school, thus transition to the clinical work of the PGY1 resident (the intern year in some countries), has been usefully described by EPAs in the USA [11] and Canada [12]. The AAMC has mapped 13 EPAs for incoming residents (Table 21.3). These speak to the generic competencies the new doctor should have, described in terms of clinical work. The new doctor is thus entrusted to be able to perform these with Level 3 (of Table 21.1) supervision, in theory, on day 1 of residency (the 1st day of medical practice).

Performance of the newly graduated doctor comes into focus in the USA in July of each year, the so-called July effect. To improve the new surgical resident's performance around the transition from medical school, many residency programs have dedicated (extra) training between April and June for the graduating medical students [13]. Others have 'boot camps' or intensive training and orientation pro-

Table 21.3 13 AAMC core EPAs for entering residency [10]

| |
|---|
| EPA 1: Gather a history and perform a physical examination |
| EPA 2: Prioritize a differential diagnosis following a clinical encounter |
| EPA 3: Recommend and interpret common diagnostic and screening tests |
| EPA 4: Enter and discuss orders and prescriptions |
| EPA 5: Document a clinical encounter in the patient record |
| EPA 6: Provide an oral presentation of a clinical encounter |
| EPA 7: Form clinical questions and retrieve evidence to advance patient care |
| EPA 8: Give or receive a patient handover to transition care responsibility |
| EPA 9: Collaborate as a member of an interprofessional team |
| EPA 10: Recognize a patient requiring urgent or emergent care and initiate evaluation and management |
| EPA 11: Obtain informed consent for tests and/or procedures |
| EPA 12: Perform general procedures of a physician |
| EPA 13: Identify system failures and contribute to a culture of safety and improvement |

grams early in that first year. Within these approaches, there is room for assessment of skill sets, so EPAs can be informative within these early programs. To use EPAs in these early days with formative intent seems appropriate followed by observation and supervision as clinical work gets underway. Boot camps are about the attendees achieving competent performance across a range of activities to enable similar safe performance, and then built upon, when starting work. Thus, EPAs for senior medical students, supplemented by boot camps, can assist with assessment of readiness for that first year of residency, should that be the preferred national approach.

When the surgical aspirant is selected after some years of clinical work, it is seen that their performance at work is at a higher level: these doctors are able to use their knowledge, skills and attributes at work, performing many tasks across the day. EPAs for this group can inform progress within the pre-surgical years and determine readiness for surgical training. EPAs can be used as part of term assessments for these doctors in their hospital workplaces as well. All of these can be observed and assessed – for that end of term assessment or to inform authentic reference writing for competitive selection processes.

Research with just-commenced surgical trainees (typically PGY5) has shown the relevance of clinical tasks to the clinical role as an early postgraduate resident as well as surgical trainee. The tasks make up much of the work role as the medical identity of the surgical resident/trainee develops – using EPA-style constructs around these tasks for authentic work-based assessment is considered valid and meaningful [14]. Working towards competency, and then developing proficiency through experiential learning with suitable supervision, observation and feedback, was well-described and accepted by the just-commenced trainees. Observation and feedback on their performance-assisted improvement enabled competence and identified readiness for surgical training [14].

RACS developed the JDocs Framework [8] to describe competency-based progression during the resident years after medical school that necessarily precede training in surgery or any other medical discipline in Australia and New Zealand. JDocs incorporates the nine RACS competencies that are utilized within SET training and also for surgeons in practice. Suggested levels are mapped, and the competencies are employed in 'key clinical tasks' (EPA-style constructs) that the junior doctor can work towards (Table 21.2). These tasks, in turn, are those expected at commencing SET training, being representative of the surgical trainee's work within the surgical team (unit, firm). Thus achieving these as reliably well-performed – often during the year of selection – marks readiness for surgical training [14] and supports transition into training. Observed performance around these 'key clinical tasks' should also support hospital/unit reports and/or work-based references towards this same selection process. The process of selection into surgical training is an enormous subject outside the remit of this chapter [15].

## 21.4 EPAs to Measure Progress Within Surgical Training

Surgical training, even when theoretically CBME, still tends to have usual or standard training times, as it did in the traditional apprenticeship/fellowship examination years. CBME has the promise of stages of training, with regular assessment based on focused observation, eventually determining readiness for practice [16]. CBME theoretically allows for variation in training time, as some individuals will take longer than 'usual time', and some trainees may reach readiness for surgical practice earlier than usual [17]. CBME intrinsically recognizes any previous related learning, as it demonstrated performance of tasks that can be structured by EPAs. CBME is thus about making the most of the training time periods, not competing with those "time" aspects. Service commitments may impose on the actual finishing date, even if readiness is established.

Should entry into surgical training be early (PGY1-2), then EPAs certainly have a role in these early years, along similar lines to the utility of the JDocs 'key clinical tasks'. As these surgical trainees progress – or for those entering training later – EPAs can measure progress within training. Such EPAs could be those entry-level tasks performed to a higher-level or specialty-specific EPAs linked to unique activities of the specialty.

In Australia and New Zealand, the JDocs 'key clinical tasks', performed to higher levels, still cover much of the generic daily work of surgical trainees. However, the specialty content and the operations that define the specialty become a major part of the trainee's learning, reflecting the specialty as currently practised. So there is room for EPAs to be constructed around the management of specific conditions and/or the specific operations of the specialty. Further, these EPAs can be used for formative feedback for informing or being documented as part of in-training term assessments. It is thought for practical purposes that these should mainly be about the common conditions and the small/medium operations of the specialty. They can be described, and commonly referenced, rather than used for frequent detailed multi-criteria recorded assessments. General surgery are piloting some in 2017–2018 [18], and paediatric surgery are referencing JDocs for the provisional first year of paediatric surgical training [18]. EPAs are being developed to align with major curriculum reviews in some surgical specialties, linking the curriculum through work-based assessment to the clinical specialty workplace. Plastic and reconstructive surgery are developing new curriculum with this approach in mind.

Thus individual performance across a group of EPAs can inform progress across the years of SET training, becoming the stages of training within some specialties. EPAs, being constructed around common work activities, arguably have more face validity than the deconstruction that is perceived about miniCEX and DOPS assessments. These comments do not claim that EPAs should replace other forms of WBA. It may be that once explained EPAs are seen to have more authenticity: thus clinical work is being assessed – service and training are intertwined.

The role of surgical supervisors and trainers, to observe and supervise the surgical residents/trainees performing clinical work, is under constant scrutiny. EPAs, once explained to these supervisors and trainers, should have much appeal, as the holistic nature of an EPA generally maps well to the clinical work tasks required, as well as providing description of aspects of the clinical educational construct. As such, what is implicit to the experienced surgical educator can now be explicit to both teacher and trainee. The competency detail (that supports the EPA) can be useful for constructive feedback and identifying next steps for improvement and progress. Faculty development is thus required for surgical educators about the principles for surgical educators, as well as the specifics of EPAs. Thus EPAs suitably applied should facilitate progress according to CBME principles within the time-based service.

## 21.5 EPAs for Completion of Surgical Training

Within surgical training programs, certification of completion of training usually involves a combination of work-based assessment through documented summative term/rotation assessments and examination. These rigorous examinations are definitely high stakes and may involve real patients with clinical problems as well as simulated patient scenarios. Operative performance is rarely directly assessed although there have been early attempts related to completion of general surgery training in the USA in a cohort then commencing fellowships in colorectal surgery. Recent literature has noted that technical performance can be reasonably assessed, building on the procedure-based assessment (PBA) approach first described within English surgical training [19]. This may have come to have application within training programs and at the time of certification [20]. The technical aspects can be built into EPAs around managing common surgical conditions according to the specialty.

In some surgical programs, EPAs have been built into training. The author has also presented within Australia and New Zealand on the concept of EPAs being required for eligibility to present for fellowship examination. These should reflect the work performance of the competent to proficient newly graduated consultant surgeon. Defining this work performance means constructing suitable EPAs for initial practice – as the examination provides certification, these EPAs enabling presentation for the fellowship should be the same as those required for initial practice. The list of proposed EPAs is provided in Table 21.4.

Some specialties will pilot some of these commencing in 2018. As surgeons do operations, the concept of proficient performance of smaller operations and procedures, competent performance of medium-level operations, competent management of common emergency conditions and an ability to recognize and manage the complex problems including referral to – or requesting assistance/advice from – senior surgeons, has so far had a wide appeal. Some of the EPAs also describe – maybe scaffold – the transition to consultant practice.

**Table 21.4** Proposed EPAs related to certification (presented by author at RACS Annual Scientific Congress, Brisbane, Australia, May 2016)

| |
|---|
| Manage a complaint |
| Supervise a trainee |
| Chair MDM, morbidity and mortality meeting |
| Advocate for minority group/community health |
| Lead a QI/quality and safety project |
| Demonstrate/lead an education project |
| Demonstrate research skills with suitable research project |
| Perform independently medium-level operation (within specialty) independently including pre- and post-operative care |
| Manage/refer suitably complex clinical problem (within specialty) |

## 21.6 Other Uses: Postsurgical Training

Surgeons recognize that practice-based experiential learning occurs throughout their careers. Much of this is careful evolution of knowledge, skills and aptitudes related to both the specialty and the location of practice. CPD programs, often provided by the surgical colleges, increasingly mention 'scope of practice' – this may be about sub-specialization or about operations performed versus those not. Therefore, EPAs being about formal learning and demonstrated performance (trainee/resident to surgeon/consultant) may be useful on the post-fellowship consultant years. However, ten Cate has raised this use across the medical education/practice continuum in international presentations including the concept of CBMP - "competency-based medical practice".

However, should a specialty undergo a major change related to its knowledge base, the management of some conditions or the allied operative management, then EPAs could be used to document the newly learned knowledge or skills. For operations, simulation and workshops, followed by proctored or supervised introduction, will often be the sensible approach. Some institutions already demand documented competent performance: EPAs may have a role to be determined in this area.

## 21.7 Conclusions

One must acknowledge the work of Prof Olle ten Cate in considering the positive aspects of the apprenticeship model, blended with the need for graded supervision around clinical work (including operations and procedures), and utilizing the competencies that the doctor brings to support clinical performance. Commencing with theatre technicians, iterative development of EPAs with obstetrics/gynaecology was then published. The detail involved has subsequently varied depending on specialty and jurisdictional context.

Surgery, with the prominence of judgement, clinical decision-making and operations, is an appropriate field for thoughtful EPA development. The clinical tasks involved with surgery often have timelines as well as observed outcomes: the trainee's emergent process within all of this should be observable and combined with suitable level of supervision. EPAs can give structure to what is otherwise sometimes intuitive or even global assessment [21]. The structure then facilitates feedback enabling explicit dialogue about next steps related to the clinical task. EPAs can give (demand) rigour around all of this, so entrustment to independent performance is an important step that should be discussed, not just inferred.

Surgical education occurs within the complex hospital system, where there is clinical service and surgical education occurring simultaneously. The author does not see 'doing the job' and 'learning as a trainee' as separate events. The supervision aspect of EPAs reinforces this, noting that good quality patient outcomes must be the common aim. General application of EPAs has been recently described by ten Cate et al. [22].

Surgeons as supervisors and trainers often spend extra time around the matters above. The author believes, as does ten Cate, that around 15–20 EPAs are useful for many surgical contexts. JDocs describes 18 for prevocational doctors to work towards, being the generic tasks for the surgical trainee role that follows if selected. In-training EPAs can then be about relevant tasks such as independent operating after hours or managing specialty-specific conditions.

Late training EPAs can be mapped towards readiness for practice as a surgeon – around ten (both generic and specialty-specific) could suitably be used to sample performance. Certification through examination should be linked to these same EPAs. Note however that the outcomes of surgical training programs are far more than ten EPAs – current systems of end-of-term assessment, logbooks and global rating by the relevant surgical unit or department should stand. Thus EPAs can usefully supplement what is currently done.

In summary, EPAs do not cover everything in surgical education. However, if thoughtfully developed, they can provide the basis for meaningful in-training assessments: it is considered that they could replace or supplement some of the approaches currently used. As described in this chapter, they can also assist with 'readiness' for training: evaluation of the JDocs framework will provide some evidence as these current prevocational doctors enter surgical and other specialty training. Projects planned around late stages of surgical training, certification and commencing consultant work will also provide much information.

## References

1. Ten Cate, O. (2005). Entrustability of professional activities and competency-based training. *Medical Education, 39*, 1176–1177.
2. Ten Cate, O., & Scheele, F. (2007). Competency-based postgraduate training: Can we bridge the gap between theory and clinical practice? *Academic Medicine, 82*, 542–547.

3. Ten Cate, O. (2006). Trust, competence and the supervisor's role in postgraduate training. *BMJ, 333*, 748–751.
4. Carraccio, C., & Englander, R. (2013). From Flexner to competencies: Reflections on a decade and the journey ahead. *Academic Medicine, 88*, 1067–1073.
5. Boyce, P., Spratt, C., Davies, M., & McEvoy, P. (2011). Using entrustable professional activities to guide curriculum development in psychiatry training. *BMC Medical Education, 11*, 96 www.biomedcentral.com/1472-6920/11/96.
6. Ten Cate, O. (2014). AM last page: What entrustable professional activities add to a competency-based curriculum. *Academic Medicine, 89*, 691.
7. RANZCP. (2012). EPA handbook. Royal Australian and New Zealand College of Psychiatrists. www.ranzcp.org.
8. RACS: JDocs Framework. (2016). http://jdocs.surgeons.org. Accessed 5 Jul 2018. Learning Outcomes and Professional Standards Royal Australasian College of Surgeons. Accessible at www.surgeons.org & www.jdocs.surgeons.org.
9. Van Loon, K., Driessen, E. W., Teunissen, P. W., & Scheele, F. (2014). Experience with EPAs, potential benefits and pitfalls. *Medical Teacher, 36*, 698–702.
10. Core Entrustable Professional Activities for Entering Residency. (2014). Accessible at www.aamc.org. https://www.aamc.org/initiatives/coreepas/.
11. Touche, C, Boucher, A, the AFMC EPA Working Group. (2016). AFMC entrustable professional activities for the transition from medical school to residency. Accessible at www.afmc.ca.
12. Ferguson, P., Kraemer, W., Nousiainen, M., Safir, O., Sonnadara, R., Alman, B., & Reznick, R. (2013). Three-year experience with an innovative modular competency-based curriculum for orthopaedic training. *Journal of Bone and Joint Surgery American, 95*(21), e166. https://doi.org/10.2106/JBJS.M.00314.
13. Antonoff, M., Swanson, J., Green, C., Mann, B., Maddaus, M., & D'Cunha, J. (2012). The significant impact of a competency-based preparatory course for medical students entering surgical residency. *Academic Medicine, 87*, 308–319.
14. Tobin, S. A. (2015). Could entrustable professional activities (EPAs) improve surgical residency programs in Australasia? Master's Thesis, University of Melbourne.
15. Maan, Z., Maan, I., Darzi, A., & Aggarwal, R. (2012). Systematic review of predictors of surgical performance. *BJS, 99*, 1610–1621.
16. Iobst, W. (2013). Competency-based medical education the basics. Presentation for American Board of Internal Medicine, Duke University.
17. Frank, J. R., Snell, L. S., Cate, O. T., Holmboe, E. S., Carraccio, C., Swing, S. R., Harris, P., Glasgow, N. J., Campbell, C., Dath, D., Harden, R. M., Iobst, W., Long, D. M., Mungroo, R., Richardson, D. L., Sherbino, J., Silver, I., Taber, S., Talbot, M., & Harris, K. A. (2010). Competency-based medical education: Theory to practice. *Medical Teacher, 32*(8), 638–645.
18. Internal communications, RACS, October 2016.
19. Marriott, J., Purdie, H., Crossley, J., & Beard, J. (2010). Evaluation of procedure-based assessment for assessing trainees' skills in the operating theatre. *BJS, 98*, 450–457.
20. Goldenberg, M., Garbens, A., Szasz, P., Hauer, T., & Grantcharov, T. (2017). Systematic review to establish absolute standards for technical performance in surgery. *BJS, 104*, 13–21.
21. Hodges, B. (2013). Assessment in the post-psychometric era: Learning to love the subjective and collective. *Medical Teacher, 35*, 1–5.
22. Ten Cate, O., Tobin, S. A., & Stokes, M. L. (2017). Bringing competencies closer to day-to-day clinical work through entrustable professional activities. *The Medical Journal of Australia, 206*, 14–16.

# Chapter 22
# Revalidation of Surgeons in Practice

Ajit K. Sachdeva

**Overview** Revalidation of surgeons in practice continues to evolve rapidly. Articulating the overall aim of revalidation as adherence to safe standards of practice, this chapter explores common goals and nuanced differences in approaches to revalidation in various countries. The different approaches are a result of disparate regulatory systems and roles of professional organizations. After describing contemporary factors affecting revalidation as an important professional consideration, its relationship to continuing professional development is explored. The author describes two types of revalidation: "Global" and "Focused." The latter relates to changes in the practices of individual surgeons and is illustrated through three case studies. Finally, strategies to support revalidation efforts are proposed.

## 22.1 Background

Myriad strong forces have coalesced in recent years to drive the movement in favor of revalidation of the knowledge, skills, and professional attributes of physicians over the courses of their careers. A variety of regulatory, social, political, and economic factors have sparked interest in this revalidation movement [1]. Satisfactory completion of training and initial certification in a specialty are no longer considered sufficient to ensure delivery of optimal patient care through the long careers of physicians, or to maintain the public trust in the medical profession. Health care delivery continues to evolve rapidly, and sharp focus is being placed on accountability, transparency, outcomes, costs, and value. The patients and the public are playing greater roles in health care decisions. Considerable variability in professional practices and technical skills of physicians has also been documented. A recent study of bariatric surgeons demonstrated wide variability in the technical skills of these surgeons, and poorer skills were associated with worse patient outcomes [2]. In addition, concerns have been expressed about the knowledge base of

---

A. K. Sachdeva (✉)
Division of Education, American College of Surgeons, Chicago, IL, USA
e-mail: asachdeva@facs.org

physicians during the later years of practice. The failure rates on the secure Maintenance of Certification (MOC) Examination of the American Board of Surgery (ABS) were found to increase with every decade beyond surgeons' initial certifications [3]. A number of high-profile adverse events have made major headlines and led to demands for greater oversight of the medical profession [1]. Further, information from licensing bodies has highlighted a number of problems relating to physician performance. Analysis of Information from the Board Action Databank of the Federation of State Medical Boards and surveys of physicians and licensing authorities have revealed that issues relating to quality of care and professionalism were important reasons for adverse actions taken by the medical boards. Communication problems were found to be critical factors in medical errors and in generating consumer complaints to the state medical boards; also, disruptive behaviors of physicians have been identified as a source of major problems in delivering optimal health care [4].

Intrinsic drivers from within the profession have influenced this revalidation movement as well. Motivation of physicians to provide the best possible patient care and to place interests of patients above all else has been founded on laudable principles of professionalism and self-regulation. This has resulted in physician-led efforts to design and implement models for revalidation and to offer continuing professional development (CPD) programs that are aimed at positively impacting physician performance and health care outcomes. Physicians continue to play important roles in addressing shortcomings of health care systems and are taking concrete steps to improve the quality of health care and promote patient safety.

In the United States, several landmark reports have helped to shape the national discourse regarding quality and safety in health care and the need to reform CPD for health professionals. The report from the Institute of Medicine, *To Err Is Human: Building a Safer Health System*, published in 2000, shed light on serious problems relating to medical errors and patient safety in health care, and highlighted the important role of systems in preventing and mitigating the impact of human errors [5]. A subsequent report in 2001 from the Institute of Medicine, *Crossing the Quality Chasm: A New Health System for the 21st Century*, defined six desirable aims for health care [6]. The report recommended that health care should be safe, effective, patient-centered, timely, efficient, and equitable. The need for transparency was also emphasized in this report.

Several other reports have focused specifically on the competencies of clinicians, and on continuing education and professional development. A report from the Institute of Medicine, *Health Professions Education: A Bridge to Quality*, in 2003 defined five competencies that all clinicians should demonstrate [7]. These are provision of patient-centered care; work in interdisciplinary teams; adoption of evidence-based practice; application of quality improvement; and use of informatics. This report also recommended that regulatory boards should require all licensed health professionals to periodically demonstrate their ability to deliver patient care based on these competencies. In 2008, a report from the Josiah Macy, Jr. Foundation, *Continuing Education in the Health Professions*, highlighted the shortcomings of the prevailing system of continuing education for health professionals and recommended that continuing education should be aimed at improving the quality of patient care, ensuring continued competency of clinicians, and demonstrating accountability to the public [8]. The report also recommended development and use of new metrics to assess the quality and effectiveness of continuing education, especially in regard to process improvement and enhanced patient outcomes.

A common thread across the aforementioned reports is the need to involve a variety of stakeholders to achieve the best outcomes. These stakeholders include the patients, the public, leaders in health care from across various disciplines, regulators, and key individuals from federal and state agencies. Other common threads are the importance of defining specific expectations, implementing changes in organizational cultures and systems of care, offering cutting-edge continuing education, and objectively assessing the impact of these endeavors. A thorough and multi-stakeholder discussion on revalidation of physicians should be conducted against the backdrop of the external and intrinsic factors previously mentioned and these important reports.

## 22.2 Revalidation and Continuing Professional Development

Revalidation should continually improve patient care; help to establish and implement high standards for practice; take into consideration the rapid changes in practice; guide continuing education activities and lifelong learning activities; and focus on the role of systems in providing optimal patient care [9, 10]. Credible revalidation needs to be continuous, rigorous, transparent, and meaningful [11]. The goals of revalidation should be to inspire physicians to reach higher levels of performance; ensure a well-trained workforce; and identify and remediate poor performers who do not meet basic standards. Revalidation should focus on both physician performance and outcomes, and encompass the broad range of knowledge, skills, and professional attributes of physicians. Valid and reliable assessment methods should be used, and factors relating to risk adjustment and case mix built into the assessment of outcomes. Patient-reported outcomes should also be included in this process of revalidation. In addition, workplace-based assessments, simulation-based assessments, multi-source feedback, and identification and analyses of adverse events and critical incidents should all be included in the revalidation process [12]. Results of these assessments should be linked with innovative CPD interventions that include state-of-the-art educational methods, such as the use of simulation, and incorporate cutting-edge technologies to facilitate learning and continuous improvement [13, 14].

Novel approaches in medical and surgical education, including rigorous assessment, offer new opportunities for revalidation of physicians and continuous improvement through CPD. The special emphasis on CPD is critical because of the potential for significant positive impact on physicians' performance and patient care outcomes, and the much longer period of professional practice during which patient care may be improved as compared to residency training and medical school education [13]. The specific strategies used to design and implement CPD programs need to be distinct from those used in residency training and medical student education; however, certain advances from residency training and medical school education may readily be applied to the CPD environment.

Major advances in CPD have included the development and use of proficiency-based education and mastery-based training models. The cycle of practice-based learning and improvement (PBLI) serves as a useful model to support design and implementation of effective CPD programs. The PBLI cycle includes four steps: definition of specific gaps through review of performance data and comparison of these data with national, regional, or local standards; participation in relevant CPD programs to address the gaps identified; application of the new knowledge and skills to professional practice; and assessment of improvement [13, 14]. Revalidation of physicians and continuing improvements in professional practice need to be founded on this four-step model. In addition to the approaches used to revalidate the knowledge and skills of all physicians, revalidation of surgeons in practice requires use of specific methods to assess surgical skills, including surgical judgment. These efforts must conform with the requirements and standards promulgated by the respective certifying boards and professional organizations. There are a variety of challenges relating to development and implementation of cutting-edge CPD programs. These result from the different needs of various specialties, dissimilar practice patterns of individuals even within the same specialty, lack of structured curricula, and logistical difficulties that deter practicing physicians from participating in longitudinal programs that focus on acquisition of new surgical skills and safe transfer of these skills to the practice environment [13]. Steps are being taken by professional organizations, such as the American College of Surgeons, to address these challenges.

Efforts aimed at revalidating physicians in practice and supporting their CPD needs should be based on a competency-based framework. In the United States, the Accreditation Council for Graduate Medical Education (ACGME) and the American Board of Medical Specialties (ABMS) defined six core competencies approximately 18 years ago [15, 16]. The ACGME accredits training programs through efforts of the Review Committees, and the ABMS is the umbrella body of all 24 certifying boards. The six core competencies are medical/surgical knowledge; patient care and procedural skills; interprofessional and communication skills; professionalism; practice-based learning and improvement; and systems-based practice. These core competencies apply to the continuum of career progression of physicians, starting with the period of initial training and spanning the entire duration of medical practice. Similarly, in Canada, the CanMEDS competency framework has been developed and is used widely both in training and for Maintenance of Competence. The CanMEDS framework addresses the physicians' roles of medical expert, communicator, collaborator, leader, health advocate, scholar, and professional [17].

Within the broad context of revalidation, two distinct but related types of revalidation need to be considered. This author has designated the first type as "Global Revalidation" and the second type as "Focused Revalidation" (Fig. 22.1). The two types of revalidation are described below.

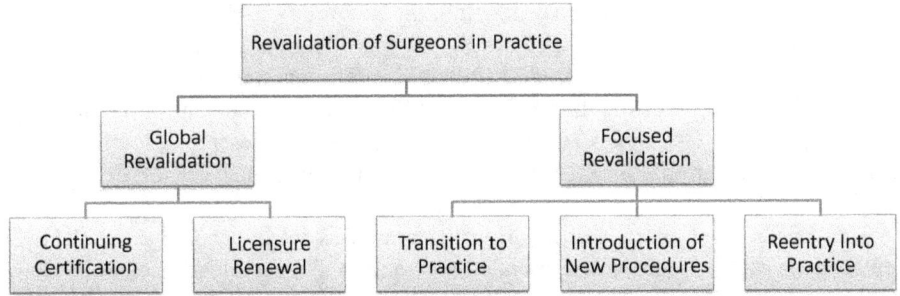

**Fig. 22.1** Model for revalidation of surgeons in practice

## 22.2.1 Global Revalidation

Global Revalidation is overarching in scope, impacts physicians throughout their professional careers, and is generally based on national and local policies, regulations, and standards. The goals of Global Revalidation should be similar across nations; however, the specific strategies employed may be different because of the specific regulatory and organizational structures within each country [18]. Such revalidation may be governed and implemented by independent professional bodies, such as certifying boards in the United States, or by professional bodies that have dual functions as certifying entities and professional organizations, such as postgraduate colleges of surgeons in certain countries. External regulatory agencies that function under authority delegated by national or local governments also play key roles in this process. Thus, Global Revalidation is composed of two elements, one that involves specialty recertification and the other involves renewal of licensure. Recertification falls within the purview of professional bodies, such as the certifying boards and postgraduate colleges; whereas, renewal of licensure is the prerogative of external regulatory agencies, such as the state medical boards in the United States. Recertification may be mandatory to practice surgery, or may be voluntary, depending upon the country. On the other hand, a valid license is generally required to practice medicine and surgery. In addition to meeting the requirements for renewal of licensure, physicians from different specialties also need to meet certain requirements to remain certified, as defined by the certifying boards or the postgraduate colleges depending upon the country where the physicians practice.

The following section focuses specifically on the revalidation of surgeons. Recertification of surgeons in the United States was introduced over 40 years ago, evolved into the program of MOC approximately three decades later, and recently evolved further into the Program of Continuing Certification, as defined by ABMS [19]. The previous MOC and now Continuing Certification have been voluntary in the United States; however, most surgeons have participated in these programs because of external pressures from the hospitals, other employers, payers, patients, and the public. All certifying boards within the umbrella of ABMS are required to design and implement a program of Continuing Certification; however, each certifying board has considerable latitude in regard to defining specific requirements to address Continuing Certification. Also, ABMS has created an online technology learning platform, CertLink®, to support the longitudinal assessment, learning, and improvement programs of certifying boards within the framework of Continuing Certification [20].

The ABS's Continuous Certification Program was introduced in 2018 [21]. It replaces the MOC Program that included the traditional recertification examination. Requirements of this Program of ABS Continuous Certification include: (i) Professional Responsibility and (ii) Education and Assessment. To address the requirement for Professional Responsibility, the surgeon must maintain a valid, full, and unrestricted medical license; hold hospital or surgical center privileges if clinically active; submit two professional references, one from the Chair of Surgery and the other from the Chair of the Credentials Committee, every 5 years; submit an operative experience report covering a 12-month period every 10 years; and participate in a local, regional, or national outcomes registry or quality assessment program, either individually or through an institution. To meet the requirements for Education and Assessment, surgeons must earn 150 Category 1 CME Credits relevant to their practices over 5 years, of which at least 50 Credits must include self-assessment, defined by achievement of 75% or higher score on an assessment linked to the CME Program. This requirement will change to 125 Category 1 CME Credits with no self-assessment credits when surgeons pass their first Continuous Certification Assessment. A new online Continuous Certification Assessment was also introduced by ABS in 2018 to replace the secure and proctored recertification examination. This is an open book assessment coupled with immediate feedback. The surgeon must achieve a score of 80% to pass within two opportunities, and the assessment needs to be taken every other year.

The second arm of the revalidation process for physicians in the United States involves periodic renewal of licenses. A valid medical license is required to practice medicine and surgery in the United States. Granting of medical licenses is a state prerogative and falls within the purview of the respective state medical board. The Federation of State Medical Boards (FSMB) is the national umbrella organization of the state medical boards. Medical licenses generally need to be renewed at 2 or 3 year intervals, which vary by state. The process generally involves answering questions about any adverse actions or liability suits during the previous licensure cycle and about the physician's health that may impact patient care. Also, most states require that physicians earn a certain number of Category 1 CME Credits during the previous licensure cycle. Certain states require Category 1 CME Credits in special domains, such as patient safety, end-of-life care, ethics, risk management, pain management, prescription of opioids, and palliative care [22].

In Canada, revalidation of physicians and surgeons is based on the Maintenance of Competence Program of the Royal College of Physicians and Surgeons of Canada (RCPSC MOC). The RCPSC MOC Program is flexible, learner-driven, and is aimed at supporting personal growth and development of the specialists, who are able to design, implement, and document their specific accomplishments [18, 23]. The Program includes development of individual CPD plans that are relevant to the specialist's practice. The RCPSC MOC Program includes three sets of activities: Group Learning; Self-Learning; and Assessment [23, 24]. Group Learning includes the more traditional CPD activities, such as accredited and unaccredited conferences, rounds, and journal clubs. Self-Learning includes personal learning projects, journal reading, and systems learning. The Assessment includes knowledge assessment through accredited self-assessment programs, and performance assessment through chart audit and feedback, multi-source feedback, simulation, and direct observation. Certain Self-Learning activities, such as personal learning projects, and all Assessment activities are assigned higher numbers of Credits for each hour spent, as compared to the other activities. Fellows are required to complete a minimum of 40 Credits per year and 400 Credits during each 5-year cycle [23, 24]. During each cycle, a minimum of 25 Credits are required in each section of the RCPSC MOC Program.

The Federation of Medical Regulatory Authorities of Canada requires all licensed physicians in Canada to participate in a recognized revalidation process and demonstrate continued competent performance that conforms to professional standards [25, 26]. Individual Canadian provinces accept the RCPSC MOC Program as a pathway for physicians to demonstrate their commitment to continuing competent performance in practice.

Revalidation in the United Kingdom is implemented under the aegis of the General Medical Council (GMC). Revalidation is aimed at driving up standards of practice as well as identifying poor performers. Goals of revalidation are to support professionalism and early identification of problems that may be remediated [27]. The process is based on the annual appraisals required by the National Health Service. These appraisals are conducted by a senior physician, usually within the same organization but not necessarily in the same specialty. During each appraisal, a portfolio of supporting information is provided by the physician being assessed to demonstrate adherence to standards of practice in four domains defined by the GMC. The domains are: (1) knowledge, skills, and performance; (2) safety and quality; (3) communication, partnership, and teamwork; and (4) maintaining trust [28, 29]. Results of audits and information relating to significant events, complaints, and feedback from colleagues and patients are reviewed as part of the appraisal process. In addition, results of the previous appraisal are examined along with information regarding participation in CPD directed at the specific needs of the individual, the individual's personal development plan, and signed statements on probity and health. The appraiser shares the assessment with the Responsible Officer (RO), who in most cases is the Medical Director of the primary care or hospital trust. The RO makes a recommendation regarding revalidation of the physician to the GMC every 5 years. All physicians, including specialists, are required to go through this revalidation process. The appraisals are conducted locally and final decisions are made at the national level. CPD and Quality Improvement activities are specific for each medical specialty [30], and specialists are required to demonstrate that they are providing quality care through audits and outcomes data that are relevant to their specialty.

Several other countries are exploring models for physician revalidation as well. For example, the Medical Board of Australia, rather than using the term revalidation, is developing a Professional Performance Framework. The framework has five pillars with responsibilities and commitments distributed across individual physicians, the medical board, and health services. The five pillars are (1) strengthening continuing professional development; (2) active assurance of safe practice; (3) strengthened assessment and management of medical practitioners with multiple substantiated complaints; (4) guidance to support practitioners; and (5) collaborations to foster a positive culture of medicine [31].

## 22.2.2 Focused Revalidation

In addition to Global Revalidation of all physicians conducted under the aegis of specific certifying bodies and regulatory authorities, there is a clear need for Focused Revalidation of the knowledge, skills, and professional attributes of surgeons in specific situations, such as during transitions in their careers. Focused Revalidation needs to be conducted locally within the context of the individual's practice using nationally accepted standards and requirements. Such revalidation and continuous improvement should include use of contemporary methods of teaching, learning, and assessment. Approaches to Focused Revalidation are described below within the context of three specific situations. Cases are used to frame the discourse.

**Case 1**

*A junior surgeon has recently completed advanced training in a surgical subspecialty Fellowship Program at a renowned academic institution. She has just joined a busy surgical practice within a large tertiary care hospital. How should her skills be revalidated to ensure delivery of optimal surgical care?*

The intake assessment of the junior surgeon should include revalidation of the knowledge, skills, and professional attributes of the surgeon. Revalidation should be based on the organizational norms and available resources at the local institution, linked to specific characteristics of the surgical practice, and aligned with the career goals of the junior surgeon. A multi-pronged assessment should be conducted by a senior surgeon or surgeons in the surgical practice using a variety of valid and reliable methods [31]. Information and data from the period of training should be reviewed and additional data collected after the surgeon joins the practice. Case logs from the period of training should be reviewed to determine the breadth of the surgeon's experience during training, but in isolation are insufficient to determine the specific levels of knowledge and skills of the junior surgeon. Additional information needs to be obtained by the senior surgeon through direct communication with the residency/fellowship director and from other surgeons within the training program who have worked previously with the junior surgeon. Also, results of the certification examinations that the junior surgeon has taken should be reviewed. Additional information collected during the selection process should be reviewed as well.

Another critical component of the intake assessment and revalidation is a detailed discussion between the senior surgeon or surgeons and the junior surgeon about her experience, confidence, and short-term and long-term career goals.

Following entry into practice, the junior surgeon's competencies need to be assessed objectively in real settings and for some situations in simulation-based environments, using a variety of valid and reliable methods. Contemporary assessment strategies and methods should be used to assess surgical knowledge, clinical and technical skills, judgment, communication skills, professionalism, interprofessional teamwork, practice management, and systems-based practice within the context of the surgical practice. Direct observations of performance through proctoring of a specific number of cases in the operating room should be conducted by a senior surgeon or surgeons. Global 360-degree workplace assessments should yield valuable information in regard to interprofessional and communication skills, professionalism, and teamwork. The 360-degree assessments should involve the entire health care team as well as the patients. Also, practice patterns of the surgeon should be monitored and objective data relating to risk-adjusted outcomes and patient-reported outcomes should be collected and reviewed. A sign-off process should be implemented to confirm proficiency and used in the process of credentialing and privileging. Feedback needs to be provided to the junior surgeon to address any weaknesses identified during the assessment and revalidation process, and preceptorship and coaching offered to address gaps and build skills aligned to future career goals. State-of-the-art technologies may be used to support telepreceptoring and coaching. Also, the junior surgeon may be paired with one or more senior surgeons in the practice, who should provide mentorship to the junior surgeon and help her settle into the practice environment and succeed professionally.

The Joint Commission (TJC) accredits and certifies health care organizations and has defined standards for Focused Professional Practice Evaluations (FPPE) and Ongoing Professional Practice Evaluations (OPPE) that need to be followed for organizations to be accredited. The aforementioned assessment and revalidation approach should help in addressing standards for FPPE as well as the privileging requirements at the institution [32]. After the initial revalidation of the knowledge, skills, and professional attributes of the junior surgeon, these should be continually revalidated using a process similar to that used for other surgeons in practice. Once again, a range of valid and reliable assessment methods should be used and specific feedback provided to the surgeon. This continuing revalidation process should help in addressing the standards for OPPE [32]. Any gaps identified through OPPE may require in-depth FPPE to collect additional data and implement specific strategies to improve performance. Early identification of problem areas and specific interventions to address any gaps identified should help in delivering optimal surgical care, and support the career goals and aspirations of the junior surgeon.

## Case #2

*A surgeon has been in practice for 10 years and has consistently demonstrated high standards of practice affirmed by routine audits of practice, and review of data relating to performance and risk-adjusted outcomes. The surgeon wants to learn a new procedure in his specialty and introduce this into his busy practice. How should the knowledge and skills of this surgeon be revalidated in regard to the new procedure to support delivery of safe surgical care?*

The revalidation process for this surgeon needs to include a number of steps. The first step involves evaluation of the efficacy and effectiveness of the new procedure and its relevance to the surgeon's practice, the needs of the patients served, and the available resources [33, 34]. The next step involves review of specific details relating to the educational program in which the surgeon participated to acquire the requisite knowledge and skills. This educational program should have been comprehensive in scope and have included an experiential course, generally conducted in a simulated environment. Multiple strategies should have been employed to support skill acquisition, such as mastery-based training, deliberate practice, specific feedback, and demonstration of achievement of pre-established standards [34]. The new knowledge and skills should have been verified using valid and reliable methods at the conclusion of the course. Following satisfactory completion of the course, the surgeon should have participated in a structured preceptorship to ensure safe transfer of the newly acquired knowledge and skills to surgical practice [34, 35]. The preceptor should have been skilled in the procedure and have worked closely with the surgeon for a period of time to provide direction, guidance, and help during the early phase of the surgeon's experience with the procedure. Because such preceptorships are difficult to arrange, details relating to the preceptorship need to be evaluated carefully. Given the focused nature of this preceptorship, it may have been offered within the surgeon's own institution if there is a surgeon skilled in the procedure and willing to offer this support. Results of assessments of the surgeon's knowledge and skills at the conclusion of the preceptorship should be reviewed, with special attention to assessment of performance and risk-adjusted patient outcomes. Following this revalidation, the surgeon may be granted privileges to perform the procedure and should undergo formal proctoring for a period of time, which should help in confirming satisfactory performance and outcomes based on established standards. This process would help to address the FPPE Standards of TJC as well.

Models for verification and revalidation of surgical knowledge and skills developed by national professional organizations may be helpful in this regard. The American College of Surgeons (ACS) Division of Education has designed a five-level Verification Model that includes the following five steps: Verification of Attendance; Verification of Satisfactory Completion of Course Objectives; Verification of Knowledge and Skills; Verification of Preceptorial Experience; and Demonstration of Satisfactory Patient Outcomes [35]. This model may be used to design the specific revalidation program for this surgeon. Also, national guidelines for granting of privileges may be of help. For example, a Study Group of the American Surgical Association has articulated specific criteria for granting of new surgical privileges, which could be useful [36].

**Case #3**
*A surgeon who has been in surgical practice for 15 years had to step away from clinical practice for three years to take care of a family member with a serious illness. He wants to return to active surgical practice. He has spent one month with a preceptor with expertise in his field of surgical practice and has performed surgery under the supervision of the preceptor. How should his skills be revalidated?*

The revalidation process for this surgeon needs to involve thorough review of the surgeon's past experience before the period of absence from active surgical practice, and steps taken by the surgeon to refresh his knowledge and skills. Detailed information regarding the surgeon's participation in a comprehensive and structured preceptorship of sufficient length under the watchful eye of an experienced surgeon needs to be examined carefully. This should include review of information relating to the conditions managed and the operations performed, the levels of involvement in operative and perioperative care, and data on risk-adjusted outcomes of patient care. The preceptor's assessment of the surgeon should provide helpful information, especially if it includes sufficient data on performance and outcomes. Preceptorial experiences are often not well structured or are of insufficient length because preceptorships of this type are difficult to arrange for a variety of regulatory, legal, and logistical reasons. The result may be a suboptimal experience for the surgeon; thus, the preceptorial experience should be scrutinized carefully. If there is a question regarding the surgeon's proficiency, the surgeon should be asked to demonstrate his knowledge and skills in a simulated setting to supplement the other available information. If results of this comprehensive assessment are satisfactory, the surgeon may be granted privileges but will need to be proctored for a period of time to assess both performance and outcomes. The reentry and revalidation plan for the surgeon should comply with reentry requirements of the ABS or other Certifying Boards [37]. These include assessment of status of practice at departure; participation in individualized reentry pathway constructed by the local physician champion to include assessment of the six core competencies; a proctoring plan; outcomes assessment; and compliance with the Continuous Certification Program.

As surgeons progress through their professional careers, their scope of practices often becomes narrow. If they want to take care of conditions they have not encountered for a period of time or perform operations they have not performed recently, a similar process of revalidation could be employed. Because the surgeon has been actively engaged in surgical practice and may have performed similar procedures, a brief period of preceptoring and proctoring may be sufficient to address this situation.

### 22.2.3 Impact of Revalidation

The positive impact of revalidation is hard to evaluate because most of the evidence reported is correlational and not causal in nature. Association between the previous MOC Examination scores and quality of care has been reported [38]. A recent review of the literature revealed that physicians reported a positive impact of MOC on knowledge, clinical care, and communication with peers and patients. Also, MOC was valued by hospitals and patients [39]. As Certifying Boards design and implement various models for Continuous or Continuing Certification to replace MOC, the impact of these new models on patient outcomes and their acceptance by various stakeholders will need to be evaluated thoroughly.

The subject of revalidation of physicians continues to generate intense discussion and often invokes strong negative reactions from physicians. This is because the benefits of revalidation have not been unequivocally demonstrated, the relevance of revalidation continues to be questioned, and the additional time and expense associated with revalidation place an additional burden on physicians in an environment when health care continues to change and physicians continually face challenges resulting from new regulations. Revalidation should reveal demonstrable improvement in performance and outcomes, and clear benefits to patients and the public to gain broad acceptance. Also, the revalidation process should be relevant to the practices of physicians. Revalidation processes should be integrated with the regular work of physicians and must be respectful of the desire for self-regulation within the profession.

### 22.2.4 Infrastructure to Support Revalidation of Surgeons

Continuing training, acquisition of new surgical skills, and revalidation of surgeons in practice require a robust infrastructure, use of effective education and training models, and the availability of trained preceptors and proctors. The ACS Division of Education has designed a program to establish such an infrastructure. The program was launched in 2005 and involves accreditation of simulation centers to support continuing training, acquisition of new surgical skills, and revalidation of surgeons in practice; offer preceptoring and proctoring; and promote interprofessional teamwork. These simulation centers are called ACS-accredited Education Institutes (ACS-AEIs) [40, 41]. As of April 2019, there are 92 ACS-AEIs located all across the United States, and in Canada, Europe, Middle East and Latin America. Multi-institutional collaborative efforts across the ACS-AEI Consortium are underway. Sharing of best practices should advance standards for revalidation and support implementation of these standards uniformly across the United States and in other regions of the world.

Another key element in the revalidation process, especially within the context of preceptoring and proctoring, is faculty development and support. Surgeons need to be trained in the latest educational methods and to serve in these distinct roles. Their skills as educators and evaluators should be validated to support implementation of robust revalidation programs. Professional organizations should play a key role in this regard. In addition to offering programs for faculty development, such as the renowned *Surgeons as Educators Course*, the ACS Division of Education has recently embarked on a new endeavor to recruit and train senior surgeons in the later years of their professional careers, when they are winding down their clinical practices or have recently retired, to serve as educators and evaluators in simulated environments [34]. This and similar faculty development efforts should be very beneficial to individuals who want to remain engaged in professional endeavors and continue to make meaningful contributions as they step away from busy clinical practices, and should benefit patients and the profession as a whole.

## 22.3 Conclusion

Various countries have taken different approaches to revalidation of physicians based on the disparate regulatory systems and roles of professional organizations. The goals of these efforts are similar and opportunities for cross-fertilization of ideas are significant. The approaches to revalidation need to be proactive rather than reactive and should support the dual goals of ensuring delivery of safe and high-quality care to patients and supporting the career goals of physicians. For revalidation to be positively received by the profession, it needs to be contextually based, relevant, and practical. Sharing of best practices from various revalidation programs should help advancing these efforts, both nationally and internationally.

**Disclaimer** The opinions expressed in this chapter are those of the author and do not necessarily represent the official position of the American College of Surgeons.

## References

1. Shaw, K., Cassel, C. K., Black, C., & Levinson, W. (2009). Shared medical regulation in a time of increasing calls for accountability and transparency: Comparison of recertification in the United States, Canada, and the United Kingdom. *Journal of the American Medical Association, 302*(18), 2008–2014.
2. Birkmeyer, J. D., Finks, J. F., O'Reilly, A., Oerline, M., Carlin, A. M., Nunn, A. R., et al. (2013). Surgical skill and complication rates after bariatric surgery. *New England Journal of Medicine, 369*(15), 1434–1442.
3. Buyske, J. (2016). Forks in the road: The assessment of surgeons from the American Board of Surgery Perspective. *Surgical Clinics of North America, 96*, 139–146.
4. Hawkins, R., Roemheld-Hamm, B., Ciccone, A., Mee, J., & Tallia, A. (2009). A multimethod study of needs for physician assessment: Implications for education and regulation. *The Journal of Continuing Education in the Health Professions, 29*(4), 220–234.
5. Kohn, L. T., Corrigan, J. M., & Donaldson, M. S. (Eds.). (2000). *To err is human: Building a safer health system*. Washington, DC: National Academy Press.
6. Committee on Quality of Health Care in America, Institute of Medicine. (2001). *Crossing the quality chasm: A new health system for the 21st century*. Washington, DC: National Academy Press.
7. Greiner, A. C., & Knebel, E. (Eds.). (2003). *Health professions education: A bridge to quality*. Washington, DC: National Academies Press.

8. Hager, M., Russell, S., & Fletcher, S. W. (2008). *Continuing education in the health professions: Improving healthcare through lifelong learning.* New York: Josiah Macy, Jr. Foundation.
9. Cuschieri, A., Francis, N., Crosby, J., & Hanna, G. B. (2001). What do master surgeons think of surgical competence and revalidation? *American Journal of Surgery, 182*, 110–116.
10. Benson, J. A., Jr. (1991). Certification and recertification: One approach to professional accountability. *Annals of Internal Medicine, 114*(3), 238–242.
11. Youngson, G. G., Knight, P., Hamilton, L., Taylor, I., Tanner, A., Steers, J., et al. (2010). The UK proposals for revalidation of physicians: Implications for the recertification of surgeons. *Archives of Surgery, 145*(1), 92–95.
12. Norcini, J., & Talati, J. (2009). Assessment, surgeon, and society. *International Journal of Surgery, 7*, 313–317.
13. Sachdeva, A. K. (2016). Continuing professional development in the twenty-first century. *The Journal of Continuing Education in the Health Professions, 36*(S1), S8–S13.
14. Sachdeva, A. K. (2005). The new paradigm of continuing education in surgery. *Archives of Surgery, 140*(3), 264–269.
15. Accreditation Council for Graduate Medical Education. Milestones annual report 2016. Available at http://www.acgme.org/Portals/0/PDFs/Milestones/MilestonesAnnualReport2016.pdf. Accessed 2 May 2019.
16. American Board of Medical Specialties. Based on core competencies. Available at http://www.abms.org/board-certification/a-trusted-credential/based-on-core-competencies/. Accessed 2 May 2019.
17. The Royal College of Physicians and Surgeons of Canada. About CanMEDS. Available at http://www.royalcollege.ca/rcsite/canmeds/about-canmeds-e. Accessed 2 May 2019.
18. Horsley, T., Lockyer, J., Cogo, E., Zeiter, J., Bursey, F., & Campbell, C. (2016). National Programmes for validating physician competence and fitness for practice: A scoping review. *BMJ Open, 6*, 1–10.
19. American Board of Medical Specialties. Continuing board certification: Vision for the future final report. Available at http://www.abms.org/media/194956/commission_final_report_20190212.pdf. Accessed 2 May 2019.
20. American Board of Medical Specialties. CertLink delivers longitudinal assessment online. Available at http://www.abms.org/initiatives/certlink/. Accessed 2 May 2019.
21. American Board of Surgery. Continuous certification. Available at http://www.absurgery.org/default.jsp?exam-moc. Accessed 2 May 2019.
22. American College of Surgeons. CME state requirements. Available at https://www.facs.org/education/cme/state-mandates. Accessed 2 May 2019.
23. Campbell, C. M., & Parboosingh, J. (2013). The Royal College Experience and plans for the maintenance of certification program. *The Journal of Continuing Education in the Health Professions, 33*(S1), S36–S47.
24. Royal College of Physicians and Surgeons of Canada. A concise guide to maintenance of certification. Available at http://www.royalcollege.ca/rcsite/documents/continuing-professional-development/moc-short-guide-e.pdf. Accessed 3 May 2019.
25. Federation of Medical Regulatory Authorities of Canada. Position statement on professional revalidation of physicians. Available at http://fmrac.ca/professional-revalidation-of-physicians/. Accessed 2 May 2019.
26. Levinson, W. (2008). Revalidation of physicians in Canada: Are we passing the test? [Editorial]. *Canadian Medical Association Journal, 179*(10), 979–980.
27. Boulet, J., & van Zanten, M. (2014). Ensuring high-quality patient care: The role of accreditation, licensure, specialty certification and revalidation in medicine. *Medical Education, 48*, 75–86.
28. Archer, J., & de Bere, S. R. (2013). The United Kingdom's experience with and future plans for revalidation. *The Journal of Continuing Education in the Health Professions, 33*(S1), S48–S53.

29. Archer, J., de Bere, S. R., Nunn, S., Clark, J., & Corrigan, O. (2015). "No one has yet properly articulated what we are trying to achieve": A discourse analysis of interviews with revalidation policy leaders in the United Kingdom. *Academic Medicine, 90*, 88–93.
30. Federation of Surgical Specialty Associations, The Royal College of Surgeons of Edinburgh, The Royal College of Surgeons of England, The Royal College of Physicians and Surgeons of Glasgow. Revalidation: Guide for surgery. January 2014.
31. Sachdeva, A. K., Flynn, T. C., Brigham, T. P., Dacey, R. G., Jr., Napolitano, L. M., Bass, B. L., et al. (2014). Interventions to address challenges associated with the transition from residency training to independent surgical practice. *Surgery, 155*(5), 867–882.
32. The Joint Commission. (2013). *Standards BoosterPak™ for focused professional practice evaluation/ongoing professional practice evaluation (FPPE/OPPE)*. Oakbrook Terrace, IL: The Joint Commission.
33. Sachdeva, A. K., & Russell, T. R. (2007). Safe introduction of new procedures and emerging Technologies in Surgery: Education, credentialing, and privileging. *Surgical Clinics of North America, 87*(4), 853–866.
34. Sachdeva, A. K., Blair, P. G., & Lupi, L. K. (2016). Education and training to address specific needs during the career progression of surgeons. *Surgical Clinics of North America, 96*(1), 115–128.
35. Sachdeva, A. K. (2005). Acquiring skills in new procedures and technology: The challenge and the opportunity. *Archives of Surgery, 140*(4), 387–389.
36. Bass, B. L., Polk, H. C., Jones, R. S., Townsend, C. M., Whittemore, A. D., Pellegrini, C. A., et al. (2009). Surgical privileging and credentialing: A report of a discussion and study Group of the American Surgical Association. *Journal of the American College of Surgeons, 209*(3), 396–404.
37. American Board of Surgery. Guidelines on re-entry to surgical practice. Available on http://www.absurgery.org/default.jsp?policypracticereentry. Accessed 2 May 2019.
38. Holmboe, E. S., Wang, Y., Meehan, T. P., Tate, J. P., Ho, S. Y., Starkey, K. S., et al. (2008). Association between maintenance of certification examination scores and quality of Care for Medicare Beneficiaries. *Archives of Internal Medicine, 168*(13), 1396–1403.
39. Lipner, R. S., Hess, B. J., & Phillips, R. L., Jr. (2013). Specialty board certification in the United States: Issues and evidence. *The Journal of Continuing Education in the Health Professions, 33*(S1), S20–S35.
40. Sachdeva, A. K., Pellegrini, C. A., & Johnson, K. A. (2008). Support for simulation-based surgical education through American College of Surgeons-accredited education institutes. *World Journal of Surgery, 32*(2), 196–207.
41. American College of Surgeons. Accredited education institutes. Available on https://www.facs.org/education/accreditation/aei. Accessed 2 May 2019.

# Chapter 23
# Demystifying Program Evaluation for Surgical Education

**Alexis Battista, Michelle Yoon, E. Matthew Ritter, and Debra Nestel**

**Overview** In this chapter, we define program evaluation, address its role in evaluating surgical education programs, describe important early steps surgical program evaluators can take to improve the usefulness of program evaluation, discuss common challenges, and offer solutions evaluators can use to overcome these challenges. The chapter is intended for those who are engaging or considering engaging in program evaluation for the first time or are doing so with limited support from a formal program evaluator. Additionally, we have included resources and examples to provide guidance beyond the scope of this chapter.

## 23.1 Introduction

There are times when policymakers, accreditation organizations, university or hospital leadership, and program and clerkship leaders will ask questions about the effectiveness of their surgical education programs and interventions. Evaluating surgical programs can answer questions such as:

---

A. Battista (✉)
Graduate Programs in Health Professions Education, Department of Medicine, F. Edward Hébert School of Medicine, Uniformed Services University of the Health Sciences, Bethesda, MD, USA

The Henry M Jackson Foundation for the Advancement of Military Medicine, Bethesda, MD, USA
e-mail: alexis.battista.ctr@usuhs.edu

M. Yoon
University of Colorado School of Medicine, Aurora, CO, USA

E. Matthew Ritter
USU/Walter Reed Department of Surgery, Bethesda, MD, USA

D. Nestel
Faculty of Medicine, Nursing & Health Sciences, Monash Institute for Health and Clinical Education, Monash University, Clayton, VIC, Australia

Faculty of Medicine Dentistry & Health Sciences, Department of Surgery, Melbourne Medical School, University of Melbourne, Parkville, Australia
e-mail: dnestel@unimelb.edu.au; debra.nestel@monash.edu

- What is the nature and scope of a surgical education program problem? Whom does it impact, how many are affected, and how does the problem affect them?
- What are the possible intervention options that are likely to ameliorate a defined problem in surgical education?
- Is the surgical residency error reduction program attaining the desired goals and benefits?
- Is a new surgical fellowship training program being implemented well?
- Is the quality improvement intervention program changing surgical outcomes?
- Is the cost of the simulation-based skills training program reasonable when compared to its effectiveness and benefits?

Seeking and providing these answers is increasingly the work of surgical program leaders, such as clerkship, residency and fellowship directors who may be asked to study, appraise, and improve surgical education programs. The purpose of this chapter is to provide a practical overview of program evaluation (PE) and how to get started. This chapter does not present a comprehensive discussion on PE but instead provides information and guidance about how to get started while pointing to additional resources that can be used to enhance evaluation efforts in the future.

## 23.2 Defining Program Evaluation

PE is the use of research methods to systematically investigate the effectiveness of social and educational programs, including surgical education and interventions, to guide future efforts, and to change or improve a program [1, 2]. *Educational evaluation* is the process of defining, gathering, analyzing, and disseminating information to guide decisions about an educational program [3, 4]. The target of an evaluation may be any organized educational program, including:

- A curriculum
- A course
- A specific instructional approach (e.g., simulation-based learning, journal club)
- Policies and guidelines
- Specific services that are part of the educational experience

PE seeks to address questions of need for, quality of, processes of, or the impact of an educational program in the context of continuous quality improvement and decision-making [5, 6]. Evaluations can focus on whether an educational program is working as intended or if there are unintended consequences [7]. In the case of surgical education, PE may be conducted on a surgery clerkship rotation, residency program, or fellowship training program. It may entail evaluating the overall program outcomes (e.g., data about satisfaction at the end of training, exam performance, job placement of graduates), as well as examining granular-level pieces such as individual teaching sessions or the teaching and learning structure or environment.

Evaluation may occur on a program that is currently in progress (formative evaluation) or on completion (summative evaluation). Both types of evaluations can help program stakeholders make decisions about what should be kept or changed in a program or even determine whether a program should continue [1, 2]. In surgical education, PE usually provides information about the effectiveness of educational training programs with the comprehensive purpose of optimizing healthcare outcomes and quality.

### 23.2.1 Why Conduct a Program Evaluation: What's in It for You?

PE can provide information that can create value at the institutional level as well as at the accreditation level. For example, assessment data, such as qualifying professional examination pass rates, can yield information about program outcomes, while PE data collected over time can provide insights into job placement and long-term program impact [7–9]. Additionally, PE findings can be used to inform or provide feedback to faculty who provide instruction in a program, which in turn, may be useful for faculty career development or promotion. Findings from a PE may also provide feedback to administrators, support staff, and others who are instrumental in maintaining a program's structure and logistic operations (e.g., library, technology, assessment). Furthermore, data generated from PE can be used to inform the design and implementation of surgical education programs which should be viewed as a cycle of *designing, implementing, evaluating, and revising*, rather than a static state [10]. PE supports this cycle because the results can inform continuous quality improvement in the instructional and curriculum design process by providing more precise information about what works, what doesn't work, and what could be altered [7, 10]. In turn, the results of PE can also support the efforts of accreditation and reaccreditation because accreditation bodies (e.g., American College of Surgeons) may require program managers to report and share student outcomes as well as demonstrate that the program engages in regular evaluation efforts.

### 23.2.2 Resources and Guidelines in Surgical Education

Highlighting the growing importance of PE in surgical education, many surgical associations offer guidance, standards, and resources for PE including the American College of Graduate Medical Education (ACGME), the Royal Australasian College of Surgeons (RACS), and the Royal College of Surgeons (RCS). It is worth reviewing and considering the guidelines from accrediting groups because they often provide specific criteria that can influence or guide your PE. Furthermore, although surgical department faculty often conduct PE, it is also important to be aware of the role the professional evaluators may play. Professional evaluators are individuals with diverse training and professional experience in the practices of evaluation. Professional evaluators can play an important role in improving the design or implementation of an evaluation, particularly if your funding agency requires it, if the PE you are planning is highly complex, or if you determine that including a professional evaluator can add credibility to the PE process or findings. For additional information about professional evaluators and their role, the American Evaluation Association (AEA) is a valuable resource.

## 23.3 Getting Started: Key Stages of Conducting a Program Evaluation

Although there are many steps included in any PE, one of the most challenging is deciding where and how to start. Importantly, a key aspect of getting started is keeping in mind that there is no "one size fits all" in PE [1]. For PE to be successful, it must be tailored to the unique needs of the organization. The most successful evaluations are ones that provide useful and credible information that support decision-making [1]. In this section, we discuss key steps of PE to support efforts in getting started and ensuring your evaluation is tailored to your organization's unique needs. These steps include identifying and involving stakeholders, developing a logic model, focusing your evaluation, and selecting an evaluation model.

### 23.3.1 Identifying and Involving Stakeholders

Identifying stakeholders early in an evaluation is a key step to ensuring the evaluation will yield useful information. Stakeholders include both people and entities, who are or may be affected by the program under evaluation [1]. Stakeholder identification sets the stage for the entire PE process and can help generate useful evaluation questions and help identify human and financial resources to conduct the evaluation and targets for dissemination of the findings.

On first pass, surgical educators new to PE may not appreciate the scope and importance of identifying and involving stakeholders. At the operational level, clerkship and program directors might quickly identify the need to respond to demands of the Chairman, regulatory bodies (e.g., ACGME, RCS, RACS), or to highlight successes to aid in the recruitment of future trainees; however, the scope and importance of stakeholder involvement extend well beyond this initial focus. Therefore, it is important that the evaluator identify a broad list and make an informed decision about each stakeholder's level of participation.

In keeping with the practical focus of this chapter, we highlight Green's (2005) conceptual framework for identifying potential stakeholders for PE [11]. Green's approach involves identifying stakeholders in one of four groups: those who have authority over the program, those responsible for the delivery of the program,

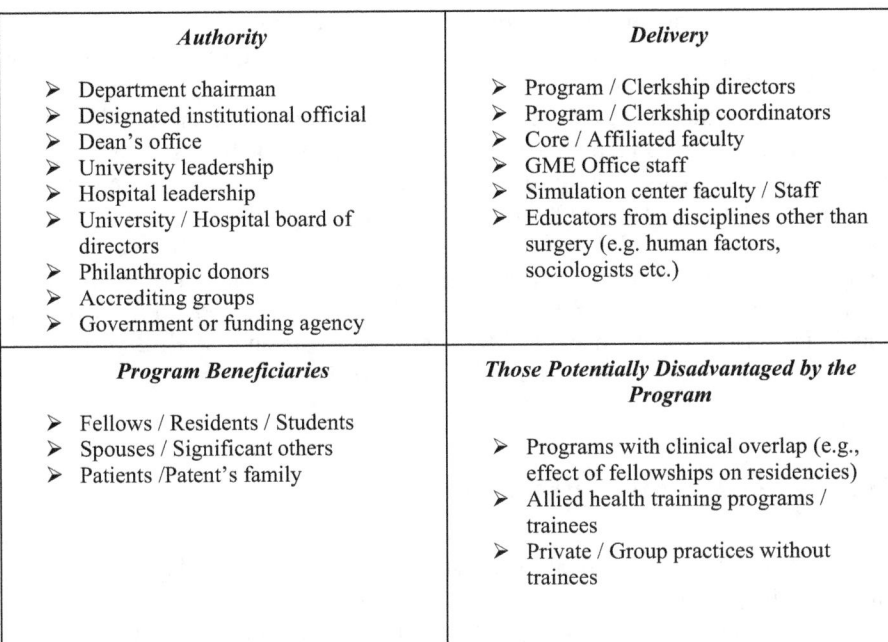

**Fig. 23.1** Examples of categorizing stakeholders drawn from Green's [11] approach to identifying potential stakeholders and their roles

intended beneficiaries of the program, and lastly and most often overlooked, those who may be disadvantaged by the program. Drawing from this model, Fig. 23.1 gives examples from surgical education for each of these categories of stakeholders.

Once identified, the role of each stakeholder in the evaluation process needs to be defined. One way to approach this is to assign a primary role to each identified stakeholder. Categorical levels of participation ranging from least involved to most involved could include awareness, policy and guidelines, input and reaction, and operational decision-making. While none of these categories need to be mutually exclusive or absolute, this organization helps the evaluator systematically consider how stakeholders may influence the evaluation. There is no correct or incorrect way to do this, but the approach should be adapted to each situation. A thoughtful approach to determining the involvement of key stakeholders will allow the PE to have the most meaningful impact.

## 23.3.2 Developing a Logic Model

Simply put, it will be difficult to evaluate how well a program is doing or working if stakeholders don't have an explicit understanding of what the program is supposed to be doing and how it is supposed to work (also called a program theory).

Therefore, when designing a PE, it can be useful to develop a *logic model*. A logic model is a graphic representation that helps visually represent the connections between the "if-then" causal relationships of the program activities (e.g., inputs such as educator time and teaching materials and outputs such as short- or long-term goals) [1, 12, 13]. By making these causal relationships explicit, stakeholders can make better judgments about programs processes or efficacy, which, in turn, can help improve the usefulness of the PE [1]. In the event that there isn't a clear understanding of the programs' theory, the focus of the PE may emphasize developing a logic model. Notably, logic models are also increasingly required in grant programs and global surgery projects. For more comprehensive details about how to develop a logic model, we refer readers to McLaughlin and Jordan (1999), Shakman and Rodriquez (2015), and Lawton and colleagues (2014), to name a few [12–14].

### 23.3.3 Focusing Your Evaluation

Once stakeholders are identified, their roles defined, and a logical model is developed, it is helpful to employ a systematic approach to further focus and plan the PE. Although there are several ways to organize and focus a PE, we highlight one framework that has been adapted from a 10-step approach presented in the American College of Surgeons "Surgeons as Educators" course. Figure 23.2 demonstrates examples of how to apply these steps.

It is important to remember that the steps outlined above help generate a *focused and comprehensive plan* for PE – a process more akin to a marathon than a sprint. For example, it is often best to generate the right questions and work to answer them, rather than only asking questions that you can answer with the data you have. Avoiding this common pitfall will result in a substantial improvement in both the evaluation and, importantly, the program itself. Once your initial plan is in place through application of the 10-step model or another framework, selecting an evaluation model that is grounded in sound measurement theory can help move the process along.

### 23.3.4 Selecting an Evaluation Model

Conducting an evaluation is a complex task, particularly if you are new to conducting evaluations, have limitations to paying for, or accessing, external resources (e.g., program evaluation professional), or, like many clinicians, are juggling evaluation efforts with your teaching and clinical responsibilities. Using and adapting an existing evaluation model can help demystify the process of conducting a PE by offering structure and support while guiding decision-making processes and methodological choices [1]. Using a model also helps assure that important steps and information are not overlooked or missed [1]. There are numerous models and approaches to PE.

|   | Step | Example |
|---|---|---|
| 1 | Identify key stakeholders | See previous section and Figure 23.1 |
| 2 | Define the evaluation purpose(s) and how the results will be used | • Identify ability of the current program to meet upcoming changes in regulatory requirements.<br>• Identify targets for cost savings without impacting quality of education. |
| 3 | Identify what should be evaluated and generate evaluation questions. (see following section on selecting an evaluation model) | • What is the percentage of high performing students who match in surgical residencies?<br>• How do fellowship directors perceive the incoming performance of residency graduates? |
| 4 | Inventory what performance evaluation data are currently being collected and by whom | • Standardized test scores, Patient satisfaction questionnaires, Individualized quality data, Centrally administered surveys |
| 5 | Match data being collected with evaluation questions and determine need for new/additional data collection | • An evaluation question of first time Board pass rates may be answered by obtaining existing data.<br>• A question about learner perception of faculty teaching effectiveness may require development of an assessment survey. |
| 6 | Develop timeline and responsibility for data collection | • Students must turn in completed clerkship patient logs before taking the subject exam.<br>• Faculty must complete trainee assessments within two weeks of the end of the rotation. |
| 7 | Specify the analysis procedure to be used for each type of data and question. | • Effectiveness of a clinical rotation could be judged by the number of defined category operative cases or by themes in the narrative comments of residents on the post rotation survey. |
| 8 | Specify criteria to be used to make judgments (i.e. define "success") | • Define an "acceptable" and "goal" for each evaluation question.<br>• This could be achieved by using percentile ranks (e.g., above 50th percentile nationally for operative trauma volume) or by quantifying frequency of categorical themes based on narrative comments (e.g., positive comments regarding faculty support). |
| 9 | Determine which evaluation questions can be answered within your timeline, budget, and resources & identify what's needed to answer all major evaluation questions | • A program director without protected time or administrative support can likely answer questions relating to case volume and first time board pass rates, but will not have the time to do in-depth analysis on faculty teaching effectiveness.<br>• Stakeholders must help provide resources to answer the questions they helped generate. |
| 10 | Communicate results and follow up with key stakeholders | Socialize the results of the program evaluation. Meetings with underperforming faculty, sites, or affiliated programs will help ensure expectations are communicated and all factors are considered. Making leadership aware of both successes and challenges can facilitate the time and resources needed for improvement. Trend important results over time. |

**Fig. 23.2** Worked example of steps for planning a surgical program evaluation. (Adapted from the American College of Surgeons as Educators Workshop)

In medical and surgical education, some common approaches include *Kirkpatrick's Hierarchy* [15]; Patton's *Utilization-Focused Evaluation* (also called "Use-Based" Evaluation) [16]; Stufflebeam's *Context, Input, Process, and Product (CIPP)* model [17]; and *Outcomes-Based Evaluation* (also see Chap. 34). Table 23.1 provides a summary of these models, their key features, and their advantages and limitations.

## 23.4 Examples of Program Evaluation in Surgical Education

Table 23.1 demonstrates that the goals and approaches to PE vary widely. In a US-based study, Torbeck et al. (2014) describe an approach to evaluating a surgical residency program using an outcomes assessment system as a component of PE [18]. They use diverse data associated with one key stakeholder – the surgical resident – to track before, during, and after the surgical residency program. Collecting data over an extended time frame and for different cohorts helped identify features of the program while also informing decisions about what program features to maintain and what to strengthen.

In a second US-based study, Gomez et al. (2014) report an evaluation of an international medical student surgery-oriented program [8]. Like Torbeck et al. [18], the PE described by Gomez and colleagues has a strong outcomes-based focus drawing data from just one stakeholder – the students enrolled in the program. The findings of the evaluation are discussed in the light of broader macro level issues such as the forecasted decline in international medical graduates applying for residencies nationally [8].

In a third example, Yu et al. (2016) report a PE designed to develop competent cataract surgeons in China [9]. The program was comprised of two phases and focused on one procedure – phacoemulsification. Surgical trainee performance data and complication rates of patients were monitored in each phase and 2 years after attending the program. Although the complication rates fluctuated, performance improved across the program. The improvements were attributed to the programs combined features – wet lab exposure, deliberate practice with patients, and regular formative feedback using the performance measurement tool.

These examples demonstrate diverse ways in which these programs tailored their evaluations by including specific stakeholders and using different types of PE approaches (e.g., learning and career outcomes, patient complication rates) which helped them demonstrate the value of their programs.

**Table 23.1** Common evaluation models used in health professions PE, key attributes, and advantages and limitations

| Evaluation model | Attributes | Advantages | Limitations |
|---|---|---|---|
| Kirkpatrick's hierarchy or four-level evaluation | Widely recognized in health professions PE | Practical way to examine different levels of learner outcomes | Does not account for factors that may influence learning (e.g., motivation) |
| | Places an emphasis on program outcomes | Outcomes measures are commonly accepted by stakeholders | Does not describe how learning outcomes are supported |
| | Often combined with other evaluation approaches | | |
| Use-based evaluations | Emphasis is on the needs and issues of the intended users, such as students, faculty, or other key program stakeholders | Focusing on intended users increases the chances that the findings will be useful and applicable | Placing the focus on the intended users can lead to other important viewpoints being overlooked |
| | Can be employed for formative and summative program evaluation | Can be used for a variety of program evaluation questions | |
| Context, input, process, and product (CIPP) | Links evaluation with decision-making and asks | Very systematic | May be very strict |
| | What needs to be done and were important needs addressed? | Comprehensive | Tends to be a "top-down" approach |
| | How should it be done? | Focuses on decision-making | May require more time to complete |
| | Is it being done? | | |
| | Is the program succeeding? | | |
| | Can be employed for formative and summative program evaluation | | |
| Outcomes-based evaluations | Sometimes referred to as impact evaluation which focuses on exploring selected effects of a program | Can help identify immediate, short-, intermediate, or long-term program impacts | May not associate links between process and outcomes and so may not identify why a program is working (or not) |
| | Usually focuses on participants of the program although secondary or indirect audiences may also be considered (similar to the level 4 of Kirkpatrick above) | May uncover unintended outcomes or consequences | |

## 23.5 Overcoming Challenges and Tensions in Program Evaluation

In the previous sections, we have highlighted and discussed key stages and processes associated with conducting PE. Although these steps suggest a linear and stepwise approach, the actual practice of PE can present a number of challenges. Some common challenges include:

- Staying the course when conducting a complex evaluation
- Considering how and where to report your PE
- Differences between PE and assessment
- Differences between PE and research

### 23.5.1 Staying the Course When Conducting a Complex Evaluation

The conduct of a PE can be overwhelming, particularly if you are new to PE or if you are juggling evaluation, teaching, and clinical duties. Additionally, some stages of PE may be more complex or take longer than others, or you may become aware of new evaluation questions and needs as your evaluation progresses. Some potential strategies for managing these challenges include:

- Use of a PE model helps guide and direct decision-making and helps minimize missed steps or stages of a PE.
- Break the PE into smaller, manageable tasks. This can offer some satisfaction that the PE is progressing while also providing you evidence of progress that can be shared with stakeholders when they request an update [1].
- When meeting with stakeholders, ask who might be available to help with the workload. As the evaluation progresses, continue to look out for additional supporters and resources.
- Develop and maintain a list of possible future evaluation questions, resources, and data sources. You may not pursue every new avenue, but keeping track of them can help you stay focused on your current evaluation plan.

### 23.5.2 Planning to Report and Disseminate Findings

It is important to think about reporting and dissemination at the outset of the PE planning process. Although most PE outcomes are reported textually, they may be accompanied by oral presentations before or after the release of a report. The sequence will vary with the purpose of the evaluation and stakeholder preferences. Additionally, there may be interim reports requested that may have different levels

| |
|---|
| I. Executive Summary |
| II. Introduction to the report |
|     a. Purpose of the evaluation |
|     b. Audiences for the evaluation report |
|     c. Limitations of the evaluation |
|     d. Overview of report contents |
| III. Focus of the evaluation |
|     a. Description of the evaluation object |
|     b. Evaluative questions used to focus the study |
|     c. Information needed to complete the evaluation |
| IV. Brief overview of evaluation plan and procedures |
| V. Presentation of evaluation results |
|     a. Summary of evaluation findings |
|     b. Interpretation of evaluation findings |
| VI. Conclusions and recommendations |
|     a. Criteria and standards used to judge evaluation object |
|     b. Judgements about evaluation object (strengths and weaknesses) |
|     c. Recommendations |
| VII. Minority reports or rejoinders (if any) |
| VIII. Appendices |
|     a. Description of evaluation plan/design, instruments, and data analysis and interpretation |
|     b. Detailed tabulations or analyses of quantitative data, and transcripts or summaries of qualitative data |
|     c. Other information, as necessary |

**Fig. 23.3** Structure of a PE Report. (Adapted from Fitzpatrick et al. [19])

of formality. Interim reporting is beneficial because it provides evaluators and stakeholders with an opportunity to engage in a dialogue about the progress of the evaluation. Interim reporting can also alert the evaluator to issues that might be important to include in the final report, which can potentially save time and increase the credibility of the findings. The audiences of the PE report may also vary, so tailoring of data may also be required in terms of the degree of detail, language style, and format. Additionally, when reporting, the evaluator must consider the ethics of PE practice to ensure accuracy, balance, and fairness [19]. Figure 23.3 highlights Fitzpatrick et al.'s (2011) structure for a written evaluation report [19].

### 23.5.3 Evaluation or Research?

In our work as program evaluators, we have often been asked, "Isn't this research? How does PE differ from research?" Confusion can occur because PE and research use similar methods. However, key differences include the purpose of the activity and the intended audience. (See Chap. 34 for further discussion of the differences.) When an evaluation reveals really interesting findings that evaluators think may be of benefit to others, they may want to share this with a wider audience. This can present challenges because, unlike research, program evaluators may not have obtained participant consent for their data. Additionally, some evaluators may not seek institutional review board guidance, which can limit how data is presented or shared. We strongly encourage evaluators to seek guidance or institutional review before beginning your evaluation. For more in-depth discussions on ethics and standards of practice, we suggest Rossi et al. (2004) and Yarbrough et al. (2010) [1, 2]. Additionally, Thomas et al. (2015) provide a detailed discussion related to ethics of PE in the health professions [20].

### 23.5.4 Evaluation or Assessment?

In addition to differences between PE and research, there are also differences between evaluation and assessment. It is not uncommon for program managers and other stakeholders to confuse these two approaches because the terms are often used interchangeably (e.g., student evaluation versus program evaluation or program assessment compared to PE). Internationally, the term "evaluation" is usually applied at the level of a program, while "assessment" is applied to an individual [1, 2]. Importantly, although program managers or evaluators may utilize student assessment data, the goal of evaluation is to examine the program's impact on its stakeholders, which can include students. Student assessment is primarily focused on a single student.

## 23.6 Conclusions

The purpose of this chapter was to provide a practical overview of systematic processes of PE and advice about how to get started. PE within and outside surgical education is a widely accepted approach used to examine the efficacy of a program, determine its impact on the designated stakeholders (e.g., students, residents, patients), and to ascertain if there are any unintended consequences. Additionally, PE within surgical education can provide program managers, program directors, and other key stakeholders with important information about how students, residents, and fellows are performing, developing, and even changing their clinical practice. Important stages of a PE include identifying and working with stakeholders, who can play an integral role in focusing the evaluation's goals and questions. Including stakeholders early and staying in touch with them is a key factor in making sure the PE adds value. Furthermore, to make the PE process easier, selection of an evaluation model can provide structure, guidance, and support while helping to ensure that you do not miss important steps along the way. Lastly, although the processes of PE can be complex, there are several resources available to help guide you: many of which we have included in this chapter.

# References

1. Rossi, P. H., Lipsey, M. W., & Freeman, H. E. (2003). *Evaluation: A systematic approach.* Thousand Oaks: Sage.
2. Yarbrough, D. B., Shulha, L. M., Hopson, R. K., & Caruthers, F. A. (2010). *The program evaluation standards: A guide for evaluators and evaluation users.* Los Angeles: Sage.
3. Stufflebeam, D. L. (1971). *Educational evaluation and decision making.* Ithaca: Peacock.
4. Cronbach, L. J. (1984). *Essentials of psychological testing* (4th ed.). New York: Harper & Row.
5. Kring, D. (2008). Research and quality improvement: Different processes, different evidence. *MEDSURG Nursing, 17*(3), 162–169.
6. Rozalis, M. L. (2003). Evaluation and research: Differences and similarities. *The Canadian Journal of Program Evaluation, 18*(2), 1–31.
7. Lovato, C., & Wall, D. (2014). Programme evaluation: Improving practice, influencing policy and decision-making. In Swanwick, T. (Ed.), *Understanding medical education: Theory and practice* (2nd ed.). Hoboken: Wiley.
8. Gomez, P. P., Willis, R. E., & Jaramillo, L. A. (2014). Evaluation of a dedicated, surgery-oriented visiting international medical student program. *Journal of Surgical Education, 71*(3), 325–328.
9. Yu, A. Y., Wang, Q. M., Li, J., Huang, F., & Golnik, K. (2016). A cataract surgery training program: 2-year outcome after launching. *Journal of Surgical Education, 73*, 761–767.
10. Dick, W., & Carey, L. (2011). *The systematic design of instruction.*
11. Greene, J. C. (2005). Mixed methods. In S. Mathison (Ed.), *Encyclopedia of evaluation.* Thousand Oaks: Sage.
12. McLaughlin, J. A., & Jordan, G. B. (1999). Logic models: A tool for telling your programs performance story. *Evaluation and Program Planning, 22*(1), 65–72.
13. Shakman, K., & Rodriguez, S.M. (2015, May). *Logic models for program design, implementation, and evaluation: Workshop toolkit.* REL 2015-057. Regional Educational Laboratory Northeast & Islands.
14. Lawton, B., Brandon, P.R., Cicchinelli, L., Kekahio, W. (2014, February) *Logic models: A tool for designing and monitoring program evaluations.* REL 2014-007. Regional Educational Laboratory Pacific.
15. Kirkpatrick, D. L., & Kirkpatrick, J. D. (2006). *Evaluating training programs: The four levels.* San Francisco: Berrett-Koehler Publishers.
16. Patton, M. Q. (2008). *Utilization-focused evaluation.* Thousand Oaks: Sage Publications.
17. Stufflebeam, D. L., & Shinkfield, A. J. (2007). *Evaluation theory, models, and applications* (1st ed.). San Francisco: Jossey-Bass.
18. Torbeck, L., Canal, D. F., & Choi, J. (2014). Is our residency program successful? Structuring an outcomes assessment system as a component of program evaluation. *Journal of Surgical Education., 71*(1), 73–78.
19. Fitzpatrick, J., Sanders, J., & Worthen, B. (2011). *Reporting evaluation results: Maximizing use and understanding. program evaluation: Alternative approaches and practical guidelines* (4th ed., pp. 453–489). Upper Saddle River: Pearson Education.
20. Thomas, P. A., Kern, D. E., Hughes, M. T., & Chen, B. Y. (2015). *Curriculum development for medical education: A six-step approach.* JHU Press.

# Chapter 24
# Simulation in Surgical Education

**Rajesh Aggarwal**

**Overview** Simulation is a tool that has been utilized for many decades in the surgical arena, from the advent of fracture fixation workshops, anatomy classes on cadavers, and practice of live animal models. The past two decades has seen an exponential growth in scientific data to support the role and impact of simulation in the surgical domain, within technical, team-based, and non-operative settings. In order to integrate simulation into surgical curricula, at student, resident, and practitioner levels, the tools, processes, and scientific outcomes of simulation need to be translated into clinical implementation, through deliberate engagement at the level of clinical departments, health systems, and professional bodies. This process needs to be underpinned by rigorous data collection and evaluation of the impact, challenges, and ongoing opportunities, for simulation in surgery to be a robust tool for health systems improvement, at a systems level.

## 24.1 Introduction

Across the developed world, it is known that despite considerable efforts to advance the quality of surgical care, about one in ten patients continue to be harmed [1]. It is an imperative that despite technological innovation such as anesthesia, antimicrobial therapy, minimally invasive surgery, and stem cell transplants, the greatest gains for the future of surgical care will be made through process innovation.

The considerable challenge is how to deliver such innovations. An important and often overlooked missing link is the responsibility to engage and train frontline clinical staff. The vast majority of current strategies in surgical education are based upon didactic teaching seminars, protocols, and "learning on the job." Education of clinical staff tends to occur in silos and less often as a multidisciplinary care team.

---

R. Aggarwal (✉)
Department of Surgery, Sidney Kimmel Medical College, Thomas Jefferson University, Philadelphia, PA, USA

Jefferson Strategic Ventures, Jefferson Health, Philadelphia, PA, USA
e-mail: rajesh.aggarwal@jefferson.edu

While the silo-based approach may be more facile from a logistics perspective, when translated to clinical work schedules, there may be poor compliance, variability in care, and even missed opportunities for clinical impact. It has been known for many decades that simulation-based training is effective to enhance clinical performance, in multiple arenas of healthcare [2].

## 24.2 Simulation in Healthcare

Healthcare simulation has continued to increase in its expanse and reach. There are a host of excellent clinical studies, which herald the benefits of simulation-based training for procedural skills such as cardiopulmonary resuscitation, central line insertion, and laparoscopic performance [3–5]. Healthcare simulation has been shown to be an effective paradigm in team skills training, with a study across the Veteran's Administration hospitals reporting an 18% reduction in mortality when introduced to 74 hospital facilities across the United States [6]. More recently, studies to evaluate the assessment and management of surgical patients in the ward setting have been undertaken, with surgical residents in a simulation-based environment [7, 8]. When trained in the simulator, there was a 25% increase in quality of patient assessment, 29% in patient management, and 31% in nontechnical skills. While overwhelmingly encouraging, despite such advances, our current focus of surgical simulation upon repetition and performance of isolated tasks in discrete environments is too simplistic and may suffer from issues of transfer to the clinical environment.

## 24.3 Learning Curves in Surgery

Within the realm of surgical education, the concept of a learning curve has been described for both real and simulated operative procedures. Such studies have reliably demonstrated an improvement in technical skill (albeit through differing metrics) as a function of procedural repetition [9]. This is further bolstered by the extensive studies that have been published in the literature with regard to volume-outcome relationships for many surgical procedures, at both the surgeon and hospital level [10]. As in other performance-related fields such as sports, music, and dance, initial improvement can be quite rapid, but improvements slowly taper toward an asymptote often described as a "plateau" in skill acquisition. There is broad interest to apply learning curves to surgical education, with regard to efforts to maximize the efficiency of training, with a keen eye upon maintaining patient safety as the top priority. Numerous efforts have attempted to define the metric by which the surgical learning curve should be measured, though the majority have employed plotting operative time, while fewer have regarded the incidence of adverse outcomes as a function of operative experience.

While trainees must obtain experience to become more skilled at performing procedures, the necessity of education must be considered in the context of patient safety. Due to increased awareness of the learning curve, surgical education has shifted away from the now defunct "see one and do one and teach one" apprenticeship model toward a more safety-driven model. The contemporary process should and often does incorporate the use of surgical simulators into training, with the intent to reduce the learning curve for surgeons in a standardized controlled setting, outside of the operating room, and away from real patients.

## 24.4 Technical Skills Simulation

Technological advances over the past two decades have fed forward the development of simulators beyond simple cadaveric animal tissue or expensive anesthetized live animals. Inanimate trainers are now available in many forms and offer varying degrees of fidelity. For example, the *Fundamentals of Laparoscopic Surgery* (FLS) box offers trainees the ability to perform basic laparoscopic tasks on simple objects such as ropes and pegs [11]. This is not only a training tool but has also been used for assessment of performance, indeed as a part of the process for all graduating general surgical residents in the United States. Other inanimate trainers utilize more complex and perhaps more realistic representations of anatomy to simulate portions of entire procedures such as laparoscopic appendectomy and cholecystectomy or more recently to consider complex procedures such as colectomy and gastric bypass procedures.

Virtual reality (VR) simulators allow surgeons to practice procedures in a computer-generated environment and provide the advantage of having built-in, automated measures of assessment such as motion and dexterity parameters, on standardized educational modules. While the initial cost of investment in VR simulators can be high, subsequent maintenance is relatively inexpensive. Importantly, trainees are able to receive instruction from modules built into the simulators, allowing them to practice skills independent of a proctor or instructor if necessary [12].

While many commercially available VR simulators come with pre-programmed curricula and suggested performance metrics, suggestions are not often based upon studies validating their use for effective surgical training. The curricula described below incorporate construct valid tasks, i.e., tasks that can distinguish the performance of novices from experienced surgeons to advance novice surgeons along the learning curve to a benchmark level of proficiency.

## 24.5 Proficiency-Based Surgical Simulation

Aggarwal et al. developed an evidence-based curriculum for training to proficiency in laparoscopic cholecystectomy using the LAP Mentor VR simulator (Simbionix Corporation, Cleveland, Ohio, USA) [13]. Construct valid metrics all showed significant learning curves, with plateaus in performance at the seventh repetition, as measured by time taken, total number of movements, total cautery time, and total cautery time without tissue contact for dissection of Calot's triangle. This validated curriculum also uses validated performance targets for proficiency rather than the time spent practicing tasks.

The goal of simulation is to shorten the learning curve for real procedures so that trainees can safely and effectively transition their education from the simulation center to the operating room. The effectiveness of a simulator can thus be assessed using the transfer effectiveness ratio (TER), first utilized by the aviation industry to assess the efficacy of virtual flight simulators in decreasing the learning curve of piloting real aircraft [14].

TER is calculated as:

$$\text{TER} = (X1 - X2)/T$$

where

$X1$ is median time required by non-simulator-trained group to reach performance criteria

$X2$ is median time required to achieve performance criterion in simulator-trained group

$T$ is total training time of the simulator-trained group ()

TER is a useful measure to determine the amount of training time that can be saved by utilizing simulation within a curriculum. For example, a TER of 2.0 would suggest that every minute spent training on a simulator is equivalent to 2 min training on the comparative model. In the context of surgical education, TER has been utilized to assess the efficacy of simulators such as the LapSim VR laparoscopic simulator where TER for proficiency training was found to be 2.28 [14]. TER calculation can be affected by the performance criteria set for users. For example, Kolozsvari et al. found the TER of the FLS peg transfer task to be 0.16 when targeting a "mastery" level of performance in preparation for learning intracorporeal suturing [15].

Just in the past decade, the importance of incorporating simulation into surgical training has been recognized by governing bodies such as the Residency Review Committee of the Accreditation Council for Graduate Medical Education (ACGME) in the United States. In 2008, there was a mandate passed that all American surgical residency programs must have access to a simulation laboratory. The intent was that the incorporation of simulation into training would reduce the length of the learning curve before trainees operate on live patients. However, the mandate was fairly nonspecific as to what constitutes a surgical simulation laboratory, until the development and implementation of the American College of Surgeons Accredited Education Institutes, which to date has accredited or reaccredited over 85 centers across the globe, through evaluation of space, equipment, personnel, curricula, and scholarly activity [16].

In 2009, Barsuk et al. reported the results of a simulation-based education program in the field of central venous catheter (or CVC) insertion and utilized central line-associated bloodstream infections (CLABSI) as their primary outcome measure of interest [17]. The two 2-hours education sessions consisting of lecture, step-by-step demonstration, and simulation-based practice with focused feedback were completed by 92 residents, in a US-based academic medical center. Of note, all residents had to meet a minimum pass score to complete the training module. Remarkably, there was a greater than sixfold decrease in CLABSI rates after simulation training (0.50 infections per 1000 catheter-days) compared with the same unit prior to the intervention (3.20 per 1000 catheter-days). The net savings were approximately $700,000 from the reduction in CLABSI rates, tempered by the annual cost of the simulation-based intervention of $112,000 [18]. This was the first study to report clinically relevant patient outcomes, in alignment with cost-benefit data of a simulation-based educational intervention.

## 24.6 The Systems Approach to Medical Error

Beyond surgical task and procedural simulation-based training, the systems-based approach to understanding the surgical process and outcomes has important implications for error reduction [19]. This approach accepts that humans are fallible and errors are to be expected, even in the best organizations. Countermeasures are based upon the building of defenses to trap errors, and mitigation of their effects should one occur. This consists of altering the attitudes between different individuals and modifying the behavioral norms that have been established in these work settings. An example of this is the specification of operating lists for training junior surgeons, ensuring that fewer cases are booked and thus reducing the pressure on both the surgeon and the rest of the team to complete all procedures in the allocated time.

Medical personnel have a good understanding of the importance of communication in the clinical environment, with over 80% reporting that pre- and postoperative discussions are an important part of safety and teamwork [20]. However, one quarter of the group questioned were not encouraged to report their safety concerns. Perhaps more alarming is the statistic that only one out of three clinicians felt that errors are handled appropriately at their hospital. When asked their top recommendations to improve patient safety, the overwhelming response from clinicians is better communication.

## 24.7 Nontechnical Skills Simulation

It has been often pointed out that a skillfully performed operation is 75% decision-making and 25% dexterity. Decision-making and other nontechnical skills are not formally taught in the surgical curriculum but are rather acquired over time. In an analogous manner, it should be possible to use the simulated operating theater environment to train and assess performance of surgical trainees at skills such as team interaction and communication. This situation will also allow surgeons to benefit from feedback, by understanding the nature and effect of their mistakes and learn from them.

It is with this background that the role of a simulated clinical environment, i.e., the operating room, over and above simulation for technical skills, was born. One of the first to be developed was at the Department of Surgery at Imperial College London, under the joint leadership of Professors Ara Darzi and Charles Vincent – a dynamic duo of an innovative surgeon and a patient safety researcher.

Briefly, the simulated operating room consists of a replicated operating room environment and an adjacent control room, separated by one way viewing glass. In the operating room is a standard operating table, diathermy and suction machines, trolleys containing suture equipment and surgical instruments, and operating room lights. A moderate fidelity anesthetic simulator (SimMan, Laerdl, UK) consists of a mannequin which lies on the operating table and is controlled by a desktop computer in the control room. This enables the creation of a number of scenarios such as laryngospasm, hypoxia, and cardiac arrhythmias. A further trolley is available, containing standard anesthetic equipment, tubes, and drugs.

The complete surgical team is present, consisting of an anesthetist, anesthetic nurse, primary surgeon, surgeon's assistant, scrub nurse, and circulating nurse. Interactions between these individuals are recorded using four ceiling mounted cameras and unobtrusively placed microphones. The multiple streams of audio and video data, together with the trace on the anesthetic monitor, are fed into a clinical data recording (CDR) device. This enables those present in the control room to view the data in real time and for recordings to be made for debriefing sessions.

In a preliminary study, 25 surgeons of varying grades completed part of a standard varicose vein operation on a synthetic model (Limbs & Things, Bristol, UK) which was placed over the right groin of the anesthetic simulator [21]. The complete surgical team was present, the mannequin draped as for a real procedure, and standard surgical instruments available to the operating surgeon. Video based, blinded assessment of technical skills discriminated between surgeons according to experience, though their team skills measured by two expert observers on a global rating scale failed to show any similar differences. Many subjects did not achieve competency levels for pre-procedure preparation (90%), vigilance (56%), team interaction (27%), and communication (24%). Furthermore, only two trainees positioned the patient preoperatively, and none waited for a swab/instrument check prior to closure. Feedback responses from the participants were good, with 90% of them agreeing that the simulation was a realistic representation of an operating theater and 88% advocating this as a good environment for training in team skills.

Practicing the skills required in a simulated environment can enable the surgical team to function in a safer and more efficient manner when the crises occur in real life, with subjective data available on the effect of CRM training in aviation and anesthetics. However, it is also important to ensure upkeep of these skills, and regular training courses in a simulated operating room can allow this to happen. Studies in aviation have led to the concept of "over learning" whereby responses to crisis scenarios become automatic. It is not inconceivable that the simulated operating theater could lead to the development of such expertise, without the necessity for this to be gained through real-life experiences on real patients. Furthermore, the simulation operating room can be used for the trial and roll-out of new technologies, such as tele-robotic surgery, novel endovascular and endoluminal approaches, and image-guided surgery too. The intent is that the modes and types of communication may differ from the standard procedures, and as such, it is important to practice in a risk-free environment, even for accomplished clinicians, in order to maintain the highest levels of performance for patient care.

## 24.8 Simulation Care Pathways

Going beyond the operating room environment, simulation care pathways (or SimCare) are a novel approach that allow for healthcare providers to practice taking care of patients through use of evidence-based care pathways, in simulated environments, with subsequent translation to the clinical setting. The pathways critically involve two or more types of healthcare professional, in two or more healthcare settings.

In 2012, at Imperial College London, the development of two simulation care pathways was heralded, one for junior surgical residents (i.e., acute appendicitis) and another for senior residents (i.e., colorectal cancer) [22, 23]. The pathways involved a resident seeing a patient in a preoperative setting (i.e., surgical clinic or emergency room), intraoperative (i.e., operating room), and postoperative (i.e., recovery room, surgical ward, emergency room, or surgical clinic). The care pathways utilized online virtual patients (or avatars) for the pre- and postoperative phases. The intraoperative phase employed virtual reality simulation for training in laparoscopic appendectomy or laparoscopic colectomy (five residents each). The training program was proficiency-based, and outcomes of interest were the impact upon clinical care of patients admitted with presumptive diagnoses of the aforementioned diseases.

For the appendix pathway, data was collected on 17 patients prior to simulation training and 21 patients following training. The patients in the post-training group had significant improvements in recovery processes (i.e., shorter time to liquid and solid diets), with reduced postoperative morbidity (unpublished data). The colorectal pathway was evaluated in ten patients pre- and post-training, which led to an 82% increase in resident participation in the operating room and improvements for patients in terms of postoperative mobilization, earlier resumption of a solid diet, and shorter length of hospital stay [24].

More recently, at the University of Pennsylvania, four further simulation care pathways were developed for training junior surgical residents. These encompassed the following surgical disease processes – biliary disease, colorectal cancer, gastric cancer, and acute appendicitis [25–27]. The pathways were similar to those at Imperial College London, though the pre- and postoperative settings involved simulated patients (or actors), and the intraoperative setting encompassed a full operating room (anesthesiologist, scrub nurse, and circulating nurse) with a suitable simulation model for hands-on operative skills (i.e., synthetic, animal-based, or virtual reality simulation). Some 18 residents completed all the simulation care pathways, and outcomes of interest for this study were ratings of performance by expert faculty. All residents performed the pathway scenario, followed by 2.5 days of a simulation-based training program. On the 3rd day, they again performed the pathway, with significant improvements in performance noted, as rated by attending surgeons.

The concept of simulation care pathways is novel and sparsely mentioned within the medical literature [28]. There is a focus of the role of simulation-based training beyond that of the novice learner to acquire discrete and clinically isolated skills. The emphasis upon patient care is paramount, and the pathways are utilized for trainees, as well as healthcare professionals in practice. Furthermore, the pathways encourage a multidisciplinary aspect to learning in a simulation environment, which once again is the exception rather than the norm. An important aspect of simulation care pathways is that as they are disease based, there is the potential to measure clinically relevant outcomes, at patient, learner, and organizational levels. This is a critical step if we are to determine the value of simulation-based training within the medical curriculum.

## 24.9 Conclusion

The adoption of novel surgical technologies and techniques requires surgeons to develop an increasingly diverse set of technical skills in a time- and cost-efficient manner. Simulation allows trainees to address difficulties in spatial awareness and psychomotor dexterity prior to advancing to more complex skills; thus, initial basic training in the skills laboratory can shorten the learning curve for more advanced procedures while decreasing the cost of training [29]. Given studies investigating the TER of laparoscopic simulators, investing trainee time in simulation learning may improve the efficiency of knowledge transfer in laparoscopy if structured, proficiency-based curricula are properly utilized. As technology continues to be integrated into modern surgical curricula, an awareness of the learning curve for skills acquisition can guide efficient, effective surgical training.

The greatest challenge in simulation is to consider the role of clinical faculty who are involved in preparation, teaching, and evaluation of simulation-based training programs, in association with simulation center administration and operations staff too. There needs to be an awareness of the need to protect time for clinicians who undertake this role and to engage associated healthcare providers such as nursing staff from the operating room and clinical ward, to deliver the educational sessions. Beyond this, simulation can also be used as a tool to undertake faculty development, either to teach in the simulation setting or to enable educators to develop and refine their skills for teaching in other clinical environments.

The role of simulation in surgical training must be underpinned by the delivery of high-quality surgical care to our patients. A patient-centered model of clinical practice is essential and can be driven toward the simulation paradigm, through the concept of multidisciplinary care pathways – the state of the art of modern simulation practice in surgery. The challenges with regard to knowledge translation from best evidence to clinical impact, innovation, and practice may be most effectively dealt with through the incorporation of all parts of simulation-based surgical training, from task trainers, simulated operating suites, and standardized patients, through the lens of simulation care pathways.

## References

1. Brennan, T. A., Leape, L. L., Laird, N. M., Hebert, L., Localio, A. R., Lawthers, A. G., Newhouse, J. P., Weiler, P. C., & Hiatt, H. H. (1991). Incidence of adverse events and negligence in hospitalized patients. Results of the Harvard Medical Practice Study I. *The New England Journal of Medicine, 324*(6), 370–376.
2. Cook, D. A., Hatala, R., Brydges, R., Zendejas, B., Szostek, J. H., Wang, A. T., Erwin, P. J., & Hamstra, S. J. (2011). Technology-enhanced simulation for health professions education: A systematic review and meta-analysis. *Journal of the American Medical Association, 306*(9), 978–988.
3. Cheng, A., Brown, L. L., Duff, J. P., Davidson, J., Overly, F., Tofil, N. M., Peterson, D. T., White, M. L., Bhanji, F., Bank, I., Gottesman, R., Adler, M., Zhong, J., Grant, V., Grant, D. J., Sudikoff, S. N., Marohn, K., Charnovich, A., Hunt, E. A., Kessler, D. O., Wong, H., Robertson, N., Lin, Y., Doan, Q., Duval-Arnould, J. M., Nadkarni, V. M., & International Network for Simulation-Based Pediatric Innovation, Research, & Education (INSPIRE) CPR Investigators. (2015). Improving cardiopulmonary resuscitation with a CPR feedback device and refresher simulations (CPR CARES Study): A randomized clinical trial. *JAMA Pediatrics, 169*(2), 137–144.
4. Barsuk, J. H., Cohen, E. R., Feinglass, J., McGaghie, W. C., & Wayne, D. B. (2009). Use of simulation-based education to reduce catheter-related bloodstream infections. *Archives of Internal Medicine, 169*(15), 1420–1423.
5. Aggarwal, R., Ward, J., Balasundaram, I., Sains, P., Athanasiou, T., & Darzi, A. (2007). Proving the effectiveness of virtual reality simulation for training in laparoscopic surgery. *Annals of Surgery, 246*(5), 771–779.
6. Neily, J., Mills, P. D., Young-Xu, Y., Carney, B. T., West, P., Berger, D. H., Mazzia, L. M., Paull, D. E., & Bagian, J. P. (2010). Association between implementation of a medical team training program and surgical mortality. *Journal of the American Medical Association, 304*(15), 1693–1700.
7. Pucher, P. H., Aggarwal, R., Srisatkunam, T., & Darzi, A. (2014). Validation of the simulated ward environment for assessment of ward-based surgical care. *Annals of Surgery, 259*(2), 215–221.
8. Pucher, P. H., Aggarwal, R., Singh, P., Srisatkunam, T., Twaij, A., & Darzi, A. (2014). Ward simulation to improve surgical ward round performance: A randomized controlled trial of a simulation-based curriculum. *Annals of Surgery, 260*(2), 236–243.
9. Harrysson, I. J., Cook, J., Sirimanna, P., Feldman, L. S., Darzi, A., & Aggarwal, R. (2014). Systematic review of learning curves for minimally invasive abdominal surgery: A review of the methodology of data collection, depiction of outcomes, and statistical analysis. *Annals of Surgery, 260*(1), 37–45.
10. Birkmeyer, N. J., Dimick, J. B., Share, D., Hawasli, A., English, W. J., Genaw, J., Finks, J. F., Carlin, A. M., Birkmeyer, J. D., & Michigan Bariatric Surgery Collaborative. (2010). Hospital complication rates with bariatric surgery in Michigan. *Journal of the American Medical Association, 304*(4), 435–442.
11. Fried, G. M., Feldman, L. S., Vassiliou, M. C., Fraser, S. A., Stanbridge, D., Ghitulescu, G., & Andrew, C. G. (2004). Proving the value of simulation in laparoscopic surgery. *Annals of Surgery, 240*(3), 518–525; discussion 525–8.

12. Aggarwal, R., Moorthy, K., & Darzi, A. (2004). Laparoscopic skills training and assessment. *The British Journal of Surgery, 91*(12), 1549–1558.
13. Aggarwal, R., Grantcharov, T. P., Eriksen, J. R., Blirup, D., Kristiansen, V. B., Funch-Jensen, P., & Darzi, A. (2006). An evidence-based virtual reality training program for novice laparoscopic surgeons. *Annals of Surgery, 244*(2), 310–314.
14. Aggarwal, R., Ward, J., Balasundaram, I., Sains, P., Athanasiou, T., & Darzi, A. (2007). Proving the effectiveness of virtual reality simulation for training in laparoscopic surgery. *Annals of Surgery, 246*(5), 771–779.
15. Kolozsvari, N. O., Kaneva, P., Brace, C., Chartrand, G., Vaillancourt, M., Cao, J., Banaszek, D., Demyttenaere, S., Vassiliou, M. C., Fried, G. M., & Feldman, L. S. (2011). Mastery versus the standard proficiency target for basic laparoscopic skill training: Effect on skill transfer and retention. *Surgical Endoscopy, 25*(7), 2063–2070.
16. Sachdeva, A. K., Pellegrini, C. A., & Johnson, K. A. (2008). Support for simulation-based surgical education through American College of Surgeons – Accredited education institutes. *World Journal of Surgery, 32*(2), 196–207.
17. Barsuk, J. H., Cohen, E. R., Feinglass, J., McGaghie, W. C., & Wayne, D. B. (2009). Use of simulation-based education to reduce catheter-related bloodstream infections. *Archives of Internal Medicine, 169*(15), 1420–1423.
18. Cohen, E. R., Feinglass, J., Barsuk, J. H., et al. (2010). Cost savings from reduced catheter-related bloodstream infection after simulation based education for residents in a medical intensive care unit. *Simulation in Healthcare, 5*(2), 98–102.
19. Vincent, C., Moorthy, K., Sarker, S. K., Chang, A., & Darzi, A. W. (2004). Systems approaches to surgical quality and safety: From concept to measurement. *Annals of Surgery, 239*(4), 475–482.
20. Sexton, J. B., Thomas, E. J., & Helmreich, R. L. (2000). Error, stress, and teamwork in medicine and aviation: Cross sectional surveys. *BMJ, 320*(7237), 745–749.
21. Moorthy, K., Munz, Y., Adams, S., Pandey, V., & Darzi, A. (2005). A human factors analysis of technical and team skills among surgical trainees during procedural simulations in a simulated operating theatre. *Annals of Surgery, 242*(5), 631–639.
22. Beyer-Berjot, L., Patel, V., Acharya, A., Taylor, D., Bonrath, E., Grantcharov, T., Darzi, A., & Aggarwal, R. (2014). Surgical training: Design of a virtual care pathway approach. *Surgery, 156*(3), 689–697.
23. Beyer-Berjot, L., Patel, V., Ziprin, P., Taylor, D., Berdah, S., Darzi, A., & Aggarwal, R. (2015). Enhanced recovery simulation in colorectal surgery: Design of virtual online patients. *Surgical Endoscopy, 29*(8), 2270–2277.
24. Beyer-Berjot, L., Pucher, P., Patel, V., Hashimoto, D. A., Ziprin, P., Berdah, S., Darzi, A., & Aggarwal, R. (2017). Colorectal surgery and enhanced recovery: Impact of a simulation-based care pathway training curriculum. *Journal of Visceral Surgery, 154*, 313–320. https://doi.org/10.1016/j.jviscsurg.2017.02.003.
25. Miyasaka, K. W., Martin, N. D., Pascual, J. L., Buchholz, J., & Aggarwal, R. (2015). A simulation curriculum for management of trauma and surgical critical care patients. *Journal of Surgical Education, 72*(5), 803–810.
26. Miyasaka, K. W., Buchholz, J., LaMarra, D., Karakousis, G. C., & Aggarwal, R. (2015). Development and implementation of a clinical pathway approach to simulation-based training for foregut surgery. *Journal of Surgical Education, 72*(4), 625–635.
27. Buchholz, J., Vollmer, C. M., Miyasaka, K. W., Lamarra, D., & Aggarwal, R. (2015). Design, development and implementation of a surgical simulation pathway curriculum for biliary disease. *Surgical Endoscopy, 29*(1), 68–76.
28. Aggarwal, R. (2017). Surgical performance: A pathway to excellence. *Annals of Surgery, 266*(2), 220–222.
29. Zendejas, B., Wang, A. T., Brydges, R., Hamstra, S. J., & Cook, D. A. (2013). Cost: The missing outcome in simulation-based medical education research: A systematic review. *Surgery, 153*(2), 160–176.

# Chapter 25
# Developing Surgical Teams: Theory

John T. Paige

**Overview** Although excellence in the care of a surgical patient depends in part on the medical knowledge and technical skill of the surgeon, such attributes are not necessarily sufficient. In addition, the expert functioning of the teams working with the surgeon in the perioperative setting is critical to a successful outcome. Developing highly reliable surgical teams, therefore, is essential for safe, effective patient care. Unfortunately, more often than not, surgical teamwork falls short of this ideal. For the surgical educator, the challenge thus becomes overcoming ingrained patterns of detrimental behavior among practicing clinicians and inculcating students in team-based competencies that will improve the quality of care. (S)he can meet such a challenge by adopting human factors (HF) principles when teaching and training inter-professional teams. The next two chapters will discuss how to develop such an approach by first addressing the theoretical underpinnings of HF concepts in the present chapter, then by demonstrating applications of these concepts to promote highly reliable team function in general and using a specific example. In doing so, they will combine to address the following objectives: (1) discussing the role of HF in promoting safe surgical care, (2) applying HF concepts to develop highly reliable surgical teams, and (3) illustrating such an application through a discussion of the development of simulation-based team training in surgery at LSU Health New Orleans Health Sciences Center.

## 25.1 Introduction

In today's dynamic, evermore complex healthcare environment in which the doubling of the sum of medical knowledge will soon approach months rather than years and disruptive technological innovations continue to change the way clinicians practice [1], surgeons can no longer rely on their own wit and talent to provide

---

J. T. Paige (✉)
Department of Surgery, Louisiana State University School of Medicine, New Orleans, LA, USA
e-mail: jpaige@lsuhsc.edu

quality care to the surgical patient. Instead, they must depend on smoothly functioning, inter-professional teams of other health professionals and disciplines who bring their own expertise within their scope of practice to assist surgeons in guiding their increasingly sick wards through surgical procedures to a successful outcome. Gone are the days in which the autonomous surgeon acted as the "captain of the ship," dictating to all around every component of the care plan. Instead, the contemporary surgeon must act more like a coach, collaborating with his teammates to ensure effective care is rendered. This fact is especially true, since advances in critical care, anesthesia, pharmacology, surgical technology, physical and occupational therapy, and the like outpace surgeons' abilities to keep abreast. The Institute of Medicine (IOM) recognized this shift in practice in *Health Professions Education: A Bridge to Quality* when it designated the ability to work in inter-professional teams as a new core competency [2]. This work was followed by the IOM's *Redesigning Continuing Education in the Health Professions* which called on the transformation of continuing education into an inter-professional activity [3].

This expanding emphasis on inter-professional teamwork and team function presents new challenges for contemporary surgical educators. In addition to teaching medical knowledge and technical skills, they must also focus on introducing learners to team-based competencies to ensure the effective development of surgical teams. Such training entails inculcating students new to the profession in teamwork concepts and principles as well as trying to overcome ingrained patterns of detrimental team behavior among practicing clinicians. By taking a human factors (HF) approach to such teaching, surgical educators can meet these challenges. This chapter will start to address how to develop highly reliable surgical teams by discussing the role of HF in promoting safe surgical care. It will do so by addressing the following objectives: (1) discussing theoretical underpinnings of HF and (2) demonstrating its need due to the current inadequacy of surgical teamwork in the clinical environment.

## 25.2 The Role of Human Factors in Promoting Safe Surgical Care

Although the term "human factors" was first coined in 1957 with the founding of the Human Factors Society, the field's origins date back to the beginning of the twentieth century and are closely tied to aviation [4, 5]. In fact, the need to identify qualified individuals for pilot training during World War I was a major impetus to the development of aviation psychology [4, 5]. With the rise of civil aviation during the interwar period, work in the field continued. In fact, it was during this time that the first flight simulator, the Link Trainer, was developed by the American Albert Edward Link in Binghamton, New York [4]. The onset of World War II provided more advances in the field as a result of two major trends: (1) the need to design processes to fit people's capabilities and minimize their limitations in the face of massive mobilization for the war effort and (2) the inability of humans to overcome poor design due to the rapid technological advances of the period [5]. In the United

States, World War II marks the birth of the discipline [5]. After World War II, the field entered a period of rapid expansion with research and development that continues to this day.

Christensen, Topmiller, and Gill have defined the term "human factors" as "…that branch of science and technology that includes what is known and theorized about human behavioral, cognitive, and biologic characteristics that can be validly applied to specification, design, evaluation, operation, maintenance of products, jobs, tasks, and systems to enhance safe, effective, and satisfying use by individuals, groups, and organizations." [6] Put another way, HF is the study of the interaction of humans with their environment. As Christensen et al.'s definition implies, this "environment" can entail the technology on which an individual works, the system processes and procedures of an individual's workplace, and the work teams with which an individual interacts.

The central axiom of the field of HF can be summed up by the following adage: "We're only human." This maxim encapsulates the HF concept that human error is *inevitable*, making the construction of an error-free system *impossible* [7]. Thus, HF is founded on "…a fundamental rejection of the notion that humans are primarily at fault when making errors in the use of a socio-technical system." [8] Instead, as James Reason [7] has posited, catastrophic errors within complex systems are the result of the combination of unnoticed weaknesses within these systems, so-called *latent conditions*, with *active failures* resulting from decisions and actions of individuals that are influenced by these systems. Consequently, multiple holes within the defenses erected to prevent a problem align, much like holes in Swiss cheese, creating a set of circumstances culminating in a catastrophic event. Recent examples of "Swiss cheese in action" can be found in multiple industries: nuclear power [9], offshore oil drilling [10], and, too frequently, healthcare [11].

One of the major goals, therefore, of work in HF is to design systems and devices with *defenses in depth* for the safe, effective use by humans [12]. In order to optimize the interaction between humans with their work environment, HF experts study human behaviors, abilities, and *limitations* in an effort to create robust systems adept at *avoiding, trapping, and mitigating* potential and real threats and errors [14]. Such an application of HF to real world situations is known as HF engineering.

In essence, HF engineers attempt to shape human behavior within a work environment through the design of systems and processes that optimize the recognition and mitigation of problems and deficiencies within those systems. According to Caffazzo and St.-Cyr [8], HF engineers pursue this goal through a two-pronged approach: (1) systems-focused and (2) people-focused (Fig. 25.1 [13–16]). The former approach is most effective in preventing error, whereas the latter approach allows for the positive impact of human judgment. Systems-based solutions to error reduction include standardization of processes, decreasing complexity and optimizing information processing within systems, the intelligent application of automation and computerization, and force functioning [17]. Of these, force functioning is the most effective, since it involves creating so-called *physical constraints* that prevents humans from committing an error. The development in anesthesia of the Pin Index Safety System (PISS), in which small cylinders of anesthetic gases can only be

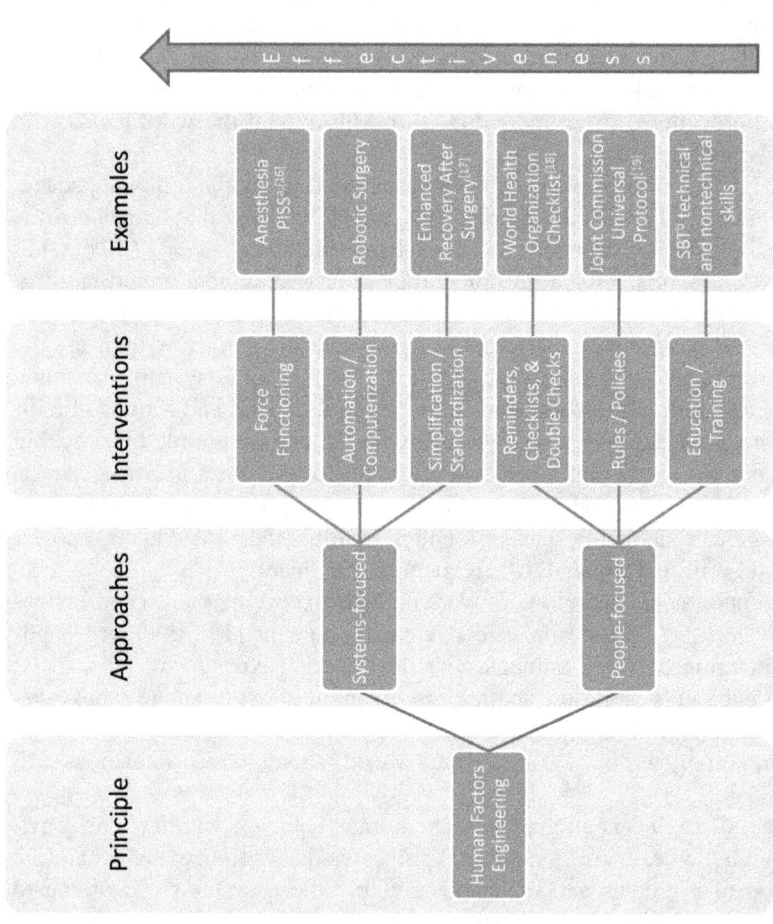

[a]PISS=Pin-Index Safety System; [b]SBT=Simulation-Based Training

**Fig. 25.1** Approaches to human factors engineering. Human factors engineers use both systems-focused and people-focused approaches in order to create robust systems adept at avoiding, trapping, and mitigating potential and real threats and errors. The effectiveness of such approaches increase moving from people-focused to systems-focused solutions

attached to the flush valve connector having that gas's unique pin orientation, is an example of this force functioning in healthcare [16]. The oversized diesel nozzle preventing its insertion in an unleaded gas tank is an everyday example.

People-focused approaches involve the application of *procedural constraints* such as the use of checklists and reminders or policies and procedures. The Joint Commission's Universal Protocol for Preventing Wrong Site, Wrong Procedure, and Wrong Person Surgery™ [19] is an excellent surgical example of such a constraint. Other people-focused interventions involve training and education to instill expected values and behaviors to be followed in the workplace. In this manner, *cultural constraints* are fostered to create an environment in which doing "the right thing at the right time" becomes the norm. In such environments, safety becomes the *primary priority*, superseding all other goals (e.g., profit, efficiency, and the like).

Such a culture of safety is the defining characteristic of a *high reliability organization (HRO)*. In *Managing the Unexpected: Assuring High Performance in the Age of Complexity* [18], Weick and Sutcliffe define the key principles and attributes of HROs that allow them to perform in a consistent and safe manner in high-risk, dynamic environments. Most notably, HROs demonstrate a *preoccupation with failure* in which they are consistently searching for weaknesses within the systems and processes of the organizational structure that may lead to threats and hazards before they surface. As a result, HROs possess *a sensitivity to operations* and *reluctance to simplify interpretations of problems* in order to avoid missing a potential latent condition. Such sensitivity to operations manifests itself in HROs' *deference to expertise* in lieu of rank or seniority when dealing with an issue. All these characteristics combine to create a *commitment of resilience* within HROs that allows them to adapt fluidly and smoothly to changing situations and conditions within their environment. In a nutshell, an HRO promotes *mindfulness* in lieu of "mindlessness" among all the individuals working within it.

Two examples outside healthcare demonstrate the benefits of having, and the perils of lacking, what Westrum [19] refers to as a *generative organizational culture*. The story of the seaman who lost a wrench on the flight deck of the nuclear aircraft carrier *USS Carl Vinson* is illustrative of how an HRO operates. Such a loss can be potentially catastrophic if the instrument gets sucked into one of the jet engines of the fighter planes taking off and landing. The seaman, therefore, spoke up to inform his superiors of the loss. Consequently, all operations were required to be halted, and the deck was systematically searched until the wrench was found. For revealing his loss, the seaman was officially recognized and rewarded the next day during a ceremony on the aircraft carrier [18].

A cautionary tale is provided by British Petroleum (BP). This energy company, which marketed itself as an environmentally friendly entity, was, in reality, anything but friendly due to an organizational culture that placed profit before safety. Even though the Macondo Well Explosion and Oil Spill in the Gulf of Mexico [11, 20] represents the most recent and costly example of the consequences of this cultural attitude, the preceding Texas City Refinery Explosion [23] and the Prudhoe Bay Trans-Alaska Pipeline Oil Spill [23] reveal that BP was prone to such catastrophic events because of it. Unfortunately, the work of several researchers have demonstrated that the cultural bent of the healthcare industry leans more toward BP than the *USS Carl Vinson* [21].

Why is achieving HRO status so difficult in healthcare? Runciman and Walton [22] have argued that its diversity of tasks and activity patterns, its lack of regulation, and its focus on sick humans with variable characteristics and outcomes are contributing factors. Given that cultural change can take up to a decade and requires a concerted, coordinated approach [23], one might consider trying to create a culture of safety in the healthcare industry a quixotic endeavor. Fortunately, such change does not need to occur at a macro-system level to ensure its existence at the clinical micro-system level. In fact, such clinical micro-systems, defined as a group of healthcare professionals working together with a shared clinical purpose to provide care to a defined patient population, can independently function like an HRO [24]. Thus, HRO practices can be fostered within an operating room (OR), postanesthesia care unit (PACU), intensive care unit (ICU), emergency department (ED), or on the patient care floor. Additionally, it might be developed within several of these at once or within a service line within an institution, such as perioperative care. Over time, the creation of such pockets of HRO-like clinical micro-systems can assist in changing the overall behavior of the institution as a whole.

The cornerstone to any HRO is having highly reliable team function within that organization [25]. Without teams of individuals performing in such a manner, the communication and resiliency needed to maintain high reliability within an organization are curtailed. Salas et al. [26] has identified key traits and coordinating mechanisms demonstrated by highly reliable teams in HRO settings that have been incorporated into the Team Strategies and Tools to Enhance Performance and Patient Safety (STEPPS)™ [27] program developed by the Department of Defense in coordination with the Agency for Healthcare Research and Quality.

## 25.3 Contemporary Surgical Teamwork

Much like the presence of a culture of safety, highly reliable team function tends to be the exception rather than the norm in healthcare. This fact is especially true in surgery and the OR where a sense of tribalism [28], fostered by a silo mentality [29] promotes multi-professional interaction instead of inter-professional teamwork [30]. Thus, the OR is characterized more as a group of experts rather than an expert team [31]. Most damaging, these behaviors are propagated from one generation of clinicians to the next through modeling by students who are influenced by this "hidden curriculum" of their training. Many factors contribute to this toxic work environment: unwanted hierarchical structures [32], role confusion [33], differing perceptions of teamwork [34], weak interpersonal skills among professions [35], and increased tension [36]. Such problems extend beyond the OR to other clinic micro-systems where surgical teams are located including the intensive care unit (ICU) and the surgical wards [37].

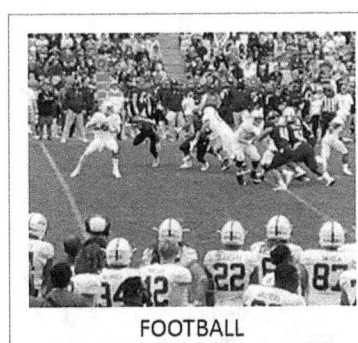
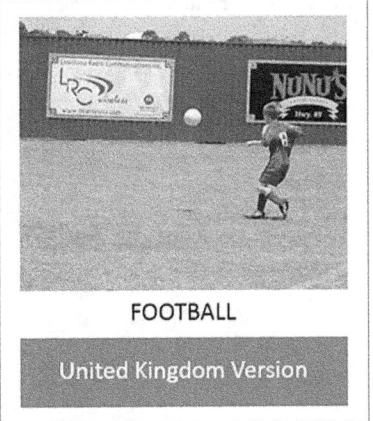
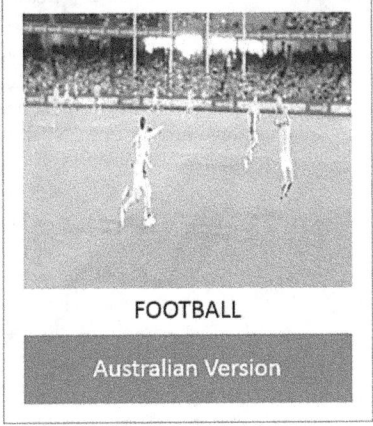

**Fig. 25.2** Separated by a common language! Much like the term "football" connotes different sports in the United States, United Kingdom, and Australia respectively, surgical team members may misunderstand or misinterpret communication between each other

Particularly remarkable is the striking lack of communication within surgical teams [38]. Such ineffective communication can be due to misunderstandings, lack of hearing, or inappropriate timing of delivery of information [39]. Unfortunately, it can occur during the management of critical events [40], and its consequences can negatively impact patient care [38]. Thus, even though members of surgical teams are speaking to one another, they are often not understanding the meaning of what is being said. Much like the citizens of the United States, the United Kingdom, and Australia, surgical team members are often separated by a common language (Fig. 25.2)!

The consequences of ineffective teamwork in surgical micro-systems are manifold. It can result in distractions that can negatively impact team function (Table 25.1 [41–44]). Thus, the dysfunctions of contemporary surgical teams have tangible consequences that can negatively impact the care given to the patient.

**Table 25.1** Disruptions in the operating room

| Group | Study description | Findings | Impact |
|---|---|---|---|
| Antoniodis et al. [41] | Observation of 65 general surgery and orthopedic cases | 9.82 ± 3.97 distractions/interruptions per hour; more disruptions during early phase of case | Equipment failures and OR environment disruptions had highest interference with OR team functioning |
| Wheelock et al. [42] | Observation of 90 general surgery cases | Most prevalent distractions were those initiated by external staff and case-irrelevant conversations | Surgeons → poorer teamwork with case-irrelevant conversations; higher stress with acoustic distractions |
| | | | Anesthesiologists → poorer teamwork with case-irrelevant conversations |
| | | | Nurses → poorer teamwork with equipment distractions; higher stress with equipment distractions |
| Weigl et al. (2015) [43] | Observation 56 cases (35 open; 21 laparoscopic) | 9.87 intraoperative interruptions per hour; people entering/exiting room and telephone-/beeper-related disruptions most common | Equipment failures and OR environment disruptions had highest interference with OR team functioning (especially in laparoscopic cases) |
| | | | Surgeons → increased distraction with procedural interruptions and case-irrelevant conversations |
| | | | Anesthesiologists → increased perceived workload with intraoperative interruptions |
| | | | Nurses → increased perceived workload with intraoperative interruptions |
| Weigl et al. (2016) [44] | Simulated disruption scenarios in OR with 19 surgeons | Increased intraoperative workload with disruptions | Telephone call caused more disruption for surgeons |
| | | | Patient discomfort increased surgeon workload |
| | | | Increase in mental workload associated with decrease in technical performance |

## 25.4 Conclusion

Surgical teams are more often ineffective than effective in contemporary clinical practice. Possessing an understanding of HF can help in addressing this gap. Key concepts of HF include the need to create defenses in depth in order to avoid, trap, and mitigate the inevitable errors that occur in a human-designed system as well as employing both systems-focused and people-focused approaches to help promote highly reliable team behavior. By doing so, HF can be applied in the surgical setting to create adaptive teams that can respond to dynamic, high-risk changes in the environment.

# References

1. Densen, P. (2011). Challenges and opportunities facing medical education. *Transactions of the American Clinical and Climatological Association, 122*, 48–58.
2. Greiner, A. C., & Knebel, E. (Eds.). (2003). *Health professions education: A bridge to quality.* Washington, DC: Institute of Medicine, National Academies Press.
3. IOM (Institute of Medicine). (2010). *Redesigning continuing education in the health professions.* Washington, DC: The National Academies Press.
4. Anonymous. *What is human factors and ergonomics?* Benchmark Research & Safety, Inc. http://www.benchmarkrs.com/main/human-factors/what.aspx. Accessed 20 Jan 2017.
5. Adams, D. (2006). *A layman's introduction to human factors in aircraft accident and incident investigation.* Australian Transport Safety Bureau (ATSB) Safety Information Paper. B2006/0094. Canberra City, ACT.
6. Christensen, J. M., Topmiller, D. A., & Gill, R. T. (1988). Human factors definitions revisited. *Human Factors Society Bulletin, 31*, 7.
7. Reason, J. (2005). Safety in the operating theatre – part 2: Human error and organisational failure. *Quality & Safety in Health Care, 14*, 56–60.
8. Cafazzo, J. A., & St-Cyr, O. (2012). From discovery to design: The evolution of human factors in healthcare. *Healthcare Quarterly, 15*, 24–29.
9. Fackler, M.. Nuclear disaster in Japan was avoidable, critics contend. *New York Times*, 3/9/2012. http://www.nytimes.com/2012/03/10/world/asia/critics-say-japan-ignored-warnings-of-nuclear-disaster.html?_r=0. Accessed 3 Feb 2017.
10. US Chemical Safety and Hazard Investigation Board. (2014). *Investigation report: Explosion and fire at the Macondo well 1 and 2* (Report No. 2010-10-I-OS). Washington, DC.
11. Associated Press. *Third wrong-sided brain surgery at R.I. hospital.* http://www.msnbc.msn.com/id/21981965. Accessed 28 Nov 2016.
12. Gawron, V. J., Drury, C. G., Fairbanks, R. J., & Berger, R. C. (2006). Medical error and human factors engineering: Where are we now? *American Journal of Medical Quality, 21*, 57–67.
13. Weinger, M. B., & Gaba, D. M. (2014). Human factors engineering in patient safety. *Anesthesiology, 120*(4), 801–806.
14. The Eras Society. http://www.erassociety.org/. Accessed 28 Nov 2016.
15. Haynes, A. B., Weiser, T. G., Berry, W. R., Lipsitz, S. R., Breizat, A. H., Dellinger, E. P., Herbosa, T., Joseph, S., Kibatala, P. L., Lapitan, M. C., Merry, A. F., Moorthy, K., Reznick, R. K., Taylor, B., Gawande, A. A., & Safe Surgery Saves Lives Study Group. (2009). A surgical safety checklist to reduce morbidity and mortality in a global population. *The New England Journal of Medicine, 360*, 491–499.
16. Joint Commission. *The universal protocol for preventing wrong site, wrong procedure, wrong person surgery™.* The Joint Commission. http://www.jointcommission.org/assets/1/18/UP_Poster.pdf. Accessed 20 Jan 2017.
17. Nolan, T. W. (2000). System changes to improve patient safety. *BMJ, 320*, 771–773.
18. Weick, K. E., & Sutcliffe, K. M. (2001). *Managing the unexpected: Assuring high performance in the age of complexity.* San Francisco: Jossey-Bass.
19. Westrum, R. (2004). A typology of organisational cultures. *Quality & Safety in Health Care, 13*(Suppl 2), ii22–ii27.
20. Cheremisinoff, N. P., & Davletshin, A. (2010). *Emergency response Management of Offshore oil Spills: Guidelines for emergency responders.* Hoboken: Wiley.
21. 2014 User Comparative Database Report. Content last reviewed March 2014. Agency for Healthcare Research and Quality, Rockville, MD. http://www.ahrq.gov/professionals/quality-patient-safety/patientsafetyculture/hospital/2014/index.html.
22. Runciman, B., & Walton, M. (2007). *Safety and ethics in healthcare: A guide to getting it right.* Aldershot: Ashgate.
23. Kotter, J. P. (1996). *Leading change.* Boston: Harvard Business School Press.
24. Mohr, J. J., & Batalden, P. B. (2002). Improving safety on the front lines: The role of clinical microsystems. *Quality & Safety in Health Care, 11*, 45–50.

25. Sanchez, J. A., & Barach, P. R. (2012). High reliability organizations and surgical microsystems: Re-engineering surgical care. *Surgical Clinics of North America, 92*, 1–14.
26. Salas, E., Sims, D. E., & Burke, C. S. (2005). Is there a big five in teamwork? *Small Group Research, 36*, 555–599.
27. Agency for Healthcare Research and Quality. Team Strategies and Tools to Enhance Performance and Patient Safety (STEPPS)™. http://www.ahrq.gov/professionals/education/curriculum-tools/teamstepps/index.html. Accessed 3 Feb 2017.
28. Weller, J., Boyd, M., & Cumin, D. (2014). Teams, tribes and patient safety: Overcoming barriers to effective teamwork in healthcare. *Postgraduate Medical Journal, 90*(1061), 149–154.
29. Bleakley, A. (2006). You are who I say you are: The rhetorical construction of identity in the operating theatre. *Journal of Workplace Learning, 18*(7–8), 414–425.
30. Bleakley, A., Boyden, J., Hobbs, A., Walsh, L., & Allard, J. (2006). Improving teamwork climate in operating theatres: The shift from multiprofessionalism to interprofessionalism. *Journal of Interprofessional Care, 20*(5), 461–470.
31. Burke, C. S., Salas, E., Wilson-Donnelly, K., et al. (2004). How to turn a team of experts into an expert medical team: Guidance from the aviation and military communities. *Quality & Safety in Health Care, 13*(Suppl 1), i96–i104.
32. Helmrich, R. L., & Davies, J. M. (1994). Team performance in the operating room. In M. S. Bogner (Ed.), *Human error in medicine* (pp. 225–253). Hillside: Erlbaum.
33. Nakarada-Kordic, I., Weller, J. M., Webster, C. S., Cumin, D., Frampton, C., Boyd, M., & Merry, A. F. (2016). Assessing the similarity of mental models of operating room team members and implications for patient safety: A prospective, replicated study. *BMC Medical Education, 16*(1), 229.
34. Makary, M. A., Sexton, J. B., Freischlag, J. A., et al. (2006). Operating room teamwork among physicians and nurses: Teamwork in the eye of the beholder. *Journal of the American College of Surgeons, 202*, 746–752.
35. Nestel, D., & Kidd, J. M. (2006). Nurses' perceptions and experiences of communication in the operating theatre: A focus group interview. *BMC Nursing, 5*, 1.
36. Lingard, L., Garwood, S., & Poenaru, D. (2004). Tensions influencing operating room team function: Does institutional context make a difference? *Medical Education, 38*, 691–699.
37. Schlitzkus, L. L., Agle, S. C., McNally, M. M., et al. (2009). What do surgical nurses know about surgical residents? *Journal of Surgical Education, 66*(6), 383–391.
38. Nagpal, K., Vats, A., Lamb, B., Ashrafian, H., Sevdalis, N., Vincent, C., & Moorthy, K. (2010). Information transfer and communication in surgery: A systematic review. *Annals of Surgery, 252*(2), 225–239.
39. Yule, S., & Paterson-Brown, S. (2012). Surgeons' non-technical skills. *The Surgical Clinics of North America, 92*(1), 37–50.
40. ElBardissi, A. W., Regenbogen, S. E., Greenberg, C. C., et al. (2009). Communication practices on 4 Harvard surgical services: A surgical safety collaborative. *Annals of Surgery, 250*(6), 861–865.
41. Antoniadis, S., Passauer-Baierl, S., Baschnegger, H., & Weigl, M. (2014). Identification and interference of intraoperative distractions and interruptions in operating rooms. *The Journal of Surgical Research, 188*(1), 21–29.
42. Wheelock, A., Suliman, A., Wharton, R., Babu, E. D., Hull, L., Vincent, C., Sevdalis, N., & Arora, S. (2015). The impact of operating room distractions on stress, workload, and teamwork. *Annals of Surgery, 261*(4), 1079–1084.
43. Weigl, M., Antoniadis, S., Chiapponi, C., Bruns, C., & Sevdalis, N. (2015). The impact of intra-operative interruptions on surgeons' perceived workload: An observational study in elective general and orthopedic surgery. *Surgical Endoscopy, 29*(1), 145–153.
44. Weigl, M., Stefan, P., Abhari, K., Wucherer, P., Fallavollita, P., Lazarovici, M., Weidert, S., Euler, E., & Catchpole, K. (2016). Intra-operative disruptions, surgeon's mental workload, and technical performance in a full-scale simulated procedure. *Surgical Endoscopy, 30*(2), 559–566.

# Chapter 26
# Developing Surgical Teams: Application

John T. Paige

**Overview** The preceding chapter discussed the theoretical underpinnings of human factors (HF) concepts and their role in promoting high reliability organizations (HROs) as well as highly reliable team function. In addition, it demonstrated that current teamwork in the clinical surgical environment is less than ideal, leading to dysfunction and the development of a silo mentality. This chapter will continue the discussion of developing surgical teams by discussing practical applications of HF concepts to develop highly reliable surgical teams and reviewing the development of simulation-based team training in surgery at LSU Health New Orleans Health Sciences Center.

## 26.1 Introduction

Today's dynamic, high-risk clinical environment, in which surgeons are required to address an ever-increasing complexity of disease processes and comorbid conditions, requires the smooth collaboration and function of a variety of care teams in order to shepherd safely surgical patients to recovery and health. Unfortunately, as demonstrated in the preceding chapter, current teamwork in the surgical setting is less than ideal, and it often results in a sense of tribalism among the various professions helping to care for the surgical patient [1]. Overcoming this situation, therefore, becomes an important challenge for surgical educators trying to develop surgical teams, especially since working in interprofessional teams is now a recognized core competency in healthcare [2]. In the United States, the Interprofessional Education Collaborative (IPEC) has worked to define major collaborative domains of interprofessional behavior with corresponding general and specific competencies within each one [3]. Such work has also been undertaken in Canada, the United Kingdom, and Australia [4].

J. T. Paige (✉)
Department of Surgery, Louisiana State University School of Medicine,
New Orleans, LA, USA
e-mail: jpaige@lsuhsc.edu

Human factors (HF), the study of the interaction of humans with their environment, have as one of its central axioms the proposition that *human error is inevitable* [5]. Its application, known as HF engineering, is devoted to improving human performance and mitigating the impact of human error in order to promote safety and effectiveness in dynamic, and at times high-risk, work environments. For surgical educators, therefore, HF principles can be brought to bear on developing surgical teams to create highly reliable function. This chapter will focus on this aspect of team development by (1) investigating how HF engineering can be employed in a practical manner to create highly reliable team behavior and (2) illustrating such an application through a discussion of the development of simulation-based training (SBT) of surgical teams at LSU Health Sciences Center New Orleans.

## 26.2 Applying HF Principles to Develop Highly Reliable Surgical Teams

By adopting an HF engineering perspective to surgical team development, the surgical educator can develop a multipronged approach to the undertaking. In this manner, both systems-focused and people-focused methods can be employed. In fact, evidence in the surgical literature suggests combining the two approaches is more effective in improving team technical and nontechnical performance as well as checklist adherence than either one alone [6].

One systems-based approach worth further discussion is the standardization of perioperative care pathways through the use of the Enhanced Recovery After Surgery (ERAS) [7] patient management strategy. ERAS is an attempt to remove variability in the surgical care of the patient through the adoption of evidence-based practices to replace traditional patterns of care. As a result, patients follow a predictable, consistent pathway of care from the first surgical office visit through the perioperative period to final discharge from the surgeon's care [8]. Such standardization of surgical care decreases complication rates across multiple surgical specialties [9].

Several people-focused approaches have been successfully employed to help develop surgical teams. The introduction of checklists, briefings, and double checks into surgical care has resulted in improvements in communication [10] and teamwork [11] as well as process [12] and outcomes [13] measures. Training and education in team-based competencies also has positive effects [14]. This training can take on a variety of forms: didactic instruction, role play, tabletop exercises, video- or web-based activities, and simulation-based training (SBT) [15]. SBT is a particularly attractive modality for teaching these competencies due to its immersive character which allows for a realistic, safe learning environment in which teams can hone skills treating rare, life-threatening conditions without harm to patients [16]. It is especially attractive to the surgical educator, since this type of experiential learning has been demonstrated to be effective in improving team-based interactions among surgical learners of all stripes, when used alone or in conjunction with other educational modalities (Table 26.1 [12, 17–35]).

**Table 26.1** Selected examples of the use of simulation-based training of surgical teams with their impacts

| Operating room (OR) teams | | | |
|---|---|---|---|
| Group | Intervention | Participant characteristics | Results |
| Paige et al. [17] | *Ex cura* high-fidelity OR team training | Senior medical students, senior undergraduate nursing students, nurse anesthesia students | Improved attitudes toward team-based competencies, improvement in individual and team-based behaviors |
| Nguyen et al. [18] | *Ex cura* laparoscopic cholecystectomy OR team training | Surgical residents, real OR team | Improved completion preoperative checklist, intraoperative ACGME[a] competencies |
| Cumin et al. [19] | *Ex cura* high-fidelity OR scenarios | Surgical residents, faculty and OR staff | Better recall of important information if given during formal communication (i.e., brief, time-out) |
| Pena et al. [20] | *Ex cura* high-fidelity OR team training in conjunction with workshop | Surgical residents and fellows | Improvement in NTS[b] between two sessions for junior and senior residents |
| Stevens et al. [21] | *Ex cura* high-fidelity cardiac surgery OR team training in conjunction with workshop | Cardiac surgeon, cardiac anesthesiologists, surgical physician assistants, cardiac OR nurse, cardiac anesthesia nurse, perfusionist | Improved concept of working as a team after intervention |
| Arriaga et al. [12] | *Ex cura* high-fidelity OR crisis scenarios | Surgical and anesthesia residents and faculty; operating room nurses, surgical technologists, certified nurse anesthetists | Increased adherence to lifesaving processes of care with the use of checklists with training |
| Arriaga et al. [22] | In situ and *ex cura* high-fidelity OR team training in crisis scenarios across a four hospital system | Surgical residents, faculty, and physician assistants; anesthesia faculty and certified nurse anesthetists; surgical technologists, operating room nurses, and biomedical engineers | Feasibility demonstrated; reduction in malpractice insurance awarded for participation |
| Dedy et al. [23] | *Ex cura* high-fidelity simulation as part of 5-day NTS[b] curriculum | PGY[c] 1 surgical residents | Improvement in knowledge, attitudes, and performance related to NTS[b] |
| Trauma teams | | | |
| Doumouras et al. [24] | *Ex cura* high-fidelity trauma team training | Surgical residents and trauma nurses | Improvement in attitudes; no decay in NTS[b] over 6 months |

(continued)

**Table 26.1** (continued)

| Operating room (OR) teams | | | |
| --- | --- | --- | --- |
| Group | Intervention | Participant characteristics | Results |
| Steinemann et al. [25] | In situ high-fidelity trauma team training | Residents, emergency medicine and trauma faculty, nurses, respiratory therapists, and emergency department technicians | Improvement in team performance; 76% increase in frequency of near-perfect task completion; 16% reduction in mean overall resuscitation time |
| Capella et al. [26] | TeamSTEPPS™[d] for trauma teams augmented by simulation | Surgery residents, faculty, nurses | Improvement in leadership, situational awareness, mutual support, communication, and overall teamwork; decrease in times to computed tomography scanner, OR, and endotracheal tube intubation |
| Zeismann et al. [27] | *Ex cura* high-fidelity trauma team training | Surgical residents, nurses, respiratory therapists | Improvement in attitudes toward teamwork principles |
| Perioperative/postoperative teams | | | |
| Nicksa et al. [28] | In situ and *ex cura* high-fidelity team training using high-risk crisis scenarios in various settings (ED, PACU, ICU, OR) | Surgical, anesthesia, medicine, critical care fellows and residents; nursing, respiratory therapy, pharmacy students, and faculty | PGY[c] 2 improvement in NTS[b]; no change PGY[c] 1 |
| Pucher et al. [29] | *Ex cura* high-fidelity training on mock surgical ward (rounds) | Surgical residents | Feasibility demonstrated |
| Arora et al. [30] | *Ex cura* high-fidelity training on mock surgical ward | Surgical residents | Improvement in communication, leadership, decision-making; improved ability to clinically recognize falling saturation, check circulatory status, reassess patient, call for help |
| Stephens et al. [31] | *Ex cura* high-fidelity training in conjunction with day long course | Practicing surgeons, anesthesiologists, nurses, other staff in perioperative care | Improved confidence related to team behaviors, recognizing different team perspectives, employing checklists |
| Doumouras et al. [32] | *Ex cura* high-fidelity crisis simulation training | Surgical residents | Improvement in NTS[b] of PGY[c] 2/3 residents with no decay in skills over year |

(continued)

**Table 26.1** (continued)

| Operating room (OR) teams | | | |
|---|---|---|---|
| Group | Intervention | Participant characteristics | Results |
| Literature reviews | | | |
| Doumouras et al. [33] | Structured literature review of simulation-based crew resource management training | Postgraduate trainees | Improvement in team-based skills; no decay at 2 months |
| Tan et al. [34] | Systematic search of literature involving simulation-based OR team training | Not stated | Positive learner response, some reported change to behavior in team environment |
| Gjeraa et al. [35] | Systematic review of simulation-based trauma team training | Pre-licensure, postgraduate, and practicing participants | Significant effect on learning; improvement in clinical performance |

[a]*ACGME* Accreditation Council for Graduate Medical Education
[b]*NTS* nontechnical skills
[c]*PGY* postgraduate year
[d]*TeamSTEPPS*™ Team Strategies and Tools to Enhance Performance and Patient Safety™

Another advantage of SBT is that it is very amenable to interprofessional education (IPE), a practice growing in popularity in health professions education. The World Health Organization (WHO) has defined IPE as follows: "…students from two or more professions [who] learn *about, from,* and *with* each other to enable effective collaboration and improve health outcomes (italics added)" [36]. IPE is now recognized as the way forward in helping to overcome the tribalism found in healthcare [1]. In addition it is seen as a means of improving communication [1] and promoting both cultural change and patient safety [37]. In addition, IPE has been demonstrated to improve collaborative team behavior within the OR micro-system [38]. Combining SBT with IPE, therefore, has the potential of accelerating the development of surgical teams by allowing learners to "deliberately work together" to promote safety and patient-centeredness [3]. Due to its large potential in transforming healthcare professional education, efforts have been undertaken around the world to help develop frameworks and competencies related to IPE [3]. By targeting such competencies, which often involve teamwork and communication, surgical educators can start building teams from the beginning of an individual's education in the health professions.

Clearly, SBT and IPE are two powerful modalities for promoting highly reliable team function, and, consequently, high reliability in healthcare. Pitfalls do exist, however, in implementation of curricula related to each. For SBT, such pitfalls can arise if the surgical educator interprets the use of simulation as the end rather than the means. Put another way, simulation is a *tool*, not a curriculum. Thus, any educational intervention employing simulation-based activities should be founded on sound principles related to curriculum development. The use of needs assessments, the creation of goals and learning objectives, the appropriate selection of teaching modalities and their delivery, the use of reliable assessment tools with evidence of validity, and the evaluation of the effectiveness of the educational program are but a few key items. In addition, scenario development for high-fidelity simulation-based sessions should follow effective, established methods of development. One accepted methodology is the event-based approach to training (EBAT) [39] that has been successfully used in scenario development for trauma team training [40]. Finally, training and expertise in debriefing is essential for surgical educators engaged in such work in order to optimize the self-reflection, gap analysis, and behavioral change that occurs during high-fidelity SBT sessions. An emphasis on "what is right" over "who is right" must be followed in this setting of immediate feedback because it opens participants to becoming more aware of patient care hazards and gives them the opportunity to help find solutions [39, 41].

IPE challenges exist as well. They often center on incongruences related to disparate professional schedules, curricula, and cultural views [42]. In addition, institutional issues, such as lack of support from leadership, entrenched cultural views hostile to IPE and/or change interventions, and faculty inadequately trained in IPE techniques, can be important impediments [42]. Often IPE and SBT challenges are similar in scope and nature. Thus, overcoming them is essential for success. Solutions can be undertaken in a variety of ways; taking a systematic approach is helpful. For example, Paige et al. [43] proposed the "5P" approach to implementing successfully surgical high-fidelity SBT. In it, potential challenges are grouped into five major categories in which strategic and tactical solutions are then developed to meet them. These categories include the following: (1) finding a *patron*, (2) developing a *plan*, (3) locating a *place*, (4) assembling the appropriate *people*, and (5) choosing effective *products*. This example illustrates that, by taking a systematic approach to the challenges faced, the necessary support, personnel, and resources can be mustered to succeed.

## 26.3 Leveraging SBT and IPE to Promote the Development of Surgical Teams: The LSU Health New Orleans Experience

At LSU Health New Orleans, SBT and IPE have both been employed across the entire continuum of professional development to promote highly reliable teams in the perioperative micro-system (Fig. 26.1). From an HF perspective, such efforts in training and education are people-focused approaches. They began over a decade ago with the development of the Virtual OR (VOR) for *ex cura* (i.e., in a center *away from the clinical environment*) training of OR surgical teams comprised of pre-licensure, postgraduate, and practicing learners [44]. Shortly following this start, training expanded with the development of the Mobile Mock OR (MMOR) and its application to in situ training of OR teams at satellite facilities within the Louisiana state hospital system [45–47]. The focus of team training then shifted to the pre-licensure level in an effort to "get them (i.e., students) while they are young." In this

## SBT for Developing Teams at LSU Health New Orleans

| Pre-licensure Education | Postgraduate Education | Continuing Professional Development |
|---|---|---|
| 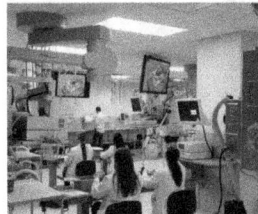 | 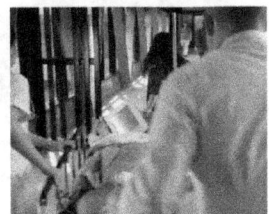 | 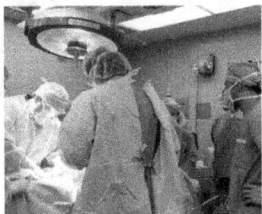 |
| • Skills and tasks training<br>• *Ex cura* inter-professional team training | • Skills, tasks, and procedures training<br>• *Ex cura* & *in situ* inter-professional team training | • *In situ* inter-professional team training |

**Fig. 26.1** Simulation-based training (SBT) for developing teams at LSU Health New Orleans. Simulation-based training activities occur across the entire continuum of professional development (i.e., pre-licensure and postgraduate education as well as continuing professional development), focusing on skills, tasks, procedures, and interprofessional team training in the clinical lab and the clinical environment

manner, students of the health professions would be afforded an opportunity to be exposed to concepts related to team-based competencies and effective teamwork that would hopefully overcome the negative modeling seen in the clinical environment. This student-based team training using high-fidelity simulation began approximately a decade ago with the Student Operating Room Team Training (SORTT) project involving senior medical students in the Senior Anatomy Elective, undergraduate nursing students in a Perioperative Nursing Elective, and nurse anesthesia students [17]. Since then, the training has expanded to the Team Training of Inter-Professional Students (TTIPS) projects [48, 49]. TTIPS currently includes both trauma team training of 3rd year medical students on their surgery clerkship with senior undergraduate nursing students taking their intensive care course and ED- and ICU-based team training of senior medical students during their Critical Concepts Course with nurse anesthesia students and various Allied Health students. In this manner, students have an opportunity to undergo distributed training in team-based competencies as they progress through these programs, reinforcing positive teamwork attitudes and behaviors.

At the postgraduate and continuing professional development level, team training using high-fidelity simulation has included *ex cura* as well as in situ examples. Multi-crew training has been undertaken *ex cura* with OR crisis scenario sessions involving general surgical and anesthesiology residents meeting about eight times

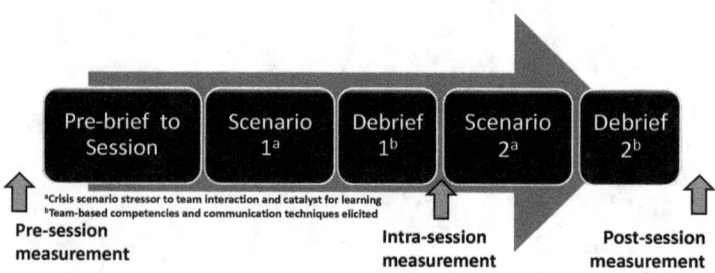

**Fig. 26.2** Dual scenario format for simulation-based training (SBT) surgical teams. Simulation-based training sessions of surgical teams begin with a pre-brief orienting learners and outlining objectives. This pre-brief is followed by a crisis scenario with after-action debrief focusing on team-based competencies and communication techniques. Learners then participate in a second crisis scenario with debriefing and summary

per year. In addition, SBT with IPE involving the *ex cura* Trauma Team Emergency Room Transfer Training (TTERTT) pilot has been successfully undertaken. In this program teams of general surgical residents, emergency medicine residents, and senior undergraduate nursing students must physically transfer computer-based mannequin "patients" needing exploratory laparotomy from a virtual trauma bay located on the second floor of the LSU Health New Orleans School of Nursing to the VOR on the fifth floor of LSU Health New Orleans School of Medicine's Simulation Center which is in a separate building connected to the School of Nursing via a sky bridge. Such team-based progressive SBT provides opportunities to discuss systems-based issues related to transfer of care. Finally, in situ OR team training has also been accomplished involving general surgical residents and practicing OR staff at the university-affiliated hospital.

Each learning session for this SBT using IPE is organized similarly for every project (Fig. 26.2) [17, 46–49, 50] and draws on Kolb's theory for experiential learning [51]. The training session begins with a pre-brief in which the facilitators introduce themselves, state the goals and objectives for the session, orient the learners to the technology, review the format of the session, and establish the ground rules for participation. This last aspect is essential to help establish the feeling of psychological safety in the learners needed for the suspension of disbelief that leads to optimal learning. Three major ground rules are emphasized: (1) treat it real (i.e., consider the mannequin as an actual patient in the clinical setting and act according to how one would act in real life); (2) treat us [the facilitators] like ghosts (i.e., act like the facilitators and mannequin operators do not exist by not addressing or acknowledging them in any manner); and (3) treat it like Vegas (i.e., what happens during the session related to the scenario type and comments made regarding others' performances and events stays in the session; team-based skills, however, are encouraged to be pursued in the clinical environment).

Following the pre-brief, a dual scenario format for training is employed in which the interprofessional team participates in a high-fidelity simulation using a computer-based mannequin patient involving a crisis event designed to place stress on team interactions. Upon completion, it is followed immediately by an after-action debriefing emphasizing reflective practice in which team-based competencies for highly reliable performance are introduced and discussed. A second, different SBT crisis scenario is then undertaken to practice targeted competencies followed by a final debrief at the end of which learners commit to adopting one teamwork behavior in clinical practice. Measurements of targeted knowledge, skills, and abilities (KSAs) using reliable instruments with evidence of validity are taken pre-, intra-, and post-session to demonstrate learning. The effectiveness of the training is evaluated using Kirkpatrick's model: participant reaction, participant learning, participant behavior change, and organizational outcomes [52]. To date, SBT using IPE to develop surgical teams at LSU Health New Orleans has yielded positive results related to promoting characteristics of highly reliable teams (Tables 26.2 [17, 46–49]).

Such SBT using IPE for teaching team-based competencies is supplemented by focused SBT in key surgical skills [53], tasks, and procedures [54] in order to ensure that team members have the requisite KSAs to provide quality care to patients. In this manner, SBT is undertaken in which all three skill sets needed for successful care in the perioperative setting are targeted: (1) technical skills, (2) cognitive skills, and (3) interpersonal skills. Surgical teams are thus developed using a comprehensive approach in an effort to promote highly reliable team function, quality of care, and patient safety.

**Table 26.2** Impact of Simulation-based Training of Surgical Teams using Inter-Professional Education at LSU Health New Orleans

| Project | STEPS[a] | SORTT[a] | TTIPS[a] | TTERTT[a] |
|---|---|---|---|---|
| Learner teams | Surgical residents, faculty, operating room personnel | Senior medical students, senior undergraduate nursing students, nurse anesthesia students | Junior and senior medical students, allied health profession students, nurse anesthesia students, senior undergraduate nursing students | Surgical residents, emergency medicine residents, and senior undergraduate nursing students |
| Training location | In situ | *Ex cura* | *Ex cura* | *Ex cura* |
| Impact of training | | | | |
| Improved attitudes toward team-based competencies | $\sqrt{}^{46}$ | $\sqrt{}^{17}$ | $\sqrt{}^{48,49}$ | $\sqrt{}^{b}$ |
| Improvement in individual and team-based behaviors | $\sqrt{}^{c}$ | $\sqrt{}^{17}$ | $\sqrt{}^{48,49}$ | $\sqrt{}^{b}$ |

(continued)

**Table 26.2** (continued)

| Project | STEPS[a] | SORTT[a] | TTIPS[a] | TTERTT[a] |
|---|---|---|---|---|
| Retention of skills up to 6 months | n/a | n/a | $\sqrt{}$[48,49] | n/a |
| Improvement in team-based attitudes over year | n/a | n/a | $\sqrt{}$[50] | n/a |
| Reinforcement of attitudinal improvements with distributed training | $\sqrt{}$[47] | n/a | n/a | n/a |

[a]*STEPS* System for Teamwork Effectiveness and Patient Safety, *SORTT* Student Operating Room Team Training, *TTIPS* Team Training of Inter-Professional Students, *TTERTT* Trauma Team Emergency Room Transfer Training
[b]Published abstract: Paige JT, Qingzhao Y, V Rusnak, Garbee DD, Kiselov V, Detiege P. Moving on up: team training for emergency room trauma transfers (TTERTT). Proceedings of the Australasian Simulation Congress 2017 (http://proceedings.simulationautralasia.com/index.html).
[c]Published abstract: Paige et al. J Am Coll Surg 207:S87–S88 (2008)

## 26.4 Conclusion

In today's evermore complex healthcare environment, developing highly reliable surgical teams is an imperative. For the surgical educator, applying HF engineering to such team development has many advantages. First, it recognizes the ubiquity of human fallibility and the need to promote a culture of safety in healthcare. Second, it provides a framework for both systems- and people-focused interventions to foster better team interaction through force functioning, automation, standardization, the implementation of checklists and policies, and training. Among the latter of these methods, the use of simulation-based techniques and IPE are powerful modalities for promoting highly reliable teamwork due to the experiential nature of simulation and the ability of members of different professions to learn with, from, and about each other. Both methodologies have been successfully integrated into surgical team training programs at LSU Health New Orleans, which can serve as an example of how to implement SBT using IPE in order to provide ultimately high-quality and safe care to the surgical patient.

## References

1. Weller, J., Boyd, M., & Cumin, D. (2014). Teams, tribes and patient safety: Overcoming barriers to effective teamwork in healthcare. *Postgraduate Medical Journal, 90*(1061), 149–154.
2. Greiner, A. C., & Knebel, E. (2003). *Health professions education: A bridge to quality*. Washington, DC: Institute of Medicine, National Academies Press.

3. Interprofessional Education Collaborative Expert Panel. (2011). *Core competencies for interprofessional collaborative practice: Report of an expert panel*. Washington, DC: Interprofessional Education Collaborative.
4. Thistlethwaite, J. E., Forman, D., Matthews, L. R., Rogers, G. D., Steketee, C., & Yassine, T. (2014). Competencies and frameworks in interprofessional education: A comparative analysis. *Academic Medicine, 89*(6), 869–867.
5. Reason, J. (2005). Safety in the operating theatre – Part 2: Human error and organisational failure. *Quality & Safety in Health Care, 14*, 56–60.
6. McCulloch, P., Morgan, L., New, S., Catchpole, K., Robertson, E., Hadi, M., Pickering, S., Collins, G., & Griffin, D. (2017). Combining systems and teamwork approaches to enhance the effectiveness of safety improvement interventions in surgery: The safer delivery of surgical services (S3) program. *Annals of Surgery, 265*, 90–96.
7. The ERAS Society. http://www.erassociety.org/. Accessed 28 Nov 2016.
8. Ljungqvist, O. (2014). ERAS--enhanced recovery after surgery: Moving evidence-based perioperative care to practice. *JPEN Journal of Parenteral and Enteral Nutrition, 38*(5), 559–566.
9. Nicholson, A., Lowe, M. C., Parker, J., Lewis, S. R., Alderson, P., & Smith, A. F. (2014). Systematic review and meta-analysis of enhanced recovery programmes in surgical patients. *The British Journal of Surgery, 101*, 172–188.
10. Hicks, C. W., Rosen, M., Hobson, D. B., Ko, C., & Wick, E. C. (2014). Improving safety and quality of care with enhanced teamwork through operating room briefings. *JAMA Surgery, 149*, 863–868.
11. Russ, S., Rout, S., Sevdalis, N., Moorthy, K., Darzi, A., & Vincent, C. (2013). Do safety checklists improve teamwork and communication in the operating room? A systematic review. *Annals of Surgery, 258*, 856–871.
12. Arriaga, A. F., Bader, A. M., Wong, J. M., Lipsitz, S. R., Berry, W. R., Ziewacz, J. E., Hepner, D. L., Boorman, D. J., Pozner, C. N., Smink, D. S., & Gawande, A. A. (2013). Simulation-based trial of surgical-crisis checklists. *The New England Journal of Medicine, 368*, 246–253.
13. Haynes, A. B., Weiser, T. G., Berry, W. R., Lipsitz, S. R., Breizat, A. H., Dellinger, E. P., Herbosa, T., Joseph, S., Kibatala, P. L., Lapitan, M. C., Merry, A. F., Moorthy, K., Reznick, R. K., Taylor, B., Gawande, A. A., & Safe Surgery Saves Lives Study Group. (2009). A surgical safety checklist to reduce morbidity and mortality in a global population. *The New England Journal of Medicine, 360*, 491–499.
14. Armour Forse, R., Bramble, J. D., & McQuillan, R. (2011). Team training can improve operating room performance. *Surgery, 150*, 771–778.
15. Hull, L., & Sevdalis, N. (2015). Advances in teaching and assessing nontechnical skills. *The Surgical Clinics of North America, 95*, 869–884.
16. Beaubien, J. M., & Baker, D. P. (2004). The use of simulation for training teamwork skills in health care: How low can you go? *Quality & Safety in Health Care, 13*, 51–56.
17. Paige, J. T., Garbee, D. D., Kozmenko, V., Yu, Q., Kozmenko, L., Yang, T., Bonanno, L., & Swartz, W. (2014). Getting a head start: High-fidelity, simulation-based operating room team training of interprofessional students. *Journal of the American College of Surgeons, 218*, 140–149.
18. Nguyen, N., Elliott, J. O., Watson, W. D., & Dominguez, E. (2015). Simulation improves nontechnical skills performance of residents during the perioperative and intraoperative phases of surgery. *Journal of Surgical Education, 72*, 957–963.
19. Boyd, M., Cumin, D., Lombard, B., Torrie, J., Civil, N., & Weller, J. (2014). Read-back improves information transfer in simulated clinical crises. *BMJ Quality and Safety, 23*(12), 989–993.
20. Pena, G., Altree, M., Field, J., Sainsbury, D., Babidge, W., Hewett, P., & Maddern, G. (2015). Nontechnical skills training for the operating room: A prospective study using simulation and didactic workshop. *Surgery, 158*(1), 300–309.
21. Stevens, L. M., Cooper, J. B., Raemer, D. B., Schneider, R. C., Frankel, A. S., Berry, W. R., & Agnihotri, A. K. (2012 Jul). Educational program in crisis management for cardiac surgery teams including high realism simulation. *The Journal of Thoracic and Cardiovascular Surgery, 144*(1), 17–24.

22. Arriaga, A. F., Gawande, A. A., Raemer, D. B., Jones, D. B., Smink, D. S., Weinstock, P., Dwyer, K., Lipsitz, S. R., Peyre, S., Pawlowski, J. B., Muret-Wagstaff, S., Gee, D., Gordon, J. A., Cooper, J. B., Berry, W. R., & Harvard Surgical Safety Collaborative. (2014). Pilot testing of a model for insurer-driven, large-scale multicenter simulation training for operating room teams. *Annals of Surgery, 259*(3), 403–410.
23. Dedy, N. J., Fecso, A. B., Szasz, P., Bonrath, E. M., & Grantcharov, T. P. (2016). Implementation of an effective strategy for teaching nontechnical skills in the operating room: A single-blinded nonrandomized trial. *Annals of Surgery, 263*(5), 937–941.
24. Doumouras, A. G., Keshet, I., Nathens, A. B., Ahmed, N., & Hicks, C. M. (2014). Trauma non-technical training (TNT-2): The development, piloting and multilevel assessment of a simulation-based, interprofessional curriculum for team-based trauma resuscitation. *Canadian Journal of Surgery, 57*(5), 354–355.
25. Steinemann, S., Berg, B., Skinner, A., DiTulio, A., Anzelon, K., Terada, K., Oliver, C., Ho, H. C., & Speck, C. (2011). In situ, multidisciplinary, simulation-based teamwork training improves early trauma care. *Journal of Surgical Education, 68*(6), 472–477.
26. Capella, J., Smith, S., Philp, A., Putnam, T., Gilbert, C., Fry, W., Harvey, E., Wright, A., Henderson, K., Baker, D., Ranson, S., & Remine, S. (2010). Teamwork training improves the clinical care of trauma patients. *Journal of Surgical Education, 67*(6), 439–443.
27. Ziesmann, M. T., Widder, S., Park, J., Kortbeek, J. B., Brindley, P., Hameed, M., Paton-Gay, J. D., Engels, P. T., Hicks, C., Fata, P., Ball, C. G., & Gillman, L. M. (2013). S.T.A.R.T.T.: development of a national, multidisciplinary trauma crisis resource management curriculum-results from the pilot course. *Journal of Trauma and Acute Care Surgery, 75*(5), 753–758.
28. Nicksa, G. A., Anderson, C., Fidler, R., & Stewart, L. (2015). Innovative approach using interprofessional simulation to educate surgical residents in technical and nontechnical skills in high-risk clinical scenarios. *JAMA Surgery, 150*(3), 201–207.
29. Pucher, P. H., Aggarwal, R., Srisatkunam, T., & Darzi, A. (2014). Validation of the simulated ward environment for assessment of ward-based surgical care. *Annals of Surgery, 259*, 215–221.
30. Arora, S., Hull, L., Fitzpatrick, M., Sevdalis, N., & Birnbach, D. J. (2015). Crisis management on surgical wards: A simulation-based approach to enhancing technical, teamwork, and patient interaction skills. *Annals of Surgery, 261*(5), 888–893.
31. Stephens, T., Hunningher, A., Mills, H., & Freeth, D. (2016). An interprofessional training course in crises and human factors for perioperative teams. *Journal of Interprofessional Care, 30*(5), 685–688.
32. Doumouras, A. G., & Engels, P. T. (2016). Early crisis nontechnical skill teaching in residency leads to long-term skill retention and improved performance during crises: A prospective, nonrandomized controlled study. *Surgery, 162*, 174.
33. Doumouras, A. G., Keshet, I., Nathens, A. B., Ahmed, N., & Hicks, C. M. (2012). A crisis of faith? A review of simulation in teaching team-based, crisis management skills to surgical trainees. *Journal of Surgical Education, 69*(3), 274–281.
34. Tan, S. B., Pena, G., Altree, M., & Maddern, G. J. (2014). Multidisciplinary team simulation for the operating theatre: A review of the literature. *ANZ Journal of Surgery, 84*(7–8), 515–522.
35. Gjeraa, K., Møller, T. P., & Østergaard, D. (2014). Efficacy of simulation-based trauma team training of non-technical skills. A systematic review. *Acta Anaesthesiologica Scandinavica, 58*(7), 775–787.
36. World Health Organization (WHO). (2010). *Framework for action on interprofessional education & collaborative practice*. Geneva: World Health Organization Available at: http://whqlibdoc.who.int/hq/2010/WHO_HRH_HPN_10.3_eng.pdf. Accessed 3 Feb 2017.
37. Firth-Cozens, J. (2001). Cultures for improving patient safety through learning: The role of teamwork. *Quality & Safety in Health Care, 10*(suppl II), ii26–ii31.
38. Reeves, S., Perrier, L., Goldman, J., et al. (2013). Interprofessional education: Effects on professional practice and healthcare outcomes (update). *Cochrane Database of Systematic Reviews, 3*, CD002213.

39. Rosen, M. A., Salas, E., Wu, T. S., Silvestri, S., Lazzara, E. H., Lyons, R., Weaver, S. J., & King, H. B. (2008). Promoting teamwork: An event-based approach to simulation-based teamwork training for emergency medicine residents. *Academic Emergency Medicine, 15*, 1190–1198.
40. Nguyen, N., Watson, W. D., & Dominguez, E. (2015). An event-based approach to design a teamwork training and assessment tool in surgery. *Journal of Surgical Education, 73*, 197–207.
41. Fernandez, R., Vozenilek, J. A., Hegarty, C. B., Motola, I., Reznek, M., Phrampus, P. E., & Kozlowski, S. W. J. (2008). Developing expert medical teams: Toward an evidence-based approach. *Academic Emergency Medicine, 15*, 1025–1036.
42. IOM (Institute of Medicine). (2013). *Interprofessional education for collaboration: Learning how to improve health from interprofessional models across the continuum of education to practice: Workshop summary*. Washington, DC: The National Academies Press.
43. Paige, J. T. (2012). Team training at the point of care. In S. Tsuda, D. J. Scott, & D. B. Jones (Eds.), *Textbook of simulation, surgical skills, and team training*. Woodbury: Cine-Med.
44. Paige, J. T., Kozmenko, V., Morgan, B., Howell, D. S., Chauvin, S., Hilton, C. W., Cohn, I., Jr., & O'Leary, J. P. (2007). From the flight deck to the operating room: Impact of a simulation based interdisciplinary team training pilot program in crisis management. *Journal of Surgical Education, 64*(6), 369–377.
45. Paige, J. T., Kozmenko, V., Yang, T., Paragi, R., Cohn, I. Jr., Hilton, C., & Chauvin, S. (2008). The mobile mock operating room: Bringing team training to the point of care. In: *Advances in patient safety: New directions and alternative approaches*. Volume 3. Performance and Tools. AHRQ Publication Nos. 08-0034 (1–4). Agency for Healthcare Research and Quality, Rockville, MD. http://www.ahrq.gov/qual/advances2/.
46. Paige, J. T., Kozmenko, V., Yang, T., Paragi Gururaja, R., Hilton, C. W., Cohn, I., Jr., & Chauvin, S. W. (2009). High-fidelity, simulation-based, interdisciplinary operating room team training at the point of care. *Surgery, 145*, 138–146.
47. Paige, J. T., Kozmenko, V., Yang, T., Gururaja, R. P., Hilton, C. W., Cohn, I., Jr., & Chauvin, S. W. (2009). Attitudinal changes resulting from repetitive training of operating room personnel using high-fidelity simulation at the point of care. *The American Surgeon, 75*(7), 584–590; discussion 590–1.
48. Garbee, D. D., Paige, J. T., Bonanno, L., Rusnak, V., Barrier, K., Kozmenko, L., Yu, Q., Cefalu, J., & Nelson, K. (2013). Effectiveness of teamwork and communication education using an interprofessional high-fidelity human patient simulation critical care code. *JNEP, 3*(3), 1.
49. Garbee, D. D., Paige, J. T., Barrier, K., Kozmenko, V., Kozmenko, L., Zamjahn, J., Bonanno, L., & Cefalu, J. (2013). Interprofessional teamwork and communication collaboration among students in simulated codes: A quasi-experimental study. *Nursing Education Perspectives, 34*(5), 339–344.
50. Paige, J. T., Garbee, D. D., Yu, Q., & Rusnak, V. (2017). Team Training of Inter-Professional Students (TTIPS) for improving teamwork. *BMJ Simulation and Technology Enhanced Learning, 3*(4), 127–134.
51. Kolb, D., & Fry, R. (1975). Toward an applied theory of experiential learning. In C. Cooper (Ed.), *Theories of group process*. London: Wiley.
52. Kirkpatrick, D. I. (1998). *Evaluating training programs: The four levels* (2nd ed.). San Francisco: Berrett-Koehler.
53. Pender, C., Kiselov, V., Yu, Q., Mooney, J., Greiffenstein, P., & Paige, J. T. (2016). All for knots: Evaluating the effectiveness of a proficiency-driven, simulation-based knot tying and suturing curriculum for medical students during their third year surgery clerkship. *The American Journal of Surgery, 213*, 362–370.
54. Paige, J. T., Yu, Q., Hunt, J. P., Marr, A., & Stuke, L. (2015). Thinking it through: Comparison of effectiveness of mental rehearsal on two types of laparoscopic cholecystectomy trainers. *Journal of Surgical Education, 72*(4), 740–748.

# Chapter 27
# Supporting the Development of Professionalism in Surgeons in Practice: A Virtues-Based Approach to Exploring a Surgeon's Moral Agency

**Linda de Cossart CBE and Della Fish**

**Overview** The intentions of this chapter are to refresh and clarify how we might construe and facilitate the continuing development of professionalism in surgical practitioners in the twenty-first century. Firstly, we consider the current concept of professionalism in surgery and then attend to two aspects of supporting the development of professionalism in practitioners who are members of a profession that serves vulnerable fellow human beings. Secondly, we share our experience of facilitating one way of beginning those deep but very sensitive considerations about the person the professional brings to their work. We conclude that all this requires members of the profession of surgery to be willing and able to articulate what it means to them to be a member of a profession and that surgical teachers take time to become well developed educators in *the moral mode* of educational practice.

## 27.1 What Does Professionalism for a Surgeon Consist of in the Twenty-First Century?

Surgeons are members of a profession that has a long history and tradition as a professional practice and which demands of the practitioner particular qualities of character and conduct. Surgery as a profession provides a public service that seeks to offer 'a good' (in this case for surgeons the best possible health) for both the individual patient and the whole community. Belonging to a profession is more than 'being professional' which today we tend to apply to anyone who does something well or to any activity done thoroughly [1–3]. It is not about 'belonging to an interest group that seeks self-interest' [4]. Indeed, the tone of irony that lurks behind the last statement indicates disappointment at the shortfall. Professional practice for a surgeon is undoubtedly an ethical practice [5–7] and as such should be engaged in

---

L. de Cossart CBE (✉) · D. Fish
Ed4medprac Ltd., Cranham, Gloucestershire, UK

by those who recognise and aspire to the unchanging principles of ethical practice because as James Drane [6] reminds us 'doctoring is through and through an ethical enterprise', and as such it is not part of the everyday activities of laymen and laywomen. Thus its practical and educational implications need deep consideration.

For some time now, professional practice in surgery (and in many other professions) has been perceived as a mere skills-based enterprise by a world that has lost its moral compass and been persuaded to adopt a technical rational view of life [5, 8–11]. We would argue that in both medicine and surgery, the technical mode of practice, while vital, is not sufficient. This is not about downgrading the importance of skills and knowledge but rather upgrading the importance of the professional's identity, personhood and humanity and their continuing flourishing throughout their professional life [7, 8, 11, 12]. Chapters 12 and 13 explore concepts around the professional identity development of surgeons and surgeon educators in greater depth.

Professionalism – for members of a profession – is about who you are, both as a person and a professional, and therefore how you conduct yourself. How you conduct yourself is more than about how you behave. Behaviour refers to your surface performance, which can be – but may not be – related to your inner beliefs and convictions. The term 'conduct' is used here to signify that visible performance is driven by inner belief about how to be and to act and about who one is as a person in life and in professional practice. Members of a profession are under scrutiny and accountable for their conduct at all times. Beyond that, however, they also recognise and accept fully that their professional practice makes demands of them that are beyond what is naturally required of those who engage in occupations other than surgery [9].

All this has profound implications for how surgeons in practice learn to become the person and the professional who can constantly aspire to the ideals of professional practice as well as to the technical accuracy and artistry of their performance in the operating theatre.

## 27.2 Aims and Intentions of This Chapter

Our aim in this chapter is to offer some provoking ideas and questions to shape and revitalise ways of thinking about and conceptualising professionalism for surgeons and ways of teaching it. Our intentions are to inspire teachers and learners in (postgraduate) surgical practice to move beyond the technical rational mode of professional practice with its emphasis on efficiency and performance and to re-engage with the moral heart of practicing medicine which is concerned with understanding the drivers of our decision-making and professional judgement (what Aristotle called *phronesis* or practical wisdom) [3, 10, 11, 13, 14]. Two of these key drivers are the person and the professional we bring to each individual patient case.

We will thus attend to two aspects of supporting the development of professionalism; firstly, we will clarify how the concept of professionalism in surgery has developed recently. Following this we will share our experience of how this might be taught and will conclude with some principles to guide teachers and learners in surgical practice.

## 27.3 Why Is All This Important?

At a national educational association seminar in 2016 for exploring virtues and values in being a doctor, we were struck by the passion of delegates (mostly senior medical practitioners) when we challenged their notions of how they saw their professional work. They talked of 'working on the shop floor', 'seeing patients as customers,' 'learning important things from marketing and industry' and aiming to 'deliver targets'. They all had pride in their work and wanted to do their best for patients despite the increasing hostility of the current environment. However, the language of trade, commerce and 'the market' had been unconsciously insinuated into their mindset and discourse. Only with some prompting did they consider the virtues and character needed to undertake the complex and moral job of being a doctor.

In medicine increasing regulation, both intrinsic and extrinsic, fuels the technical mindset with the laudable aim of reassuring the public about professionals' 'fitness to practice'. 'Fitness to practice', with its assumption of mastery, is inappropriate in a medical world where knowledge and understanding is always incomplete and where everyday practice can only call on best endeavours rather than the achievement of perfection.

How does all this influence teaching and learning professionalism? How should this be approached in the postgraduate surgical curriculum and how might this look with respect to real practice today? How do we balance the increasing technical mode of professionalism with the endemic ideals of the moral heart of medicine?

## 27.4 Towards Reconceptualising Professionalism and Professional Education

We argue here that education in professionalism for surgeons ought to begin with seeing the responsibilities of being a member of the profession of surgery as a major permeating theme throughout all aspects of professional development and not as an add-on extra [7]. This means taking account of the past traditions, current challenges and future trends of the current social and political environment. Further, we do not see it as merely a matter of changing the definition of professionalism or adding on a new assessment process [15, 16]. We see it as a matter of identifying and retaining certain inescapable fundamental principles (and character development) that need to shape a *doctor's* practice [2, 6, 17].

Fish and Coles [2], extrapolating from Freidson's work [17], offer the notion that membership of a profession:

- Is an occupation exercising 'good' in the service of another
- Is a specialised work in that it cannot entirely be understood by the layman
- Is not measured by financial reward alone
- Is ethically and morally based
- Has an esoteric and complex knowledge base
- Requires the capacity for and the exercise of discretion and depends upon wise professional judgement

Indeed, *being a member of the profession of surgery* goes far *beyond* complying with the standards and the codes of good practice set down in regulatory documents. It requires the doctor to be a moral agent for their own practice, with accountability for their discretionary judgements as practitioners [4, 11, 13]. The importance of this most crucial ability has been echoed by the hundreds of doctors we have taught who recognise this as a never-ending quest.

The Keogh report in 2013 highlighted that young doctors in the UK are undervalued and receive inadequate supervision and support, particularly when dealing with complex issues [18]. But despite the claim Pringle makes that '[doctors] have a strong internal sense of appropriate and good behaviours, based on a robust set of inbuilt values and virtues', we argue that these capacities need to be explicitly appreciated, nurtured and strengthened throughout professional life [19].

Engaging in *the moral mode of educational practice* requires the postgraduate teacher to put their learner's growth as a person and a professional at the centre of the teaching transaction, so that the learning is worthwhile and the teaching encourages the learner's flourishing as exemplified in their maturing capability, confidence and effectiveness as a practitioner [3, 5, 20]. This requires recognising the learner's own humanity as well as developing their clinical expertise. We argue that this means attending to their *being, knowing, thinking, doing and becoming* a better doctor [5, 13]. Developing professionalism is therefore far more than role modelling, which leaves implicit the conduct modelled. It requires intentional and explicit teaching to foster learning.

Educating surgeons for all this demands a rigorous approach to help them to understand themselves, their values and what specific virtues they have, in order to nurture, develop and enrich their role as a doctor and surgeon [18]. It would seem reasonable therefore to claim that these themes should permeate the whole postgraduate surgical curriculum, and beyond, because they influence and will always influence the very heart of a surgeon's actions. Currently the curriculum does not explicitly require this to be attended to. Further, teachers are not aware of how to recognise in their own practice and develop in others' an awareness and understanding of *phronesis* and how and why it goes beyond technical and procedural ability [1, 5]. This starts with knowing yourself and having the language to discuss these matters with all learners.

## 27.5 Exploring a Surgeon's Moral Agency and Professionalism in Practice: An Illustration of a Virtues-Based Approach

Working together for 16 years, as a surgeon with 40 years of experience and a teacher educator with more than 30 years of experience in teacher education and postgraduate medical education, we have explored, written about and taught on these matters in real clinical practice since 2005.

Our most recent blended learning series *Medical Supervision Matters* is aimed at the worthwhile education of supervisors in postgraduate medical education (PGME) in the UK and contains the permeating themes *teaching as a practice in its own right, the moral mode of practice, epistemology and ontology, the importance of reflection, and the importance of being, knowing, doing, thinking and becoming* [9, 21–23]. Table 27.1 shows the themes specifically relevant to preparing supervisors to explore and develop with supervisees the virtues endemic to professional practice. An evaluation of this programme reported that teachers were now more likely to focus on the professional development and well-being of learners, having completed the programme [24]. Evaluations of similar programmes we have designed and taught have found similar evidence [25, 26].

The process leading up to our specific example involved teachers/supervisors working through an initial set of learning materials (Booklet One) [9] to explore their own thinking and understanding about matters ontological and the distinctions between values and virtues [27]. This was achieved through distance learning materials and a face-to-face day session. Part of this included sharing together the results of their work with a junior doctor in charting and exploring what qualities of

Table 27.1 Curriculum themes for teaching virtues and values in PGME

| |
|---|
| *Booklet one: starting with myself as a doctor and supervisor* [9] |
| 1. What as a person do I bring to my supervision of doctors? |
| 2. What is required of me as a clinician who supervises doctors? |
| 3. How do I construe the nature of clinical practice and why does it matter? |
| 4. How do I see virtues, values, character education and professionalism? |
| 5. How do I view the nature and status of medical knowledge? |
| 6. How do I see patients and the relative priorities of patient care and supervision? |
| 7. Review: How do I now see supervision? |
| *Booklet two: practical dilemmas about supervision and teaching* [21] |
| 1. How does and how should clinical supervision work in practice for doctors? |
| 2. What is teaching, what is education and how would I characterise good teaching? |
| 3. How, in the moral mode of practice, should I engage in teaching my supervisee? |
| 4. What do I see as the basis of my authority and my agency as a supervisor? |
| 5. How can I cultivate character, virtue and moral reasoning in my supervisee? |
| 6. What is education theory and what do I need to know about it as a supervisor? |
| 7. What do I need to understand about the role of language in supervision? |
| 8. How should I prepare, as a teacher, and what is involved in the appreciation of my practice? |

character they each brought to a shared clinical case. Montgomery argues that '[case narrative] is the principal means of thinking and remembering – of *knowing* – in medicine' and rigorously exploring clinical judgement [11]. We strongly support this approach because real cases from practice are the source of key learning opportunities.

The similar and differing ideas about the case that teacher/supervisor and junior doctor each brought to their discussion proved a highly enlightening experience for both and is one useful starting point for introducing and making explicit the thinking needed and the language used in developing professionalism as well as the virtues and wise judgement of surgical practice.

Further distance learning and a second face-to-face teaching day introduced what we call *The Moral Reasoning Pathway*. Table 27.2 provides an exemplar framework for exploring the qualities of character demanded in a second clinical

**Table 27.2** An excerpt from, and example of, how to explore the virtues and moral reasoning endemic to a real clinical case

| Column I: virtues identified | Column II: the outline of the clinical case | Column III: dilemmas in moral reasoning in this case |
|---|---|---|
| Respect for others and the system | At the 8 am handover on a Saturday morning, I (an SpR year 3) received a case of a young adult who had been admitted at 3am drunk and smelling of urine with a laceration on his arm. The arm had been sutured but the youth had been surly and uncommunicative. He had received antibiotics and a tetanus injection. He was deemed likely to be ready for discharge later | Respect for patient |
| | | Critique of handover diagnosis |
| Honesty | | Enforcing zero-tolerance policy |
| Integrity | | A drunk or a human being? |
| Uprightness | I began the ward round on the acute admissions ward. I was nearing the bed of the young man when a nurse approached and said that his mother was outside and wanted a word before she saw her son. The boy had obviously heard this and nodded his consent to me that I should see her | Moral responsibility to patient |
| Commitment | | Being non-judgemental |
| Respect | | |
| Compassion | I left the ward with the nurse and headed for the visitor's room. The nurse filled in more of his story saying that he had been found slumped in an alley way in the town and had been rather rude. He had been warned of the zero-tolerance policy with respect to abuse of staff. I entered the visitor's room ahead of the nurse | Patient confidentiality |
| Fairness | | Following protocols or not |
| Non-judgemental | | |
| Curiosity | A woman in her mid-40s was sitting on the couch and was crying. She was being comforted by a man who I assumed was her husband. She stood up as we entered | Being cognisant of the wider circumstances |
| Kindness | She thanked us for seeing her and asked anxiously if he was *ok*. I confirmed that he did not have any serious injury and would be fine | Being caring or expedient |

The moral reasoning pathway for a patient case [9]

case and the moral dilemmas it created for the doctor. The use of this second clinical case entailed the supervisor and supervisee completing column one independently of each other. The supervisor also completed column three, identifying the moral dilemmas faced during this case. Then, during a planned professional conversation together lasting about 45 min, they shared and critiqued their varying results in column one and explored the moral issues identified by the supervisor in column three. This extended the understanding of *phronesis* related to this case. A written reflection created after the meeting by the junior doctor, on the learning stimulated by this event, served as hard evidence of what was achieved. Later versions of this activity put greater responsibility on the learner, requiring the supervisee/junior doctor to both fill in column three before the meeting. This whole process is suitable for cases from all areas of surgical practice (clinic, ward and operating theatre) and can be adapted to respect the level of experience of the surgeon.

Those we have worked with have found that their learners engaged enthusiastically with the exercise, shared a much deeper and more meaningful discussion than expected about professional matters and showed remarkable thoughtfulness. The flourishing of the learner was also evident in their new confidence and interest in their work. It also engaged each in a more meaningful and collaborative educational partnership between teacher and learner and broadened their shared language and understanding of why these things are important.

## 27.6 Conclusions

### 27.6.1 The Educational Principles for Teaching Professionalism Including Character Development and the Virtues Development of Character

In concluding this chapter, we summarise the principles offered.
These are that:

- Surgical practice is a moral enterprise.
- Surgeons are members of a profession with a long and valuable tradition.
- Teaching professionalism needs well-prepared teachers who understand ontology and *phronesis* and can make their own judgements explicit.
- Teaching professional capacities and characteristics is an *intentional* activity and should not be left to chance.
- The moral mode of education and of professional practice can enable the young to flourish in a sustainable way.
- Learning these matters is possible with teachers who have set out and shared with learners their well-considered and worthwhile educational intentions for their work together.

All this requires both that members of the profession of surgery are willing and able to articulate what it means to them to be a member of a profession and also that surgical teachers take time to become well-developed educators in the moral mode of practice.

## References

1. Fish, D., & de Cossart, L. (2007). *Developing the wise doctor*. London: Royal Society of Medicine Press.
2. Fish, D., & Coles, C. (Eds.). (1998). *Developing professional judgement in health care: Learning through the critical appreciation of practice*. Oxford: Butterworth Heinemann.
3. Carr, D. (2000). *Professionalism and ethics in teaching*. London: Routledge.
4. Hilborne, N. (2015) Jackson: 'Professional negligence' could disappear as attitudes to professionals change. *Legal Futures* (Online). Available at: http://www.legalfutures.co.uk/latest-news/jackson-professional-negligence-could-disappear-as-attitudes-change. Accessed 7 Oct 2016.
5. Fish, D. (2012). *Refocusing postgraduate medical education: From the technical to the moral mode of practice*. Cranham: Aneumi Publications.
6. Drane, J. F. (1995). *Becoming a good doctor: The place of virtues and character in medical ethics* (2nd ed.). Kansas: Sheed and Ward.
7. The Jubilee Centre for Character and Virtues' statement on character, virtue and practical wisdom in the professions. http://www.jubileecentre.ac.uk/userfiles/jubileecentre/pdf/Statement_Character_Virtue_Practical_Wisdom_Professional_Practice.pdf. Accessed 15 Oct 2015.
8. Blond, P., Antonacopoulou, E., & Pabst, A. (2015). *In professions we trust: Fostering virtuous practitioners in teaching, law and medicine*. London: ResPublica Available via: http://www.respublica.org.uk/wp-content/uploads/2015/02/In-Professions-We-Trust.pdf.
9. Fish, D. (2015). *Starting with myself as doctor and a supervisor. Booklet 1 of Medical Supervision Matters*. Cranham: Aneumi Publications.
10. Cruess, R. L., Cruess, S. R., & Steinert, Y. (2010). *Teaching medical professionalism*. Cambridge: Cambridge University Press.
11. Montgomery, K. (2006). *How doctors think: Clinical judgment and the practice of medicine*. Oxford: Oxford University Press.
12. Gelhaus, P. (2012). The desired moral attitude of the physician: 1 empathy. *Medical Healthcare and Philosophy, 15*(2), 103–113. https://doi.org/10.1007//s11019-011-9366-4 Published 14 December 2012.
13. de Cossart, L., & Fish, D. (2005). *Cultivating a thinking surgeon: New perspectives on clinical teaching, learning and assessment*. Shrewsbury: TfN Publications.
14. Eraut, M., & du Bouley, B. (2000). *Developing the attributes of medical professional judgement and competence: A review of the literature* (Cognitive Sciences Research Paper 518). University of Sussex, 2000. Online version. Sections 3.1 and 3.2 reprinted on CD as part of Module 1 of the Human Face of Medicine. London: BMJ Publishing Group.
15. Canter, R. (2016, January). The new professionalism. *98*(1), 10–13.
16. Non-technical skills for surgeons (NOTSS). http://www.notss.org/. Accessed 13 Oct 2016.
17. Freidson, E. (2001). *Professionalism, the third logic*. Chicago: University of Chicago Press.
18. Keogh, B. (2013). *The Keogh review*. NHS England. http://www.nhs.uk/NHSEngland/bruce-keogh-review/Documents/outcomes/keogh-review-final-report.pdf. Accessed 15 Oct 2016.
19. Arthur, J., Kristjansson, K., Thimas, H., Kotzee, B., Ignatowicz, A., & Qui, T. (2015). Virtuous medical practice: Research report Birmingham University Jubilee Centre. www.jubileecentre.ac.uk/userfiles/jubileecentre/pdf/Research%20Reports/Virtuous_Medical_Practice.pdf. Accessed 13 Oct 2016.

20. Hansen, D. (2001). *Exploring the moral heart of teaching: Towards a teacher's creed*. London: Teachers College Press.
21. Fish, D., de Cossart, L., & Wright, T. (2015). *Practical dilemmas about supervision and teaching. Booklet 2 of Medical Supervision Matters*. Cranham: Aneumi Publications.
22. Fish, D., de Cossart, L., & Wright, T. (2015). *Practical dilemmas about the learner and learning. Booklet 3 of Medical Supervision Matters*. Cranham: Aneumi Publications.
23. Fish, D., de Cossart, L., & Wright, T. (2015). *Practical dilemmas about assessment and evaluation. Booklet 4 of Medical Supervision Matters*. Cranham: Aneumi Publications.
24. Brown, J., Leadbetter, P., & Clabburn, O. (2016). Evaluation at East Lancashire Hospitals Trust (ELHT) of the impact of the project: 'Supervision Matters: Clinical Supervision for Quality Medical Care'.
25. Thomé, R. (2012). *Educational practice development: An evaluation (An exploration of the impact on participants and their shared organisation of a postgraduate certificate in education for postgraduate medical practice 2010–2011)*. Cranham: Aneumi Publications.
26. Thomé, R. (2013). *Educational practice development: An evaluation of the second year 2011–12 (An exploration of the impact on participants and their shared organization of year two of the postgraduate masters in education for postgraduate medical practice)*. Cranham: Aneumi Publications.
27. Annas, J. (2011). *Intelligent virtue*. Oxford: Oxford University Press.

# Chapter 28
# Managing Underperformance in Trainees

**Jonathan Beard and Hilary Sanfey**

**Overview** Managing surgical trainees who underperform can place significant demands on surgeons responsible for training. And it is not just trainees who underperform. In some specialities, more than 50% of surgeons can expect suspension from clinical duties pending the outcome of an investigation at some point in their career! This underperformance and its management can have a profound impact on the individual, patients, other surgeons and colleagues and the health service. This chapter explores some of the common categories of underperformance, the underlying causes and strategies for remediation.

## 28.1  Introduction and Scale of the Problem

While the number and percentage of underperforming trainees is low, more than 50% of problems are associated with about 10% of trainees [1], and those with behaviour problems consume substantial programme director and staff time, adversely affect patient care and disrupt team function [2]. Furthermore, if such unsatisfactory behaviours are not addressed in training, they often continue in practice [3]. Thus there is a strong argument for identifying and remediating underperforming trainees sooner rather than later. In this chapter, we explore some of the more common categories of underperformance and the underlying causes and suggest strategies for remediation.

A national US study identified the cumulative risk of termination as 3% for surgical trainees with a 19.5% cumulative risk of voluntary resignation. However, the nature of the deficiency leading to terminations was not identified [4]. The UK data based on the Annual Review of Competence Progression (ARCP) indicate that the

---

J. Beard (✉)
Faculty of Medicine, University of Sheffield, Sheffield, UK

H. Sanfey
Department of Surgery, Southern Illinois School of Medicine, Springfield, IL, USA
e-mail: hsanfey@siumed.edu

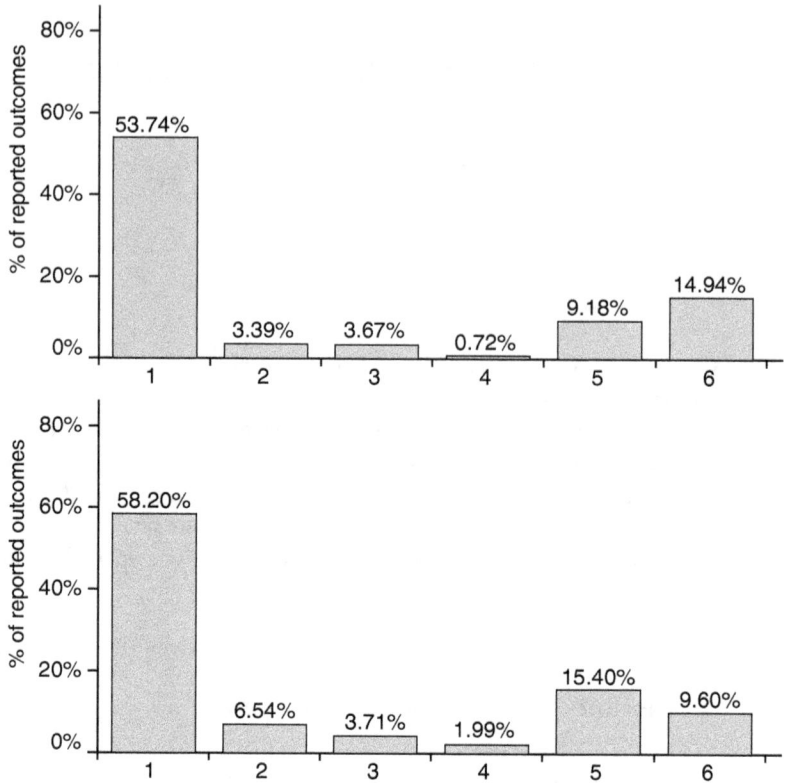

**Fig. 28.1** Annual Review of Competence Progress (ARCP) outcomes for all UK trainees (top) compared to surgical trainees (bottom) [18]. Outcome 1 = satisfactory progress – continue with training programme. Outcome 2 = development of specific competencies required – additional training time not required. Outcome 3 = development of specific competencies required – additional training time is required. Outcome 4 = released from training programme with or without specified competencies. Outcome 5 = incomplete evidence presented – additional training time may be required. Outcome 6 = all required competencies acquired – training programme completed

annual proportion of trainee surgeons in significant difficulty (i.e. none, one or six outcomes) is higher at 12%, compared to the 8% national average for all doctors in training (Fig. 28.1). The National Clinical Assessment Service (NCAS) data indicate that senior (i.e. certificated) surgeons in the UK also get into difficulty more frequently than most other doctors, along with emergency doctors, psychiatrists and obstetricians [5]. The annual investigation rate for senior surgeons is higher at 0.8% compared to an average of 0.5% for all other senior doctors (Fig. 28.2). This of course is an annual rate, but in some high-risk specialties like cardiac surgery, more than 50% of surgeons can expect suspension from clinical duties pending the outcome of an investigation at some point in their career. This is an alarming figure, which adversely impacts patients, surgeons, other colleagues and the health service.

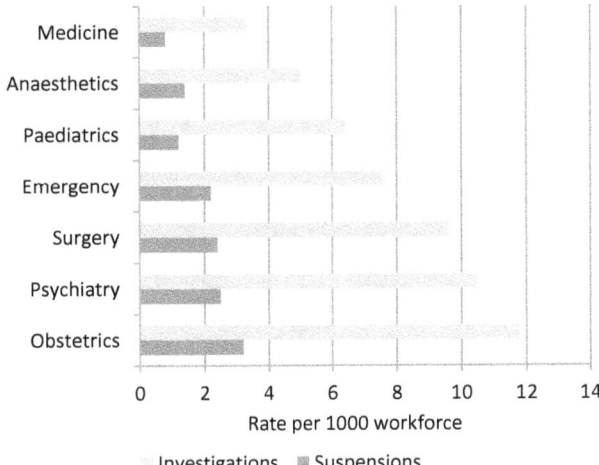

**Fig. 28.2** Annual rate of investigations and suspensions for UK consultants. (Source: 2014 data from NCAS (unpublished))

Anecdotal data suggest that allowing trainees to graduate on time without adequate remediation is not unusual, particularly when the deficiency involves poor communication or professional behaviour. Some explanations include the lack of assessment standards and unproven remediation options. In addition, programme directors (PDs) are often faced with scanty or conflicting documentation. Frequently there is inadequate oversight of trainee performance at the bedside or in clinic by trainers resulting in delayed identification of problems that are obvious to other healthcare professionals. Occasionally lapses in professionalism may be tolerated in the surgical trainee who is well liked and has excellent technical skills. Furthermore, the system often inadvertently enables and rewards bad behaviours. For example, staff working around uncooperative trainees overburden the more "pleasant" individual with tasks, thus "rewarding" bad behaviour.

## 28.2 Types of Underperformance

Underperformance can be classified within the domains of competence and performance that define surgical practice. In the UK Intercollegiate Surgical Curriculum Programme, these include knowledge, clinical skills, technical skills, decision-making and professional behaviour [6].

A single institution study in the USA noted that only 3 of 20 trainees with marginal performance had deficient technical skills [7]. A second single institution study of trainees graduating over two decades identified 17 of 78 with serious performance problems; but a technical skill deficiency was noted in only 6 of the 78 cases [8]. In interviews with a cohort of PDs, none of those interviewed had ever

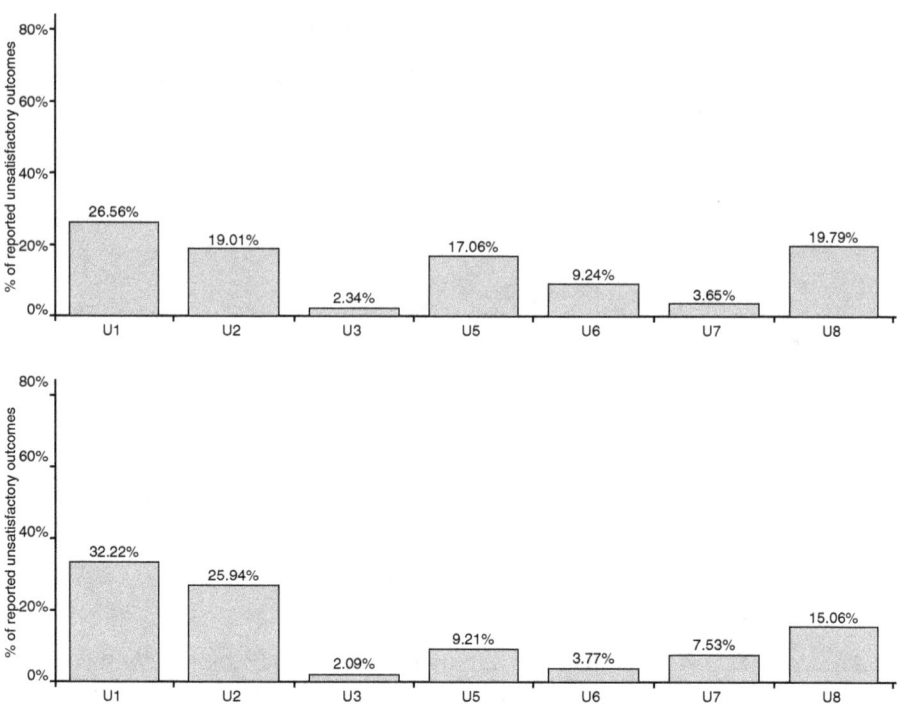

**Fig. 28.3** Reason for unsatisfactory Annual Review of Competence Progress (ARCP) outcome for all UK trainees (top) compared to surgical trainees (bottom) [18]. U1 = unsatisfactory record keeping and evidence. U2 = inadequate experience. U3 = no engagement with supervisor (trainer). U4 = supervisor (trainer) absence. U5 = single exam failure. U6 = continual exam failure. U7 = trainee requires Deanery support (poor professional behaviour). U8 = other

terminated or denied promotion because of poor technical skills [9]. Therefore in the USA, the dominant problem would appear to be in the area of *non-technical skills*.

In the UK, the majority of unsatisfactory outcomes for all trainees are due to poor maintenance of their training portfolio, lack of engagement with their supervisor, slow acquisition of knowledge/clinical/technical skills and/or exam failure. These problems are more common in the early years of training, are usually temporary and respond well to targeted training, with or without additional time and/or placements [10]. Echoing the US studies, behavioural deficiencies, including deficits in communication skills and professional conduct, explain unsatisfactory outcomes for 3.5% of all UK trainees, but this rises to 7.5% for those in surgical specialty training (Fig. 28.3). This pattern continues with seniority, with poor behaviour accounting for more than 70% of senior surgeons who are suspended from clinical duties (unpublished data from NCAS). The differences between surgeons and other doctors raise the question of whether the problem is due to the surgeons themselves, their training or their work. This is addressed in the next section.

## 28.3 Factors That May Affect Performance

Underperformance can be classified according to the attributes of the trainee, personal/social pressures, the training programme and the working environment. Identification of the underlying cause, particularly in instances where underperformance represents a change in behaviour, is key.

### 28.3.1 Attributes of the Trainee

Stable, conscientious, extraverted doctors, who are agreeable to others and open to new experiences, tend to have successful and enjoyable careers, whatever specialty they enter [11]. In the past, surgery has been rather unique in emphasising the importance of the individual *heroic* surgeon rather than the team as a whole. There is certainly something strange about encouraging individuals to assault patients with sharp objects and expecting them to live with the consequences! This requires a degree of self-belief that, for some, can be associated with maladaptive behaviours and might explain why some surgeons have difficulty in communication, empathy and/or team working and may become angry when criticised [12]. Conversely, surgeons lacking in self-confidence and resilience and those with high neuroticism scores on psychometric testing may suffer from guilt, depression and burnout when things go wrong [13].

Rigorous selection and adequate support mechanisms have vital roles to play in this respect, but too often we select surgeons on the basis of attributes that are easy to measure (e.g. manual dexterity or test scores), rather than those that are important. Hospitals rarely provide adequate support to individuals when things go wrong [14], preferring a blame rather than a learning culture, as highlighted by the Berwick Report [15]. Chapter 15 on *Recruitment and Selection into Surgical Training* explores some of these aspects in more detail.

Unsatisfactory ARCP outcomes are higher for women and those training part-time. This is a difficult area to untangle, because most part-time surgical trainees are women who have to train in a workplace culture that is predominantly male and full-time. Ali et al. (2015) evaluated gender differences in the acquisition of surgical skills through a systematic literature review [16]. They noted that gaming experience and interest in surgery correlated with better acquisition of surgical skills, regardless of gender. The differences in assistance-seeking behaviour between male and female surgeons may also play a part in assigning gender differences in outcome as women are more prepared to ask for help than men [17].

In the UK, the situation is much worse for graduates from overseas universities, especially in the early years of surgical training: with 50% having unsatisfactory ARCP outcomes compared to only 18% of UK graduates [18]. This may well be due to cultural differences, as reassuringly, there is little evidence for any effect of race for those doctors graduating from UK universities. The question of whether training programmes can or should make reasonable adjustments for the needs of overseas trainees is addressed below.

## 28.3.2 Personal and Social Pressures

For many trainees, postgraduate training coincides with a number of life-events including moving house, entering into relationships, raising children, looking after elderly parents and financial worries. This struggle for work-life balance particularly impacts women [19] and may help explain declines in performance. A busy job combined with the pressures of training, CV building and taking exams can leave little time for relationships with family and friends, eating well and taking regular exercise. To promote well-being and effective performance, it is vital that senior surgeons provide good role models with respect to a healthy work-life balance and encourage trainees to confront any social, mental or physical health problems at an early stage [20].

## 28.3.3 The Training Programme

A good training programme will have a framework to support the education of every trainee, as well as support the continuing education of its faculty of senior surgeons, thus creating a learning culture for all. Key elements of such a culture include a comprehensive induction programme, well-trained educational supervisors who meet regularly with their trainees and the availability of pastoral support including career advice and counselling services. These aspects are dealt with in more detail in Chap. 14 on *Designing Surgical Education Programmes*.

Whenever possible, the programme should be tailored to the needs of the individual trainee, the legal term being *reasonable adjustment*. Ali et al. [16] recommended that surgical curricula should consider developing personalised programmes that accommodate more mentoring and one-on-one training for female physicians while giving male physicians more practice opportunities to increase the acquisition of technical skills. Obvious differences such as gender, religion, race, disability and part-time working are rightly the subject of anti-discrimination legislation, but many aspects of equality and diversity are more nuanced, and legislation is often focussed on work rather than training. The key question is whether the training programme can make reasonable adjustment to accommodate the needs of an individual trainee without affecting patient safety or overly inconveniencing colleagues.

## 28.3.4 The Work Environment

To succeed, surgical training requires a culture of supervision and feedback and a balance between training and service. The dangers of excessive hours and sleep deprivation for both doctors and patients are well recognised and have been the subject of working-hour regulations [21]. The question of whether or not the reduction in hours of work, whether 48 hours in Europe or 80 hours in North America, has a deleterious effect on patient safety or the quality of training is the subject of debate [22]. In a recent US study, 117 programmes were randomly assigned to current Accreditation Council for Graduate Medical Education (ACGME) [23] duty-hour policies or more flexible policies that waived rules on maximum shift lengths and time off between shifts. Outcomes included the 30-day rate of post-operative death or serious complications and resident perceptions and satisfaction regarding their well-being, education and patient care. Flexible, less-restrictive duty-hour policies were not associated with an increased rate of death or serious complications. Residents under flexible policies were less likely than those under standard policies to perceive negative effects of duty-hour policies on multiple aspects of patient safety, continuity of care, professionalism and resident education but were more likely to perceive negative effects on personal activities. As compared with standard duty-hour policies, flexible, less-restrictive duty-hour policies for surgical residents were associated with non-inferior patient outcomes and no significant difference in residents' satisfaction with overall well-being and education quality [24].

The Americans with Disabilities Act [25] mandates that educators must make reasonable accommodation to ensure that a trainee with a disability can complete the curriculum; however, this accommodation must be requested before a deficiency occurs. Disability legislation is similar in the UK, and there is increasing recognition of the challenges faced by surgeons with autism spectrum disorder (ASD). Deficiencies should be addressed as a performance problem and not as a health issue. For example, stress must be discussed as it relates to poor performance—not mental health. In addition, the ADA limits when a psychiatric evaluation can be required and is usually restricted to decisions about fitness to practice. A physician-patient relationship does not, and should not, exist between a trainee and PD; therefore, these concerns must remain confidential and separate from the academic file. After such evaluations, the PD should receive notification that appropriate follow-up is occurring but should not receive medical details. Future employers should not be told about impairment except to the extent that it involved misconduct (or lack of fitness for practice) that resulted in employment action [26].

Regardless of the origin of difficulties for trainees, faculty have a vital leadership role to play. They need to act as advocates for surgical training and fiercely protect the quality of their training programmes from erosion by service pressures. They also need to maintain the structure of their team from the ravages of duty rotas and ensure that trainees feel valued and supported as members of that team. Awareness of the individual and environmental factors that can impact performance can aid PD in tailoring such support to specific trainees. This may require some time and effort, but there is good evidence that paying careful attention to training opportunities in the same way as service commitments can dramatically improve training without compromising the service [27].

## 28.4 Recognition of the Underperforming Trainee

The underperforming trainee is "one who fails to meet the standard of performance in one or more ACGME competency" [28]. Deficits may exist in the competency domains of knowledge, skill or behaviour. Performance in any of these domains can be impaired by internal factors, such as fatigue or stress, and external factors, such as workload and poor work environment [29]. Behaviour problems are further defined as "personal conduct, whether verbal or physical, that negatively affects or potentially affects patient care including conduct that interferes with one's ability to work with members of a health care team [AMA]," [30] as "behavior that undermines a culture of safety" [31]. These behaviours include verbal outbursts and physical threats and/or exhibit an uncooperative attitude. Institutional leaders are required to have policies that address such behaviours whether caused by impairment due to substance abuse or other psychiatric disorder, external life stressors, personality characteristics, lack of training or system factors.

There is a spectrum of problem behaviour that extends from a single unprofessional event at the less serious end to misconduct at the most extreme. Determining whether to call such behaviours unprofessional or misconduct is often at the discretion of the PD; however the difference is important as the consequences for misconduct are more severe.

## 28.5 Analysing Underperformance Using Evidence

Norfolk and Siriwarden [32] offer a method for diagnosing performance issues, coined SKIPE that involves careful and comprehensive evidence collection. The first step involves identifying the level of *skill* demonstrated and the *knowledge* underpinning it. Then *internal* factors and *past* factors that might be having an impact are determined. Finally, *external* factors should be examined. It is helpful to have as much information as possible, both verbal and written, depending on the severity of the problem. In the UK, previous educational supervisors' reports, logbook data, exam results, untoward incidents and multisource feedback (360) are available for scrutiny in the trainee's portfolio.

Evaluation may include a review of all letters, e-mails, patient complaints [33] and incident reports, the trainee's portfolio as well as input from multiple team members and previous trainers [34]. Setting up a confidential hotline is another means of collecting data, but this is open to abuse through retaliatory reporting. Effective evaluation includes setting standards to measure resident performance, providing rater training and enforcing consequences for not completing evaluations of the trainee in a timely manner. Narratives are often more useful than numeric ratings in identifying issues [35], and all evaluations should be based on direct observation.

While investigating clinical supervision practices, Kennedy et al. [36] identified four factors that affect supervisor perception of trainee trustworthiness: knowledge/skill, discernment of limitations, truthfulness and conscientiousness. Two techniques used to assess trustworthiness included double-checking trainees' clinical findings and identifying cues from the trainees' use of language. Language cues included the structure of delivery during case presentations and the ability to anticipate needed information before it was solicited by the supervisor. In an internal medicine study, Yao et al. (2000) [37] noted that 60% of PDs identified problem behaviours through critical incident reports, for example, a patient complaint. In addition, 75% of PDs most frequently became aware of problem trainees because of verbal complaints from faculty and only 31% from written faculty evaluations. Thus, all notifications, regardless of formality, are valuable in assessing difficulty. Faculty members with only occasional contact with residents tend to be more generous with their ratings; thus, these ratings need to be interpreted with caution.

After scrutinising the information, the PD should arrange to meet with the trainee on neutral territory (e.g. the medical education centre) and inform the trainee of the reason for the meeting. At the meeting, it is helpful to give them time to reflect on the allegation, invite them to comment and document the discussion.

All incidents of alleged misconduct should be investigated, and a report generated that considers extenuating circumstances, particularly if this represents a change from previous behaviour. If found culpable, they do not have to be given an opportunity to repeat misconduct, depending on its severity, as long as the final decision is made through a reasonable process. There are often red flags that appear early in a trainee's career and these must be taken seriously. Early indicators that an individual may be in difficulty include the "disappearing act" [12]. The individual may arrive late, leave early and take excessive poorly explained days off or is hard to track down. The causes include relationship challenges, financial difficulties, mental or physical health problems and substance abuse or loss of confidence. Outbursts in patient care settings may indicate stress. Trainees in difficulty may seem not to fit in with the group, either because they are loners or because others are isolating them [10]. If others notice lack of competence or confidence, this may marginalise an individual, escalating the feeling of self-doubt. Because behavioural problems are frequently identified early in training, there is a case for conducting quarterly reviews of new residents [8, 33]. Any problem arising at any time should be brought to the attention of the PD for full investigation and the creation of a documented action plan with timeline for further evaluation.

## 28.6 Remediation

Residents with a *growth* mindset believe their success is based on hard work and learning, while those with a *fixed* mindset attribute their success to innate ability and their failures to the actions of others [38]. The latter are challenging to successfully remediate. Because a growth mindset is essential for self-improvement, evaluations should note the extent to which individuals take responsibility for improvement. How the trainee responds to feedback provides useful information about their insight and willingness to improve. The best response will be from the recipient who understands that he or she is being presented with a learning opportunity and therefore acknowledges a need for improvement. The more defensive the individual becomes and the more he/she argues, the more likely it is that this person has a fixed mindset and will be a challenge to remediate.

Trainees' deficit in medical knowledge should be prescribed a remedial reading schedule and encouraged to prepare for each case by developing a *flight plan* (mental rehearsal) of critical steps. Deficiencies in either basic or advanced technical skills are best remediated in the skills laboratory under expert guidance to ensure that juniors have the basic skills necessary to participate in surgical procedures and to permit a focus on more complex patient care issues in the operating theatre [9]. If a trainee is unable to answer "what if/what next questions", this could be addressed by prescribing a remedial reading plan along with developing a preoperative flight plan of critical steps (i.e. mental rehearsal) for discussion with the surgeon in advance. Further ideas for aiding a trainee's operative skill development can be found in Chap. 16, *Models of Teaching and Learning in the Operating Theatre*, and Chap. 17, *Supporting the Development of Operative Skills*.

With the current focus upon patient safety, the operating theatre is not an ideal environment for remediation to occur; the use of structured scenarios in a simulation laboratory allows trainees to acquire skills that transfer to the operating theatre in a safe environment that permits independence and the introduction of more challenging scenarios as the trainee's skill level improves.

Once any performance deficit is suspected, the trainee should be provided with a notice of deficiency that defines the expected behaviour, the timeline for improvement and the consequences for noncompliance. He/she needs to understand that such behaviour is unacceptable and detrimental to the individual, the programme and patients. The Vanderbilt Promoting Professionalism Pyramid (Fig. 28.4) for managing unprofessional behaviour is a useful approach for residents/trainees with behaviour problems. This four-step programme was developed primarily for disruptive faculty but has been expanded to unprofessional trainees. The large base of the pyramid conveys that most physicians rarely exhibit unprofessional behaviour. The next block is *single unprofessional incidents*. These could be isolated events unlikely to recur or the first observation of a pattern of behaviour. They are treated as anomalies and are the subject of an informal cup of coffee conversation. If the behaviour is repeated, then the next level up is a confidential non-punitive awareness intervention, followed by an authority intervention if problems continue. Finally, there is disciplinary action. Using this approach about 60% of physicians improve after level 1 interventions. Recidivism is less than 2%. Another 20% require additional help at level two authority interventions to improve [34]. If efforts at remediation are unsuccessful, PDs must follow through on the previously discussed consequences of probation, failure to promote or dismissal. Failure to enforce consequences has a negative effect on the behaviour and morale of all trainees and the care delivery system.

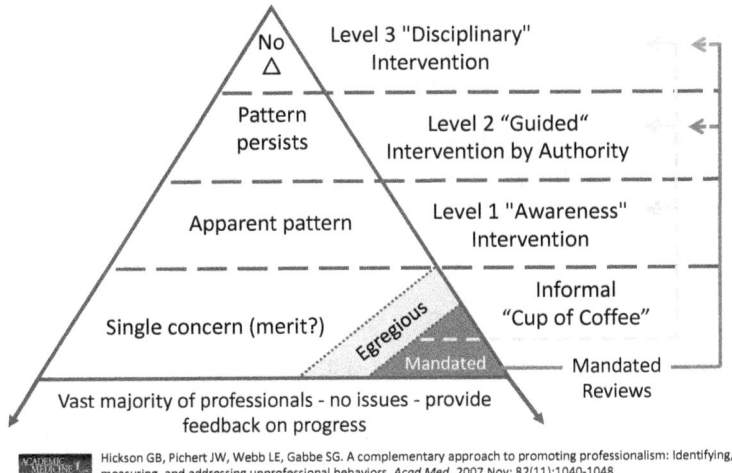

**Fig. 28.4** Promoting professionalism pyramid
https://www.cms.gov/Regulations-and-Guidance/Guidance/Manuals/downloads/som107ap_q_immedjeopardy.pdf
http://www.compass-clinical.com/hospital-accreditation/2011/05/19/deciphering-tjc-condition-level-findings/

The most effective method of ensuring fair decisions is to use a clinical competency committee. Problems are often identified in committees that are not raised by individuals [39], permitting the identification of patterns of behaviour. Roberts and Williams [40] suggest that committees consider whether the trainee's performance can be improved sufficiently to perform effectively as a member of the healthcare team and whether this improvement is likely to be sustained. Other considerations are the cost of remediation in time, effort and resources, as well as the hidden cost of retaining a trainee in terms of the increased workload on colleagues necessitated by *work-arounds*, double-checking and low morale [40].

From a legal stand point, the US courts have generally agreed that as long as the individual was provided with "notice and an opportunity to cure and the faculty decision is conscientious and deliberate", courts will not second-guess the academic decision [41, 42]. Misconduct must be distinguished from academic deficiency. By definition, misconduct is a behaviour that is wrong and that one knows (or should know) is wrong and therefore will not be *cured* by remediation. Treating misconduct as academic deficiency could be legally precarious by holding trainees to different legal and performance standards than other employees. Misconduct includes dishonesty, patient abandonment, criminal activity and covering up mistakes. All incidents should be investigated with probing of extenuating circumstances, if present. In assessing the culpability of an individual accused of such misconduct, Hickson et al. [34] recommend using the Reason [43] criteria and asking whether the team member intended to cause harm and came to work impaired and knowingly and unreasonably increased risk and whether another team member in the same situation would act in a similar manner. In certain situations, recommending a multidisciplinary evaluation can be helpful in elucidating contributing factors and remediation potential. In the USA, final decisions about the trainee are made by the PD, regardless of the majority opinion or the unpopularity of the decision. The trainee may request a review. In the UK, the final decision about continuation of training is made by the postgraduate dean.

## 28.7 Conclusions

A key element to avoid underperformance is trainee orientation with clarification of roles and responsibilities and educational objectives. Skilled surgical performance requires both technical and non-technical skills. Basic skills training should provide juniors with a foundation of motor skills for further learning in the operating room. The assessment of these basic skills is critical in juniors to identify and correct deficiencies before these become ingrained. However, the assessment of non-technical skills is even more important for senior residents. Centres of simulation can serve as safe and efficient environments for trainees to acquire proficiency in new skills and for remediation.

It is essential to set clear expectations for professional behaviour with both faculty and trainees and to describe problem behaviours as a deficiency in one or more competencies and not as a character flaw. PDs should incorporate an assessment of trustworthiness and ability to take responsibility for personal behaviour into evaluations and note system problems that enable unprofessional behaviour by providing secondary gain for such activities. Any complaint or critical incident, particularly in a new trainee, should be investigated and addressed promptly. Once a problem has been identified, the trainee must be provided with a notice of deficiency and an opportunity to improve. Consequences must be enforced for failing to address the deficiency. While the responsibility for improvement rests with the trainee, he/she will need guidance in locating appropriate resources. Whatever final decision is made about the trainee, as long as the process is fair and the decision was not arbitrary or capricious, it should be upheld in court. Finally, legal proceedings and grievance hearings are costly and time-consuming, so prevention is better than a cure. Therefore, early intervention is paramount.

## References

1. Hickson, G. B., Pichert, J. W., Webb, L. E., et al. (2007). A complementary approach to promoting professionalism: Identifying, measuring, and addressing unprofessional behaviors. *Academic Medicine, 8*, 1040–1048.
2. Williams, B. W., & Williams, M. V. (2008). The disruptive physician: A conceptual organization. *Journal of Medical Licensure and Discipline, 94*(3), 12–20.

3. Papadakis, M. A., Arnold, G. K., Blank, L. L., et al. (2008). Performance during internal medicine residency training and subsequent disciplinary action by state licensing boards. *Annals of Internal Medicine, 148*(11), 869–891.
4. Yeo, H., Bucholz, E., Sosa, J., et al. (2010). A national study of attrition in general surgery training: Which residents leave and where do they go? *Annals of Surgery, 252*(3), 529–536.
5. NCAS page specifics, year. NHS National Clinical Assessment Service. [online] Available at: http://www.ncas.nhs.uk/about-ncas. Accessed 5 Oct 2017.
6. Intercollegiate Surgical Curriculum Programme, V10. www.iscp.ac.uk. Accessed 19 Dec 16.
7. Naylor, R. A., Reisch, J. S., & Valentine, R. J. (2008). Factors related to attrition in surgery residency based on application data. *Archives of Surgery, 143*(7), 647–652.
8. Williams, R. G., Roberts, N. K., Schwind, C. J., et al. (2009). The nature of general surgery resident performance problems. *Surgery, 145*(6), 651–658.
9. Sanfey, H., Williams, R. G., & Dunnington, G. (2012). Recognizing residents with a deficiency in operative performance as a step closer to effective remediation. *JACS, 216*(1), 114–122.
10. Paice, E. (2009). Identification and management of the underperforming surgical trainee. *ANZ Journal of Surgery, 79*(3), 180–184.
11. McManus, I. C., Keeling, A., & Paice, E. (2004). Stress, burnout and doctor's attitudes to work are determined by personality and learning style: A twelve year longitudinal study of UK medical graduates. *BMC Medicine, 2*, 29.
12. Paice, E., & Orton, V. (2004). Early signs of the trainee in difficulty. *Hospital Medicine, 65*, 238–240.
13. Hubbard, E. (2004). The business case for diversity. In E. Hubbard (Ed.), *The diversity scorecard: Evaluating the impact of diversity on organizational performance* (pp. 3–27). Burlington: Elsevier Butterworth – Heinemann.
14. Seys, D., Scott, S., Wu, A., et al. (2013). *International Journal of Nursing Studies, 50*, 678–687.
15. National Advisory Group on the Safety of Patients in England. (2013). *A promise to learn – A commitment to act*. www.gov.uk/government/uploads/system/uploads/attachment_data/file/226703/Berwick_Report.pdf. Accessed 19 Dec 16.
16. Ali, A., Subhi, Y., Ringsted, C., et al. (2015). Gender differences in the acquisition of surgical skills: A systematic review. *Surgical Endoscopy, 29*, 3065.
17. Sanfey, H., Fromson, J. A., Mellinger, J., et al. (2015). Surgeons in difficulty: An exploration of differences in assistance seeking behaviors among male and female surgeons. *Journal of the American College of Surgeons, 221*, 621–627.
18. General Medical Council: National Training Survey. (2016). http://www.gmc-uk.org/education/surveys.asp. Accessed 19 Dec 2016.
19. Dyrbye, L., Shanafelt, T. D., Balch, C. M., et al. (2011). Relationship between work-home conflicts and burnout among American surgeons: Comparison by sex. *Archives of Surgery, 146*(2), 211–217.
20. Paice, E., Heard, S. R., & Moss, F. (2002). How important are role models in making good doctors? *British Medical Journal, 325*, 707–710.
21. Nurok, M., Czeisler, C. A., & Lehmann, L. S. (2010). Sleep deprivation, elective surgical procedures and informed consent. *The New England Journal of Medicine, 363*, 2577–2579.
22. Moonesinghe, S. R., Lowery, J., Shahi, N., et al. (2011). *BMJ, 342*, d1580. https://doi.org/10.1136/bmj.d1580.
23. ACGME. *ACGME programme requirements for graduate medical education in general surgery*. http://www.acgme.org/. Accessed 19 Dec 2016.
24. Bilimoria, K. Y., Chung, J. W., Hedges, L. V., et al. (2016). National cluster-randomized trial of duty-hour flexibility in surgical training. *The New England Journal of Medicine, 374*, 713–727.
25. Americans with Disabilities Act (ADA). http://www.ada.gov/American with Disabilities Act (ADA). http://www.ada.gov/. Accessed 24 July 2012.

26. Sanfey, H., DaRosa, D., Hickson, G., et al. (2012). Pursuing professional accountability: An evidence based approach to addressing residents with behavior problems. *Archives of Surgery, 147*(7), 642.
27. Marriott, J. C., Millen, A., Purdie, H., et al. (2011). The lost opportunities for surgical training in the NHS. *Annals of the Royal College of Surgeons of England (Suppl), 93*, 202–206.
28. Lucey, C. R., & Boote, R. (2008). Working with problem residents: A systematic approach. In E. S. Holmboe & R. E. Hawkins (Eds.), *Practical guide to the evaluation of clinical competence* (pp. 201–216). Philadelphia: Mosby Elsevier.
29. Rethans, J. J., Norcini, J. J., Baron-Maldonado, M., et al. (2002). The relationship between competence and performance: Implications for assessing practice performance. *Medical Education, 36*, 901–909.
30. American Medical Association. *AMA code of medical ethics: Opinion 9.045: Physicians with disruptive behavior.* http://www.ama-assn.org/ama/pub/physician-resources/medical-ethics/code-medical-ethics.page. Accessed 9/2016.
31. Joint Commission. (2008). Behaviors that undermine a culture of safety. Sentinel Event Alert. Issue 40.
32. Norfolk, T., & Siriwarden, A. N. (2013). A comprehensive model for diagnosing the causes of individual medical performance problems: Skills, knowledge, internal, past and external factors (SKIPE). *Quality in Primary Care, 21*(5), 315–323.
33. Sullivan, C., & Arnold, L. (2009). Assessment and remediation in programmes of teaching professionalism. In R. L. Cruess, S. R. Cruess, & Y. Steinert (Eds.), *Teaching medical professionalism* (pp. 124–149). Cambridge: Cambridge University Press.
34. Hickson, G. B., Federspiel, C. F., Pichert, J. W., et al. (2002). Patient complaints and malpractice risk. *JAMA, 287*, 2951–2957.
35. Schwind, C. J., Williams, R. G., Boehler, M. L., et al. (2004). Do individual attendings' post-rotation performance ratings detect residents' clinical performance deficiencies? *Academic Medicine, 79*(5), 453–457.
36. Kennedy, T. J., Regehr, G., Baker, G. R., et al. (2008). Point-of-care assessment of medical trainee competence for independent clinical work. *Academic Medicine, 83*(suppl), S89–S92.
37. Yao, D. C., & Wright, S. M. (2000). National survey of internal medicine residency programme directors regarding problem residents. *JAMA, 284*(9), 1099–1104.
38. Dweck, C. S. (2006). *Mindset: The new psychology of success.* New York: Random House.
39. Williams, R. G., Schwind, C. J., Dunnington, G. L., et al. (2005). The effects of group dynamics on resident progress committee deliberations. *Teaching and Learning in Medicine, 17*(2), 96–100.
40. Roberts, N., & Williams, R. (2011). The hidden costs of failing to fail residents. *Journal of Graduate Medical Education, 3*(2), 127–129.
41. Board of Curators of the University of Michigan v Horowitz. (1978). 435 US 78, 98 S Ct 948.
42. Richard, K., & Padmore, J. (2006). Does "fair hearing" = "due process" in residency programmes? *Health Law News, 10*(12), 16–17.
43. Reason, J. T. (1997). *Managing the risks of organizational accidents.* Aldershot: Ashgate Publishing.

# Chapter 29
# Patient Safety and Surgical Education

S. D. Marshall and R. M. Nataraja

**Overview** In recent times, simulation has played an increasingly prominent role in the acquisition of surgical skills. The association of patient safety with a surgeon's optimal technical operative skills is self-evident. However an educational experience in a simulation setting adds more than just skills training to enhance patient safety. Simulation is also valuable for developing the essential non-technical skills required working as part of a multidisciplinary team. Leadership skills, situation awareness and decision-making are all enhanced by simulation, particularly when uncommon, life-threatening events are replicated. Simulation allows the testing of both processes and protocols that leads to a system change. It also allows the duplication of situations from previous clinical events requiring further investigation. A more comprehensive understanding of the events and processes leading to adverse events allows training and redesign for future prevention. Measuring the effects of simulation-based interventions to improve safety can be challenging. Nevertheless, there is a growing evidence base of improved patient outcomes related to this.

---

S. D. Marshall (✉)
Department of Anaesthesia and Perioperative Medicine, Central Clinical School, Monash University, Melbourne, VIC, Australia

Department of Medical Education, University of Melbourne, Melbourne, VIC, Australia

Australian Centre for Health Innovation, Alfred Health, Melbourne, VIC, Australia

R. M. Nataraja
Department of Paediatric Surgery, Monash Children's Hospital, Melbourne, VIC, Australia

Department of Paediatrics, School of Clinical Sciences, Faculty of Medicine, Nursing and Health Sciences, Monash University, Melbourne, VIC, Australia
e-mail: ram.nataraja@monash.edu

## 29.1 Introduction

Surgery is one of the most complex of human endeavours. Unlike other high-reliability industries such as aviation, nuclear power and manufacturing, the significant components of the system, namely, the patient and their pathologies, have not been purposefully designed by an engineer. As such, knowledge is always imperfect, and decision-making, experience and technical skills have significant roles to play in ensuring a safe result.

'Safety science' is a relatively new branch of engineering that encompasses aspects of psychology, design and organisational quality improvement to reduce the risk of harm. Overlapping with this is the multidisciplinary science of 'human factors' or 'ergonomics', which uses the same techniques to ensure the design of equipment, processes and education optimally support the human working in the environment. Again, in human factors engineering, the goal is a safer, more efficient system of working.

The Institute of Medicine boosted interest in safety science in health in 1999 with the release of the report *To Err is Human* [1]. This report suggested that up to 98,000 patients every year in the USA lost their lives as a result of preventable mistakes. The figure has been both disputed and corroborated by many studies since, but despite the controversy, the suggested countermeasures are still valid today. These included the development of reporting systems and team training and simulation for those specialties, like surgery, that work in teams.

Indeed, the ultimate aim of any surgical education programme is to improve patient outcomes. These improved outcomes may be achieved not only through the training of individuals to a high degree of technical proficiency but also by teaching the non-technical skills and team processes that are associated with high quality in surgical care. In this chapter, we will explore how simulation-based surgical education can contribute to patient safety at system, individual and team levels.

## 29.2 System

Despite all of the interventions that optimise patient safety, incidents will still occur. How we deal with these is paramount, and the process should be analysed to prevent recurrence. The terms 'medical error' and 'adverse events' are commonly confused and often incorrectly interchangeably used. Medical error may be defined as either an error of either execution or planning of a medical intervention. These errors are essentially no different to other slips, lapses and mistakes that occur in everyday (non-clinical) life. However, the consequences of error in a health setting are of course are much greater. Adverse events are defined as a circumstance where harm or potential harm may occur. Errors do not in themselves lead to adverse events as there are usually many protective mechanisms or barriers that prevent the patient coming to harm. These barriers are conceptualised as slices of Swiss cheese in the famous model by psychologist James Reason [2], imperfect obstacles that may occasionally be circumvented.

When human operator errors are thought to have occurred, they can be classified into skill-based, rule-based or knowledge-based errors. In a skill-based error, the practitioner has failed to complete the task such as commencing the oxygen flow after fitting the facemask. These are the most common errors in skilled individuals through simple task omissions, often termed 'slips' or 'lapses'. A rule-based error relates to an inadequate application of a rule or poor planning such as the failure to follow an established protocol, such as the identification band check of the patient prior to starting a blood transfusion. Knowledge based is usually secondary to inadequate training of a clinician in an unfamiliar environment, e.g. failure to prescribe the correct dose of a medication to a paediatric patient. By understanding the type of errors that could occur, preventative strategies can be constructed. There are also a number of modifying factors that influence these errors such as stress levels, distraction and tiredness. Simulation plays a key role in developing an understanding about when errors are likely and to generate strategies to identify and navigate error-prone conditions. This awareness of error in clinical practice is termed 'error wisdom' and includes an appreciation of how their own limitations, their team and environment may contribute to adverse events in any given situation.

Most adverse events, as noted earlier, are due to a number of often unrelated failures at a system and individual level. In order to determine the nature of these failures, root cause analyses (RCAs) are undertaken. RCAs are system-wide investigations that attempt to determine where the barriers to harm broke down in any particular adverse event. Essentially three questions are asked:

1. What happened?
2. Why did it happen?
3. What can be done to prevent it from happening again?

There should also be an overview of the whole organisation in terms of clinical governance and risk management, so that if different departments have had similar events, this can be detected and rectified.

In addition to the education of clinical staff about potential errors, simulation can be used to test out approaches to harm and error prevention through a range of mechanisms. Equipment design, clinical processes and knowledge gaps may be identified that can be rectified and tested in realistic clinical settings. Merely re-creating previous events that led to patient harm can generate new solutions in education, process and equipment design leading to reminders and prompts where needed. An example of this is the World Health Organization's (WHO) Safe Surgery Checklist ('time out') [3]. Implementation of these tools has been demonstrated to improve hazard detection, surgical complications and team communication [4]. Simulation has been shown to play a key role in implementing these interventions through both testing and education with best practice guidelines now available to enable this [5–7]. Each health service may adapt and refine the checklist for the clinical and cultural context of the organisation, such that it has the desired effect of building teamwork and capturing important information that might otherwise be missed.

It is essential for patient safety and also the continuous quality of healthcare improvement that there is an open culture of medical errors and adverse events reporting. There should also be the avoidance of a "blame culture" in which there is a shift from highlighting individual clinician failings to a systems-based change. There has to be a widespread culture of medical error reporting as suggested by the IOM report *To Err Is Human* [1]. Without this appropriate disclosure and attitudes, appropriate analysis cannot occur, and hence future critical events be prevented. For a successful system of error reporting, there needs to be anonymity and confidentiality as well as independence of the investigating team. Without this there will be reluctance to error reporting in the clinical setting.

## 29.3 Technical Skills

Surgical simulation allows the acquisition of technical skills in an environment outside of the operating room, such that patients are not exposed to the initial learning curve of junior surgeons. Recent technological advancements have extended the scope from low complexity skills such as suture tying, to more sophisticated skills required for minimally invasive surgery (MIS) and endoscopy. This has aided the introduction of simulation into routine surgical educational practice. Simulation-based training is now accepted as a safe alternative to the traditional 'Halstedian' apprenticeship model of training using only patients as teaching material.

While simulation was once the reserve of only specialised educational centres, technology has now evolved to include devices such as home-based MIS box trainers with motion tracking. This increased accessibility of advanced surgical simulation has led to increased exposure and an increase in self-directed learning without the potential risk to patients. These advanced technologies have several advantages. The incorporation of mandatory simulation programmes into surgical curricula, as well as the application of the principles of mastery learning, deliberate practice and competency-based learning, has led a more standardised, efficient acquisition of surgical skills prior to actual patient contact. Progress can be monitored remotely with regular formative and summative assessments.

The ultimate question with technical skills training is whether the surgeon's individual performance plays a role in the prevention of errors, and therefore has a potential effect on patient safety. There is growing evidence of the educational value of a variety of simulated procedural interventions and part task trainers [8–12]. These are either using endoscopic, virtual reality (VR) or box trainers in simulation-based educational programmes. In these programmes learners are able to acquire skills that are transferable to the operating room environment. This skill transfer has been demonstrated by a number of different randomised controlled trials and systematic reviews, and the evidence base for this is expanding but not well established [13–16]. The majority of published evidence demonstrates improved performance on a simulator after training rather than transference of skills to the clinical setting. Overcoming the initial part of the learning curve in a safe environment has obvious patient safety implications. However, there is a limit to the fidelity and realism of surgical simulation tasks in regard to the tissue responsiveness, tensile strength and handling with haptic feedback. In addition, the complexity of anatomical variations and unexpected challenges might not be able to fully replicate. For these reasons simulation-based educational activities will not in the foreseeable future be able to completely replace patient-based training models, but patient safety is ensured by maximisation of skill acquisition in a safe environment.

## 29.4 Non-technical Skills

There is a significant focus in the literature on technical rather than non-technical skills (NTS) in surgical education. Non-technical skills have been defined as "the critical cognitive and interpersonal skills that underpin technical proficiency" [17]. Failure of these skills such as communication [18–20], team coordination [21–23], leadership [24, 25], decision-making [26, 27], situational awareness [28], perception [29] and clinical judgement [30, 31] has been demonstrated to be the causative factors in the majority of adverse clinical events [32, 33]. These skills are also critical in emergency situations when individual team members assemble in a crisis having not necessarily worked together before [34]. This has led to a focus on the development of these skills in recent years.

### *29.4.1 Situation Awareness*

Situation awareness is perhaps simultaneously one of the most important and the most difficult NTS to determine. Situation awareness is the development and maintenance of a dynamic awareness of the situation in the operating theatre by assessing environmental data (patient, team, time, monitors, equipment) and then interpreting them to predict future events [28]. Fixation on a particular aspect of a situation and exclusion of other information is a common feature of performance under stress [29]. Simulation education may help counteract these fixation errors, or loss of situation awareness, by developing strategies surgeons can use to help their decision-making under stress. These strategies may include stress management and mindfulness, communication with other colleagues or decision-making ('cognitive de-biasing') strategies [35].

### *29.4.2 Decision-Making*

Decision-making is the process by which a surgeon determines the optimal intervention or procedure for the best patient outcome. This may include judgements before, during or after surgery and is influenced by the prior experience of the surgeon. Most clinical decisions are based on pattern matching and previous experience and are termed 'recognition primed decisions' [36]. When novel situations arise, surgeons revert to other strategies such as those related to heuristics or 'rules of thumb', or from a synthesis of existing knowledge and evidence-based medicine [37]. It is important to appreciate what basis the decisions are being made on and to recognise that they are likely to be affected by personal experience rather than empirical evidence. Decision-making strategies and cognitive de-biasing techniques mentioned above can be taught to improve the decision-making process.

### 29.4.3 Leadership and Teamwork

Communication and teamwork is essential for ensuring patient safety, and with this it is also important to create an environment that is nonthreatening and non-confrontational allowing all team members to voice any concerns [38]. The implementation of the "time out" at the start of a theatre session with the individual introduction of all team members is crucial for this to occur. A breakdown or lack of communication is often the causative factor for an adverse event. Leadership is closely aligned to this and needs to be defined although may originate from the surgeon, anaesthetist or nursing team leader depending on the circumstances.

The Non-Technical Skills for Surgeons (NOTSS) instrument was developed to assess individual surgeons NTS [39]. It was developed by a multidisciplinary team of psychologists, surgeons and anaesthetists in 2003 and has four NTS categories that are assessed (situation awareness, decision-making, communication and teamwork and leadership). In each of these categories, there are three elements that are then scored on a scale of 1 (poor) to 4 (good), resulting in four domain scores (e.g. situation awareness domain score – SDS) and a global score. This NOTSS instrument has been successful applied to the clinical setting and has been shown to be both procedure independent and also achieve good reliability.

One of the advantages of the NOTSS approach is that it allows a framework for the assessment of intra-operative clinical decision-making. The majority of the literature is focused on the preoperative phase, whereas the cognitive and interpersonal skills demonstrated by a surgeon in the intra-operative phase are paramount to patient safety. This instrument may also be used in the simulation scenario setting for trainees to develop their NTS in a safe environment. When this technique is combined with a video debriefing, it can become a powerful tool to enhance the surgeon's self-awareness and perception of their own abilities with the corresponding improvement in patient safety.

Surgical NOTECH (NOn-TECHnical, adapted from aviation) and OTAS (Observational Teamwork Assessments for Surgery) instruments [40] have also been developed to focus on the performance of the entire surgical team. These tools use the team itself rather than the individual team members as the unit of measure. They rely on the processes within the team such as communication and coordination being improved.

## 29.5 Team Training

Rather than merely teaching individuals the non-technical skills required for effective teamwork and hoping that these principles are applied, in some circumstances it may be more appropriate to educate the whole team. Whole team training is generally beneficial when the composition of the team is relatively stable [41]. Goals of the education include creating team processes that improve coordination and communication and safety and learning cultures to ensure sustainability of the changes. Several simulation methods can be used to achieve this, most commonly using immersive, mannequin-based simulation techniques [42]. Team training has been shown to translate to improved team processes in health [43] and other industries [44]. These processes have also been linked to indices of improved safety and job satisfaction.

A few particular forms of whole-team training have specifically been suggested to improve patient safety.

### 29.5.1 Team Coordination Training

Crisis (crew or clinical) resource management (CRM) training is a form of team coordination training originally developed in the aviation industry [45]. The philosophy of this training is to improve the communication, leadership and coordination of teams by comparing their performance in simulation or clinical work with the ideal performance. In most cases this is used to improve the non-technical skills of individuals. However, when stable teams are included, it can also have the effect of setting the cultural norms of safety for these teams.

### 29.5.2 Team Self-Correction Training

This type of team training involves observation of teams' performances usually in simulation settings but occasionally using recordings of real cases. A skilled facilitator guides the discussion of the actions undertaken in order to generate a learning culture within the team. Over a period of time, the facilitator takes a reduced role in debriefing the team as the ability of the team to learn from the different members improves. This particular form of training may be useful when new teams are created, or when new procedures are being implemented with the same team members for every case. Limited team self-correction training may also be seen with simulation-based 'mission rehearsals' of single, one-off procedures as has been performed with neonatal surgery [46].

### 29.5.3 In Situ Scenario-Based Training

More extensive whole-team training in the actual clinical setting can have additional effects on safety processes. Draycott and colleagues implemented an in situ team-training course in obstetrics [47]. Their aim was for teams to derive their own local solutions to common problems in the labour ward and obstetric theatres based on existing clinical structures and processes. Impressively, a halving of hypoxic ischaemic encephalopathy and low 5-min APGAR score rates were observed in the groups that undertook the team training sessions. This latter approach demonstrates that the opposite approach to CRM training can also work; by concentrating on the clinical work of the team rather than how the team functions. In situ training also lends itself to an examination and modification of the clinical environment to provide cues and equipment that improves clinical outcomes in emergencies.

## 29.6 Measurement of Safety Interventions

In order to determine if patient safety is truly improved by the educational intervention, a number of direct and indirect measures can be used. It is tempting to count the numbers of errors and extrapolate this to a measure of safety, but this is fallacious and ignores not only the important narrative detail of safety but the subjective nature of errors.

Safety itself is a difficult concept to measure. Just as health is not merely an absence of disease, so safety is not merely an absence of morbidity or mortality. The problem with measurement of any patient outcome is the number and complexity of other factors that may confound the results. As a result, surrogate measures such as observed technical errors or speed of completion of tasks in simulation are commonly measured and the conclusions extrapolated to patient outcomes.

In contrast, McGaghie and colleagues [48] describe a framework that goes beyond measures of the effects on the learners and on to changes in patient treatment, patient outcome and population-wide effects. Many of these effects are particularly relevant for patient safety such as complication rates and patient discomfort. Nevertheless, some aspects of safety are still difficult to measure. 'Resilience' in safety science refers to the ability of an organisation to adapt to prevent and mitigate adverse events in the face of difficult circumstances. From a practical perspective, this includes both the daily efficiencies and cutting of corners of clinicians to get the job done as well as additional fail-safes they put in place to ensure safety is maintained. These resilient strategies are often difficult to identify, but once they have been, they can be demonstrated in education sessions, brought into regular care and measured in the clinical setting. The example of the WHO safer surgery checklist is again instructive. Team briefings prior to an operating list or procedure were noted to be resilient strategies used by high-performing teams to prevent adverse events. The application and adoption only became widespread when it was described in a clinical process and cognitive tool in the form of a checklist.

Patient outcomes are clear areas in which safety may be measured. Rate of complications before and after an education and/or process intervention are well-recognised indices of safety. Nevertheless, morbidity and mortality rates may be very low and require surrogate measures of safety such as features associated with the risk of complications. Examples may include estimated blood loss or duration of tourniquet use. Other patient outcome measures include satisfaction surveys relating to the surgery such as quality of recovery scores for anaesthesia. The importance of the role of the patient's involvement in both education and safety assessment cannot be overstated.

Measures from staff members may also be used as indices of safety. There are now a number of safety climate scores used in health that have been shown to correlate with other safety measures. Over time these safety climate surveys can build a detailed picture of the effects of education and process interventions. Staff satisfaction surveys have also been used in surgery to determine the effectiveness of team training and safety within the operating theatre.

The most common measures of improvement in safety from educational intervention are more distant, surrogate measures. These measures are often undertaken in simulation and include time to perform a procedure, number of omissions, slips and lapses and technical proficiency. Although easy to measure, these do not always transfer to improved safety for patients.

## 29.7 Conclusions

Surgical education, particularly in association with simulation, has a high potential for improving patient safety. These improvements come not only from the training of individual technical skills but also from creation of effective teams, new processes at organisational levels and the dissemination of resilient, safe behaviours.

## References

1. Kohn, L. T., Corrigan, J. M., & Donaldson, M. S. (1999). *To err is human: Building a safer health care system*. Washington, DC: National Academy Press.
2. Reason, J. T. (2000). Human error: Models and management. *BMJ, 320*, 768–770.
3. Haynes, A. B., Weiser, T. G., Berry, W. R., et al. (2009). A surgical safety checklist to reduce morbidity and mortality in a global population. *The New England Journal of Medicine, 360*, 491–499.
4. Treadwell, J. R., Lucas, S., & Tsou, A. Y. (2014). Surgical checklists: A systematic review of impacts and implementation. *BMJ Quality and Safety, 23*, 299–318.
5. Goldhaber-Fiebert, S. N., & Howard, S. K. (2013). Implementing emergency manuals: Can cognitive aids help translate best practices for patient care during acute events? *Anesthesia and Analgesia, 117*, 1149–1161.
6. Marshall, S. D. (2017). Helping experts and expert teams perform under duress: An agenda for cognitive aid research. *Anaesthesia, 73*, 289–295.

7. Keane, M., & Marshall, S. D. (2010). Implementation of the WHO surgical safety checklist: Implications for anaesthetists. *Anaesthesia and Intensive Care, 38*, 397–398.
8. Nataraja, R. M., Webb, N., & Lopez, P. J. (2018). Simulation in paediatric urology and surgery, part 2: An overview of simulation modalities and their applications. *Journal of Pediatric Urology, 14*, 125–131.
9. Ljuhar, D., Alexander, S., Martin, S., & Nataraja, R. M. (2018). The laparoscopic inguinal and diaphragmatic defect (LIDD) model: A validation study of a novel box trainer model. *Surgical Endoscopy, 32*, 4813–4819.
10. Fonseca, A. L., Evans, L. V., & Gusberg, R. J. (2013). Open surgical simulation in residency training: A review of its status and a case for its incorporation. *Journal of Surgical Education, 70*, 129–137.
11. Hamdorf, J. M., & Hall, J. C. (2000). Acquiring surgical skills. *British Journal of Surgery, 87*, 28–37.
12. Hennessey, I. A. M., & Hewett, P. (2013). Construct, concurrent, and content validity of the eoSim laparoscopic simulator. *Journal of Laparoendoscopic & Advanced Surgical Techniques Part A, 23*, 855–860.
13. Marshall, S. D., & McKarney, L. (2015). Section 1: A focused review of simulation to improve patient outcomes. In *Simulation, patient outcomes and mental health review* (pp. 1–9). Melbourne: Victorian State Government, Department of Health and Human Services.
14. Aggarwal, R., & Darzi, A. (2006). Technical-skills training in the 21st century. *The New England Journal of Medicine, 355*, 2695–2696.
15. Nagendran, M., Toon, C. D., Davidson, B. R., & Gurusamy, K. S. (2014). *Laparoscopic surgical box model training for surgical trainees with no prior laparoscopic experience. The Cochrane Library* (pp. 1–75). Chichester: Wiley.
16. Okrainec, A., Soper, N. J., Swanstrom, L. L., & Fried, G. M. (2011). Trends and results of the first 5 years of Fundamentals of Laparoscopic Surgery (FLS) certification testing. *Surgical Endoscopy, 25*, 1192–1198.
17. Flin, R., O'Conner, P., & Crichton, M. (2008). *Safety at the sharp end*. Aldershot: Ashgate.
18. Manser, T., Harrison, T. K., Gaba, D. M., & Howard, S. K. (2009). Coordination patterns related to high clinical performance in a simulated anesthetic crisis. *Anesthesia and Analgesia, 108*, 1606–1615.
19. Cadogan, M. P., Franzi, C., Osterweil, D., & Hill, T. (1999). Barriers to effective communication in skilled nursing facilities: Differences in perception between nurses and physicians. *Journal of the American Geriatrics Society, 47*, 71–75.
20. Fischer, U., McDonnell, L., & Orasanu, J. (2007). Linguistic correlates of team performance: Toward a tool for monitoring team functioning during space missions. *Aviation, Space, and Environmental Medicine, 78*, B86–B95.
21. Entin, E. E., & Serfaty, D. (1999). Adaptive team coordination. *Human Factors, 41*, 312–325.
22. Hall, P. (2005). Interprofessional teamwork: Professional cultures as barriers. *Journal of Interprofessional Care, 19*, 188–196.
23. Dickinson, T. L., & RM, M. I. (1997). A conceptual framework for teamwork measurement. In M. T. Brannick, E. Salas, & C. Prince (Eds.), *Team performance assessment and measurement* (pp. 19–43). Mahwah: Lawrence Erlbaum Associates.
24. Cohen, S. G., & Bailey, D. E. (1997). What makes teams work: Group effectiveness research from the shop floor to the executive suite. *Journal of Management, 23*, 239–290.
25. Salas, E., Sims, D. E., & Burke, C. S. (2005). Is there "big five" in teamwork? *Small Group Research, 36*, 555–599.
26. Kuhlmann, S., Piel, M., & Wolf, O. T. (2005). Impaired memory retrieval after psychosocial stress in healthy young men. *Journal of Neuroscience, 25*, 2977–2982.
27. deLeval, M. R., Carthey, J., Wright, D. J., Farewell, V. T., & Reason, J. T. (2000). Human factors and cardiac surgery: A multicenter study. *Journal of Thoracic and Cardiovascular Surgery, 119*, 661–672.
28. Endsley, M. R. (1995). Measurement of situation awareness in dynamic systems. *Human Factors, 37*, 65–84.

29. Fioratou, E., Flin, R., & Glavin, R. (2010). No simple fix for fixation errors: Cognitive processes and their clinical applications. *Anaesthesia, 65*, 61–69.
30. Cox, T. (1987). Stress, coping and problem solving. *Work and Stress, 1*, 5–14.
31. Serfaty, D., Entin, E. E., & Volpe, C. E. (1993). *Adaptation to stress in team decision-making and coordination. Human Factors and Ergnomics Society 37th annual meeting* (pp. 1228–1232). Santa Monica: Human Factors and Ergonomics Society.
32. Greenberg, C. C., Regenbogen, S. E., Studdert, D. M., et al. (2007). Patterns of communication breakdowns resulting in injury to surgical patients. *Journal of the American College of Surgeons, 204*, 533–540.
33. Mishra, A., Catchpole, K., Dale, T., & McCilloch, P. (2008). The influence of non-technical performance on technical outcome in laparoscopic cholecystectomy. *Surgical Endoscopy, 22*, 68–73.
34. Andreatta, P. (2009). *A typology for healthcare teams. SimTect Health*. Melbourne: SIAA.
35. Crosskerry, P., Singhal, G., & Mamede, S. (2013). Cognitive debiasing 2: Impediments to and strategies for change. *BMJ Quality and Safety, 22*, ii65–ii72.
36. Klein, G. (1999). *Sources of power: How people make decisions*. Cambridge, MA: MIT Press.
37. Tversky, A., & Kahneman, D. (1974). Judgement under uncertainty: Heuristics and biases. *Science, 185*, 1124–1130.
38. Lingard, L., Espin, S., Whyte, S., et al. (2004). Communication failures in the operating room: An observational classification of recurrent types and effects. *Quality and Safety in Health Care, 13*, 330–334.
39. Yule, S., Flin, R., Paterson-Brown, S., Maran, N., & Rowley, D. (2006). Development of a rating system for surgeons' non-technical skills. *Medical Education, 40*, 1098–1104.
40. Undre, S., Healey, A. N., Darzi, A., & Vincent, C. A. (2006). Observational assessment of surgical teamwork: A feasibility study. *World Journal of Surgery, 30*, 1774–1783.
41. Marshall, S. D., & Flanagan, B. (2010). Simulation-based education for building clinical teams. *Journal of Emergencies, Trauma and Shock, 3*, 360–368.
42. Weller, J., Nestel, D., Marshall, S. D., Brooks, P. M., & Conn, J. J. (2012). Simulation in clinical teaching and learning. *MJA, 196*, 594.
43. Schmutz, J., & Manser, T. (2013). Do team processes really have an effect on clinical performance? A systematic literature review. *British Journal of Anaesthesia, 110*, 529–544.
44. Salas, E., DiazGranados, D., Klein, C., Shawn-Burke, C., Stagl, K. C., & Goodwin, G. F. (2008). Does team training improve team performance? A meta-analysis. *Human Factors, 50*, 903–933.
45. Gaba, D. M., Howard, S. K., Fish, K. J., Smith, B. E., & Sowb, Y. A. (2001). Simulation-based training in anesthesia crisis resource management (ACRM): A decade of experience. *Simulation and Gaming, 32*, 175–193.
46. Auguste, T. C., Boswick, J. A., Loyd, M. K., & Battista, A. (2011). The simulation of an ex utero intrapartum procedure to extracorporeal membrane oxygenation. *Journal of Pediatric Surgery, 46*, 395–398.
47. Draycott, T., Sibanda, T., Owen, L., Akande, V., Winter, C., & Reading, S. (2006). Does training in obstetric emergencies improve neonatal outcome? *BJOG: An International Journal of Obstetrics and Gynaecology, 113*, 177–182.
48. McGaghie, W. C., Draycott, T. J., Dunn, W. F., Lopez, C. M., & Stefanidis, D. (2011). Evaluating the impact of simulation on translational patient outcomes. *Simulation in Healthcare, 6*(supp), S42–S47.

# Part IV
# Research in Surgical Education

Surgical education must be advanced by research. In this part, we share approaches to undertaking surgical education research. Matthews et al. (2016) conducted a bibliometric analysis of publications in surgical education [1]. The technique enables examination of cited works offering some insight to the nature of surgical education and scholarship. Influenced by the search terms, the top 100 articles were published in 31 journals, 1 book series with the most published in Annals of Surgery ($n = 16$) [1]. Simulation training was the topic most widely reported, closely followed by assessment and clinical competence. Reliability and validity of assessment tools and transferability of training regimens made up the focus of 15 articles, and 8 articles reported developments in clinical skills training. Most articles were research papers ($n = 76$) and reviews ($n = 16$). Of the 76 research papers, 8 were randomized controlled trials, 5 were systematic reviews, and 3 were consensus guideline statements.

This fourth part of the book is intended to orient readers to key concepts and practices in order to give them the tools and skills to both evaluate the surgical educational literature critically as well as to provide tasters into how worthwhile and thoughtful contributions can be made to it. In this manner, they will be able to consider how they would go about developing effective curricula using best practices as well as to move the field of surgical education forward through innovation and research.

This part opens with both theoretical and practical advice. Ajjawi and McIlhenny provide an overview of surgical education research through an exploration of three paradigms of research commonly used (Chap. 30). Next, Liang, a surgeon and educator, provides a surgeon's perspective related to challenges moving from a bench model paradigm for research to the multi-paradigm formats of surgical educators, adding pragmatic solutions and advice (Chap. 31). Colville and Green *clear the air* with an insightful discussion of how surgical educators new to educational research can overcome apparent barriers to contribute to the field (Chap. 32).

We then offer insights to salient topics in surgical education research. D'Souza and Wong describe how to perform a literature review for framing a research project or as an independent systematic review (Chap. 33). Martin addresses the critical topic of accurate measurement of educational interventions through the proper selection and implementation of quantitative measures (Chap. 34). Next, two editors of this book, Dalrymple and Nestel, address key concepts and guidelines for conducting qualitative research in surgical education, a topic with which many surgeons are completely unfamiliar (Chap. 35). Kingsbury describes ethical considerations in conducting research in surgical education and assists readers in navigating the sometimes labyrinth of human research ethics review (Chap. 36).

We then move to three shorter chapters that document examples of surgeons conducting educational research. We asked them to focus on their experiences of the research rather than detailed reporting of their research. We hope this approach inspires other surgeons to consider undertaking surgical education research. Kokelaar shares his experiences of using qualitative research techniques to explore the concept of community of practice in laparoscopic surgery (Chap. 37). Alderson challenges convention with an example of presenting research findings creatively through drama and its impact on the reach and audience (literally and figuratively) (Chap. 38). Miyasaka concludes the section with a discussion of how an innovative simulation-based, experiential training program was successfully incorporated into a first-year general surgical curriculum to allow trainees a comprehensive exposure to treatment of targeted surgical diseases across the continuum of care (Chap. 39).

In summary, this part progresses from the general to the specific in an effort to provide foundational knowledge and, at the same time, concrete examples for making meaning of and/or conducting research in surgical education. That is, paradigms for conducting research are followed by more in-depth discussions of key aspects of the research process. Personal experiences are then provided of specific projects that were undertaken and their lessons and results. In this way, we hope to make research in surgical education more accessible and productive for our readers.

# Reference

1. Matthews, A. H., et al. (2016). Surgical education's 100 most cited articles: A bibliometric analysis. *Journal of Surgical Education, 73*(5), 919–929.

# Chapter 30
# Researching in Surgical Education: An Orientation

**Rola Ajjawi and Craig McIlhenny**

**Overview** This chapter provides an orientation to research approaches in surgical education. Education research seeks to deepen the knowledge and understanding of learning and pedagogy. We start with highlighting common research paradigms. Beliefs about knowledge and reality influence research questions and design, and so it is important to be aware of these and to actively consider these assumptions in the research design process. We then outline the link between conceptual frameworks and research questions. A brief audit of published surgical education research highlights that most of the research in this field is quantitative in nature, single site and atheoretical. We conclude with a discussion of the challenges and opportunities for surgical education research. Surgical education offers a rich and exciting setting for conducting education research. We urge surgical education researchers to go beyond their comfort zones, to use theory and to consider alternative research paradigms.

## 30.1 Introduction

In their classic text, *Handbook in Research and Evaluation*, Isaac and Michael [1] emphasise the importance of research in education as "the only way to make rational choices between alternative practices, to validate educational improvements, and to build a stable foundation of effective practices as a safeguard against faddish but inferior innovations". With this in mind, in this chapter we provide an orientation to surgical education research (SER). In particular, we consider four broad paradigms of research – positivism (typically encompasses quantitative research),

R. Ajjawi (✉)
Centre for Research in Assessment and Digital Learning (CRADLE), Deakin University, Melbourne, Australia
e-mail: rola.ajjawi@deakin.edu.au

C. McIlhenny
Scottish Centre for Simulation and Clinical Human Factors, Larbert, UK

Royal College of Surgeons of Edinburgh, Edinburgh, UK
e-mail: c.mcilhenny@nhs.net

post-positivism (typically encompasses mixed methods research), constructivism and critical theory (typically encompass qualitative research). We describe trends in SER and consider challenges to and opportunities for developing education research expertise.

## 30.2 What Is Education Research?

The primary objective of all research is to generate new knowledge. The purpose of education research "is to deepen the knowledge and understanding of learning and education by studying phenomena, relations and how and why and what works for whom" [2]. Education research is not primarily about answering local, concrete questions or improving local practice. The local context is where *researchable problems* about education are studied [2]. This notion of addressing gaps in the literature to add to the knowledge base of the community and to address problems that go beyond the local context is what differentiates research from evaluation.

## 30.3 Paradigms of Research

Whether you choose to produce research or not, your role as a surgical educator means that you must be able to consume it judiciously. In order to understand, judge and apply knowledge from education research to your education practice, as described in our opening quote, requires an understanding of research paradigms. Further, because the aim of research is to generate knowledge, researchers need to be aware of what knowledge is and the different ways it can be generated and verified in order for it to become accepted. Knowledge of the philosophical underpinnings of various research paradigms helps to facilitate the design and implementation of a good research project and to maintain consistency between the questions and the approach; alignment is an important requirement for all credible research [3].

Research paradigms provide a framework for understanding, describing and justifying research strategies. They represent sets of beliefs and practices shared by communities of researchers [4]. Guba and Lincoln [5] defined a paradigm as "the basic belief system or worldview that guides the investigator, not only in choices of method but in ontologically and epistemologically fundamental ways". Epistemology is the theory of knowledge; it is about the relationship between the knower (i.e. the researcher) and what can be known (i.e. the phenomenon of study) [6]. Ontology is the theory of what really exists and is concerned with the nature of reality and the nature of human beings in the world [6]. These grand theories dictate what you choose to do and how you interpret the outcomes and results, whether the researchers are conscious of them or not [4]. Methodologies are also typically considered within a research paradigm. Methodology is the theory that guides the choice and use of particular data collection and analysis methods [7]. The actual methods used

**Table 30.1** Common paradigms in SER

|  | Positivism | Post-positivism | Constructivism | Critical theory |
|---|---|---|---|---|
| **Ontology:** what is the nature of reality? | Naïve realism: reality is static and fixed. There is a single truth that can be discovered | Critical realism: reality is static and fixed but can only be imperfectly and probabilistically accessible | Relativism: reality is subjective and multiple. Human actions continuously constructing social life | Political, ideological factors, power shaping behaviour |
| **Epistemology:** what is the nature of knowledge | Objective, generalisable knowledge is neutral or value-free | Knowledge is objective but can only be approximated. Seeks to establish probable truth | Knowledge is subjective, constructed. Multiple and diverse interpretations exist | Knowledge is co-constructed and collective, mediated by power relations and constantly under revision |
| **Methodology:** what is the nature of the approach? | Typically quantitative, e.g. RCT[a], experimental | Can be pragmatist, e.g. mixed methods | Typically qualitative, e.g. grounded theory, ethnography | Dialogic/dialectical. Focus on emancipation and participation, e.g. PAR[b], VRE[c] |
| Researcher position | Research conducted from the outside | Research conducted from the outside | Personal involvement of the researcher | Collaborative research with participants as researchers |

Adapted from Lincoln et al. [6]
[a]*RCT* randomised controlled trial
[b]*PAR* participatory action research
[c]*VRE* video-reflexive ethnography

(e.g. observation, survey, interviews) are just tools and should not be associated with any one particular form of research.

Four common paradigms in health professions education research are positivism, post-positivism, constructivism and critical theory [4]. Table 30.1 highlights the grand theories (ontology and epistemology), methodologies and researcher positioning common to each of these paradigms. These are by no means exhaustive of existing paradigms, and by necessity we have simplified the understandings presented here. We contend that none of these research paradigms is inherently superior. The choice of paradigm is determined by the research phenomenon of interest and is influenced by (and also influences) the specific research questions.

## *30.3.1 Positivism*

Positivist research assumes that reality exists independently apart from our consciousness, and it is there to be discovered [8]. This stance assumes that reality is observable and can be measured. The researcher and the object of the research are independent entities, and so the object may be studied without being influenced by the researcher [5]. Knowledge is commonly presented as time- and context-free generalisations, which can be in the form of cause-effect [5]. Quantitative research tends to be conducted within the positivist paradigm. Research processes common to quantitative research include experimental studies and randomised controlled trials (RCTs). These are difficult to do well in education due to the myriad of contextual features that influence learning. Cook [9] has suggested a framework for surgical RCTs: *exploratory studies* for the early assessment of new techniques or theories, *explanatory studies* to assess the intervention in favourable conditions and *pragmatic studies* to inform clinical decision making through evaluation of the intervention in a realistic clinical setting; this may open up quantitative SER findings to the broader surgical audience.

### 30.3.2 Post-positivism

A positivist perspective of reality is rigid and cannot be considered as the only valid one [8]. To assume that reality can be fully known is not how we experience the world, and therefore it has given way to post-positivism with modest claims of probability rather than absolute certainty. Common to this paradigm is the use of mixed methods where research involves the collection, analysis and integration of both qualitative and quantitative data in a single study [10]. Mixed methods research upholds the importance and value of both qualitative and quantitative methods to the study design [11] and attempts to integrate them based on the assumption of mutual relevance [12]. It rejects the rigidity of knowledge claims of other paradigms and strives for practical solutions to practical problems. It is driven by its research questions and uses pluralistic approaches to derive knowledge about the problem – the methods become secondary. The benefits of using mixed methods include exploring complex interventions with multiples stakeholders, triangulating research findings to deepen understandings of the research phenomenon and creating a dialogue between different ways of seeing, interpreting and knowing [10, 12].

### 30.3.3 Constructivism

Constructivist research assumes that human beings construct meanings as they engage with the world they are interpreting [8]. In this way knowledge is both time- and context-dependent rather than universal and objective. Because knowledge is constructed, it is neither objective nor truly generalisable, with scientific knowledge representing just one form of constructed knowledge designed to serve particular purposes [8]. Human beings construct meaning from their engagement with the world (rather than being passive recipients of meaning); even when they experience the same objects, people experience them in different ways. This is the notion of multiple constructed realties. That is, the ontological perspective is subjective and multiple, such that there are several versions of reality. Therefore, there is no one true or valid interpretation. Qualitative research within health professions education is typically conducted using constructivist frameworks where it seeks to understand complexity taking into account context (including social, cultural, political, physical and technical).

Qualitative research assumes "that all knowledge, and therefore all meaningful reality as such, is contingent upon human practices, being constructed in and out of interaction between human beings and their world, and developed and transmitted within an essentially social context" [8]. In this type of research, findings are generated through the interactions between the researcher and the participants as the research progresses. Therefore, subjectivity is valued. Qualitative researchers acknowledge that humans are incapable of total objectivity because they are situated in a reality constructed by subjective experiences. Further, the research is value-bound, by the nature of the questions being asked, the values held by the researcher and the ways data are co-produced and interpreted. Therefore, findings are not generalisable because there is no single truth or one way of seeing things.

Considering the value-bound nature of interpretive research and the assumption of multiple realities, the criteria of reliability and validity become irrelevant. Yet, it is common to see positivist researchers judging qualitative research using the criteria of reliability, validity and generalisability. For example, they might calculate inter-coder reliability coefficients to show that the coders identified a common truth in the data rather than subjectively interpreted, discussed and developed a coding framework. Several introductory articles and frameworks are available to guide researchers through constructivist paradigm research [13, 14].

## *30.3.4 Critical Theory*

Critical theory research denotes several alternative theoretical perspectives including feminism, materialism and participation inquiry. Research in this paradigm assumes that over time social, political, cultural, economic, ethnic and gender factors form "a series of structures" that are inappropriately taken as "real", i.e. natural and immutable [5]. Knowledge is viewed as subjective, co-constructed and value mediated (knowledge is not neutral). Research within this paradigm seeks to effect change and is often political and emancipatory [4]. Although both constructivist and critical theory research are broadly termed 'qualitative', the former seeks to understand research phenomena, whilst the latter seeks to change structures and situations that may be invisible to the participants themselves but become visible and open to change through co-participation in the research. Critical theory research is thus transformative; using participatory and reflective dialogic approaches allows the researcher and the participants to challenge the status quo and the structure mechanisms for order maintenance. Issues such as how power is produced and reproduced within a surgical setting and what are legitimate forms of knowledge and who benefits may be explored within this research paradigm.

## 30.4 Where Do Research Questions Come from?

Earlier we said that the research paradigm, research questions and methods should be in alignment. The process of designing these is iterative, and often the phenomenon of interest and gaps in the literature drive the research questions and approach [15]. The first step in generating a researchable problem is situating the idea or problem within a conceptual framework. Conceptual frameworks "represent ways of thinking about a problem or a study, or ways of representing how complex things work" [16]. The conceptual framework is composed of the following three components [2]:

1. Suitable theories of learning and education that can clarify the underlying mechanisms pertaining to the idea or problem
2. A critical synthesis of information from the empirical literature identifying what is already known and what is not known about the idea to inform the development of a concrete research topic
3. The researcher's individual thoughts and ideas

This vital first step of constructing a coherent conceptual and theoretical framework is often lacking in SER. Bordage [16] uses the analogy of a lighthouse – shining light on a phenomenon to illuminate and magnify certain aspects that you make a stand for and claim to be important in your research. For everything you choose to shed light on, there are other things that remain in the dark (some by design others through ignorance).

Conceptual frameworks can come from theories that have been confirmed by observations or experiments; models derived from theories, observations, or sets of concepts; or evidence-based best practices derived from outcome and effectiveness studies [16]. There are a number of reasons why we might be motivated to embrace the idea of conceptual frameworks perhaps chief amongst them are clear indications from journal editors that they prioritise these articles. Conceptual frameworks enable researchers to move beyond mere descriptions of "what" to explanations of "why" and "how", they provide an explanation that helps to define the research questions and make sense of the data, they enable selection of appropriate data collection and analysis methods, and they identify boundaries of work.

## 30.5 Trends in Surgical Education Research

We conducted an audit of SER articles published in the *Journal of Surgical Education*, *Medical Education*, *Advances in Health Sciences Education*, *BMC Medical Education* and *Academic Medicine* from January 2016 to August 2016. A manual search of all articles relevant to SER identified that about 87% of these used quantitative research approaches, 6% used mixed methods, 3% were systematic reviews and meta-analyses and 3% used qualitative research methods. Within the (broad) medical education journals, less than 5% of published articles focused on

SER. The majority of the research we reviewed was single site and interventional with pre- and post-measures; many used surveys and included Likert scales to measure participants' self-perception such as improved confidence following an educational intervention. Participants were typically surgical trainees or a mixture of surgical trainees and surgeons; few targeted undergraduate medical students and even less were interprofessional. Only a handful of articles mentioned theory and these were primarily qualitative studies. This paints a picture of an emerging discipline that is applying principles of biomedical (positivist) clinical research to answer what are in their very nature social type problems. Indeed others have critiqued this approach, instead aligning medical education research with the social sciences [17].

Our quick audit accords with findings in the literature around SER approaches and quality. In a 10-year analysis of SER (1988–1998), the authors concluded that there was a lack of theory-based research, and most (77%) of the studies took a quantitative approach [18]. A more recent audit of postgraduate SER (1991–2009) found that 74% ($n = 28$) were evaluation studies [19]. In 2003, the *American Journal of Surgery* published 19 original quantitative medical education research studies. The main areas requiring improvement were that the research methodologies were weak in more than 50% of these articles, only a minority of these articles reported evidence of validity with their measurement instruments, and only 5% of the articles reported healthcare outcomes [20].

In terms of trends in the content of SER, there are also published similarities with our findings. An audit published in 2000 found that curriculum and teaching were the most frequent topics studied (40%), followed by assessment (23%) and programme evaluation (18%) [18]. Similarly, a 2016 review of the 100 most cited articles in surgical education identified the two top topics of research as simulation (45%) and surgical skills competence and assessment (40%) [21]. A recent priority setting exercise conducted in the USA for SER identified the following top five priorities: teaching methods and curriculum development, assessment and competency, simulation, faculty development and impact of work-hour restrictions [22].

## 30.6 Challenges to Surgical Education Research

### 30.6.1 The Challenge of Credibility of SER

Perhaps our biggest challenge is ensuring that our SER informs the practice of surgical education. This is not a problem that lies purely within the surgical domain. The general acceptance that education research has borne little in the way of applicable results has multiple roots; but poor quality of research being carried out and a negative perception of education research as being less academically challenging than other fields are key points. The perception that because SER is not carried out in the proud tradition of basic science research and clinical trials means that a whole hidden curriculum where education practice and research are seen as academically inferior to research rooted in the biomedical tradition continues to flourish. This false perception amongst surgeons of education research lacking credibility has been quoted as the number one barrier to carrying out research into surgical education [23]. Linked to perceptions of credibility is the lack of funding for SER compared with biomedical or clinical research which signals lack of valuing from the top. Incidentally, lack of funding for SER was the second most quoted barrier [23].

### 30.6.2 The Challenge of Quality of SER

As educators we would agree that high-quality research to advance the evidence base for education is imperative, yet the quality of SER has been examined and found wanting. This is an issue that has also been debated in the wider medical education research arena [24, 25].

Norman [26], as editor of the journal *Advances in Health Sciences Education*, although tongue-in-cheek, wrote an article on how to *not* get your article published. He argued that having an educational intervention (something) against no intervention (nothing) is meaningless (and therefore "useless") as any educational intervention will have intended and unintended consequences. This was something we saw published in SER where a one group pretest-posttest design was commonly used to infer the success of an educational intervention. Indeed, Reed et al. [20] found that nearly half (47.4%) of the SER studies they reviewed used single-group cross-sectional or single-group posttest-only designs. Another feature of poorly designed studies was the reliance on self-reported measures such as satisfaction or confidence as self-assessment abilities are uncorrelated with actual performance [27]. Finally relying on p-value alone is not enough as this does not confer educational importance, its direction and why there might have been significance.

Often researchers evaluate complex educational interventions asking does "x" work when x is made up of multiple sub-interventions and without questioning the likely mechanism for why and how it might work, for whom and in what circumstances [28]. Learning is a function of the interplay between the learner, the teacher, the educational design and the context (or educational milieu) so treating educational interventions as if they are context-free and easily standardised and generalisable is too reductionist and simplistic to be meaningful. And although such articles do get published, their educational impact and hence value to the broader community are often limited.

### 30.6.3 The Challenge of Paradigm

SER has been dominated by a preference for quantitative rather than qualitative studies with variations of cohort designs and nonexperimental studies predominating. Surgeons are very firmly set in the traditional biomedical research mindset;

however, one of the distinctive qualities of education research methodology is its diversity. Although this is expected and welcomed by social scientists, it can be quite overwhelming to surgeon researchers especially if they have previously performed clinical or basic science research.

## 30.7 Opportunities for Surgical Education Research

### 30.7.1 Improving Credibility of SER and Building Research Capacity

Changes in the landscape of the delivery of surgical care and therefore surgical training have been well described previously [29]. Reduced opportunities for training have resulted in greater awareness of the need for more effective training. This is evidenced by increased focus and resource on how we deliver training [30]. In turn, this has led to increased awareness within the community of education research as a foundation for pedagogical decision making [23]. Along with these changes, and often driving them, research in surgical education has seen an unprecedented growth [22]. This can be seen in a great increase in the number of articles published within the SER domain [18]. Interestingly, this main increase has been in surgical journals, while there has actually been a decrease in those published in medical education journals [18].

The increase in frequency of SER literature in peer-reviewed surgical journals has positive implications. This may reflect a heightened sensitivity of surgeons to educational issues and a need to better educate ourselves on how best to both teach and learn. Conceivably this describes the path that peer-reviewed surgical journals are taking, which is towards accepting more education research articles. This may also be influenced by an increased number of surgeons leading SER.

Credibility by peers is slowly increasing as the subject matter and design of education research improves in quality. A generation of surgeons, such as Richard Reznick and Teodor Grantcharov, have legitimised education research as an academic pursuit and inspired young surgeons to consider it as an academic path. A study [23] of the top 15 published surgeons in SER identified the top three factors contributing to success were chair support, collaboration with peers and mentors and participation in a surgical education community such as the Association for Surgical Education (USA), the Faculty of Surgical Trainers (UK) or the Academy of Surgical Educators (Australia). These associations also offer dedicated funding opportunities for SER. Opportunities for collaboration between education researchers and practitioners can enhance the quality of SER as well as surgical education programmes.

## 30.7.2 Promoting Diversity of Method and Quality in SER

We clearly need to address and expand the focus and quality of SER. It should span any aspect of surgical education, yet our focus seems to be fairly narrow in topic and method [18, 21, 22]. While assessment of competence is obviously a vital aspect of surgery, and surgical education, SER ignores large swathes of unexplored territory in the wider landscape of surgical education. Regehr [31] urged researchers to shift from a narrow focus of trying to prove their intervention works to trying to understand complex educational phenomena. He argued for: "Reorienting education research … from a problematic search for proofs of simple generalisable solutions to our collective problems, towards the generation of rich understandings of the complex environments in which our collective problems are uniquely embedded". However, for those who wish to conduct interventional research then we urge you to: develop a conceptual framework of what is to be learned, actively consider the educational theories and principles that underpin the interventional design and reframe the question to does the educational intervention work, for whom, how and in what circumstances.

Aggarwal [32] has called for a coordinated approach to high-quality SER and a move towards multi-institutional collaborative studies that have relevant outcomes. These need to be multicentre studies, designed in a prospective manner, using validated tools with outcome measures of relevance to multiple stakeholders and impact upon patient care. As education researchers, however, we must bear in mind that when Aggarwal talks of "outcome measures of relevance", we should not revert to our biomedical research paradigm of patient outcomes being the only outcomes of import. As cited by Cook and West [33], "an emphasis on patient outcomes in medical education would be akin to focusing clinical research outcomes on mortality, which would neglect other outcomes important to patients". We need to be more nuanced in our choices of educational outcomes, and these stem from our conceptual, theoretical and philosophical frameworks.

## 30.8 Conclusion

Surgical education offers a rich and exciting setting for conducting education research. Surgical educators need to understand common research paradigms in order to design and conduct research studies as well as to become critical consumers of journal articles that report education research findings. Clinical research in surgery is seeing an exponential increase in multisite coordinated trials and SER needs to follow suit. Furthermore, we urge surgical education researchers to go beyond their comfort zones, to use theory and to consider alternative research paradigms. We end with another quote: Gawande [34] argued that training for the twenty-first century needs to change "it requires that surgeons learn not just how to operate but how to create good working systems of care". We argue that in order to do this, SER must shift from a heavy quantitative focus on individualistic acquisition of knowledge and skills to broader naturalistic and political understandings of complex ways of working and systems of care.

## References

1. Isaac, S., & Michael, W. B. (1997). *Handbook in research and evaluation: For education and the behavioral sciences* (3rd ed.). San Diego: EdITS.
2. Ringsted, C., Hodges, B., & Scherpbier, A. (2011). 'The research compass': An introduction to research in medical education: AMEE Guide No. 56. *Medical Teacher, 33*(9), 695–709.
3. Carter, S. M., & Little, M. (2007). Justifying knowledge, justifying method, taking action: Epistemologies, methodologies, and methods in qualitative research. *Qualitative Health Research, 17*(10), 1316–1328.
4. Bunniss, S., & Kelly, D. R. (2010). Research paradigms in medical education research. *Medical Education, 44*(4), 358–366.
5. Guba, E. G., & Lincoln, Y. S. (1994). Competing paradigms in qualitative research. In N. K. Denzin & Y. S. Lincoln (Eds.), *Handbook of qualitative research* (pp. 105–117). Thousand Oaks: Sage.
6. Lincoln, Y. S., Lynham, S. A., & Guba, E. G. (2011). Paradigmatic controversies, contradictions, and emerging confluences, revisited. In N. K. Denzin & Y. S. Lincoln (Eds.), *The SAGE handbook of qualitative research* (4th ed., pp. 97–128). Thousand Oaks: SAGE Publications.
7. van Manen, M. (1997). *Researching lived experience: Human science for an action sensitive pedagogy* (2nd ed.). Ontario: The Althouse Press.
8. Crotty, M. (1998). *The foundations of social research: Meaning and perspective in the research process*. Sydney: Allen & Unwin.
9. Cook, J. A. (2009). The challenges faced in the design, conduct and analysis of surgical randomised controlled trials. *Trials, 10*(1), 1–9.
10. Schifferdecker, K. E., & Reed, V. A. (2009). Using mixed methods research in medical education: Basic guidelines for researchers. *Medical Education, 43*(7), 637–644.
11. Maudsley, G. (2011). Mixing it but not mixed-up: Mixed methods research in medical education (a critical narrative review). *Medical Teacher, 33*(2), e92–e104.
12. Morgan, D. L. (2014). *Integrating qualitative and quantitative methods: A pragmatic approach*. Thousand Oaks: SAGE Publications.
13. Tai, J., & Ajjawi, R. (2016). Undertaking and reporting qualitative research. *The Clinical Teacher, 13*(3), 175–182.
14. O'Brien, B. C., Harris, I. B., Beckman, T. J., Reed, D. A., & Cook, D. A. (2014). Standards for reporting qualitative research: A synthesis of recommendations. *Academic Medicine, 89*(9), 1245–1251.
15. Lingard, L. (2015). Joining a conversation: The problem/gap/hook heuristic. *Perspectives on Medical Education, 4*(5), 252–253.
16. Bordage, G. (2009). Conceptual frameworks to illuminate and magnify. *Medical Education, 43*(4), 312–319.
17. Monrouxe, L. V., & Rees, C. E. (2009). Picking up the gauntlet: Constructing medical education as a social science. *Medical Education, 43*(3), 196–198.
18. Derossis, A. M., DaRosa, D. A., Dutta, S., & Dunnington, G. L. (2000). A ten-year analysis of surgical education research. *The American Journal of Surgery, 180*(1), 58–61.
19. Toumi, Z., & Lightbody, K. (2011). Systematic review of postgraduate surgical education in the last two decades. *Webmed Central Surgery, 2*(5), WMC001941.

20. Reed, D. A., Beckman, T. J., & Wright, S. M. (2009). An assessment of the methodologic quality of medical education research studies published in The American Journal of Surgery. *The American Journal of Surgery, 198*(3), 442–444.
21. Matthews, A. H., Abdelrahman, T., Powell, A. G. M. T., & Lewis, W. G. (2016). Surgical education's 100 most cited articles: A bibliometric analysis. *Journal of Surgical Education, 73*, 919–929.
22. Stefanidis, D., Cochran, A., Sevdalis, N., Mellinger, J., Phitayakorn, R., Sullivan, M., et al. (2015). Research priorities for multi-institutional collaborative research in surgical education. *The American Journal of Surgery, 209*(1), 52–58.
23. Dutta, S., & Dunnington, G. L. (2000). Factors contributing to success in surgical education research. *The American Journal of Surgery, 179*(3), 247–249.
24. Cook, D. A., Bordage, G., & Schmidt, H. G. (2008). Description, justification and clarification: A framework for classifying the purposes of research in medical education. *Medical Education, 42*(2), 128–133.
25. Shea, J. A., Arnold, L., & Mann, K. V. (2004). A RIME perspective on the quality and relevance of current and future medical education research. *Academic Medicine, 79*(10), 931–938.
26. Norman, G. (2014). Data dredging, salami-slicing, and other successful strategies to ensure rejection: Twelve tips on how to not get your paper published. *Advances in Health Sciences Education, 19*(1), 1–5.
27. Eva, K. W., & Regehr, G. (2005). Self-assessment in the health professions: A reformulation and research agenda. *Academic Medicine, 80*(10), S46–S54.
28. Wong, G., Greenhalgh, T., Westhorp, G., & Pawson, R. (2012). Realist methods in medical education research: What are they and what can they contribute? *Medical Education, 46*, 89–96.
29. Reznick, R. K., & MacRae, H. (2006). Teaching surgical skills—changes in the wind. *New England Journal of Medicine, 355*(25), 2664–2669.
30. Sachdeva, A. K., Blair, P. G., & Lupi, L. K. (2016). Education and training to address specific needs during the career progression of surgeons. *Surgical Clinics of North America, 96*(1), 115–128.
31. Regehr, G. (2010). It's NOT rocket science: Rethinking our metaphors for research in health professions education. *Medical Education, 44*(1), 31–39.
32. Aggarwal, R. (2015). Surgical education research: An IDEAL proposition. *Annals of Surgery, 261*(2), e55–ee6.
33. Cook, D. A., & West, C. P. (2013). Perspective: Reconsidering the focus on "Outcomes Research" in medical education: A cautionary note. *Academic Medicine, 88*(2), 162–167.
34. Gawande, A. A. (2001). Creating the educated surgeon in the 21st century. *The American Journal of Surgery, 181*(6), 551–556.

# Chapter 31
# Researching in Surgical Education: A Surgeon Perspective

**Rhea Liang**

**Overview** This chapter draws on perspectives gained as a surgeon undertaking education research. It begins by addressing three questions that surgeons may ask regarding the relationships between themselves, educationalists, and surgical practice. *What is the place of education research in surgical practice? What is the place of surgeons in education research? What is the place of educationalists in surgical education research?* It then discusses three threshold concepts which may prove problematic for surgeons – moving from one dominant research paradigm to multiple potential paradigms, thinking outside the apprenticeship model, and moving from a neutral stance to an examined (and declared) stance. Finally, five practical suggestions for undertaking education research are offered – finding or developing a community of practice, narrowly defining the research, proper consideration for ethical aspects, finding the balance between being 'far enough in' and 'far enough out', and time management with surgical practice.

## 31.1 Introduction

This chapter draws on perspectives gained as a surgeon undertaking education research. It begins by addressing three questions that surgeons may ask regarding the relationships between themselves, educationalists, and surgical practice. It then discusses three threshold concepts which may prove problematic for surgeons – moving from one dominant research paradigm to multiple potential paradigms, thinking outside the apprenticeship model, and moving from a neutral stance to an examined (and declared) stance. Finally, five practical suggestions for undertaking education research are offered – finding or developing a community of practice,

R. Liang (✉)
Gold Coast Health, Southport, QLD, Australia

Bond University, Gold Coast, QLD, Australia

Royal Australasian College of Surgeons, Melbourne, VIC, Australia
e-mail: Rhea.Liang@health.qld.gov.au

narrowly defining the research, proper consideration for ethical aspects, finding the balance between being 'far enough in' and 'far enough out', and time management with surgical practice.

## 31.2 Three Questions

### 31.2.1 What is the Place of Education Research in Surgical Practice?

Fry and Kneebone (2011) identify 'craft' as a defining characteristic of surgery [1]. In the craft tradition, which remains the predominant educational paradigm in surgery, there is an emphasis on technical learning within a relationship between trainer and apprentice. The novice gradually becomes proficient, and finally an expert, through imitation and repetition.

Why should surgeons choose to do research into a system of education that has ostensibly performed well for many years? Surgeons increasingly find themselves in an environment that is rapidly changing in many ways – techniques, technologies, health systems, societal expectations, and training programmes. It is no longer sufficient to judge teaching and learning against a historical benchmark, or perhaps even against 'what it is now', and even less sufficient to judge teaching and learning solely against a surgeon's personal belief or experience. In order to make sound educational provision for an unpredictable future, robust evidence and theory are required.

### 31.2.2 What is the Place of Surgeons in Education Research?

The practicalities of 'how to teach' are seldom explicitly taught in surgery training, creating a cohort of consultant surgeons who feel educationally naïve. More abstract ideas about 'how trainees learn' or 'theories about education' are often perceived to be the domain of either consultant surgeons with a special interest in education or educationalists with a special interest in surgery. It is tempting to think that the 'average' practising surgeon cannot contribute good research in this setting.

Surgeons, however, have access to the 'business' of surgery. The distinctive characteristics of surgery which makes it so interesting to educationalists, such as the specialised knowledge, the kinaesthetic skills, and the need for sterility, also make surgical settings difficult for non-surgeons to access. Surgeons provide access to and intimate knowledge of the operating theatre, the outpatient clinic, the inpatient ward, the research laboratory, the tutorial room, and the lecture theatre. They are familiar with the constraints of time and urgency, the unpredictability of daily work, and the sometimes devastating effect of errors. They teach trainees and are simultaneously learning and perfecting their own craft.

Surgeons are therefore engaged in a sort of private educational research enquiry all the time. It is the moments when they wonder 'can the medical students think critically without their electronic devices?' or 'why is this trainee so disorganised in their case presentation?' or 'would a workshop or online video be the best way for me to learn this new technique?' Such private musings become the seeds of surgical education research when they are stated explicitly and made 'visible' for investigation and analysis. When combined with their existing professional development skill set (task-focused enquiry, literature review, data collection, and complex reasoning), all surgeons can be assured that they are capable of high-quality surgical education research.

### 31.2.3 What is the Place of Educationalists in Surgical Education Research?

The process of becoming familiar with education and education theory is a significant cognitive and affective change for many surgeons. The fields of surgery and education can appear 'mutually mysterious' in their world view, culture, practice, and lexicon. They are sufficiently different that 'mastering education' can become a threshold towards a 'Masters of Education'.

It is vitally important that surgeons embarking on education research collaborate with expert educationalists. Educationalists scaffold the learning of surgeons embarking on education research in the same way that expert surgeons provide scaffolding for the learning of the surgical trainee. For example, surgeons may be surprised that problems which they considered unique to the surgical setting often have well-developed and readily accessible corollaries in educational theory, even if the theory has been developed in another setting. Research which translates existing educational theories into surgical practice, such as cognitive load theory or Wenger's communities of practice, has been very productive [2, 3]. (See Part II – *Theories Informing Surgical Education*.) Without collaborating with educationalists, it is unlikely that surgeons will make these linkages fortuitously or develop equivalent theories on their own.

## 31.3 Three Threshold Concepts

### 31.3.1 Moving from One Dominant Research Paradigm to Multiple Potential Paradigms

The vast majority of clinical surgical research occurs within a positivist or post-positivist paradigm and utilises quantitative methods. The conduct of research is quite rigidly defined with a clear hierarchy designated as 'levels of evidence' from systematic reviews (Level 1) and randomised controlled trials (Level 2) downwards

[4]. Implicit in this hierarchy is an assumption that the 'best' research design is one which minimises variability by focusing on measurable parameters and aggregating large amounts of data.

Education research is very different. The ontology and epistemology is chosen to match the intention of the research, and the methodology can be quantitative, qualitative, or mixed. Relatively small numbers of study subjects may be required in order to assure quality, for example, by reaching saturation in a grounded theory analysis. The phenomena being studied are not always measurable. Variability is valued, with outliers often considered to be very informative. The field of education research is also developing rapidly compared to the already codified methods of clinical biomedical research. At all times within education research, there are multiple competing schools of thought, new research methods being proposed, and existing research methods being refined.

For many surgeons who have expended much effort conducting the 'perfect' research trial (large numbers, clean data, few confounders, small p-values), the 'softness' and sheer variety of education research can be challenging. It is tempting to revert to familiar quantitative methods, to try to find measurable proxies for phenomena which would be better researched by other means. As an example, the percentages of women who choose to leave surgical training and the percentages who quote various factors (long hours, pregnancy, etc.) as the reasons for leaving [5, 6] are well described. But the numbers have not been sufficient to suggest effective strategies to address the issue. They do not explain the complex interactions between factors and the sociocultural milieu in which the issue arises. They are unable to explore the time course and critical events, internal dialogues, and conflicts experienced by the women which lead them to finally leave surgical training.

Exploring these aspects requires qualitative methods. Surgeons need encouragement to think in 'nonquantitative' ways and specific training to implement qualitative methods such as interviews and focus groups. The skills required are quite different to the repetitive, and sometimes mechanistic, process of collecting the same items of data on large numbers of subjects in a quantitative research project. Learning to perform qualitative research may initially be challenging, but eventually it is very rewarding – even liberating – to realise the increased breadth and flexibility of approach which characterise education research.

### *31.3.2 Thinking Outside the Apprenticeship Model*

As a craft, surgery still ascribes to an apprenticeship model of imitation and practice. Within this model, learning is seen as a 'natural process' where the learner becomes more proficient by repeatedly performing a given procedure as closely as possible to the pattern demonstrated by the expert consultant. This traditional view of apprenticeship is still prevalent, as seen in conference biographies and curricula vitae where the location of training and the identity of consultant trainers are emphasised. There is an inherent assumption that excellent teachers and institutions provide the optimal model for an apprentice and therefore produce an excellent surgeon.

This rather passive view of learning is at odds with modern educational theory. Ideas such as the conscious use of strategies for learning, the modification of teaching techniques for specific learning needs, and the use of scenario and simulation training, experiential learning, and reflective practice all imply an agency in both the learner and teacher which have not been present in surgical education until recently. As a result, surgeons can initially be resistant to the idea that surgical learning can be made explicit, problematized, and examined. Educational theories and innovations may be regarded by surgeons as unnecessary or an upset of the 'natural process' or 'the way things have been done'.

A related problem with the apprenticeship model is the emphasis on technical learning, at the expense of a great deal of socially constructed learning that is neither made explicit nor examined. This is compounded by an attitudinal tendency to diminish the importance of 'non-technical' skills [7]. A common example is the excusing of undesirable behaviours such as bullying or poor communication skills with '…but they are an excellent operator…' While there is growing recognition of the importance of 'non-technical' surgical competencies, such as the nine competency framework of the Royal Australasian College of Surgeons [8], surgeons are still more likely to initially comprehend educational theory that can be applied to technical learning, such as deliberate rehearsal and simulation. Theory that applies to 'non-technical' competencies, particularly the more abstract or overarching theories, can take longer to learn and assimilate.

### 31.3.3 *Moving from a Neutral Stance to an Examined (and Declared) Stance*

The surgical environment is geared towards the surgeon's understandings and world view. Surgeons are accustomed to working in settings that conform to them and not the other way around. A surgeon's personal stance is therefore often unexamined.

It may take effort and practice for a surgeon to be able to 'step outside' and purposefully examine their personal stance. Becoming aware of personal stance can be a troubling process, especially if cognitive biases are identified which need to be addressed in order to progress with research. This process is aided by interaction with non-surgical research colleagues and reflective observation. By crossing this threshold, key qualitative research skills are enabled, such as being able to shift perspectives (e.g. when using different theories as lenses for data analysis) and becoming aware of things that are 'invisible' to the surgeon researcher or taken for granted.

Particularly careful attention should be paid to stance during the write-up phase. Surgical research literature is conventionally written from a neutral third person stance, consistent with a positivist or post-positivist paradigm where the researcher's experiences, emotions, and views are minimised in the search for perfectly objective (usually quantitative) data. The convention in education research of declaring a personal stance, often in the first person, is a new and unfamiliar requirement. The keeping of a reflective diary during research can help a surgeon to find their personal 'voice' and to become familiar with writing in the first person prior to the formal write-up.

## 31.4 Practical Considerations

### 31.4.1 A Community of Practice

One of the most rewarding aspects of surgical education research is the inbound trajectory into a community of surgical education practice, and it is highly recommended that surgeons undertaking education research find or develop a suitable community. Such a community enables dialogue with like-minded surgical and non-surgical colleagues and provides an opportunity to jointly contribute to a rapidly developing field. It is an environment where a novice surgical education researcher can gradually become more expert.

Increasingly there are now formalised structures such as higher-degree programmes and academies which function as communities of practice and are easily accessed in the digital age regardless of a surgeon's physical location. Examples include the Master of Surgical Education offered by Melbourne University and the Academy of Surgical Educators [9, 10].

### 31.4.2 Defining the Research

Surgical education research is newly developing field, with large gaps in the current knowledge base. It is relatively easy to find an education question arising from practice for which there is no clear answer, and it is tempting to formulate an ambitious research project that will fill the largest gap. This tendency is not helped by years of training in the surgical philosophy of addressing the most consequential deficit first.

Defining a research project should err on the side of narrowness, because far more projects are hampered by being too broad than the converse. A well-refined research question and an achievable study design are essential. The surgeon's relative lack of knowledge in educational literature should be acknowledged, and the guidance of education colleagues sought, as their ability to place some educational 'signposts' into the formulation of a research project can certainly prevent a great deal of 'wandering in the wilderness'.

Surgeons should also not underestimate the time commitment required, especially for qualitative research methods. The axiom that 'each hour of interviewing results in eight hours of analysis' is not the exaggeration it initially appears to be.

Surgeons should not be seduced into thinking that a qualitative research project of 'only' a small number of participants (compared to quantitative research projects) is an invitation to expand the scope of the research.

### 31.4.3 Ethical Aspects

Ethics in education research differs from ethics in clinical research in significant ways. For example, the material risks in a clinical trial are often physical (treatment side effects, operative complications, death), while the risks in education research are more likely to be psychological (though of no lesser severity). Another example is that the relation between the surgeon and the patient in a clinical trial entails a fiduciary responsibility, which tends to mitigate the power imbalance in the relationship, but there may not be the same responsibility between a surgeon and a participant in an education research trial. Given the traditional hierarchy within surgery, any surgeon who wishes to involve junior colleagues, trainees, or medical students as research participants needs to pay careful attention to the ethical implications of a perceived power imbalance.

One particular ethical problem is that behaviours which are problematic to educationalists, such as bullying and discrimination, are prevalent and may persist in surgery because they are imbued with some utility by surgeons and trainees [11, 12]. The surgeon may face a personal ethical dilemma when their educational self tries to assess the 'harm' in such behaviours at the same time that their surgical self ascribes 'benefit'. Surgeons should be aware of the same dilemma in the potential audience for the results of such research. Education research which examines surgical culture needs to be undertaken with sensitivity towards the meanings ascribed to such behaviours (while still recognising the behaviours as being less than ideal) if the conclusions of the research are not to engender resistance by being perceived as an attack on surgical culture itself.

A final practical consideration is that education research often falls under a different department or institution to clinical research. Surgeons must allocate sufficient time to navigate an unfamiliar ethical process with different application portals, documentation requirements, key contact persons, and timeframes from those which they customarily use for clinical research.

### 31.4.4 Finding Balance: Being 'Far Enough In' and 'Far Enough Out'

Surgical culture is mediated by shared knowledge, language, symbols, and actions. These can be highly idiosyncratic, sometimes specific to small subspecialties and geographical locations or within a particular craft group. Surgeons who choose to research a topic arising from their own practice will usually enjoy being 'far enough in' to understand the relevant pithy sayings, contextual clues, and hidden meanings which may arise during data collection. This may be particularly important in a real-time setting such as interviews and focus groups, where the direction of questioning relies on the ability to simultaneously 'read' the emerging data.

Surgeons may find that they are not 'far enough in' where the research design requires data collection from participants in other specialties or groups, or where there is a difference in seniority (such as a senior surgeon interviewing residents). It may be necessary to specifically recruit research collaborators who have the relevant knowledge or group membership.

There is, however, a tension between being 'far enough in' while simultaneously being 'far enough out' to be able to see and problematize themes arising from data. Surgeons may find that the surgical world is so familiar to them that they are relatively blind to phenomena which are apparent to others. Awareness of personal stance, collaboration with a diverse research team, triangulation of themes between research team members, and the conscious use of different theories as lenses to view data are strategies which can help the surgeon researcher to position themselves 'far enough out'.

### *31.4.5 Time Management with Surgical Practice*

Much has been made of the difficult 'work-life balance' in surgery, and 'work-research balance' can pose the same challenges. While data collection in clinical research is often built into workflow of providing clinical care, the data collection in educational research is often separate. Even when research design allows for data collection within the daily workflow, qualitative data analysis in particular demands sufficient time outside of 'work' – not only for the time to read, re-read, discuss, and ponder the emerging themes but also because it takes time for the cognitive processes that lead to proper data formulation and the emergence of theory.

Recognising that there is great diversity amongst surgeons, it would be presumptuous to offer any advice about how to best manage the many competing demands on a surgeon's time. However it is worth noting that delays during data analysis due to workload can be a 'cloud with a silver lining', because the time spent thinking (or fretting) about the education research data within the context of ongoing work can bring new insights, as can the revisiting of data after a short absence at work. The important thing is not to become discouraged, and to recognise that the quality of research output is very much about the process, which takes time.

## 31.5 Conclusion

Surgeons bring specific 'surgical' perspectives which need to be taken into account when they undertake education research. Some arise because of the differences between the disciplines of surgery and education, others arise because surgeons are more familiar with the conventions of clinical biomedical research, and still others arise from the limitations imposed by the fact of being surgeons, particularly with regard to time management. By describing surgeon perspectives, it is hoped that readers will be able to anticipate issues and more easily enjoy the rewards of undertaking surgical education research.

## References

1. Fry, H., & Kneebone, R. (Eds.). (2011). *Surgical education: Theorising an emerging domain.* London: Springer.
2. Bharathan, R., Vali, S., Setchell, T., Miskry, T., Darzi, A., & Aggarwal, R. (2013). Psychomotor skills and cognitive load training on a virtual reality laparoscopic simulator for tubal surgery is effective. *European Journal of Obstetrics, Gynecology, and Reproductive Biology, 16*(2), 347–352. https://doi.org/10.1016/j.ejogrb.2013.03.017.
3. Hill, E., & Vaughan, S. (2013). The only girl in the room: How paradigmatic trajectories deter female students from surgical careers. *Medical Education, 47,* 547–556. https://doi.org/10.1111/medu.12134.
4. National Health and Medical Research Council. (2000). *How to review the evidence: Systematic identification and review of the scientific literature.* Canberra: Commonwealth of Australia.
5. Gifford E, Galante J, Kaji AH, et al. Factors associated with general surgery residents' desire to leave residency programs: A multi-institutional study. *JAMA Surg* 2014;149: 948–53. doi: 10.1001/jamasurg.2014.935
6. Khoushhal Z, Hussain MA, Greco E; Mamdani M, Verma S, Rotstein O et al. Prevalence and causes of attrition among surgical residents: a systematic review and meta-analysis. *JAMA Surg* 2017;152:265–272. doi: 10.1001/jamasurg.2016.4086
7. Arora, S., Sevdalis, N., Suliman, I., Athanasiou, T., Kneebone, R., & Darzi, A. (2009). *American Journal of Surgery, 198,* 726–732. https://doi.org/10.1016/j.amjsurg.2009.01.015.
8. Dickinson, I., Watters, D., Graham, I., Montgomery, P., & Collins, J. (2009). Guide to the assessment of competence and performance in practising surgeons. *ANZ Journal of Surgery, 79,* 198–204. https://doi.org/10.1111/j.1445-2197.2008.04839.x.
9. The University of Melbourne. Graduate programs in surgical education. https://www.surgeons.org/media/20261799/gp_surgical_education_2014_final.pdf. Accessed 10 Aug 2016.
10. Collins, J. P., & Gough, I. R. (2010). An academy of surgical educators: Sustaining education- enhancing innovation and scholarship. *ANZ Journal of Surgery, 80,* 13–17. https://doi.org/10.1111/j.1445-2197.2009.05170.x.
11. Crebbin, W., Campbell, G., Hillis, D. A., & Watters, D. A. (2015). Prevalence of bullying, discrimination and sexual harassment in surgery in Australasia. *ANZ Journal of Surgery, 85,* 905–909. https://doi.org/10.1111/ans.13363.
12. Musselman, L. J., MacRae, H. M., Reznick, R. K., & Lingard, L. A. (2005). 'You learn better under the gun': Intimidation and harassment in surgical education. *Medical Education, 39,* 926–934. https://doi.org/10.1111/j.1365-2929.2005.02247.x.

# Chapter 32
# From Dense Fog to Gentle Mist: Getting Started in Surgical Education Research

**Deb Colville and Catherine Green**

**Overview** Understanding and conducting surgical education research can be difficult for the beginner. The idea that prompted this chapter is that it is useful to break down some initially opaque concepts into steps. In this chapter, the reader is taken on a journey that provides an explanation of some signposts for the novice qualitative surgical researcher. These include scoping a broad list of "burning questions" down to asking a potentially answerable question and choosing a research paradigm that aligns with researcher perspective and the research setting. Some visual tools to aid the research process are presented.

## 32.1 Introduction

An increased focus on the generation of robust research in medical and surgical education has led to rapid change in the professionalization in this field [1, 2]. For the researcher, getting started in surgical education research may be simultaneously exciting and daunting. Many surgical educators are well trained in the operational aspects of education and training, but may need guidance and mentorship to develop their research skills [3]. As members of the surgical profession, they are usually familiar with research conducted using a positivist paradigm, but may only just be getting to grips with theories, concepts, and paradigms found in the social sciences and education literature that they have may not encountered previously, at the same time as embarking on research in this field.

---

D. Colville (✉)
Ophthalmology, Eye and Ear Hospital, Faculty of Medicine, Dentistry and Health Sciences, The University of Melbourne, Melbourne, Australia

Department of Ophthalmology, Royal Children's Hospital, Melbourne, Australia
e-mail: colville@unimelb.edu.au

C. Green
Royal Australian and New Zealand College of Ophthalmologists, Surry Hills, Australia

Royal Victorian Eye and Ear Hospital, East Melbourne, Australia

© Springer Nature Singapore Pte Ltd. 2019
D. Nestel et al. (eds.), *Advancing Surgical Education*, Innovation and Change in Professional Education 17, https://doi.org/10.1007/978-981-13-3128-2_32

The authors of this chapter are both experienced practicing ophthalmic surgeons. DC has a PhD in ophthalmic surgical education, a qualitative study of the apprenticeship nature of Australasian ophthalmology education. CG is completing a Master of Surgical Education, including a research project in in ophthalmic workplace-based assessment.

In his paper, Total Internal Reflection, Kneebone (2002) describes his experiences of moving beyond a positivist paradigm, entering this previously unexplored territory, and the challenges he encountered grappling with a new literature with unfamiliar language [4].

His experience is echoed by a novice researcher, who comments:

> *I read Kneebone's 'Total Internal Reflection' at the beginning of my course: I thought: how hard can it be? But it was more difficult than I thought: I didn't believe it at first! Now I affirm Kneebone: surgical education research is about unfamiliar ways of thinking, leading to a personal transformation. After three days of writing in "Education Land", when I go back to real life (in surgical practice), I feel as though I come back from a different country, where the pace, the words the thinking and the people are all different.. CG*

The experience of a surgeon embarking for the first time on education research could also be likened to being in thick fog, with the road ahead seemingly opaque without any identifiable landmarks. In this chapter, we hope to provide signposts that will allow the fog to lift to a gentle mist of unexplored territory open for discovery. We write for surgeons getting started in surgical education research.

## 32.1.1 Prepare for the Journey

While most people conducting surgical education scholarship are experienced professionals, many with advanced degrees, some additional preparation for the different demands of education research may be required. Training in research design, survey development, program evaluation, and statistical analysis is useful [5]. Enrolling in a postgraduate program (e.g., Graduate Certificate, Graduate Diploma, and/or Masters of Medical or Surgical Education) and attending workshops and conferences (e.g., the Association for Medical Education in Europe (AMEE), the Ottawa Conference, the Association of American Medical Colleges (AAMC), the Asia-Pacific Medical Conference, and, in Australia and New Zealand, ANZAHPE) present opportunities to expand your own knowledge and understanding and also to develop a network of potential supervisors, mentors, and collaborators.

When embarking on any research project that is curiosity-led, a list of priorities in relation to current knowledge gaps, in combination with evaluating personal strengths and areas for self- development, will provide fertile motivation for sustained attention to a surgical educational project.

At the start of a research project, Smith et al. (2002) describe the "Research Spider" [6], a method of measuring one's current education research skills while identifying gaps that may need to be filled, either before, or through, the project:

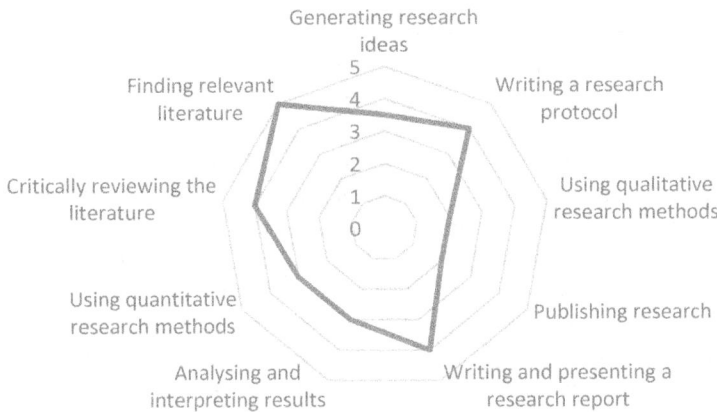

**Fig. 32.1** The "Research Spider": preparing to explore your skill strengths and gaps with your peers, supervisor or mentor

> *Using this tool, I identified knowledge gaps in several areas, allowing me to develop strategies for addressing deficiencies/weaknesses. Use of the tool also gave me the opportunity to acknowledge areas of strength and to reflect on my progress in developing surgical education research skills.* CG

An example of the Research Spider comprises Fig. 32.1. For instance, based on her prior biomedical research experience, a researcher self-reported her need for skills acquisition in quantitative research methods as merely two. By contrast, she then self-rated as five her need for skills in the topics new to her, such as finding the relevant surgical education literature. She also self-rated her own learning needs as quite high, four, in critically using qualitative methods.

Such a Research Spider diagram can be a useful visual prompt for a discussion of strategies that will better equip you. The Research Spider provides a visual prompt to explore the elements of the spider's web with a mentor or supervisor, to enable you to embark more effectively on a surgical research project. The spider arrangement leaves room too for you or your mentor to insert self-ratings of some other skills that either might want to discuss. Those not considered relevant can simply be deleted from the diagram.

You should read widely to develop ideas for research questions and strengthen familiarity with the concepts, language, and protocols of education research. There are myriad medical and surgical education journals, each with slightly different foci and emphases. The *Journal of Surgical Education* offers an accessible portal into the literature, as many of the articles are framed in a format familiar to biomedical researchers, using quantitative methodology aligned with a positivist paradigm. Other journals, such as *Academic Medicine*, *Advances in Health Sciences Education*, *Medical Education*, *Medical Teacher*, and *The Clinical Teacher*, offer a wider range of perspectives and an introduction to qualitative and mixed-methods research.

## 32.1.2 Identify a Mentor or Supervisor

For the researcher, having support and guidance is critically important. The invaluable role a mentor can play includes guiding the researcher in obtaining the correct training, asking the right questions, designing a project to yield defensible results, sharing results with others, and establishing connections in the field [5]. Mentors may also offer opportunities for discussing career development, political and cultural navigation strategies, and more personal matters too such as balancing work and family life, dealing with difficult colleagues, etc. [7].

The choice of supervisor/mentor will be determined by the purpose of the arrangement, the professional needs of both supervisor and researcher, and a compatible approach [8]. It may be helpful to have several mentors, each meeting a specific need. Explicit conversations about expectations and finding alignment will ensure a successful mentor-mentee relationship [7]. You may wish to clarify such assumptions with your supervisor early on in your project:

> As a researcher, embarking on a Masters research project, I had intended to explore the topic using qualitative research. Unexpectedly, my supervisor was firmly planted in a positivist paradigm and I found my project morphing to a quantitative project. DC

## 32.1.3 Ask an Answerable (and Important) Question

The goal of education research is to create new knowledge. When framing a research question, it is important that the topic chosen is of interest to you; it is very difficult to maintain the momentum to complete a project without this. A useful technique for brainstorming ideas is to write down all your many possible areas of research interest. Next, turn the "curiosity" items on this "burning problems" list into some answerable research questions. In qualitative research, each question needs to be converted in due course into exploratory questions, rather than wording that signifies that there is to be a single "right" answer. Making them into open questions is often the next task. For example, "how do surgical trainees learn their surgical craft in the theater setting?"

Your list of main and subsidiary questions can include a methods research question, as well as the substantive question. For instance, a methods question might be "in what ways can qualitative methods be used to generate new knowledge about ophthalmic training?" where the main substantive question might be 'how do ophthalmic surgical trainees learn their craft?'

The next step is to generate some of your ideas about your solution to the problem. Often these seem sweeping or very general. The advantage of this approach is that your own experience drives your research, and you will learn more about your own conceptualization of the problem. This is called using the "researcher as instrument" during several iterations of research data collection. You will (inadvertently at times) refine your statement of what the problem is via your reflections on the data. Puzzling over why this problem exists, why the solution might seem obvious to you, yet at the same time has not already been solved, is a useful way to proceed with a research project. It is also useful to brainstorm with a colleague or expert in the field you plan to research. DC reflects on this process:

> *I observed that the ophthalmic tradition of apprenticeship posed difficulties for ophthalmic surgical educators in incorporating two historical developments into its current curriculum form, and curriculum practices. These two developments comprised firstly the changing composition of the ophthalmic profession, including older, graduate entry medical practitioners, and a higher portion of women doctors, within Australia's diverse medical practitioner composition. Secondly, the developing recognition of the vital role of chronic, as distinct from acute or single disease approaches to improve medical practice posed a problem to the apprenticeship form of training. The research puzzle I found myself with was to define the underpinning educational basis of the current curriculum, its form, in the light of these two developing challenges to ophthalmic education. From this basis, I developed my PhD research proposal. DC*

### 32.1.4  Review the Literature

The next step is to investigate what is already known on the topic through a diligent literature review, as outlined in Chap. 33 – Reviewing Literature for and as Research. This will identify whether the answer is already known and help to refine additional aspects that could potentially be explored. When conducting the literature review, you should consider what paradigm would be most suited to the research question. Consider the ontology and epistemology relating to this topic (see Chap. 30 – Research in Surgical Education: An Orientation), as this will illuminate the relevant paradigm and provide clues to the ideal methodology for the research question [9]. The result of the literature review should be your own list of the key concepts that others have defined as the main ideas about solving your research puzzle. Read these critically, and identify what disparities or logical inconsistencies form the basis for arguing the place for your own research. Highlighting and quantifying the gap in understanding will demonstrate how answering your question will advance the field, help frame your research question, and define the scope of the study.

While conducting your literature review, it is helpful to ask questions that enable improvements and application in new contexts. Cook (2010) recommends classifying education questions or studies into three groups: description, clarification, and justification [5]. Rather than simply describing, clarification studies go further by helping explain why or how things work and how to make them better. It is observed that clarification studies are uncommon in medical education: an appeal has been made for education scholars to reflect on the purpose of inquiry and the research questions we ask and to strive to ask more clarification questions [10].

If you read with an open mind, you will find many useful precedents for your research outside medical literature. Keep in mind Kneebone's metaphor of total internal reflection. This refers to the "blindness" that the biomedical literature has adopted toward counting qualitative understandings of surgical healthcare as "real."

The contribution that social sciences can make has been neglected in surgical practice, and yet education itself and hence surgical education are social sciences.

It is as if we, as surgeons, view the outside world not with benefit of the light of day but rather from the bottom of a pond. Optically, light from the floor of the pond is reflected to the bottom of the pond from the interface of air with the water's surface. We have difficulty seeing the outside "real" world above the depth of a pond: we as surgeons are positioned "underwater," and we take our stand as surgeons from there. An example might be that surgeons have largely been blind to the extensive field of linguistics and rhetoric, which has much to offer us in understanding the exchanges between surgeons and surgical team in an operating theater [11].

### 32.1.5  Refine Your Research Question

Having completed this process, it is important now to write your research question clearly. This can interchangeably take the form of a research hypothesis or study goals and purpose. The question should be "FINER" – feasible, interesting (to you and others), novel, ethical, and relevant to practice [5].

An alternative approach is to use Swales' "Creating a Research Space (CARS)" model of research introductions [12]. Although described in the context of writing a research paper, it is also relevant in the planning stage. The model involves three steps:

1. *Establishing a territory*: set the context for the research, providing necessary background for the topic. This involves placing the research in the context of what is and is not known.
2. *Establishing a niche*: outline the open "niche" in existing research, and outline how the research will fill this.
3. *Occupying a niche*: turn the niche in step 2 into the research space that will be filled, demonstrating how the gap identified will be filled, answering questions asked, and continuing a research tradition.

Figure 32.2 shows a way of representing your project as a research space diagram [21].

### 32.1.6  Scope Your Project

The next task is to scope your project. It is advisable to "start small and grow" [5]. This allows you to develop skills in a sustainable way, be able to measure tangible progress, and gain a sense of achievement as projects are completed.

For smaller projects, only one or two quite specific research questions are feasible, whereas larger projects tend to have a main and some subsidiary questions. A process of devising a series of sub-studies that match a list of subsidiary questions is the often the rule for the projects with a larger scope.

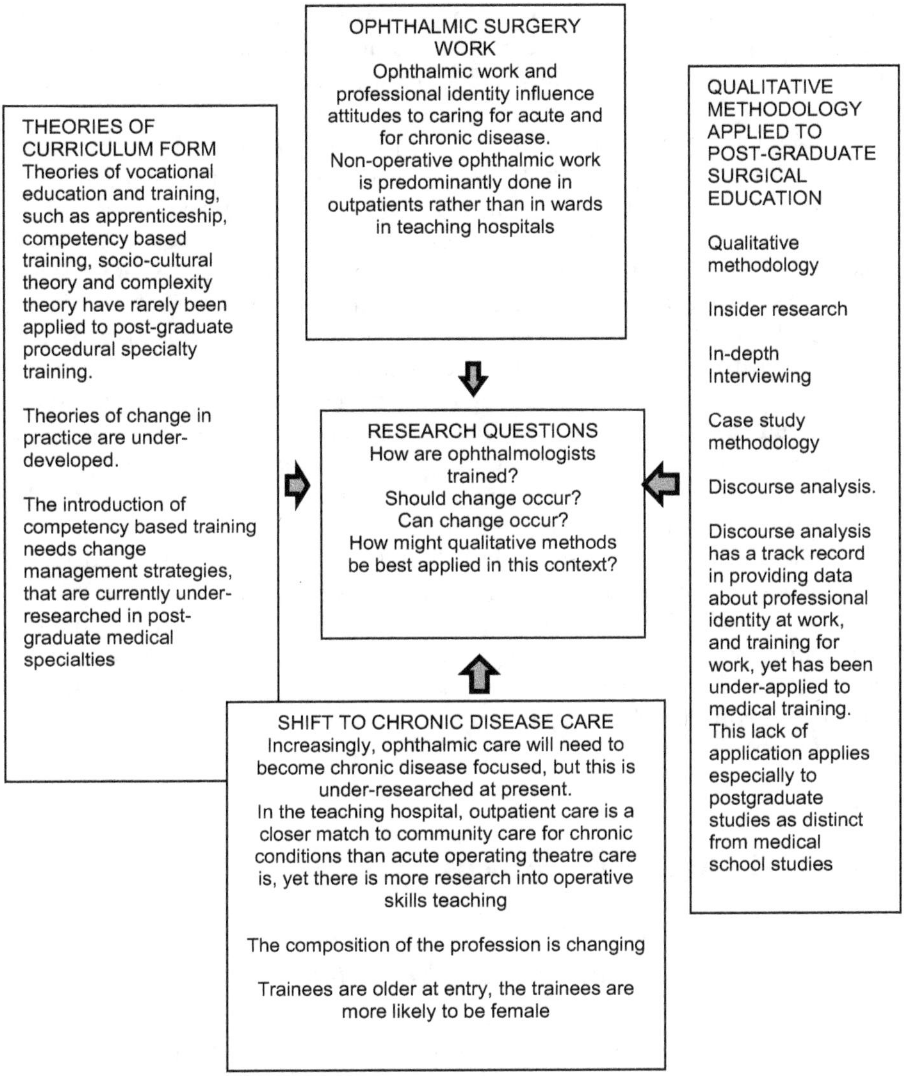

## OPHTHALMIC SURGERY WORK

Ophthalmic work and professional identity influence attitudes to caring for acute and for chronic disease.

Non-operative ophthalmic work is predominantly done in outpatients rather than in wards in teaching hospitals

## THEORIES OF CURRICULUM FORM

Theories of vocational education and training, such as apprenticeship, competency based training, socio-cultural theory and complexity theory have rarely been applied to post-graduate procedural specialty training.

Theories of change in practice are under-developed.

The introduction of competency based training needs change management strategies, that are currently under-researched in post-graduate medical specialties

## RESEARCH QUESTIONS

How are ophthalmologists trained?
Should change occur?
Can change occur?
How might qualitative methods be best applied in this context?

## QUALITATIVE METHODOLOGY APPLIED TO POST-GRADUATE SURGICAL EDUCATION

Qualitative methodology

Insider research

In-depth Interviewing

Case study methodology

Discourse analysis.

Discourse analysis has a track record in providing data about professional identity at work, and training for work, yet has been under-applied to medical training. This lack of application applies especially to postgraduate studies as distinct from medical school studies

## SHIFT TO CHRONIC DISEASE CARE

Increasingly, ophthalmic care will need to become chronic disease focused, but this is under-researched at present.
In the teaching hospital, outpatient care is a closer match to community care for chronic conditions than acute operating theatre care is, yet there is more research into operative skills teaching

The composition of the profession is changing

Trainees are older at entry, the trainees are more likely to be female

**Fig. 32.2** The research space diagram: an evolving visual representation of the research space (Swales) can be used to represent and refine the key pillars of the research project

The feasibility of a project includes factors such as the time allowed for the project, the funding, the numbers of surgeons and trainees accessible for the research, and the ethical considerations, such as equity, including traditionally under-included participants in surgical education research.

Funding and institutional support are required. It is acknowledged that funding for educational research can be difficult to source and secure [13]. This should not dissuade you from trying. Blanco and Lee [13] provide a comprehensive summary of how to optimize opportunities for obtaining funding. Their tips include identifying funding agencies and resources, getting to know the funding agency, and submitting clearly written, detailed grant proposals according to the instructions provided.

It is useful to jot down your "idealized" project, as above, and then "operationalize" the project according to all the feasibility factors that you can identify. Often this involves stating what would be ideal, naming the feasibility issues, and balancing all the mitigating factors to make the best compromise. The process of stating these feasibility issues can be assisted by a diagrammatic representation of your project.

Limiting a project to make it doable requires a mindset that is sometimes difficult to master. The challenge is to convert your eagerness to solve a large problem into effort expended toward solving a small but significant aspect of the overall problem. This may be unfamiliar to those unused to conducting research, and this is particularly difficult while at the same time training oneself in a social science paradigm. The process involves a shift in ambition: discarding any notion of entirely solving a big problem within the scope of a small project. This process of shedding for the sake of intellectual clarity is tough emotional work for many surgeons. To make such a change in thinking goes against the tide: clinicians are trained toward a global, action-oriented view, and a sense of loss may be experienced.

Scoping includes stakeholder identification. This leads you to explicitly consider the potential impact of your research project on stakeholders. This forms part of the introduction to, and scoping of, your project report. Later the discussion section of your report will list the potential implications of your research project to stakeholders.

## 32.2 Methodology and Methods

### 32.2.1 Methodology: Adopt a Social Science Paradigm, and State the Researcher Perspective

Methodology is the strategic approach to answer the research question and to gain knowledge; it is essentially the research design [9]. Having framed and refined the research question, the next step is to determine which methodology will be most suited to answering the question (see Chaps. 30, 32, 33, and 34).

In adopting a social science paradigm, it is customary in education research to identify your own perspective and background. This flies in the face of traditional surgical research, which in the guise of unproblematic scientific "hypothesis testing," adopts what social scientists identify as a pretense of scientific objectivity, whereby the researcher's own identities are deemed irrelevant and hence undeclared. Developing the skills of generating and presenting an up-front statement of one's own background and methodological position, the process of "reflexivity," can sometimes be the most difficult transition to make in becoming a qualitative surgical education researcher. However, when a surgeon uses the technique of "researcher as instrument," this is a very powerful research paradigm for surgical education "hypothesis generation."

### 32.2.2 Obtain Human Research Ethics Board Approval

The National Health and Medical Research Council of Australia describes four ethical pillars: research integrity, beneficence, justice, and consent [14]. Peer-reviewed publication of surgical education research usually requires evidence of a formal ethics approval process. Since educational programs are an institution-wide affair, often an institutional letter of support is expected. All relevant stakeholders should be identified in the research ethics proposal. Samples of interview schedules should be appended. For Australian and New Zealand postgraduate medical colleges, the ethical issues involved in transnational privacy need to be acknowledged. Ethics committees more accustomed to evaluating biomedical research projects may be less familiar with the issues pertaining to qualitative research, for example, the ethical debates around interview techniques, and the researcher may need to highlight these to ensure appropriate ethical approval is provided. A critical examination of distinctions between surgical education research and regular audit data around teaching hospital clinical activities may need to be outlined (see Chap. 36 – *Ethical Issues in Surgical Education Research*).

Patient safety should be an extremely high priority for surgical educators. Surgical research ethical issues are "high stakes," since surgical education research involves human participation, and high stakes healthcare in vulnerable populations of sick or potentially sick individuals. Despite being highly trained doctors, research participants may nonetheless find themselves in an hierarchical teaching environment, in which patronage may often be the basis for ongoing approval for either continuation of training, or professional approval where scrutiny is already high. Female trainees may find themselves in double ethical jeopardy as both trainees and females in a male-dominated profession [15]. Gender issues apply as both researcher and as participant. Females leading surgical education research challenge the notion that they are less traditionally understood as prime generators of surgical knowledge in many cultures around the world [16]. Female participants may be inadvertently but still unjustly excluded since they tend to be treated in a disprivileged way in the culture of surgery at large [17].

### 32.2.3 Research Methods

The choice of methods useful to surgical education research is vast. Examples of qualitative methods are focus groups, semi-structured in-depth individual interviews, observations, visual methodologies, and qualitative survey research. For recruitment, posters, flyers, advertisements, and emails to membership lists are some options for recruitment tools. Often institutional support is necessary to do this. Research recruitment can be at arm's length to insider researchers in the profession of surgery. Recruitment techniques should ensure subjects are able to consent freely to participate.

## 32.3 Write

### 32.3.1 Write Your Proposal and Develop a Project Plan

Writing a research proposal will include all the steps discussed above. Diagrammatic representations of your project framework are helpful in ensuring you have considered all relevant components.

A worked example of aligning the elements of methodology, research question, and methods is shown as in Fig. 32.3 [21]. The logic of the project can also be usefully laid out using a phase diagram such as in Fig. 32.4 [21].

A critical part of the planning process is to develop a detailed project plan with anticipated timelines. This will ensure that the project is feasible and able to be performed within a realistic timeframe. The development of a Gantt chart or similar project-planning tool is extremely helpful in listing the various stages of the project, identifying stakeholders, and committing to achievable timeframes. If it becomes

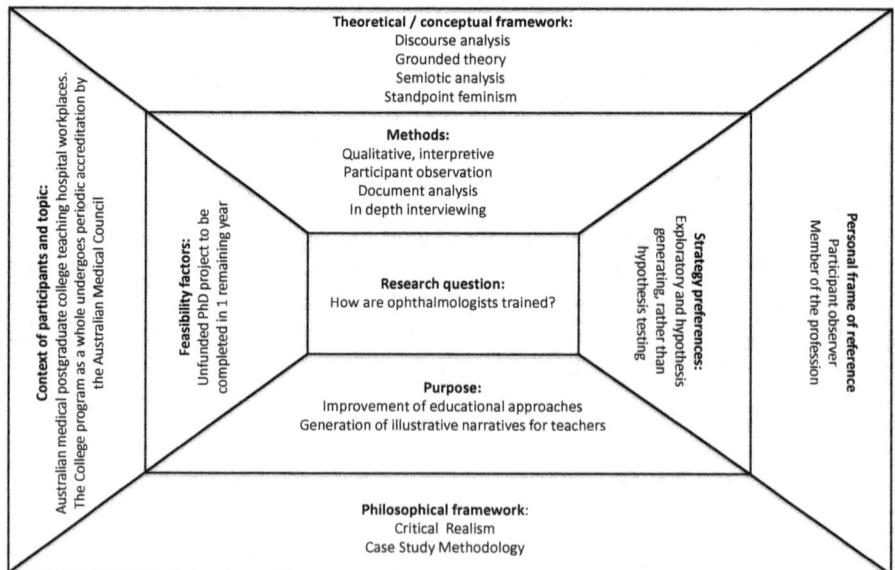

**Fig. 32.3** Framing research questions (frameworks dimensions). (Adapted from [8, 21 22, 23, 24]

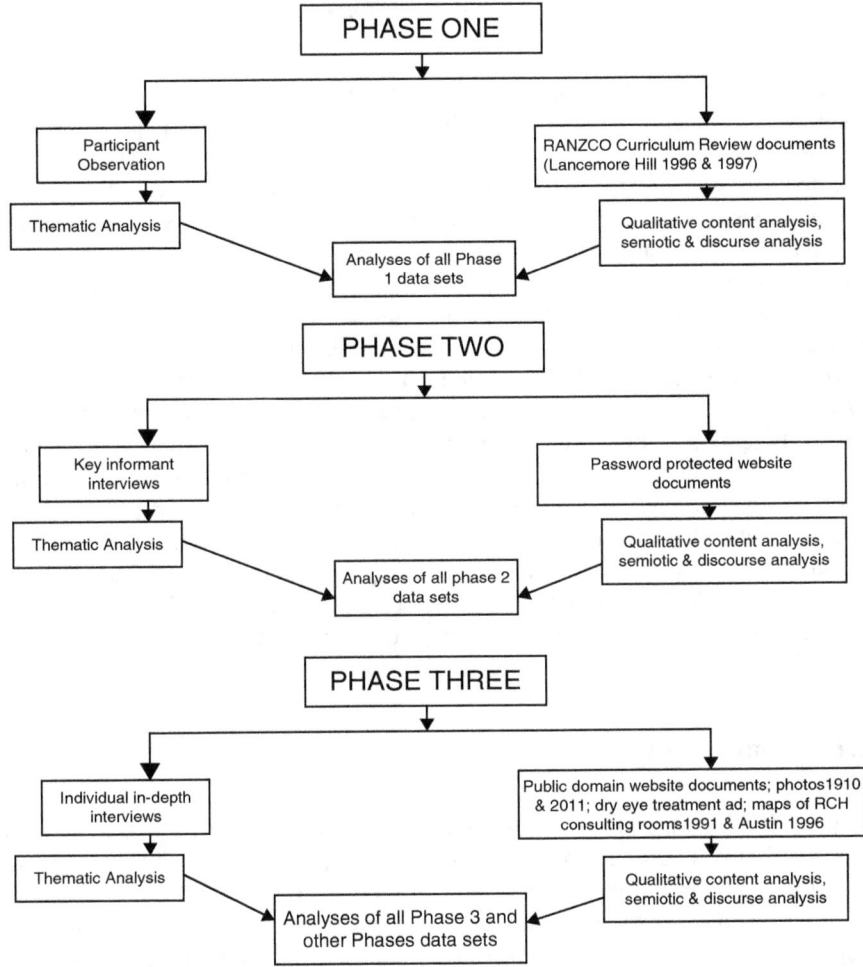

**Fig. 32.4** Phase diagram of a more complex surgical education research project. This demonstrates an iterative process that includes initial participant observation and later individual in-depth interviews

apparent that the project is too ambitious, either in terms of scope or timelines, this is the opportunity to review your approach. The project plan should, at a minimum, provide for time allocation for the literature review, planning for methodology and methods, development of research tools, recruitment, data collection, data analysis, application for ethics approval, writing up, and planning for dissemination of results, including publication.

## 32.3.2  Write Up and Disseminate Results

Academic report writing is a new and sometimes difficult genre for aspiring surgical education researchers. Follow expert advice on writing for publication in medical education [12, 18–20]. It is advisable to start writing your manuscript early [3]. It is possible to start writing the paper before data collection is complete, especially the literature review, methodology, and methods. The representations you may use can be narrative or pictorial. A project mind map is also useful tool that provides a clear framework of your project.

Learning how to argue a case is a skill required to effectively conduct and disseminate your research. The "CARS" framework, discussed earlier, provides a useful approach to planning [12]. Translating your research report from an insider to an outsider audience can be challenging. Insider and outsider research are both useful ways to disseminate your research findings. Expect (and relish) that your identity will inexorably alter: the transition from your insider role as a surgeon to becoming a surgical education researcher will inexorably alter you. It can be difficult to convince surgical colleagues who are firmly entrenched in a positivist paradigm of the value and validity of your research. Depending on your dissemination plan, you may need to decide if you wish your research to be more readable to surgeons, in the first instance, or more readable to non-surgeon education academics or others.

## 32.4  Conclusion

The journey from surgeon to surgical education researcher may seem daunting at the outset, but it is both rewarding and transforming. There are many steps in conducting your research project. This starts with a list of your research interests and narrows to a small doable project. Consideration of research paradigm, researcher perspective, and identifying a list of stakeholders is important. The research methods available are wide. Writing your proposal requires a method that matches your paradigm.

Publication of high-quality research strengthens the argument for funding and resourcing education research. Surgical training that is based on sound education research will result in better surgeons; safer, more efficient, and cost-effective training; better surgical educators; financial savings; and ultimately, better health outcomes for patients.

## References

1. Davis, M. H., & Ponnamperuma, G. G. (2006). Medical education research at the crossroads. *Lancet, 367*(9508), 377–378.
2. Gill, D., Griffin, A., Woolf, K., & Cave, J. (2009). Twelve tips for studying medical education at doctoral level. *Medical Teacher, 31*(7), 601–604.

3. Markert, R. J. (2010). Getting started on your research: Practical advice for medical educators. *Teaching and Learning in Medicine, 22*(4), 317–318.
4. Kneebone, R. (2002). Total internal reflection: An essay on paradigms. *Medical Education, 36*(6), 514–518.
5. Cook, D. A. (2010). Getting started in medical education scholarship. *The Keio Journal of Medicine, 59*(3), 96–103.
6. Smith, H., Wright, D., Morgan, S., Dunleavey, J., & Moore, M. (2002). The 'research spider': A simple method of assessing research experience. *Primary Health Care Research & Development, 3*(3), 139–140.
7. Cristancho, S., & Varpio, L. (2016). Twelve tips for early career medical educators. *Medical Teacher, 38*(4), 358–363.
8. Siddiqui, Z. S., & Jonas-Dwyer, D. R. (2012). Twelve tips for supervising research students. *Medical Teacher, 34*(7), 530–533.
9. Bergman, E., de Feijter, J., Frambach, J., Godefrooij, M., Slootweg, I., Stalmeijer, R., et al. (2012). AM last page: A guide to research paradigms relevant to medical education. *Academic Medicine: Journal of the Association of American Medical Colleges, 87*(4), 545.
10. Cook, D. A., Bordage, G., & Schmidt, H. G. (2008). Description, justification and clarification: A framework for classifying the purposes of research in medical education. *Medical Education, 42*(2), 128–133.
11. Lingard, L., Reznick, R., Espin, S., Regehr, G., & DeVito, I. (2002). Team communications in the operating room: Talk patterns, sites of tension, and implications for novices. *Academic Medicine: Journal of the Association of American Medical Colleges, 77*(3), 232–237.
12. Swales, J., & Feak, C. B. (2004). *Academic writing for graduate students: Essential skills and tasks* (2nd ed.). Ann Arbor: University of Michigan Press.
13. Blanco, M. A., & Lee, M. Y. (2012). Twelve tips for writing educational research grant proposals. *Medical Teacher, 34*(6), 450–453.
14. National Health and Medical Research Council. Health and research ethics 2015 [cited 2016 31 October]. Available from: https://www.nhmrc.gov.au/health-ethics
15. Hill, E., & Vaughan, S. (2013). The only girl in the room: How paradigmatic trajectories deter female students from surgical careers. *Medical Education, 47*(6), 547–556.
16. Franco-Cardenas, V., Rosenberg, J., Ramirez, A., Lin, J., & Tsui, I. (2015). Decadelong profile of women in ophthalmic publications. *JAMA Ophthalmology, 133*(3), 255–259.
17. Parle, G., & Parle, J. (2015). Summary report: Expert Advisory Group advising the Royal Australasian College of Surgeons. Discrimination, bullying and sexual harassment prevalence survey.
18. Bordage, G. (2001). Reasons reviewers reject and accept manuscripts: The strengths and weaknesses in medical education reports. *Academic Medicine: Journal of the Association of American Medical Colleges, 76*(9), 889–896.
19. Lingard, L. (2015). Joining a conversation: The problem/gap/hook heuristic. *Perspectives on Medical Education, 4*(5), 252–253.
20. Ramani, S., & Mann, K. (2016). Introducing medical educators to qualitative study design: Twelve tips from inception to completion. *Medical Teacher, 38*(5), 456–463.
21. Colville, D. J. (2011). 'We need you to be able to do this operation': Continuity and contradiction in the training of ophthalmologists. Monash University http://arrow.monash.edu.au/hdl/1959.1/530686
22. Higgs, J. (1988). Structuring Qualtiative research theses. In J. Higgs (Ed.), *Writing qualitative research* (pp. 137–150). Sydney: Hambden Press.
23. Byrne-Armstron, H., Higgs, J., & Horsfall, D. (Eds.). (2001). *Critical moments in qualitative research*. Oxford: Butterworth Heinemann. (Diagram is page 61).
24. Higgs, J. (Ed.). (1988). *Writing qualitative research* (pp. 137–150). Sydney: Hambden Press.

# Chapter 33
# Reviewing Literature for and as Research

**Nigel D'Souza and Geoff Wong**

**Overview** The literature review has become an important tool to summarise and synthesise knowledge from the growing volume of research in medical education. The diversity of literature review methodologies has proliferated to an extent that can appear bewildering, particularly within qualitative and mixed methods approaches, some of which originate from non-medical disciplines. Matching the appropriate review technique to the research question(s) will determine its success. This chapter describes the breadth of quantitative, qualitative and mixed methods review techniques which may be used in educational research and looks at their strengths and weaknesses. Case scenarios are used to illustrate how specific review techniques can be used to address different research questions. Common essential steps to conducting a literature review, regardless of review technique, are described to provide some practical guidance.

## 33.1 Why Search

The literature review has become ubiquitous in all realms of medical literature including clinical medicine and medical education. It is commonly carried out to establish the background of a primary study or as a review to consolidate knowledge from primary studies. Many research studies have performed a literature review to establish that the study is useful by:

- Identifying gaps in the literature that show the study is novel, timely or relevant
- Contrasting results that highlight the controversy of the study's findings
- Establishing that it builds on previous results (including inconsistencies) to advance the scientific method by following a line of inquiry

---

N. D'Souza (✉)
Wessex Deanery, Winchester, United Kingdom

G. Wong
Nuffield Department of Primary Care Health Sciences, Oxford, UK
e-mail: geoffrey.wong@phc.ox.ac.uk

A literature review can become a study in its own right when performed to synthesise evidence. The research question should govern the choice of review methodology.

## 33.2 Which Search Technique

A wide variety of review techniques exist that may evaluate data that is solely quantitative, quantitative and qualitative, or solely qualitative. It may be challenging to choose the appropriate literature search technique with over 25 described [1].

> *The following example illustrates the methodological options available. Ali is a trainee starting a fellowship in robotic colorectal surgery. After a meeting with his supervisor, they come up with the following research questions to study:*
>
> *Research question 1: To what degree does operative experience with robotic colorectal surgery influence operative outcomes?*
> *Research question 2: What factors influence a patient to elect for a robotic approach over a laparoscopic or open one in colorectal surgery?*
> *Research question 3: How might training techniques be incorporated into a robotic training programme in order to optimise trainee progress?*

The above three research questions focus on examining different types of data sets, and, as such, require different methodologies for review of the literature. Literature review techniques can be broadly divided into three methodologies: quantitative, qualitative and mixed methods.

### 33.2.1 Quantitative Evidence Synthesis

A quantitative approach such as a systematic review would be the optimal technique for research question 1 to compare measurable outcomes such as operative time or complications. Systematic reviews synthesise results from primary studies most commonly used to inform decision-making in evidence-based medicine.

Where the primary studies are sufficiently similar (i.e. there is homogeneity), this may involve a meta-analysis, which is a statistical aggregation of quantitative results from these studies. The most widely recognised systematic review is the Cochrane review, which has been in existence for over 20 years.

Systematic reviews are based on the **PICO** model, comparing outcomes of an intervention on two (or more) populations: one that underwent the intervention and one that did not. In our example:

- *P*opulation: patients undergoing robotic colorectal surgery
- *I*ntervention: robotic colorectal surgery performed by trainees
- *C*omparison: robotic colorectal surgery performed by consultants
- *O*utcomes: complications of surgery, operative time

If Ali chooses to investigate this question with a Cochrane review, he will find that the methodology for this technique has been operationalised in a step-by-step format published in the *Cochrane Handbook* [2]. Reporting standards have been clearly outlined in the preferred reporting items for systematic reviews and meta-analyses (PRISMA) statement [3]. Workshops, online learning [4] and postgraduate qualifications [5] are available to carry out systematic reviews. Furthermore, there is an international network of experienced Cochrane authors and statistical support available to novices embarking on their first review.

Meta-analysis is regarded by many as the highest level of medical evidence [6]. As the methodology and analysis are clearly laid out, each step is transparent and reproducible. Every included primary study undergoes assessment for risk of bias and methodological quality. Prior to publication, a Cochrane review undergoes peer review by senior editors for feedback and quality assurance.

When systematic reviews are not performed robustly, they can yield misleading information if, for example, issues such as bias or heterogeneity are not adequately or transparently reported [7]. While systematic reviews can measure heterogeneity (variance), they lack a means by which to explain it and can result in decontextualised lessons [8]. This approach is generally considered to be unable to discover or explain the causal processes underlying findings that occur under certain circumstances – that is, why outcomes occur and when (please see Quantitative and Qualitative Evidence Synthesis below for more on this).

### *33.2.2 Qualitative Evidence Synthesis*

Ali is interested in the preferences and beliefs patients have regarding robotic surgery for research question 2. He doesn't believe this question fits the PICO model and thinks a qualitative approach may be more appropriate.

Qualitative research can build understanding by describing how any why things occur. In clinical medicine, it has been defined as aiming "to identify the essential component parts of clinical phenomena" and being "especially suited to areas that have both social and clinical dimensions" [9]. Identification and description of these phenomena can then lead to an understanding on the values, perceptions and experiences of patients. There are many forms of qualitative review – up to 25 have recently been described [1] – and there is little consensus as to which approach is better than another. There are also some overlaps between the terms, assumptions and methods used: "critical interpretive synthesis, critical review, interpretive approach, interpretive synthesis, meta-interpretations" [1].

It may be challenging for a clinician to select a qualitative synthesis technique, particularly, since many are rooted in potentially unfamiliar disciplines such as philosophy, psychology or education. Without an academic background in these areas, or access to academic supervisors with expertise, clinicians may find it easier if they select a method that has been more operationalised.

For research question 2, Ali decided to utilise meta-ethnography: an approach that is "suited to conveying patients' views and experiences and informing implementation of services and interventions" [10]. Although guidelines for meta-ethnography approaches are still under development [11], Ali finds worked examples of meta-ethnography approaches [12] and guidance on appraising study quality in this technique [13].

While the review methodology is undoubtedly appropriate to answer the research question, as a newcomer to this technique, Ali has a few concerns.

The subjectivity of qualitative reviews can be both a strength or a weakness. Immersion, through reading and rereading of the literature, may enable him to gain unique insights into nuanced or subtle aspects of the research topic (or may not). The reviewer's values and interpretive skills will determine the quality of the process and insight of the review. As a result, the process is not reproducible and potentially opaque, if not reported transparently, with no clear distinction between data findings and author(s) interpretation.

For most of the qualitative evidence syntheses, the subjectivity of the process is compounded by a lack of guidance and protocols for many reviews. Since over 95% have been established since 2000 [1], these are methodologies that have not been refined, developed or disseminated like the Cochrane review. While some have been more operationalised (meta-synthesis), only 12 of the 25 methodologies (such as meta-ethnography) can be used for the entire process of literature review [14]. There is commonly no systematic appraisal of the quality of included studies, which might further diminish the reliability and plausibility of the review findings.

The use of "purposeful sampling" of studies rather than an exhaustive literature review can result in sampling error. This may lead in a failure to capture diversity and a bias towards uniformity and generalisations that may not be applicable to a wider context or broader population. However, new purposeful sampling strategies have been devised to make this process more systematic and transparent [15].

### 33.2.3 *Quantitative and Qualitative Evidence Synthesis*

For research question 3, Ali wants to investigate what training techniques can be used to optimise the development of operative skills in a robotic fellowship. Although a meta-analysis may show what outcomes can be achieved by trainees in robotic surgery, Ali is concerned it will not yield adequate information on what contextual factors in these training programmes enable good trainee outcomes.

To account for these contextual factors, he decides to employ a mixed methods review technique that integrates both qualitative and quantitative data. Options for this include realist review, narrative synthesis, integrative review or critical interpretive synthesis. These methods hope to combine the strengths of both qualitative and quantitative techniques – to address complex questions and produce evidence while accounting for context. When choosing a methodology, Ali elects to opt for a review technique that has been more operationalised with guidelines and training materials – realist review [16].

Realist review seeks to answer, "What works for whom under what contexts, how and why?" Ali hopes to find out how training affects outcomes in certain contexts and whether those lessons can be extrapolated into his own training programme. Many factors affect surgical outcomes, which may be unpacked by a realist review. Ali might find that some trainees might have better outcomes than others for reasons including:

- They have access to simulation facilities.
- They are allocated of sufficient operating time per case to train.
- They are allocated cases of appropriate complexity.
- They operate on an adequate volume of cases.
- They perform cases under the appropriate level of supervision.
- Their consultant supervisors have sufficient operative skill.
- Their consultant supervisors have sufficient teaching skill.
- There is little risk of litigation from patients following complications.

A superficial understanding may lead to a flawed interpretation of results. For example, trainees involved in a high volume of cases may have poor outcomes when further investigation reveals that these trainees only assist in these cases due to litigation risk from potential complications. Understanding context fully is key to unpacking the causal relationships that underpin realist inquiry (more details at www.ramesesproject.org).

Realist review is an emerging systematic review methodology that bridges the worlds of academic research, implementation and policy. Reporting standards and guidelines have been issued for each step to help new authors [16]. It can be particularly useful in complex interventions such as education to understand the multiple social/human components which interact to produce outcomes that are highly context dependent.

Meta-analysis may not identify or account for the complexity of the interactions between these components and context and find substantial heterogeneity. Although realist review seeks to explain the influence of context on outcomes, it acknowledges that to make a review feasible, it needs to be focused down, for example, by limiting the range of outcomes of interest, the territory covered by each review, the nature and quality of information retrieved and the extent of expected recommendations [17].

"Dilution (the progressively attenuated impact of education as filtered through other health care providers and systems)" and "failure to establish a causal link" are concerns that realist methodology is better placed to explain and address, with its careful examination of context and its influence on causal processes (i.e. something realists call *mechanisms*) [18, 19].

Immersion and interpretation of quantitative papers can yield [20] this information, but still miss other informal data relating to communities of practice, or values (social/political/cultural/economic/ethnic), hence the need to include qualitative data as well. However, the process of integration of qualitative and quantitative data can be labour-intensive and "intellectually enormously challenging" [21].

## 33.3 How to Perform a Literature Search

All literature searches have a generic structure, the steps of which we have outlined below. Different approaches may have variations on these steps, or additional steps. If these have not been described in guidelines, it may be worthwhile booking a course or doing further research before attempting to utilise the search methodology.

1. *Carefully Consider the Research Question*

The research question is the beginning (and end) of every research paper; many aspects of the study hinge on it. In any study, the research question must be important, timely and relevant, in addition to other considerations [22]. While qualitative techniques may be suitable for answering exploratory or complex questions, it is worth first considering whether the question is "researchable". That is, there is data available to synthesise.

2. *Choose the Appropriate Review Technique*

The appropriate review technique (quantitative, qualitative or mixed methods) must be selected if the research question is to be successfully addressed. An approach can be chosen given the review question. In other words it is the review question that should guide which review approach you use.

An important consideration is whether the technique will work for the author's own expertise and resources. If one particular technique looks appropriate, but has not been used by the authors before, it would be wise to read the guidance for the selected literature review technique as well as previous published reviews that have employed the same methodology. The authors then need to decide whether they agree with the various assumptions (implicit and explicit) that underpin the review technique and if they possess the necessary skills. Kastner et al. have recently identified a range of qualitative review techniques and matched them to review objectives [13]. Further description of these approaches can be found in the links (http://www.cihr-irsc.gc.ca/e/36331.html, https://www.york.ac.uk/crd/SysRev/!SSL!/WebHelp/6_5_SYNTHESIS_OF_QUALITATIVE_RESEARCH.htm).

If the technique is not fully operationalised, they may need to seek out supervisors or collaborators with sufficient expertise and/or go on a training course – it might be difficult to use the technique as a novice without any guidance. If one of the less established literature review methods is employed, the authors will need to understand any methodological limitations and expect that others might question their choice of technique and later on challenge their findings.

Some common review techniques of each methodology are described in the table below.

| Data set | Methodology | Description | Strengths and weaknesses |
|---|---|---|---|
| Quantitative | Systematic review | A review and analysis of multiple research studies to answer a research question | Strengths: well-established methodology, fully operationalised, more likely to be reproducible |
| | | | Weakness: omits data on context, less able to arrive at firm conclusions when data heterogeneous |
| | Meta-analysis | Systematic review that employs statistical methods to combine data from multiple studies | Strengths: as per systematic review, can quantify effect sizes form different studies |
| | | | Weaknesses: as per systematic review, requires statistical expertise |
| Qualitative | Meta-ethnography | Translate concepts across studies, explores and explains contradictions to create new interpretations or theory | Strengths: generates theory while focusing on context and experience on individual level |
| | | | Weaknesses: subjective, findings may require further interpretation to inform policy |
| | Meta-synthesis | Develops new theory through interpretation of qualitative data | Strengths: generates theory |
| | | | Weaknesses: not operationalised, subjective |
| | Other qualitative methodologies: critical interpretive synthesis, concept synthesis, meta-study, meta-interpretation | | |
| Mixed | Realist review | Uses theory to explain how context influences outcomes through mechanisms | Strengths: accounts for context and heterogeneity |
| | | | Weaknesses: subjective, only partially operationalised, can be more time-consuming |
| | Metanarrative | Assesses topics from the perspective of paradigms held by academic disciplines | Strengths: can explain theoretical and conceptual conflicts and evolution |
| | | | Weaknesses: subjective, only partially operationalised, requires expertise across disciplines |
| | Other mixed methodologies: integrative review, meta-summary, mixed studies review, narrative synthesis | | |

3. *Assemble a Team*

Frequently a team will require the following members (as a minimum):

- Protocol/write-up: one author
- Methodology: one experienced author
- Search: one author with search expertise
- Data extraction: two authors
- Data analysis: two authors (qualitative), one author with statistics expertise (quantitative)

A systematic review is a significant and frequently laborious piece of work. Practically, there are usually two junior authors who drive the review, carry out the bulk of work and consult with experienced authors who are experts in searches, methodology, analysis and/or write-up. If only one junior author is driving the process, there is a risk of burnout from the workload but also of avoidable errors that will occur during search filtering and data extraction. Qualitative reviews are especially labour-intensive and benefit from the knowledge, insights and discussion from an additional author. Collaborating as a team is key to producing a high-quality review.

4. *Write a Study Protocol*

The goal of the protocol should be to a priori describe and justify all steps of the process. This can ensure that all work is transparent – i.e. others can see and understand what you did and why. Keeping a "paper trail" can prevent or correct mistakes which inevitably occur with large volumes of information. This data is most easily stored electronically, and the advent of cloud storage makes it easier for authors to access and collaborate on shared data. Reporting guidelines – e.g. PRISMA P [23] – exist to facilitate the preparation of a protocol.

5. *Search for Eligible Studies*

A literature search takes place after composing search terms to retrieve relevant articles from selected electronic databases. Expert assistance from research librarians and or authors with search expertise is invaluable, particularly to junior researchers with little experience.

Database selection will depend on the review topic area and methodology. Most medical papers will be archived within MEDLINE and EMBASE. Further articles can be accessed on Scopus or Web of Science. To retrieve studies from other disciplines, particularly those associated with education, ERIC (Educational Resources Information Centre), CINAHL, PsycINFO, Social Sciences Abstracts, Library and Information Science Abstracts and Philosopher's Index may yield papers not found in other databases.

The research team will also need to decide whether to search the grey literature. This is a source of non-peer-reviewed research including postgraduate dissertations, presentations at conferences, reports or other unpublished work. Personal and expert contacts or textbooks may also yield other sources of data. While not always peer-reviewed, they may still contain relevant data, particularly of a qualitative nature.

All literature searches are a compromise between broad and narrow search terms. The broadest search terms will be more sensitive (i.e. not miss any relevant studies) but will likely have too many irrelevant papers to feasibly filter and check. The narrowest search terms will be more specific (i.e. return a higher percentage of eligible studies) but at the possible expense of missing other relevant papers that might contain relevant data. Creating a search strategy is an iterative process that balances sensitivity, specificity and feasibility. Each set of search terms and the numbers of studies yielded should be recorded so that the search can be reproduced but also to justify the breadth of the search.

Before the search, the authors should check that important relevant (landmark) papers on their topic are returned with the search terms. As even the best design searches may miss eligible studies, a process known variously as "snowballing", "citation tracking" or "pearling" can significantly improve the yield of relevant papers [24]. This involves checking the reference lists of all relevant studies for potentially eligible studies or using citation tracking databases. Finally, asking colleagues and experts about potential sources can also reveal valuable results.

6. *Filter Studies*

Study selection will be governed by the inclusion and exclusion criteria created by the author during the protocol. These will be primarily designed to retrieve studies and other documents that are likely to contain relevant data. To make the searching and review feasible, many authors will also use exclusion criteria. Examples of exclusion criteria might be language, publication date or non-peer-reviewed studies.

Ineligible studies will be filtered out during the process of study selection.

This is accomplished in several stages. During the first stage, study titles alone are scanned – they are only excluded if clearly irrelevant. If potentially relevant, the abstracts are retrieved. If the contents of the abstract do not meet inclusion criteria, it is excluded and the reason documented. Full texts of the remaining studies are then retrieved. Again, if the study does not meet inclusion criteria, it is excluded and the reason documented.

In many of the review techniques, the recommendation is that the process of study selection is best accomplished by at least two authors in duplicate and independently. This reduces the possibility of eligible studies being excluded and ineligible studies being included in error and ensures consistency. If this is unfeasible, an acceptable compromise is that a 10% random sample of results may be checked by a second author to check for consistency. Documenting this process on spreadsheets will keep a record of study flow, which is required for most reporting guidelines. Any disagreement between authors should be noted before proceeding to the next stage of study selection. A process for settling disagreements should be in place. For example, if the authors are unable to resolve their disagreement, the senior author may arbitrate to resolve the issue.

## 7. Extract Data

Data extraction for systematic reviews is often performed on predesigned proformas, which capture data on study characteristics, variables and/or other data of interest. Dedicated software for qualitative and mixed methods techniques such as NVivo™ and AtlasTI™ can help manage data to facilitate analysis. As a rule of thumb, for quantitative review techniques, risk of bias and study quality should be assessed using the relevant study tool. With regard to qualitative and mixed methods review techniques, quality assessment requirements and the tools used vary. None have been accepted as gold standard, with over 100 tools in existence for qualitative data alone (Please find examples here: https://www.york.ac.uk/crd/SysRev/!SSL!/WebHelp/6_4_ASSESSMENT_OF_QUALITATIVE_RESEARCH.htm).

Whatever tool is used, the authors must be able to capture and describe study quality. The proforma or any other data extraction processes used should be piloted on several studies and refined to ensure fitness for purpose. As with study selection, data extraction ideally should be carried out in duplicate to minimise errors. Again as a compromise, a 10% random sample of results may be checked for consistency by a second author. A process for settling disagreements should be in place.

## 8. Synthesise Data

At the time of data synthesis, findings can be analysed and explored. In quantitative analysis, this is a two-stage process of statistical analysis, followed by interpretation of results. Each qualitative review technique will have its own processes for analysis and synthesis. In both situations, the aim of synthesis is to produce a clear message or "bottom line", supported by data, that is insightful and explicit in its appraisal of the literature for "relevance, rigour and significance" [25]. This requires authorial interpretations and judgements not only of content, but of the weaknesses (and strengths) of the research methodologies of the included studies. The review's own methodology will need to be transparent and defensible, which will necessitate, in some review techniques, an exploration of sources of bias and threats to validity, as well as complete reporting of the review's methods. Readers' questions should be anticipated; these might centre on the assumptions of the review or its choice of methodology.

## 9. Reporting + Write-Up

While adhering to guidelines can be seen as cumbersome, they enable transparent reporting. Transparent reporting enables readers to assess the strengths and weaknesses of the review and hence make judgements as to whether findings are credible and useful for their purpose(s). It may be advisable to look at the guidelines for the finished study at the protocol point, to ensure that all the relevant data is being captured and reported prospectively. For meta-analysis, the PRISMA guidelines [26] and its variants are the gold standard and similarly the RAMESES guidelines [16] for realist reviews. While no guidelines exist for meta-ethnography, authors can adapt guidelines for other methodologies or refer back to previous studies, particularly worked examples [12]. A good place to look for reporting guidelines for reviews and other research techniques is the EQUATOR Network (http://www.equator-network.org/).

## 33.4 Future Developments

Methodological research is ongoing in quantitative, qualitative and mixed methods review techniques. For qualitative and mixed methods review techniques, in the future, it is likely that further methodologies will be better operationalised and refined. When more established, they may be more accessible to researchers in surgical education. However, in the interim, it can be daunting and perhaps even unwise for a clinician to embark on literature reviews in these techniques without adequate training or support.

## 33.5 Conclusion

Well-executed, insightful and defensible evidence synthesis can sift and make sense of the growing volume of data in surgical education to advance best practice. Researchers will need to choose from a large variety of literature review techniques. The Cochrane Collaboration has established the systematic review as the most widely used approach to quantitative data. A large variety of approaches exist for solely qualitative or mixed quantitative and qualitative data. While some have been more fully operationalised, other techniques are still undergoing development. Choosing the correct research technique depends not only on the research question but also on the training and support available to the researcher to use newer techniques.

## References

1. Tricco, A. C., et al. (2016). A scoping review identifies multiple emerging knowledge synthesis methods, but few studies operationalize the method. *Journal of Clinical Epidemiology, 73*, 19–28.
2. Higgins, J. P. T., & Green, S. E.. *Cochrane handbook for systematic reviews of interventions*. The Cochrane Collaboration.
3. Moher, D., et al. (2009). Preferred reporting items for systematic reviews and meta-analyses: The PRISMA statement. *Annals of Internal Medicine, 151*(4), 264–269.
4. Training, C. (2016). *Learn how to conduct, edit, and read systematic reviews*. Cited 2016. Available from: http://training.cochrane.org/
5. Portsmouth, U.o. (2016). *PgCert systematic reviews in health*. Cited 2016. Available from: http://www.port.ac.uk/courses/health-sciences-and-social-work/pgcert-systematic-reviews-in-health/

6. Group, O.L.o.E.W. (2011). *The Oxford 2011 levels of evidence.* Oxford: Oxford Centre for Evidence-Based Medicine.
7. Walker, E., Hernandez, A. V., & Kattan, M. W. (2008). Meta-analysis: Its strengths and limitations. *Cleveland Clinic Journal of Medicine, 75*(6), 431.
8. Pawson, R. (2002). Evidence-based policy: In search of a method. *Evaluation, 8*(2), 157–181.
9. Berkwits, M., & Aronowitz, R. (1995). Different questions beg different methods. *Journal of General Internal Medicine, 10*(7), 409–410.
10. France, E. F., et al. (2015). Protocol-developing meta-ethnography reporting guidelines (eMERGe). *BMC Medical Research Methodology, 15*(1), 1–14.
11. France, E. F. (2016). *The eMERGe project – developing a meta-ethnography reporting guideline.* Available from: https://www.stir.ac.uk/emerge/
12. Britten, N., et al. (2002). Using meta ethnography to synthesise qualitative research: A worked example. *Journal of Health Services Research & Policy, 7*, 209–215.
13. Kastner, M., Tricco, A., Soobiah, C., Lillie, E., Perrier, L., Horsley, T., et al.. What is the most appropriate knowledge synthesis method to conduct a review? Protocol for a scoping review. *BMC Medical Research Methodology, 12*(1).
14. Tricco, A. C., et al. (2016). Knowledge synthesis methods for integrating qualitative and quantitative data: A scoping review reveals poor operationalization of the methodological steps. *Journal of Clinical Epidemiology, 73*, 29–35.
15. Benoot, C., Hannes, K., & Bilsen, J. (2016). The use of purposeful sampling in a qualitative evidence synthesis: A worked example on sexual adjustment to a cancer trajectory. *BMC Medical Research Methodology, 16*, 21.
16. Wong, G., et al. (2013). RAMESES publication standards: Realist syntheses. *BMC Medicine, 11*, 21.
17. Pawson, R. (2006). *Evidence-based policy. A realist perspective.* London: Sage.
18. Astbury, B., & Leeuw, F. L. (2010). Unpacking black boxes: Mechanisms and theory building in evaluation. *American Journal of Evaluation, 31*(3), 363–381.
19. Dalkin, S. M., et al. (2015). What's in a mechanism? Development of a key concept in realist evaluation. *Implementation Science, 10*(1), 1.
20. Wong, G., Greenhalgh, T., & Pawson, R. (2010). Internet-based medical education: A realist review of what works, for whom and in what circumstances. *BMC Medical Education, 10*, 12.
21. Pawson, R., & Tilley, N.. (1997). *Realist evaluation.* Los Angeles: Sage.
22. Bordage, G., & Dawson, B. (2003). Experimental study design and grant writing in eight steps and 28 questions. *Medical Education, 37*(4), 376–385.
23. Moher, D., et al. (2015). Preferred reporting items for systematic review and meta-analysis protocols (PRISMA-P) 2015 statement. *System Review, 4*, 1.
24. Greenhalgh, T., & Peacock, R. (2005). Effectiveness and efficiency of search methods in systematic reviews of complex evidence: Audit of primary sources. *BMJ, 331*, 1064–1065.
25. Bearman, M. (2016). Quality and literature reviews: Beyond reporting standards. *Medical Education, 50*(4), 382–384.
26. Moher, D., et al. (2009). Preferred reporting items for systematic reviews and meta-analyses: The PRISMA statement. *Annals of Internal Medicine, 151*, 264–269.

# Chapter 34
# Measuring the Impact of Educational Interventions: A Quantitative Approach

**Jenepher A. Martin**

**Overview** This chapter will discuss impact evaluation, an important method of measuring the effectiveness of an educational intervention. This form of evaluation represents a subset of program evaluation and focuses on outcomes and consequential events related to an educational intervention. In doing so, it incorporates several different quantitative methods and is typically reserved for stable, long-standing educational programs/curricula. Many of these methods are also used as part of program evaluation as a whole and in surgical research. Readers are directed to Chaps. 23 ("Demystifying Program Evaluation for Surgical Education", Battista et al.) and 30 ("Researching in Surgical Education: An Orientation", Ajjawi and McIllhenny) for more information on these subjects. In addition to providing a working definition of impact evaluation, this chapter will help define key concepts related to its successful use as well as aid in delineating the most useful quantitative methods to employ.

## 34.1 Introduction

The distinction between evaluation and research is important to reiterate in the context of this chapter. Patton [1] reminds us that evaluation research is a subset of program evaluation and more knowledge-oriented than decision and action oriented. He points out that systematic data collection for evaluation includes social science research methods and, in addition, other sources of data about programs. In the surgical education context, these may include statistics relating to training programs, assessment information and practice observation. Patton's views help us to get over our fixation on experimental method and desire for generalizability of

---

J. A. Martin (✉)
Medical Student Programs, Eastern Health Clinical School, Box Hill, Australia

Faculty of Medicine Nursing and Health Sciences, Monash University, Clayton, Australia

School of Medicine, Deakin University, Melbourne, Australia
e-mail: jenepher.martin@monash.edu

evaluation results and value the usefulness of evaluation in our own context. This in turn promotes a pragmatic approach of making the best judgements and decisions with the available information.

This chapter will discuss impact evaluation, and specifically quantitative methods for contemporary evaluation practice. A working definition of impact evaluation will be developed, followed by a discussion of impact evaluation design and specific applicable quantitative methods. Examples from surgical education will highlight quality of education measurement in research and evaluation. Throughout this chapter the term 'program' will be used in a generic way for any educational event, intervention or course.

## 34.2 What Is Impact Evaluation?

Impact evaluation focus is on outcomes and consequential effects [2], and impact evaluation is usually undertaken for an established program and with summative intent. By their very nature, impact evaluations are retrospective and assume program stability over time sufficient to have observable impacts. In the context of this chapter, the impact must also be measurable.

Impact evaluation designs are also suitable for evaluation of pilot interventions and for comparisons of two or more interventions, providing the interventions are in steady state for the period of evaluation. Thus, the findings of impact evaluation may also be useful for formative purposes in program evaluation. For example, if unintended outcomes are uncovered that are undesirable then even a stable program may be revised and improved. Attempting impact evaluation too early in program implementation, or during program development, risks unreliable and untrustworthy results, with incorrect inferences being made about the program in question and, ultimately, poor decision-making.

Impact evaluation is applicable to both large and small educational programs or interventions, when intended outcomes are clearly understood and defined. Of worldwide relevance to surgical practice, implementation of the World Health Organization (WHO) Surgical Safety Checklist from 2009 had measurable positive impacts on patient outcomes reported within 3 years [3]. On a smaller scale, Evers et al. [4] used a combined process and impact evaluation design to examine a social marketing campaign to increase asthma awareness among older adults in an Australian community. At your own local level, the immediate change in attitudes or behaviour for education participants could be the focus for impact evaluation and unintended outcomes you uncover may need to be addressed for ongoing implementation.

Your evaluation may relate to a small educational workshop you have developed and implemented, an aspect of a national surgical training program at local, regional, or national level, or the local impact of a worldwide program. Common principles apply at all levels, and the remainder of this chapter will address:

- Impact evaluation design
- Focusing impact evaluation
- Quantitative methods for impact evaluation

## 34.3 Designing Impact Evaluation

A practical evaluation design framework has been introduced in Chap. 23 ("Demystifying Program Evaluation for Surgical Education", Battista et al.), and the design flow diagram below (Fig. 34.1) complements the framework. When considering an impact evaluation, three key aspects require clarification:

(i) Is impact the most suitable form of evaluation?
(ii) What outcomes/impacts are of interest?
(iii) Which methods are required for the evaluation?

(i) *Is Impact the Most Suitable Form of Evaluation?*

Before launching into your impact evaluation design, determine if the program you are intending to evaluate is ready for impact evaluation and if the evaluation questions you are interested in relate to impact or another aspect of the program.

Characteristics of the program that indicate readiness for impact evaluation include full implementation, stability and a temporal duration that is sufficient for impacts of interest to have occurred [1, 2]. Clearly these criteria may be met sooner for small, local educational interventions such as a student workshop than for large and complex programs such as surgical training. Even if a program meets the criteria for impact evaluation, this may not be the preferred focus. You may need to spend some time considering this and discussing with program stakeholders just what it is they want to know about the program and for what purpose. Remember, impact evaluation can be formative, but may not be the best approach for programs in development or early implementation. On the other hand, for an established program under review, the question of impact is highly relevant.

(ii) *What Outcomes/Impacts Are of Interest?*

Once the decision to undertake an impact evaluation has been reached, the questions for evaluation are defined. In medicine, research that is valued often has an unashamedly positivist perspective, where objective reality can be quantified and defined by measurement. Tavakol and Saunders [5] remind us that in education a post-positivist approach often sits more comfortably and allows for mixed methods. To use quantitative measures in educational evaluation, however, questions related to output, outcome, or impact measures are required. In considering your evaluation questions the 'distance to target' or 'reach' of the program is a useful concept (Fig. 34.2). Is the evaluation interested in immediate effects on participants, or the longer-term outcomes and impacts on patient care for example? The impact of the implementation of the WHO Surgical Safety Checklist has been evaluated at indi-

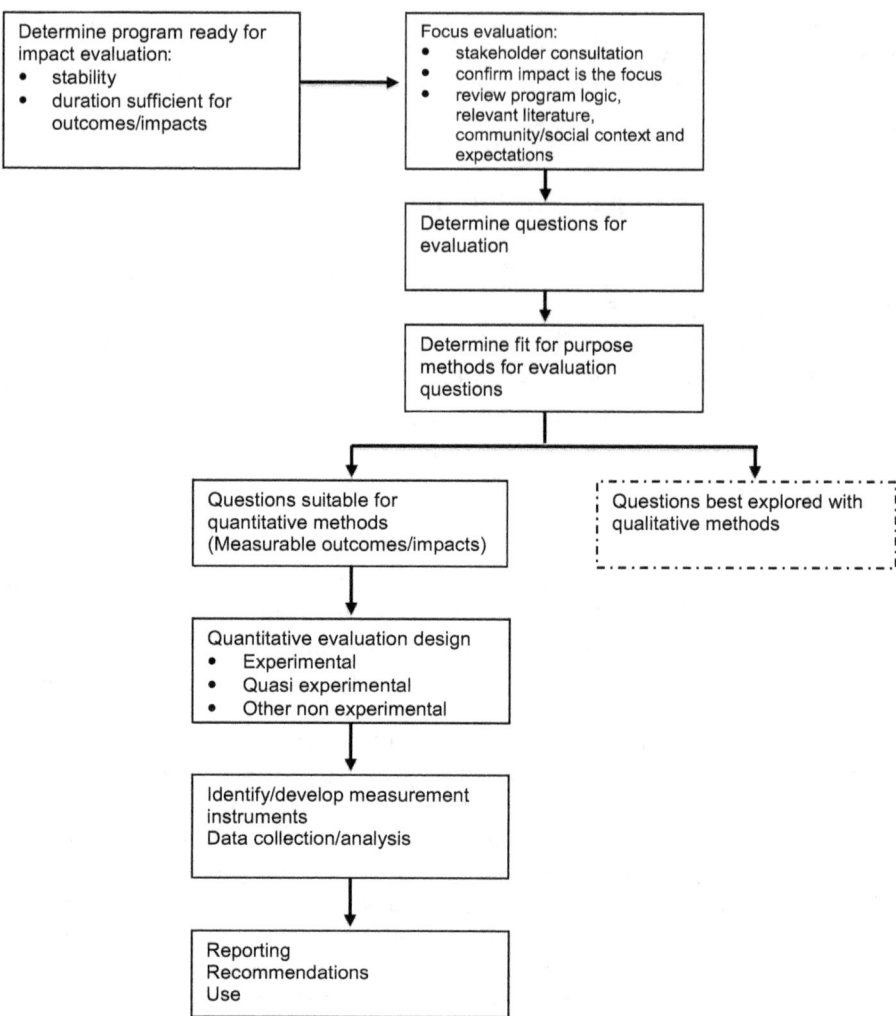

**Fig. 34.1** Impact evaluation design

vidual [6] and patient outcome levels [3]. As noted in Chap. 30 ("Researching in Surgical Education: An Orientation", Ajjawi and McIllhenny), longer-term and distant impacts from educational interventions, such as patient outcomes, may be inaccessible to local researchers or evaluators. Information about more immediate outcomes for participants in the local context, such as changes in surgical team members' awareness of patient safety after checklist introduction described by Papaconstantinou et al. [6], informs the local program and supports the positive global impact objective of WHO.

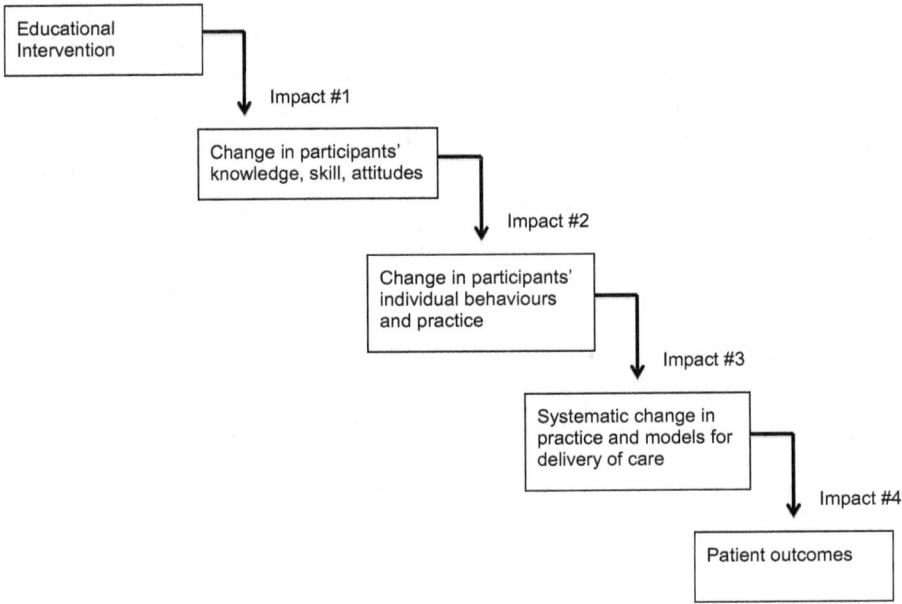

**Fig. 34.2** Distance to impact

The critical step of stakeholder consultation may result in a range of evaluation questions, especially if there are competing interests for various stakeholders. For example, in multi-site specialty training programs, hospital-based supervisors may be primarily interested in consistency of implementation across sites or equity of access to learning resources and opportunities, and impact evaluation may not be the most suitable approach. On the other hand, the surgical college faced with prioritizing funding for the overall program may be seeking information about the impact of the program in terms of training outcomes. For a small local intervention such as a suturing workshop, the workshop facilitator may be interested in the immediate impact of the intervention on participants' surgical skills and/or their subsequent opportunities to put these into practice. The questions for the evaluation determined through stakeholder consultation will determine methodology, data collection and analysis.

In addition to stakeholder consultation, the 'logic' or 'theory' of the program will inform the evaluation questions, as this defines the planned outputs, outcomes and impacts [2]. As good quantitative research is driven by theory [5], so is good quantitative impact evaluation.

(iii) *Which Methods Are Required for the Evaluation?*

Ideally, methodology is considered after determining the questions for the evaluation, leading to an approach where 'fit for purpose' methods are matched with evaluation questions and there are no resource constraints. In practice, this stage of the design is often one of compromise and reality checking. There may be existing 'good enough' sources of data available for low cost; tight time lines may preclude longitudinal data collection; or small numbers of participants limit statistical power. Your aim is to conduct rigorous evaluation within local constraints to make the best judgements and decisions about your program under the circumstances.

The remainder of this chapter will focus on quantitative methods for impact evaluation studies, with an emphasis on the development and validation of measurement instruments.

## 34.4 Quantitative Approaches for Impact Evaluation

Many of the concepts for the design of impact evaluation for educational interventions using quantitative methodology will be familiar to surgeons and surgical trainees as there are similarities with clinical research methods. For impact evaluation, important considerations include:

- The study design
- Sources of data, sampling and surveys
- Data analysis and reporting
- Measurement instruments

### 34.4.1 Quantitative Evaluation Design

Quantitative designs range from experimental to descriptive [5] and are summarized in Table 34.1. What best suits your program evaluation will be determined by multiple factors including your evaluation questions, any hypotheses you put forward, available resources, the structure of the program being evaluated, and the context of the educational program.

Experimental design for program evaluation purposes is not common in the surgical education literature. There are, however, some illustrative studies with a research purpose. Seymour et al. [7] conducted a randomized, double blinded study exploring the effect of virtual reality (VR) training on operating performance of surgical trainees. This demonstrated benefits of VR training over standard training of decreased operative time and fewer errors in the experimental group. Although this study is described as double-blinded, the participants in the education intervention were, of course, aware of their randomization status, in contrast to many therapeutic trials. The two sets of assessors were blinded to participant status in this case. Other randomized studies of interest include the examination of three different education conditions on transfer of operative skills to a cadaver model [8] and work by Moulton et al. [9] on the role of distributed practice in surgical skill development. These studies have contributed new knowledge to surgical education; however, in

**Table 34.1** Designs for quantitative impact evaluation

| | |
|---|---|
| Experimental | Random assignment to intervention (experimental) and non-intervention (control) groups |
| | Participants/assessors may be 'blinded' to intervention – single (participants) or double (participants and assessors) blinding |
| | Crossover designs are sometimes used |
| | Advantage: strong causal inferences |
| | Disadvantage: experimental conditions may not reflect the real world, design not practical for many evaluations |
| Quasi experimental | Non experimental design, |
| | Assignment to intervention/non intervention not random |
| | Single group design can be utilized (e.g., pre/post-intervention evaluation of participants) |
| | Participants/assessors may be 'blinded' to intervention – single (participants) or double (participants and assessors) blinding |
| | Advantage: practical design option for real world settings |
| | Disadvantage: complex statistical analysis often required; causal inferences made with caution |
| Correlational | Non experimental design |
| | Explores the associations between features of education programs (the variables). Can be used where assignment to a group of interest is not possible. Data can be quantitative or nominal, and exploration of relationships between two or more variables conducted |
| | Advantage: Suitable for most contexts. Exploration of associations can lead to further evaluation of important program aspects |
| | Disadvantage: Limited use when relationship is not linear, range is restricted or outliers in data. No causal inferences possible |
| Descriptive | Detailed documentation of program outcomes/impacts using descriptive statistics (frequencies, percentages, etc.), and graphics |
| | Applicable for all impact evaluation and provides overview |
| | Often required for reporting to stakeholders |
| | Advantage: Facilitates clarification of the program and explicit understanding of outputs and outcomes of interest. May identify unintended outcomes/impacts |
| | Disadvantage: No causal inferences possible |

the context of impact evaluation of established programs, randomization of participants may be impractical, particularly so if the education is high stakes and there could be any perception of benefit or disadvantage for participants to randomization status. For 'near target' and low-stakes education programs, experimental impact evaluation design may be possible and helpful for comparing interventions under consideration.

Quasi-experimental designs [5, 10], on the other hand, are often very practical for program evaluation, although less familiar to surgeons. Quasi-experimental designs are described comprehensively in Cook and Campbell's [10] classic work on the subject, and interested evaluators are encouraged to explore further. Practical and commonly used quasi-experimental options suitable for your initial practice include single group or control group pre-test/post-test designs, and interrupted time-series designs. These designs fall into the category of non-randomized intervention studies. Because randomization to intervention status is not used, causal inferences are not as robust as in experimental designs. However, the suitability of quasi-experimental designs for real world clinical practice and surgical education settings where randomization may be precluded due to ethical, logistic or cost considerations offsets the weaker certainty about causal inferences in these designs. Despite limitations, useful and timely information from complex and uncontrolled contexts is often acquired, facilitating decision-making.

- Pre-test/post-test designs.

The choice between single group or control group pre-test/post-test evaluation is often pragmatic. The use of a control group, even though selection bias is not managed by randomization, does enhance validity of findings. Obviously, demographic data and context details can be used to establish how closely matched control and intervention groups are. An issue you may face when using control group designs, randomized or not, is the perception of 'fairness' when some students have access to an intervention and others don't. In some situations this can be managed by delivering your intervention to the control group post hoc; in others, a single group design is the most acceptable solution. Documented change in surgical team members' perspectives before and after the introduction of the WHO Surgical Safety checklist [6] is an example of this design.

- Interrupted time series designs.

These designs are cohort studies, either cross-sectional or longitudinal, a concept familiar to many surgical educators from clinical epidemiology. Integral to these designs are multiple measurements over time, both before and after an intervention of interest. As with other quasi-experimental designs, inferences about the intervention causing observed effects must be made cautiously. Examples of this design include some studies discussed by Fudickar [3] in relation to the WHO Surgical Safety checklist and the study by Martling et al. [11] of the effect of surgeon training on rectal cancer outcome.

Non-experimental correlational designs are very common in evaluation practice. Exploring associations between variables is important; however, it does not imply causation of observed effects. In impact evaluation, correlational studies may be very useful in uncovering unintended outcomes or impacts, which may then require further study. In thinking about the use of correlational designs in your practice, the concept of 'natural experiments' may be useful, [10] where there is very little manipulation of the environment and/or no specific intervention. Exploration of the association between video game experience and laparoscopic skill is one such example [12], raising interesting questions for further research.

## 34.4.2 Sources of Data, Sampling and Surveys

The data required for your impact evaluation will be determined by your evaluation questions, and identifying sources of data is part of the planning process (Chap. 23, "Demystifying Program Evaluation for Surgical Education", Battista et al.). Selecting sources of data, gaining access to these and obtaining the data for analysis constitutes the assembly of evidence on which your ultimate judgements and recommendations are based [2].

Accessing the data you want is not always straightforward. For example, performance data from health services, universities and surgical training organizations may require formal application. Negotiation with third parties to distribute surveys may be required. Existing databases, while useful, may not have all the information you want, leading to modification of your plans. Ethical, logistic, financial and political considerations will also come into play. Bear in mind that when you obtain outcome/impact data from others you will be relying on the quality of measurement that generated those data without necessarily knowing how robust that measurement is.

For some impact evaluations, it will be possible to predictably obtain outcome/impact measures from all program participants. In other evaluations the population of interest may require sampling, and your approach to sampling should be determined and made explicit in the evaluation planning. The aim is to achieve a representative sample of your program participants. You will most likely use non-probability sampling methods such as convenience sampling, purposive sampling and quota sampling [13].

Data collection often involves surveys and these may include multiple forms of data including demographic information as well as embedded measurement instruments. Artino et al. [14] offer practical advice about survey design for medical education research, underpinned by sound theory [15, 16]. Underlying measurement principles are discussed further below.

## 34.4.3 Data Analysis and Reporting

The purpose of analysis is to make sense of the data, to construct meaning and ultimately answer your evaluation questions. Data management and analysis as described by Owen [2] involves constructing 'an organized assembly of information' or 'data display', data reduction to simplify and transform raw information and then drawing conclusions that relate to evaluation questions.

Quantitative evaluation designs require statistical analysis, and it is critical you seek advice about this in the planning stages. As evaluators, we want to make the best judgements and decisions we can with the available evidence even if the evidence would not meet clinical decision-making standards. Remember, evaluation research is a subset of program evaluation, and statisticians familiar with analysis of experimental data in biomedical research may not be familiar with some of the more sophisticated analyses in quasi-experimental and correlational designs [10]. Clinical epidemiologists may well be able to advise about analysis of data for interrupted time-series designs. Educational measurement and associated analyses is a separate area of expertise and briefly discussed below.

Intended users of your evaluation are ideally involved during data analysis, interpretation, making judgements, and recommending consequent actions [1]. This co-construction of the evaluation outcome between evaluator and stakeholders is a distinct difference between research and evaluation and promotes use of your evaluation.

### 34.4.4 Identifying Measures

Measurement of outcomes, impacts and consequences is central to quantitative approaches described above, and precision of measurement underpins the robustness of the results. Precise, accurate measurement depends on reliable and valid measurement instruments.

Some outcome measures, such as mortality, numbers of errors or time are clear; however, many are more complex. The two key concepts of reliability and validity underpin your choice of measurement instrument, and these will be outlined now. For in depth information about measurement theory, further reading is recommended. An additional consideration in designing evaluations is the feasibility of implementing your measure. Reliability is a pre-requisite for measurement validity and so will be discussed first.

- Reliability

Measurement reliability refers to the consistency of scores; however, on its own, it is not sufficient to provide evidence for validity [17, 18]. Measures of reliability may quantify internal consistency of the instrument, reproducibility over time or inter-rater agreement (Table 34.2). High reliability indicates consistency with little error in the measurement, considered important when the stakes are high.

For the assessment of non-technical skills of surgeons, the Non-Technical Skills for Surgeons (NOTSS) Behaviour Rating System was developed, and reliability information is available for this relating to internal structure and inter-rater reliability [19]. In assessments of operative skill in surgical trainees, comparative reliability of global ratings and checklist scoring systems has been examined [20]. Reliability information such as this is helpful in selecting measurement instruments with the caveat that the reliability of a measure is not inherent in the instrument itself, but relates to the scores obtained, and using an instrument under different conditions (e.g. context, population or rater training status) may change the reliability. Reliability studies such as those discussed are often the first published information about measurement instruments in surgical education; however, further validity evidence is required for confident use in research and evaluation.

**Table 34.2** Types of reliability

| Type of reliability | | Methods for reliability calculation |
|---|---|---|
| Internal consistency | Commonly used for tests that relate to a single construct such as 'knowledge' or 'empathy' where each item in the test should be well correlated with other items. High internal consistency supports the single construct | Split half reliability |
| | | Kuder Richardson |
| | | Cronbach's alpha |
| Stability of the measurement | These measures assess 'in-person' stability of measures either across time (test-retest) or equivalent versions of the test (parallel forms). There is an assumption that the subject remains stable with respect to the measured construct between test occasions or forms | Test-retest reliability |
| | | Parallel forms reliability |
| Inter-rater reliability (IRR) | These measures assess the agreement between different raters of the same subject test performance using the same rating instrument. The most appropriate measure for IRR calculation will be determined by factors such as the form of measurement data (rank, dichotomous, continuous) and number of raters | Percent agreement |
| | | Phi (correlation) |
| | | Kappa |
| | | Kendall's Tau |
| | | Intraclass correlation |
| Generalizability of the measure | Assigns the variance of test scores to multiple possible sources (subjects, raters, items, etc.). Understanding where score variance is attributed is helpful in planning interventions to improve assessment such as rater training | Generalizability coefficient |

APA [17, 18] and Cook and Beckman [21]

- Validity

For educational evaluations, you will often want to measure outcomes in terms of knowledge, skills and attitudes of participants in the program or of others impacted by the program. To do this, you will require a measurement instrument of some type that you are confident is actually measuring the construct of interest. The types of instruments you could consider include educational tests and examinations, observed performance ratings, attitude rating scales, psychological tests, and questionnaires. So how do you know the instrument you are considering does actually measure the construct you are interested in? After all, for many constructs, the measure is a proxy as the underlying construct is not directly measurable [21]. For example, empathy can be inferred from physicians' self-reported perceptions and behaviours [22].

Validity, as defined by the APA standards is 'the degree to which evidence and theory support the interpretations of test scores entailed by the proposed use of tests' and that validation is the 'process of constructing and evaluating arguments for and against the identified interpretation of test scores and their relevance to the proposed use' [17, 18]. This definition highlights that validation of a measurement instrument requires supporting evidence, that meaning is derived from measurements and not inherent to scores in themselves, and that validity of a specific measure is context specific. So, validation of a measurement instrument uses multiple sources of evidence, is cumulative and takes time. One contemporary view of validity is that all sources of evidence relate to construct validity, with five broad categories identified [17, 18, 21, 23] (Table 34.3).

**Table 34.3** Evidence to support validity of measurement

| Evidence category | Question answered | Criteria to consider |
|---|---|---|
| Content | How well does the content of the measurement represent the underlying construct? | Construct definition |
| | | Intended purpose of the measurement |
| | | Process for instrument development (blueprinting, sampling, item development, etc.) |
| | | Item quality, wording |
| | | Qualifications of item writers and review process |
| Response process | Is the response process/behaviour of the subject to the test item(s) consistent with the underlying construct being measured? | Theoretical and /or empirical analysis of the processes test takers use in their response to item(s). (e.g. in a test of clinical reasoning, are they undertaking this process or simply applying a learned algorithm?) |
| | Are the judgement-making processes of the raters consistent with the intended use of the test scores? | Empirical analysis of the criteria used to arrive at judgements. (e.g. clinical performance assessment should not be influenced by unrelated student factors such as gender or race) |
| Internal structure | Are the relationships between test items consistent with the underlying construct? | Internal consistency as evidence for homogeneity and single construct vs multifactorial structure |
| | | Factor structure alignment to theoretical construct(s) |
| | How well does test performance reflect predicted performance of particular subgroups with respect to the underlying construct? | Differential performance aligned with construct prediction. E.g. more senior trainees perform better |
| Relation to other variables | Is the relationship with other variables as expected based on the predicted relationship between the constructs measured? | Positive correlations between two measures that are either expected to co-vary (e.g. engagement with clinical learning and clinical performance), or are measuring the same construct (e.g. knowledge tests of common content in different formats,) |
| | | Negative or no correlation between measures consistent with expectations based on the underlying constructs being measured (e.g. eye colour and surgical skill) |
| Consequences | What are the consequential effects, intended and unintended, of the assessment? | Behaviours of test takers in response to the format of the assessment. (E.g 'OSCE practice' vs authentic patient/student interactions; rote learning vs deep learning) |
| | | Methods and criteria used to determine categorization of test takers leading to subsequent consequential outcomes for them. (E.g. pass/fail cut scores, degree of depression, level of intelligence) |

APA [17, 18], Cook and Beckman [21], and Cook and Hatala [23]

**Table 34.4** Example constructs and potential measurement methods in surgical education

| Construct | Type of assessment | Candidate measurement methods |
|---|---|---|
| Knowledge (e.g. clinical sciences, disease specific information) | Written or oral tests of knowledge | Multiple choice tests, short answer or essay questions. Viva tests |
| | Written or oral tests of applied knowledge/problem solving (note: item construction and format must be matched to intended level of knowledge testing) | Simulation- or clinical-based objective structured clinical examination |
| | Performance-based assessment of applied knowledge/problem solving (note item construction matched to this assessment objective) | Observed clinical practice |
| Clinical skills (e.g. history, examination) | Performance-based assessment of applied knowledge/problem solving (note item construction matched to this assessment objective) | Simulation- or clinical-based objective |
| Communication skills | | Observed clinical practice |
| Teamwork | | |
| Procedural skills | Performance-based assessment of applied knowledge/problem solving | Direct observation procedural skills (DOPS), |
| | | Objective structured assessment of technical skills (OSATS), |
| | | Time and motion analysis, |
| | | Error analysis |
| | | Product quality assessment |

- Selecting a measurement instrument.

Be clear about the constructs you want to measure and specify these as precisely and accurately as possible. The construct definitions will determine what measurement instruments are appropriate. For example, a written test of anatomy measures knowledge, not surgical skill (Table 34.4). The caveat here regarding validity evidence is for the interpretation of measurement for which it was established. If you are using a measurement for an alternative interpretation then validity should be established for that use [21, 23].

As surgical educators, we are often interested in student or trainee outcomes, and the following practical examples will illustrate the common options for choosing measurement instruments: (i) use existing data, (ii) use an 'off the shelf' instrument or (iii) design a new instrument.

Examination scores are one of the most frequently used sources of existing data for education outcomes/impact evaluation. If you are using these data, endeavour to assure yourself of the validity of the measurement. One disadvantage of using existing test scores is that validation studies may not have been undertaken.

An 'off the shelf' test may be the best choice for psychological constructs such as empathy or self-efficacy. Many of these instruments have been used in large and/or diverse populations and norms are established. Checking what validation evidence is available and in what use contexts can help you decide if an 'off the shelf' test is suitable. If you were interested in surgeon empathy, you might choose the Jefferson Scale of Physician Empathy [22].

When you are unable to identify a suitable measurement instrument, it may be necessary to develop one, or modify an existing one. In both cases pilot studies to validate the measure are required. The objective structured assessment of technical skills (OSATS) is an example of a new instrument developed when no suitable measure was available [24, 25]. Since its development, OSATS has become an established measure in surgical education research, evaluation and training.

## 34.5 Conclusion

Impact evaluation is a specific evaluation form applicable to stable programs, large or small, with defined impacts and outcomes. Quantitative methodology for impact evaluation includes experimental, quasi-experimental and non-experimental design. Measurement of outcomes/impact for evaluation must be reliable and valid for credible judgments and well-founded decision-making.

## References

1. Patton, M. Q. (1997). *Utilization-focused evaluation* (4th ed.). Thousand Oaks: Sage Publications.
2. Owen, J. M. (2006). *Program evaluation: Forms and approaches* (3rd ed.). Crows Nest: Allen and Unwin.
3. Fudickar, A., et al. (2012). The effect of the WHO Surgical Safety Checklist on complication rate and communication. *Deutsches Ärzteblatt International, 109*(42), 695–701.
4. Evers, U., et al. (2013). 'Get your life back': Process and impact evaluation of an asthma social marketing campaign targeting older adults. *BMC Public Health, 13*, 759–768.
5. Tavakol, M., & Sanders, J. (2014). Quantitative and qualitative methods in medical education research: AMEE Guide No 90: Part I. *Medical Teacher, 36*(9), 746–756.
6. Papaconstantinou, H. T., et al. (2013). Implementation of a surgical safety checklist: Impact on surgical team perspectives. *The Oschner Journal, 13*, 299–309.
7. Seymour, N. E., et al. (2002). Virtual reality training improves operating room performance. Results of a randomized, double-blinded study. *Annals of Surgery, 236*(4), 458–464.
8. Anastakis, D. J., et al. (1999). Assessment of technical skills transfer from the bench training model to the human model. *American Journal of Surgery, 177*(2), 167–170.
9. Moulton, C. E., et al. (2006). Teaching surgical skills: What kind of practice makes perfect? A randomized, controlled trial. *Annals of Surgery, 244*(3), 400–409.
10. Cook, T. D., & Campbell, D. T. (1979). *Quasi-experimentation: Design & analysis issues for field settings* (1st ed.). Chicago: Rand McNally.

11. Martling, A. L., et al. (2000). Effect of a surgical training programme on outcome of rectal cancer in the County of Stockholm. *Lancet, 356*(9224), 93–96.
12. Rosser, J. C., et al. (2007). The impact of video games on training surgeons in the 21st century. *Archives of Surgery, 142*, 181–186.
13. Tavakol, M., & Sanders, J. (2014). Quantitative and qualitative methods in medical education research: AMEE Guide No 90: Part II. *Medical Teacher, 36*(10), 838–848.
14. Artino, A. R., et al. (2014). Developing questionnaires for educational research: AMEE Guide No.87. *Medical Teacher, 36*(6), 463–474.
15. DeVellis, R. F. (2014). *Scale development: Theory and applications* (2nd ed.). Newbury Park: Sage Publications.
16. Dillman, D., et al. (2009). *Internet, mail and mixed-mode surveys: The tailored design method* (3rd ed.). Hoboken: Wiley.
17. American Educational Research Association, American Psychological Association, & National Council on Measurement in Education. (1999). *Standards for educational and psychological testing*. Washington, DC: American Educational Research Association.
18. American Educational Research Association, American Psychological Association, National Council on Measurement in Education. (2014). *Standards for educational and psychological testing*. Washington, DC: American Educational Research Association.
19. Yule, S., et al. (2008). Surgeons' non-technical skills in the operating room: Reliability testing of the NOTSS behaviour rating system. *World Journal of Surgery, 32*, 548–556.
20. Regher, G., et al. (1998). Comparing psychometric properties of checklists and global rating scales for assessing performance on an OSCE-format examination. *Academic Medicine, 73*(9), 993–997.
21. Cook, D. A., & Beckman, T. J. (2006). Current concepts in validity and reliability for psychometric instruments: Theory and application. *The American Journal of Medicine, 119*, 166. e7–166.e16.
22. Hojat, M., et al. (2002). Physician empathy: Definition, components, measurement and relationship to gender and speciality. *American Journal of Psychiatry, 159*(90), 1563–1569.
23. Cook, D. A., & Hatala, R. (2016). Validation of educational assessments: A primer for simulation and beyond. *Advances in Simulation, 1*, 31.
24. Martin, J. A., et al. (1997). Objective structured assessment of technical skill (OSATS) for surgical residents. *British Journal of Surgery, 84*, 273–278.
25. Reznick, R., et al. (1997). Testing technical skill via an innovative 'bench station' examination. *American Journal of Surgery, 173*(3), 226–230.

# Chapter 35
# Understanding Learning: A Qualitative Approach

**Kirsten Dalrymple and Debra Nestel**

**Overview** Building on ideas from Chaps. 30 to 36, we offer worked examples of high-standard qualitative research in surgical education to illustrate key concepts *underpinning their design, execution and presentation* but also essentially *how they achieve coherence through these activities.* A key goal is to forward the idea that a significant proportion of surgical education is about humans and social interaction and hence influenced by context, time, place, individual experience and background. There are myriad configurations that create educational success or difficulty and multiple interpretations and explanations for their existence. Qualitative research aims to explore this complexity to answer questions, as argued in Chap. 30, of the how, why, where, when and for who our education practices work. Given the complexity, variability and instability of surgical education, we argue that researchers should embrace the subjective and expand their approaches to creating and evaluating the quality of knowledge gained through research whilst upholding an overarching scientific ethos of being principled and systematic in designing and carrying it out. Engaging in qualitative research entails elevating the concept of 'coherence' above that of 'proof' when evaluating quality and justifying design. We write this chapter for surgeons who are coming to educational research for the first time.

---

K. Dalrymple (✉)
Faculty of Medicine, Imperial College London, London, UK
e-mail: k.dalrymple@imperial.ac.uk

D. Nestel
Faculty of Medicine, Nursing & Health Sciences, Monash Institute for Health and Clinical Education, Monash University, Clayton, VIC, Australia

Faculty of Medicine Dentistry & Health Sciences, Department of Surgery, Melbourne Medical School, University of Melbourne, Parkville, Australia
e-mail: dnestel@unimelb.edu.au; debra.nestel@monash.edu

## 35.1 Introduction

Qualitative research methodology, as described by Denzin and Lincoln [1] and elaborated by Ajjawi and McIlhenny in Chap. 30, stems from a constructivist view of reality and knowledge as being multiple and influenced by unique, complex contexts (e.g. an operating theatre replete with modern technology, a M&M meeting, an A&E department, a breast clinic, etc.), inhabited by unique individuals (e.g. members of a theatre team with different healthcare backgrounds, of varying seniority, trained in different countries, with different personal backgrounds and values, not to mention patients, families, managers) who are active interpreters of their reality. Of critical note, the researcher, who is exploring some aspect of this natural phenomenon, is considered part of the research, not as a measurer but as an interpreter and 'co-constructer' of findings. This has significant implications for the way in which a qualitative study, regardless of its particular methodology and methods, is carried out. It means, as Lichtman [2] describes, that *natural settings* (or context) should be sought after and, by corollary, the people who have knowledge of these settings and the phenomena that occur there should be *purposely recruited*. It means that *researcher and researched* come with insights and views of the phenomena and that these are indeed influenced by values and beliefs. It means that the findings drawn from what we see our research participants do and say represents one of *many possible interpretations* of the phenomena that may or may not hold up in a different setting. Given there are often power differentials between the participants in education research (namely, teacher and student) and that mistakes and failure represent particularly sensitive topics (even more so in the context of learning surgery!), *ethical treatment of research participants* is not only a moral imperative; it has a direct impact on the quality of participants' responses and hence the validity of data. In Chap. 36, Kingsbury describes how consideration of these ethical considerations are built into research design.

In this chapter, we present three published reports of research that highlight frequently employed qualitative constructivist approaches and which contribute relevant and significant knowledge to surgical education. Although we simply scratch the surface in terms of design possibilities, we hope it will highlight how coherence and quality are achieved through various aspects of a qualitative research study. This includes, as previous authors have argued, *defining a research focus for the education phenomena of interest in concert with locating a gap in the literature, developing research questions, considering a relevant conceptual/theoretical framework, seeking appropriate study environments and participants, justifying approaches to data collection and analyses, considering the nature of the study's findings and its implications for surgical education and, perhaps most importantly and most unusual to those who have been schooled in biomedical research traditions, reflecting on your role* in the research process.

To maximize learning, we suggest the three articles profiled are read before, during and after working through this chapter. The first reading to provides a view of concrete qualitative research reports of a high standard. The second reading enables greater insights from the primary source as to how qualitative methodologies and principles inform design decisions and then lead to particular kinds of knowledge. The third reading allows you to consider what you now understand relative to your first reading. Each section is devoted to one article and is headed by the research question/s under investigation.

## 35.2 What Are the Beliefs and Values About Intraoperative Teaching and Learning That Are Held by Surgical Teachers and Trainees? [3]

### 35.2.1 Framing the Research Topic, Questions and Basic Design

Ong, a surgeon and surgical educator, and colleagues describe, based on personal experience and the literature, that trainers and trainees feel satisfaction when a trainee completes an operation with limited intervention by the trainer. They share a common interest in the trainee's operative development. Operative complexity and variability however often prompt trainers to take control of the operation for the sake of patient safety. Ong et al. sought to explore how trainers' and trainees' beliefs and values of teaching and learning in theatre would influence their respective behaviours particularly around this control dynamic [3].

Ong's team chose a multiple, paired case study design to explore their research question. Case study methodology can take many forms but usually looks at specified, real-life phenomena or a case (e.g. an event, process, individual, group or institution) and attempts to explore, explain or make sense of it. Ong's team defined, what Yin [4] calls, the 'unit of study' for their 'case' to be the shared experience of intraoperative teaching and learning between trainer and trainee. Case study methodology draws on methods that illuminate the case and hence can combine qualitative methods (such as interviews, observation, documentary analysis) with quantitative ones (e.g. exam data, numeric survey data) in order to see the phenomena from different perspectives and shed light on the research question. As the research question in this study sought to explore what values and beliefs about teaching and learning underpin behaviour, both observation of the shared intraoperative teaching and learning experience and a semi-structured, interview-based exploration of the trainers' and trainees' views were sought. Employing two qualitative methods alongside one another allowed the team to compare observed behaviour from the observations with espoused values and beliefs revealed in the interviews, providing the researchers with insight into how these align (or not). This represents a type of 'triangulation' of methods that, in qualitative research terms, serves as quality criteria (Table 35.1) contributing to the study's 'credibility' [5].

**Table 35.1** Establishing 'trustworthiness' in qualitative research: a view of quality criteria

| Criteria | Criteria demonstrates | Some measures to develop |
|---|---|---|
| Credibility | Confidence in the 'truth' of the findings | Triangulation, negative case analysis, member checking, long-term engagement and observation |
| Transferability | Applicability of findings in other contexts | Thick/rich description of methods and research context |
| Dependability | Findings are consistent and could be repeated | Audit trail, external review |
| Confirmability | Findings exhibit a degree of 'neutrality', showing findings are strongly shaped by respondents and not overly influenced by researcher bias, motivation or interest | Audit trail, external review, triangulation and reflexivity |

Adapted from Lincoln and Guba [5]

## 35.2.2 Use of Theory

Theory, as Ajjawi and McIlhenny argue in Chap. 30, can inform various aspects of a qualitative study and can serve to bring greater coherence to the whole. In Ong et al.'s work, we see theory used in several ways. *Firstly, theory is used as a tool to frame and focus the study* around the essential areas of interest, namely, the social interactions between trainer and trainee and the cognitive activities being emphasized by the trainer to support the execution of the operation. For Ong et al., Lave and Wenger's [6] social constructivist ideas of situated learning as well as cognitive apprenticeship theory [7] were selected as relevant frameworks. This framing is part and parcel of clarifying the educational problem of interest. Framing helps establish where the study sits relative to the literature, in terms of what has been studied, using what theoretical/conceptual lenses, and with what research methods. Lingard's [8] proposal of the Problem-Gap heuristic describes this process concisely, clearly and convincingly and, alongside Chap. 33, shows the surgical education researcher how he/she might carefully unpick their educational problem. Problem clarification alongside wider reading improves clarity and justifies research design, a process mirroring, in many respects, that undertaken in quantitative research.

Ong et al.'s *second use of theory* in their research design was to *use concepts from both situated learning and cognitive apprenticeship to structure data collection*, for example, in selecting the foci for their intraoperative teaching and learning observations and in how they phrased questions asked during their interviews. The chosen theories were woven through subsequent stages of the research process, namely, as part of the analysis where an 'a priori' coding template drawing on concepts from these theories was applied to the data and in the researchers' interpretation of their findings. Weaving theory through multiple aspects of the research process promotes a stronger, more coherent design that, in turn, and in combination with other practices used in qualitative research, enhance the relevance and rigor of the findings.

## 35.2.3 Research Participants and Setting

Having made use of theory to define the nature and scope of the educational problem, Ong et al. went about purposeful selection of study participants and the context for observation. They recruited, active and well-regarded trainers from their own institution to participate on a voluntary basis. Trainees of these trainers were then approached to provide the partner for the 'paired' cases. In a similar vein, an uncomplicated operative list was chosen as the observational focus for the likelihood that trainees would be able to complete the operations undertaken. These are deliberate decisions that serve to focus the study on the research questions and on the individuals who are best placed to 'inform' the researchers about the phenomena. It is a decidedly non-random sampling approach but one that makes sense given the study's qualitative aim.

## 35.2.4 Role of the Researcher

'Researchers know that they influence the research and results', claims Lichtman [2] p22) with both qualitative and quantitative paradigms deploying devices to manage this influence. Quantitative, positivist approaches seek to manage this influence by stripping out the subjective influence of the researcher through placing experimental controls, randomized sampling, reducing variables, applying statistical tests and even writing in the third person – devices all intended to remove human influence and 'values' as a source of bias. Qualitative research, as described in Chap. 30, takes the researcher as an instrument of data collection, on the backdrop of a philosophy that reality and knowledge of it is co-constructed and multiple. Assumed to have values and unique experience, the researcher is argued to also bring value to the research process. Ong, for example, is a staff surgeon in the institution where the study took place, carried out the recruitment, data collection and primary analysis of her data. She declares and critically justifies her role as an 'insider' arguing that it would facilitate recruitment and aid the analysis of data generated from a context where specialist language conveys meanings that are unfamiliar to the non-surgical layperson. Her values and the influence they might exert on the research however do not go unexamined. The team put into place measures to enhance the quality and validity of the research process, made visible through declaring her position and justifying her design choices as part of the methodology and discussion. The researchers describe how they mitigated potential over (or mis)-interpretation of the findings. For example, Ong subjected her coding designations to challenge by her 'outsider' coinvestigators until the coding set was agreed by the team. The data was analysed, and adjusted where necessary, through iterative team discussion. In these ways, the benefits and the risks associated with having the value-laden researcher as an explicit part of the process are attended to. Many of these methods draw on quality criteria described in Table 35.1.

## 35.2.5 Bringing It All Together: Presenting the Analysis and Interpretation

Ong et al. present their findings in a table based on five cases [i.e. specific trainer and trainee(s) pairs]. Here they bring together what Lincoln and Guba [5] describe as a 'thick description' of their analysis and provide illustrations through quotes. This offers the reader not with proof that all the participants did or said similar things but rather that the interpretation is based on themes they marshalled from the data and that the reader can inspect. The presentation draws attention to the comparisons and contrasts between trainers and trainees within and across cases.

What Ong et al. note most strongly of the 'shared experiences' is that this 'sharing of perspectives' centred on technical aspects of the operation and was limited to satisfaction in the knowledge that trainees had completed it. Trainers and trainees had markedly different perceptions around non-technical domains of practice in terms of what was emphasized and seen as important (e.g. in surgical judgement). Though feedback practices varied, from haptic to verbal, not all of the latter registered with the trainees. These disparities were revealed through comparison of observation with interview data.

Through their application of cognitive apprenticeship concepts in analysis, Ong et al. draw further conclusions about teaching and learning in the operating theatre noting that whilst a number of practices were present, reflection and articulation, for example, were not. Given the discordances between trainer and trainee perceptions, the authors argue that the full complement of teaching and learning practices associated with cognitive apprenticeship be drawn upon to help bridge this gap. They also argue that the benefits of learning in the naturalistic setting of the operating theatre be emphasized and protected. Not only is it a site that offers diverse feedback modalities, but it is a place where expert surgical judgement can be revealed. The theatre's value is not then in providing efficient and standardized learning but rather as a place, when optimized, is rich in context and where surgical judgement is exacted under uncertain conditions. The challenge to the educator then is to make surgical judgement more visible and open to contemplation by the learner.

## 35.3 How Do Experienced Surgeons Perceive and Handle Uncertainty During Challenging Intraoperative Situations [9]?

Where Ong et al. chose to focus on alignment of the teaching and learning relationship between trainers and trainees, and selected straightforward cases to guide their design, Cristancho et al. [9] focus on how experienced surgeons manage uncertainty in challenging cases. Though the latter may initially look like a study examining clinical practice and patient safety, its aim is also educational in that they wish to explore an area of expert practice, in depth, for how it might inform the training of surgeons. Like Ong et al., Cristancho et al.'s study highlights the use of theory as a means to structure and provide coherence to a qualitative research project. Both research groups also use the methods of observation and interviewing to answer their research questions and employ other qualitative strategies that have significant overlap. Whilst it is worth exploring the differences in approaches, there is merit in seeing that the overlap stems from the upholding of key tenets associated with qualitative research.

### 35.3.1 *Framing the Research Topic, Questions and Basic Design*

Cristancho et al. describe uncertainty as a dominating, inevitable feature of surgical practice and one that is weakly understood in terms of how it is perceived and handled in practice by surgeons. This lack of understanding has implications for patient safety and innovation as well as for education. Insight into how uncertainty is recognized and decision-making influenced in response, they argue, would provide surgical education with a conceptual map and list of descriptors that reveal the tacit knowledge of experts to those who are developing themselves as surgeons. The idea of making explicit the recognition and response to operative uncertainty is treated as a systemic concern by the authors, and hence, they anticipate that the conceptual map should also shed light on how the variety of decisions taken in moments of uncertainty can lead to adaptive (innovation) and maladaptive (patient safety breaches) surgical outcomes. The focus then is to highlight decision-making under uncertainty and challenge, with the findings being of relevance educationally and in practice.

Looking for conceptual frameworks of relevance takes the group outside education, to ideas of greater relevance for the problem at hand. This entails not only wide reading in, around and outside, surgical education; it benefits from lateral thinking, an idea Kneebone refers to as looking for new kinships [10]. If a surgeon sees themselves as a professional who makes frequent, complex, high-stakes decisions in the real world, they may see the world of executives as kin to their own. Organizational psychology, for one, offers a rich literature and conceptual thinking on the topic of decision-making in conditions of uncertainty (referred to as naturalistic decision-making, NDM) [11], and it is this domain that the authors use to shape their study design and bring new insights to surgical education.

The authors do not adopt a specific methodology to answer their question, taking instead what they refer to as a generic qualitative constructivist approach. Lichtman's notions [2] of qualitative research being holistic, grounded in real settings and informed by participants with knowledge of the phenomena are visible features of Cristancho et al.'s study design. The research team looks, in depth, at a particular facet of surgical practice, by observing complex operative cases selected and carried out by experienced surgeons and then talking to them about these same cases via in depth interviews.

Cristancho et al.'s study demonstrates other qualities associated with a qualitative research paradigm and design, namely, that it is flexible, can combine different approaches in different phases of the study and is iterative. An important demonstration of this flexibility is in the author's integrated use of observation and interviews. Elements of the field notes taken by the non-participant observer are used as probes to query the surgeons they interview later. This practice addresses concerns about hindsight bias because of the interview's retrospective nature. The specific interview technique they employ, critical decision-making [12], accommodates generation of question probes in this way and is coherent conceptually with NDM. Together the selection and combination of specific methods in the study design serve to enrich the quality of the data gathered.

### 35.3.2 Use of Theory

Cristancho et al.'s study draws on both psychologic and social theories around decision-making to frame the research, in particular, NDM. Lipshitz and Strauss's [11] NDM describes decision-making in uncertainty as featuring:

- An inadequate understanding of a situation
- Incomplete information
- Conflicting alternatives

Though their model emanates from a different domain, its concepts are recognizable to the world of surgical decision-making. Beyond this framing function, principles from NDM are used at subsequent stages of the study. In the analysis of their interview and observation transcript data, the researchers apply an existing template, namely, the principles of NDM above, to identify (or 'code') episodes of uncertainty. The template analysis is supplemented by inductive analysis (i.e. developing new concepts directly from the data) allowing them to 'test' the applicability of NDM in surgical practice without being hemmed in excessively by the existing theory. The inductive analysis complements and responds to the unique setting in which NDM theory is being applied, that of intraoperative decision-making in response to uncertainty.

### 35.3.3 Research Participants and Setting

Like Ong et al., Cristancho et al. employ observation and interviewing as complementary data collection tools. The study's observation component is carried out in the 'naturalistic' setting of the theatre in a single teaching hospital. The 'informants' of the phenomena are seven staff surgeons representing different specialties. Those who agreed to take part were asked to deliberately select their own difficult cases for observation on the basis that these would present multiple instances of uncertainty to examine. Participation also entailed being willing to reflect on the cases under observation. Twenty-six operative cases were examined in total, producing a large qualitative data set for analysis, and one, that some, but importantly not all, would argue, facilitates the likelihood of reaching saturation and stronger knowledge claims [13].

### 35.3.4 Role of the Researcher

Cristancho and the research team consisted of professional education researchers and surgeons who carried out distinct aspects of the study. Unlike Ong, Cristancho, an experienced researcher, but not a clinician, carried out the observations and interviews and in this sense is a non-participant researcher. Though experienced in observing operations, she would not have had the same depth of insight into what was taking place or what was being said compared to Ong in her study. The group's response to this is to build in features to mitigate the potential shortcoming of not having 'insider' knowledge and to reflect on the overall impact on the findings. In conducting the analysis, Cristancho and another education researcher carried out the initial coding of the data. The full research team, including its surgical members, then scrutinized and adjusted the resulting themes and conceptual models through discussion. Analytic findings were relayed to 'surgeon' research participants, a process known as 'member-checking'. Such measures serve as qualitative rigor checks on the researcher, and similar to the Ong et al. study, they are declared and examined by the researchers as a part of the reflexive process of undertaking qualitative research and are responsive to the particulars of the study at hand [5]. In Ong et al. seeking non-surgical perspectives from the team serves to balance the surgical views. In Cristancho et al., seeking surgical perspectives from the team and the surgical research participants achieves a similar aim by stretching analysis and interpretation in a different direction.

### 35.3.5 Bringing It All Together: Presenting the Analysis and Interpretation

Before considering the nature of the 241 'instances of uncertainty' that were identified in the 26 observed operations, it is worth not only pausing on the sheer numbers but also defining what flags up such an instance. Viewed through an NDM lens, Cristancho describes this as a moment when, 'the surgeon experienced a sense of doubt while trying to make a decision for which there was no clear "best" answer [9]'.

The analytic moves by Cristancho et al. combine findings from the NDM-driven template analysis with the more data-driven inductive analysis to produce an integrated model that elaborates and provides a descriptive surgery-specific language for the overarching themes of 'recognizing' and 'responding' to uncertainty. The subthemes they describe draw, in part, on surgical examples linked directly to the principles of NDM, whilst others fall outside it. Novel subthemes under 'responding to uncertainty' included 'prioritizing alternatives' and 'reevaluating and adapting the plan'. In the former, for example, the authors describe how surgeons contemplated action in light of balancing potential risks and benefits to the patient. They draw on the following quote from their data to illustrate the subtheme:

> So [the decision] was are we going to give him an ostomy which is the safe thing to do or are we going to remove the rest of the colon and do an anastomosis which is maybe slightly riskier but would give him a better quality of life? (S1-I16) [9]

Grounding themes in examples is an essential component of presenting qualitative results. Examples bring themes to life and contribute to transparency of analysis [2] (p301). Unlike quantitative research, the authors do not need to present similar quotes from multiple interviewees under this subtheme to prove to the reader their data is reliable and valid.

Description of what has been found, through examples, is useful but not sufficient. Qualitative researchers should also seek to interpret and derive meaning from data analysis. To this end, the authors' main themes and subthemes are woven together to produce a model that attempts to explain relationships between uncertainty in decision-making, innovation, patient safety and training. In their model, the authors argue that standardized practice might be better conceptualized as a spectrum where uncritical 'drift' in one direction could yield lapses to patient safety whilst reacting to uncertainty when standardized practice is insufficient could be considered an adaptive, and at times, innovative response.

Cristancho and colleagues' interpretation is strengthened by a host of measures described earlier but also by 'locating' their findings within wider literatures, not only around patient safety but, given the readership for the article in a medical education journal, to that of education. Whilst the study itself does not focus on education, the implications to training are prioritized and elegantly justified by linking them to educational theories related to cultivating adaptive expertise in situations of uncertainty and complexity. They argue that their study serves as a starting point for making explicit a high-level feature of expert decision-making, one that is, as they describe, often taking place at times when the theatre is at its most quiet and inscrutable for learners [9].

## 35.4 Slowing Down to Stay Out of Trouble in the Operating Room: Remaining Attentive in Automaticity [14]

A notable feature of this research question is that it is not one; rather, it is a study title. We will explore this point as part of discussing Moulton's (2010) study, one which employs grounded theory as its research methodology. The study builds on earlier work where Moulton et al. presented a model for expert judgement in surgery that continues to resonate strongly with educators and healthcare professionals for its messages about how experts adapt their thinking and behaviour to fluid and complex circumstances [15]. Its credibility was heightened by the topic it addressed, the messages it delivered and the research team, led by a surgeon who had undertaken a doctorate in education and who worked with an established and respected team of research collaborators. Though not the first study in medical education to draw on Glaser and Strauss's [16] grounded theory methodology, the 2007 article broke important ground in attracting and, consequently, familiarizing a wider community of surgeons with a powerful qualitative approach to research.

Like the inductive, constructivist methodologies employed in the Ong and Cristancho studies, grounded theory also draws on general principles upheld in qualitative research (e.g. reflexivity, naturalistic settings, purposeful sampling of research participants) as well as the common data collection methods of observation and interviewing. Where it differs, and where Lichtman [2] suggests it holds special appeal to researchers, is in its more systematic approach to design and analysis. Above these principles and processes, a key feature of grounded theory is that it aims to build explanations of complex phenomena (i.e. theory) from the ground (i.e. the data) up. This is to say that applying preconceived ideas, principles or theories to the data through, for example, coding templates, or in the phrasing of research questions or in interview prompts, as in Ong or Cristancho's studies, is not well-aligned with grounded theory. Though many well-considered critiques to this claim exist [17], grounded theory aims to let the data do the talking! For the moment put aside your misgivings that your previous knowledge about Ericsson's expertise development or Lave and Wenger's communities of practice domains might creep in to what you do in your grounded theory study. Key components for employing grounded theory include:

Theoretical sampling and saturation

> A process of choosing what to sample (e.g. interviewees, observation sites, etc.) and analysing data, alongside collecting it, until new ideas fail to appear (i.e. we claim our sample is 'saturated')

Constant-comparative method of coding

> Includes *open, axial* and *selective coding*, which are distinct albeit overlapping processes. Open coding serves as the first attempt to identify relevant categories, followed by axial coding where grouping of like categories and establishing relationships between them is undertaken. Selective coding aims to reduce the data further by identifying central categories that bring together the preceding ones. Codes derived from initial samples are compared to newly collected data to add and refine the iterative coding processes.

We will examine implementation of these processes, in brief, through the discussion of Moulton's 2010 study. Those setting out to do a grounded theory study would be wise to read up on the approach and its procedures in greater detail [18, 19].

### 35.4.1 Framing the Research Topic, Questions and Basic Design

In Moulton et al.'s 2010 follow-up study, the focus of research hinges on deeper examination of the 'slowing down' phenomena as a part of expert decision-making in areas of uncertainty. Having already described that surgeons appear to 'slow down' in response to (or in anticipation of) difficulty and do things in order to free up their cognitive resources, the 2010 study becomes a deeper examination and theorizing of the 'slowing down' phenomenon, in particular, around the switch from automated to attentive and deliberative behaviour.

The researchers again use grounded theory to evince these new concepts. In keeping with the iterative nature of grounded theory, they pick up where they left off from the 2007 interview study. The substantive addition to the study design was the inclusion of observation as a method that would contribute to the study's theoretical sampling around the phenomenon. Interviews were carried out alongside observation to explore the central theme and emergent ones in greater depth and the coding carried out through constant comparison of their growing data set.

Framing the topic on a narrower area promotes deeper investigation with the authors aiming to produce a detailed model that maps onto critical junctures in operations and the concordant behaviours associated with effortful surgical practice. Like Cristancho, an important educational aim of charting out expert practice is that it helps make explicit what expert performance consists of and thereby makes concrete what trainee surgeons should work to develop.

### 35.4.2 Use of Theory…

As the primary goal of grounded theory is to produce 'theory' from data to explain a phenomenon, views around how to 'use' existing theory around the methodology are inconsistent, even thorny. Glaser and Strauss originally suggested that clouding one's thoughts with existing theory through carrying out a literature review in advance would interfere with the generation of new theory [20]. Critics reject this 'blank slate' view, along with many other tenets of grounded theory, arguing it is folly to think one can put aside existing beliefs, knowledge, and values to allow one to 'survey the data unencumbered by the grip of those beliefs' [17]. Rather than pretend oneself out of existence, it would be better to acknowledge how other ideas and one's values sensitize one to the current research and put limits to what one can claim as being novel. Though difficult to know what stance Moulton's research team took, given the study followed related work, it seems more likely the group operated with such sensitizing ideas in mind and that were presented in their introduction and returned to in the discussion.

## 35.4.3 Research Participants and Setting

Moulton's theoretical sampling consists of different elements that, combined, illuminate the phenomenon more clearly. As we will explain below, some of this sampling is aimed at gathering diverse views (e.g. by including different hospitals, interviewing surgeons from a range of specialties), some at drilling down on strong or well-developed views and some at heightening what could be observed. In the main interviewing phase of the study, 28 surgeons, known for having expert judgement, and coming from a range of specialties, were interviewed. Eight of these were interviewed again because of strong views they had expressed rejecting the claim that surgeons operated on 'autopilot'. Following up on these eight participants in this way aids the researchers in expanding on the phenomena of interest and again reflects the iterative and flexible nature of grounded theory, in particular, and qualitative research, in general. Design is not set in stone, and it is this ability to respond to what happens during data collection through sampling of extreme, deviant or unexpected views that allows for deeper insights to be uncovered [21].

Observations were completed for 29 operations, across 4 hospital sites, but from a single area of specialty practice, hepatopancreatobiliary surgery (HPB). These operations were performed by five HPB surgeons who were not involved in the first set of interviews in an attempt to have their performance not be influenced by ideas from the study. Some of these surgeons were also interviewed after the observations took place. One surgeon took a particular interest in the phenomenon, noted as a 'key informant' by the research team, and provided additional interviews and participated in the coding and emerging theory being developed by the research team. Interacting with research subjects may seem peculiar and undesirable in a quantitative paradigm, but as described earlier, the qualitative paradigm's view of knowledge as being co-constructed makes this practice coherent, even sensible, provided it is accounted for through quality measures such as those noted in Table 35.1.

## 35.4.4 Role of the Researcher

Of special note for this study, the HPB surgeons chosen for observation were from the same specialty and were possibly colleagues of the lead investigator. The interviews and observations were carried out by both her and a research assistant (who had an anthropology background and was further 'trained' by the lead investigator to carry out intraoperative observations in the specific specialty); the rationale for this choice was likely aimed at gleaning the maximum amount of meaning from the setting whilst working pragmatically around the resources available. As in the Ong and Cristancho studies, multiple instances of cross-checking the coding and emerging concepts were carried out amongst the two lead researchers and the whole research team to refine and challenge analysis. In addition to taking coding regularly to the research team, other measures, such as keeping an audit trail and engaging in reflexivity, serve to heighten the quality of the research and mitigate unhelpful bias in the research (Table 35.1).

### 35.4.5 Bringing It All Together: Presenting the Analysis and Interpretation

By drilling down into a specific area with more targeted interviews, making comparisons with observation data, employing a strategic sampling approach and working with a 'key informant', Moulton et al. developed a model to further explain the phenomena of automaticity in the operating theatre. They describe a 'spectrum' of behaviour associated with moving from 'automatic' to 'attentive' modes of practice in response to situational cues and enacted, they argue, to free up cognitive resources and redirect attention. Responses, ranging from complete stoppage of a procedure to removing distractions, to more subtle 'fine-tuning', and to 'drifting off', were described. The authors and surgeons interviewed make an important distinction between acting in an unthinking, automatic mode and engaging in what the researchers call 'baseline surveillance'.

Grounded theory's methodologic features provided tools for the researchers to better investigate the phenomenon and add an important dimension to their analysis. Through 'theoretical sampling' the team not only delves deeper into the topic of 'staying attentive'; it drives the sampling of 'extreme' views, in this case, surgeons who strongly deny working on autopilot. The notion of engaging in 'baseline surveillance' is useful and may help individuals rationalize and defend their behaviour, but it is not the full story. In examining the interview themes against the behaviour observed in theatre, Moulton et al. produce a more balanced, insightful account that questions what individuals can or are willing to see in their practice.

From this analysis, implications for learning follow. Educators should make explicit the situations and resulting adaptive behaviours that lead experts to change their intraoperative approach. Doing so would serve to model constructive metacognitive behaviour associated with expert surgical judgement as well as highlight potentially unhelpful or unsafe behaviours associated with 'drifting off'.

## 35.5 Final Thoughts

Qualitative research seeks to better understand relationships in the complex social world where values and beliefs vary and are of consequence. There are many ways to go about undertaking research in this paradigm, as is demonstrated, but are by no means limited to the differing approaches taken in the three examples above (Box 35.1) [22]. Regardless of the particular methodology, several ideas underpin them: the role of interpretation, gaining understanding through deliberate and deep

**Box 35.1 Five qualitative methodologies described by Creswell [22] with references of surgical and health professional education studies**

**1. Narrative research**

Gordon LJ, Rees CE, Ker JS, Cleland J. Leadership and followership in the healthcare workplace: exploring medical trainees' experiences through narrative inquiry. BMJ Open. 2015 Dec 1;5(12):e008898. doi: https://doi.org/10.1136/bmjopen-2015-008898

Bleakley, A. (2005). Stories as data, data as stories: making sense of narrative inquiry in clinical education. *Medical Education, 39,* 534–540

**2. Phenomenological research**

Tseng, W. T., & Lin, Y. P. (2016). "Detached concern" of medical students in a cadaver dissection course: A phenomenological study. *Anat Sci Educ, 9*(3), 265–271. doi:https://doi.org/10.1002/ase.1579

Pinto, A., Faiz, O., Bicknell, C., & Vincent, C. (2013). Surgical complications and their implications for surgeons' well-being. *Br J Surg, 100*(13), 1748–1755. doi:https://doi.org/10.1002/bjs.9308

**3. Grounded Theory research**

Apramian, T., Watling, C., Lingard, L., & Cristancho, S. (2015). Adaptation and innovation: a grounded theory study of procedural variation in the academic surgical workplace. *J Eval Clin Pract, 21*(5), 911–918. doi:https://doi.org/10.1111/jep.12398

Apramian, T., Cristancho, S., Watling, C., Ott, M., & Lingard, L. (2016). "They Have to Adapt to Learn": Surgeons' Perspectives on the Role of Procedural Variation in Surgical Education. *J Surg Educ, 73*(2), 339–347. doi:https://doi.org/10.1016/j.jsurg.2015.10.016

Moulton, C., Regehr, G., Lingard, L., Merritt, C., & MacRae, H. (2010). Slowing down to stay out of trouble in the operating room: Remaining attentive in automaticity. *Academic Medicine, 85*(10), 1571–1577

**4. Ethnographic research**

Cleland, J., Walker, K. G., Gale, M., & Nicol, L. G. (2016). Simulation-based education: understanding the socio-cultural complexity of a surgical training 'boot camp'. *Med Educ, 50*(8), 829–841. doi:https://doi.org/10.1111/medu.13064

Lingard, L., Espin, S., Rubin, B., Whyte, S., Colmenares, M., Baker, G. R., ... Reznick, R. (2005). Getting teams to talk: development and pilot implementation of a checklist to promote interprofessional communication in the OR. *Quality & Safety in Health Care, 14*(5), 340–346.

**5. Case Study Research (in addition to Ong et al. [3])**

Quinn, E. M., Cantillon, P., Redmond, H. P., & Bennett, D. (2014). Surgical journal club as a community of practice: a case study. *J Surg Educ, 71*(4), 606-612. doi:https://doi.org/10.1016/j.jsurg.2013.12.009

Source: Creswell [22]

exploration of natural settings and perspectives of people who 'operate' in them, reflecting on one's role as a researcher and, generally speaking, seeking coherence over proof. Accepting these premises is not straightforward. Engaging with them often introduces a new type of uncertainty for novice educational researchers, leaving them unclear as to when they have 'done enough' and 'well enough' to warrant stopping data collection or to believe they have developed a valid interpretation from the findings. Though this guidance came in response to a question about how to know whether 'saturation' had been achieved, the response from Mayan [23] is reassuring to new educational researchers and goes beyond this:

> There comes a point when you believe you can say something about the phenomena, in whatever form you choose (e.g. art, performance, text). You keep going until you are convinced you can do this. (p. 64) [23]

Engaging in qualitative research for the sake of understanding learning, teaching and education in ways that are different to familiar positivist, empirical research approaches can be a significant challenge but one that offers major potential for personal growth as a surgical educator. Wrapped up in many years of immersion in the biomedical sciences and its beliefs about knowledge and how it is generated and trusted, it is no surprise that amending these values is not easily accomplished and can evoke rather strong (sometimes negative) reactions on initial exposure. Solely as a pragmatic step, engaging in qualitative research can help you diversify your research and appraisal skills in a different research paradigm. If, through engagement, you also expand your views of how and where 'legitimate' knowledge is generated, then this epistemologic shift stands to have a greater impact, one that we would argue can also feed into your practice as an educator and clinician. In this respect, you may also add new layers to your identity as researcher, teacher and surgeon.

## References

1. Denzin, N., & Lincoln, Y. (2005). Introduction: The discipline and practice of qualitative research. In *The Sage handbook of qualitative research* (3rd ed., pp. 1–32). Thousand Oaks: Sage.
2. Lichtman, M. (2013). *Qualitative research in education: A user's guide* (3rd ed.). Thousand Oaks: Sage.
3. Ong, C. C., Dodds, A., & Nestel, D. (2016). Beliefs and values about intra-operative teaching and learning: A case study of surgical teachers and trainees. *Advances in Health Sciences Education: Theory and Practice, 21*(3), 587–607.
4. Yin, R. K. (2003). *Case study research: Design and methods* (3rd ed.). Thousand Oaks: Sage.
5. Lincoln, Y. S., & Guba, E. G. (1985). *Naturalistic inquiry*. Newbury Park: Sage.
6. (cited in Ong)Lave, J., & Wenger, E. (1991). *Situated learning: Legitimate peripheral participation*. New York: Cambridge University Press.
7. (cited in Ong)Collins, A., Brown, J. S., & Holum, A. (1991). Cognitive apprenticeship: Making thinking visible. *American Educator, 15*(6–11), 38–46.
8. Lingard, L. (2015). Joining a conversation: The problem/gap/hook heuristic. *Perspectives on Medical education., 4*(5), 252–253.

9. Cristancho, S. M., Apramian, T., Vanstone, M., Lingard, L., Ott, M., & Novick, R. J. (2013). Understanding clinical uncertainty: What is going on when experienced surgeons are not sure what to do? *Academic Medicine, 88*(10), 1516–1521.
10. Kneebone, R. (2016). Simulation reframed. *Advances in Simulation, 1*, 27. https://doi.org/10.1186/s41077-016-0028-8.
11. Lipshitz, R., & Strauss, O. (1997). Coping with uncertainty: A naturalistic decision-making analysis. *Organizational Behavior and Human Decision Processes, 69*, 149–163.
12. (cited in Cristancho)Crandall, B., Klein, G. A., & Hoffman, R. R. (2006). *Working minds: A practitioner's guide to cognitive task analysis.* Cambridge, MA: MIT Press.
13. Baker, S. E., Edwards, R., & Doidge, M. (2012). How many qualitative interviews is enough? Expert voices and early career reflections on sampling and cases in qualitative research. In: *Research and enterprise.* University of Brighton. http://eprints.brighton.ac.uk/11632. Accessed 14 Sept 2017.
14. Moulton, C. A., Regehr, G., Lingard, L., Merritt, C., & MacRae, H. (2010). Slowing down to stay out of trouble in the operating room: Remaining attentive in automaticity. *Academic Medicine, 85*(10), 1571–1577.
15. Moulton, C. A., Regehr, G., Mylopoulos, M., & MacRae, H. M. (2007). Slowing down when you should: A new model of expert judgment. *Academic Medicine, 82*(10 Suppl), S109–S116.
16. Strauss, A. (1998). *Basics of qualitative research: Techniques and procedures for developing grounded theory.* London: Sage.
17. Thomas, G., & James, D. (2006). Reinventing grounded theory: Some questions about theory, ground and discovery. *British Educational Research Journal, 32*(6), 767–795.
18. Charmaz, K. (2006). *Constructing grounded theory: A practical guide through qualitative analysis.* Thousand Oaks: Sage.
19. Watling, C. J., & Lingard, L. (2012). Grounded theory in medical education research: AMEE Guide No. 70. *Medical Teacher, 34*(10), 850–861.
20. Glaser, B. G., & Strauss, A. L. (1967). *The discovery of grounded theory: Strategies for qualitative research.* Chicago: Aldine Transaction.
21. Patton, M. Q. (2002). *Qualitative research and evaluation methods* (3rd ed.). Thousand Oaks: Sage.
22. Creswell, J. (2013). *Qualitative inquiry and research design: Choosing among five approaches* (3rd ed.). Thousand Oaks: Sage.
23. Mayan, M. (2009). *Essentials of qualitative inquiry.* Walnut Creek: Left Coast Press.

## Further Reading

Braun, V., & Clarke, V. (2013). *Successful qualitative research: A practical guide for beginners.* London: Sage.
Charmaz, K. (2014). *Constructing grounded theory: A practical guide through qualitative analysis* (2nd ed.). London: Sage.
Creswell, J. (2012). *Educational research: Planning, conducting, and evaluating quantitative and qualitative research* (4th ed.). Boston: Pearson.
Creswell, J. (2013). *Qualitative inquiry and research design: Choosing among five approaches* (3rd ed.). Thousand Oaks: Sage.
Miles, M., Huberman, A., & Saldana, J. (2014). *Qualitative data analysis: A methods sourcebook* (3rd ed.). Los Angeles: Sage.
A valuable website on resources for qualitative research methods is: https://www.methodspace.com/resources/methods-links/links-qualitative-research-methods-and-analysis/

# Chapter 36
# Ethical Issues in Surgical Education Research

**Martyn Kingsbury**

**Overview** This chapter introduces some elements of moral philosophy in order to contextualise the ethical review process and provide a framework for the ethical consideration necessary to successfully negotiate ethical review and be an ethical researcher. Given its complexity and lack of consistency, it is impossible to provide unequivocal pragmatic advice suitable for local ethical review processes. However, this chapter discusses ethical issues inherent in some research approaches and considers the three ethical principles of respect for persons, beneficence and justice and the common ethical issues of confidentiality, consent, power and positionality. There are seldom simple answers when considering such issues, and the chapter also includes short vignettes to facilitate the reflective deliberation of ethical issues and how they might be addressed in the conduct of educational research practice.

## 36.1 Introduction

Ethics can be complicated. It may be considered in a general philosophical sense: the various codes and constructs of moral philosophy that debate ethical questions in order to address the very broad question of how one should behave in society. It can also be considered on a more personal level; 'What are the set of concepts and principles that guide me?' At this level it is sometimes conflated with morality or the moral principles of a particular tradition and with behaving in accordance with social conventions, religious beliefs and the law. Finally, ethics may be considered as the procedural, regulatory 'gate keeping' process required before undertaking research. Detailed consideration of the moral philosophy of ethics at a general or personal level is outside the scope of this chapter, and while the regulatory procedures of ethical review process may seem more pragmatically useful, the various

M. Kingsbury (✉)
Educational Development Unit, Imperial College London, London, UK
e-mail: m.kingsbury@imperial.ac.uk

processes are by no means universal. This chapter will therefore discuss some relevant ethical issues that need consideration in order to be an ethical researcher and successfully negotiate ethical review. The chapter will introduce some moral philosophy but only to contextualise the ethical review process and provide a framework for ethical thinking. For those who want a little more information, the ethics textbook by Noel Stewart provides a straightforward and very approachable introduction to moral philosophy [1]. Given that there are seldom simple answers when considering ethical issues in research and much depends on a careful consideration of the issues in context, the chapter also includes short vignettes to facilitate the reflective consideration of some ethical issues.

## 36.2 What Is Ethics?

The word 'ethics' is derived from the Greek noun êthos meaning 'character' or 'disposition' and is defined in the dictionary both as the moral principles that govern a person's behaviour or conduct and as the branch of knowledge that deals with those moral principles. In this chapter, I adopt a more pragmatic view of ethics as the common human ability to think about ethical problems rather than viewing it through the lens of any particular moral philosophy or theory. As bioethicist Larry Churchill wrote: 'Ethics, understood as the capacity to think critically about moral values and direct our actions in terms of such values, is a generic human capacity' [2].

Thinking about research ethics is 'situated', a consideration of the relative ethical costs/benefits of an issue in a particular context. What should I do? The various ethical theories and moral philosophies are more about thinking about ethics in a general way. What does society find acceptable, and what framework is useful for testing and explaining that? I briefly consider three broad approaches to moral philosophy that inform the principles of research ethics and the ethical approval process. Some understanding of these philosophical traditions may also help individual researchers frame their thinking when planning and performing research and lend a more informed perspective to decision making.

## 36.3 Utilitarianism

At its simplest, utilitarianism examines the foreseeable consequences of any action and judges on the utility of these consequences. An action is considered in terms of its possible consequences, and one attempts to maximise benefit and minimise harm. In this philosophical tradition, the actual act is inherently neither good nor bad but judged purely on its outcomes. While actions may potentially result in both benefit and harm, they are judged in terms of what gives the maximum 'net benefit' to the majority. Thus, it may be considered ethically 'right' to harm one person in order to benefit many.

The difficulty is knowing how to define and 'measure' the relative benefits and harms. How does one judge the utility? Are benefit and harm considered in terms of happiness, pleasure, material gain or a combination of such things? If they are by some combination, what is the relative worth of the component factors? Similarly, while the idea of an optimum 'net benefit' for the majority is a relatively easy concept, whose benefit counts or counts more? One also has to be careful to consider as many foreseeable consequences as possible and perhaps to form some contingency for unforeseen outcomes.

Despite these difficulties, utilitarianism does have a degree of practical commonsense appeal. When considering research, contemplating the consequence of actions and attempting to minimise harm and maximise benefit for the majority and justifying the decision whether to weigh the judgement in terms of particular outcomes or stakeholders is a reasonable approach to deliberating the ethical implications.

## 36.4 Deontology

In contrast to the 'end justifies the means' approach of utilitarianism, in deontology, acts are considered intrinsically right or wrong, irrespective of motivation or consequence. This philosophy hypothesises that there are certain things a 'purely rational agent' will always do, to do otherwise would mean they were not rational. It is a system based on categorical imperatives and the universal principle that every person has equal value and deserves equal consideration. Thus, if the act of harming an individual is 'wrong', it is 'wrong' no matter what the motivation and no matter whether the individual or many others benefit as a result of that act. The act of harm is in itself 'wrong'.

Deontology is often criticised for overemphasising rationality and the freedom to do what reason dictates. It is a system based on 'universal laws' and takes no notice of context of the freedom or power of individuals to act. It is arguable that this approach lends itself better to consider the more absolute world of scientific research rather than the contextual and relativistic world of educational research. Despite these criticisms this philosophy has led to the prima facie assumption of beneficence (doing good), non-maleficence (not doing harm), justice (being fair) and fidelity (being truthful). These principles underlie most ethics processes and are a good basis for an ethical approach to any research.

## 36.5 Virtue Ethics

While both deontology and utilitarianism are action orientated, that is to say it is the actions or their potential implications that are judged, virtue ethics is agent based. In virtue ethics, rather than assessing the action or its consequences, it is the person acting that is the basis of the ethical decision. Virtue ethics considers our motivations and simply requires that we try to be a 'good' person and act accordingly. Specific virtues and a definition of good or bad are less important than our efforts to become good and act accordingly. Thus, a person sincerely seeking to be virtuous and do 'good' is acting ethically even if the consequences are unintentionally harmful.

The strengths and weaknesses of this philosophy largely both stem from the fact that 'virtue' is not defined. This allows the philosophy to be readily adapted to context and different cultural perspectives but also leads to criticism for being vague. Virtue ethics recognises that an individual's capacity to act virtuously in an ethical manner depends on upbringing, opportunity and education, which together form our 'character'. The role of guides and role models is also important in supporting the development of appropriate virtuous behaviour. The explicit importance of education in this ethical philosophy makes it of interest to educationalists, and many educational ethics review processes seek to not only act as a gatekeeper for appropriate ethical behaviour but also as a guide to encourage researchers to behave in a virtuous way.

## 36.6 Theories of Ethics

While deontology and utilitarianism have been influential in informing ethical thinking and the principles of research ethics guidance and many ethical approval processes, virtue ethics have provided a flexible way of considering ethics in contexts that are challenging when restricted by the more formalised codes. There are other theoretical perspectives that are relevant. There is a rights-based approach that postulates ethical behaviour is about respecting the rights of individuals, such as the right to liberty, equality and privacy, which apply equally to everyone and should not be removed by an individual or by society. There is also a care-based ethical approach that relies on caring for others and maintaining a caring network of relationships with a reciprocal obligation for cooperation, empathy and compassion. Finally, there are Foucauldian ethics that recognise that knowledge has both ethical and power dynamics and that, in research, the perception of power is mobile and modifiable and is often crucial to ethical behaviour. Foucault therefore considered 'truthful speaking' as being central to ethical behaviour [3].

This consideration of ethical theories and philosophical approaches is necessarily brief with the intention of informing the rest of the chapter and framing the consideration of the later vignettes. A fuller but approachable consideration of these ideas can be found in ethics textbooks and the peer-reviewed, scholarly online resource *The Internet Encyclopaedia of Philosophy* (ISSN:2161-0002).

## 36.7 Ethics Approval Processes

The Belmont Report [4] is generally regarded as the first formalising guidelines for research with human subjects and still forms the primary research ethics framework in the USA. Although focussed on biomedical and behavioural research, the principles and procedures generated from this report have been applied in Social Science research, including education. The three ethical principles, 'respect for persons', 'beneficence' and 'justice', and the three key processes, 'informed consent', 'risk/benefit assessment' and 'selection of subjects', form, with some modification, the basis for human research ethics across the English-speaking world. However the scope and application of these commonly accepted principles vary considerably. In Australia, the National Health and Medical Research Council has national responsibility for ethical guidelines across all disciplines and for regulating the research ethics committees that apply them. In contrast, in the UK, there is no cross-disciplinary ethical body, and different disciplinary professional associations have their own guidelines. For education, the British Educational Research Association (BERA) guidelines are often used, but British Sociological Association or the Social Research Association guidelines may be equally valid. Furthermore, not all countries have such comprehensive ethical guidelines, and even with those that do, the implementation of the codes and ethics review processes varies between discipline areas and between institutional committees and processes.

In some circumstances educational research is considered using the same criteria and processes as used for human biomedical research, where the risks are arguably considerably greater. This can lead to an unnecessarily heavy administrative burden and prolonged process. Committees more familiar with reviewing scientific biomedical studies can tend to favour a deontological approach with its 'logic' and 'universal rules' and often take a consequentialist stance to examining risk and benefit. This can lead to misunderstanding, inconsistent advice and poor recommendation when considering more contextual and nuanced educational studies, particularly those taking a less fixed and systematic, context-specific ethnographic approach [5]. Equally unhelpfully, such scientific, biomedical focussed institutional review processes can dismiss educational research as evaluation or of insufficient 'risk' to warrant ethical review. While this may not seem problematic, work then fails to benefit from robust ethical review and may struggle to find a publisher, who are increasingly demanding evidence of ethical review. Perhaps more typically, research with human participants is considered with a stratified approach to review depending on perceived risk. Thus 'high-risk' studies such as clinical trials or educational studies that focus on sensitive issues or vulnerable groups are subject to full review at institutional or national level. Lower 'risk' studies, more typical of educational research, are subjected to expedited panel review or if 'low risk' perhaps online review rather than full committee consideration.

In addition to appropriate ethical review, there may also be additional gatekeeping processes aimed at management awareness and approval for access to institutions and potential participants. Examples include medical school approval processes for access to medical students and National Health Service management approval for studies involving hospital premises and staff. Such bureaucratic processes are often required for access and institutional insurance cover.

This complexity and lack of clear, pedagogically appropriate ethical review processes have led some to question the utility of ethical review in qualitative pedagogic research [5–8]. However, in addition to addressing issues of public accountability and moral, social and legal responsibility, a robust, fair and appropriate ethical review process promotes good research [9].

Given its complexity and lack of consistency, it is impossible to provide unequivocal pragmatic advice for local ethical review processes. However, researchers would be wise to consider the following questions:

- What are the local ethical review processes, practices, expectations and deadlines?
- Is the research question clearly articulated and aligned with research methods to provide answers?
- Is there access to appropriate participants, and has inclusion of any vulnerable groups been minimised, justified and described?
- What are the risks and benefits; are they appropriately described in ethics process and research documentation?
- Is the research designed to protect participants, minimise risks and maximise benefits in an ethically appropriate way?

The answers to these questions should be carefully considered and clearly articulated; they will likely form the basis for ethical review AND for good research.

## 36.8 Ethical Issues

Given the complexity of ethical review, it may be tempting to view the process as an 'administrative hurdle' in tension with research. But by considering basic ethical issues and managing the review process in good time, the ethical process is integrated with and facilitates good quality research.

All ethical review processes are essentially a 'risk/benefit' exercise. While educational research is unlikely to result in physical risk, pain or harm, there may potentially be psychological harm such as embarrassment, loss of self-esteem, guilt or depression. These can be transitory or potentially longer lasting or recurring. There is also potentially the risk of a less than optimal educational experience and reduced 'learning' for either participants or for others not involved in the research. Even if these risks do not feature, there are always risks associated with the time commitment for both participants and researchers. All risks must be minimised and balanced with the potential educational benefits arising from the research, thus the quality of the research should be maximised so as, at the very least, the time of those involved is not wasted.

## 36.9 Research Design

The choice of topic, formulation of a hypothesis or research question and the methodological approach taken are not politically or ethically neutral decisions. The US, UK and Irish governments, amongst others, have all promoted a more 'evidence-based' educational research and have favoured more quantitative, randomised, controlled trial approaches. Goldacre commissioned by the UK government to write a report on experimental methods within education [10] noted:

'Where they are feasible, randomised trials are generally the most reliable tool we have for finding out which of two interventions works best' (p26). A randomised controlled trial design may also prove more publishable in medical and scientific journals where editors and reviewers are more familiar with the approach. Indeed, Ellis comments that researchers using qualitative approaches are more likely to have the quality of their research called into question by research ethics committees more familiar with a quantitative paradigm [11].

A quantitative or mixed-methods approach following a randomised controlled trial design comparing educational interventions can be ethically appropriate if well aligned with the research question. Consider, are there observable outcomes that can be measured and controlled? Is there an 'honest ignorance' of benefit between interventions? Or, does the situation lend itself to a crossover design where groups experience interventions at different times? (Although care must be taken that delayed access to the more 'effective' does not disadvantage participants). Are there relatively large numbers of representative subjects that can be randomly assigned to

> **Vignette 1**
> Julie is a surgical trainee doing a part-time Master's in education. She is contemplating a research project about how surgeons 'learn from their mistakes' and thinking of interviewing colleagues from her specialty who have been through a disciplinary process and/or a significant delay in their training progression. As recruitment may be challenging, she will attempt to recruit nationally from her specialty and will interview participants in their local hospitals for convenience. Time is limited as her project deadline is looming.
>
> **Consider:**
> *What are the likely issues that may make ethical approval difficult?*
> *How may the research be reframed to minimise these issues?*

groups? The most appropriate approach ethically, and in terms of research quality, is to align the methods with the research question and context. If the research question is answerable in terms that are measureable and there is appropriate access to subjects, then a quantitative design may be best. However, in education, measurable outcomes are often limited, data is context dependent and subjective and therefore qualitative approaches are often preferable.

While it is helpful to be mindful of the local ethical review process [12], '… the choice of research methods should not be driven by assumptions about the priorities and preferences of research ethics committees' (p67). Ultimately research quality and ethics are not well served by compromising research design to appease a potentially poorly informed ethics review process. It is the researchers' responsibility to put a clearly evidenced justification of their chosen methods and how they are aligned to their research question(s) and context to the ethical review process [12]. It is the research ethics committee's responsibility to facilitate good research with appropriately informed expert review and constructive feedback. That said, it is normally more efficient to get this 'right' first time rather than engage in an extended dialogue with the ethics committee process.

## 36.10 Action Research

Action research, where practitioners research their own practice, has become increasingly common and is often a starting point for those new to educational research, especially those bridging practitioner and educational roles. In action research, researchers have multiple roles, surgeon (practitioner), educator and researcher; inevitably one has to acknowledge and use these relationship(s) to gain insight and depth and thus power and validity. However researching one's own practice, students or colleagues means this has to explicitly acknowledge this position and carefully consider the complexity of power relationships [13].

## 36.11 Research Location

The location of educational research is often determined by the research question. While action research and ethnographic studies are normally co-located with the practice under investigation, there may be some choice of location. This choice is not neutral; it may exacerbate or mitigate power relationships and influence subjects and data. Location may affect ease of participation and thus influence recruitment and time commitment and potentially impact participant and researcher safety. Researchers have an ethical obligation to protect themselves and their subjects and collect data in a way that maximises validity and quality. Pragmatic issues such as the ability to protect privacy and record data also have to be considered. These issues have to be 'balanced'; for example, while a public space may be safer and more neutral, it may limit privacy and the ability to record an interview.

Locating research in the virtual space of the internet can be an attractive option. Increased technology-enhanced learning provides opportunity to use metrics of technology engagement. This can provide useful data and a safe and anonymous space; however there are potential issues of data reliability and quality. The abstract nature of such metrics may imply levels of accuracy and fidelity that, while they might be accurate for interaction with the technology, are only a surrogate measure of the learning. Also, while some data on the internet may be regarded as being public, there are ethical issues concerning identity and privacy. In the virtual space of the internet, people may not be who they claim or appear to be, it can be hard to interpret context, and consent processes are challenging [14].

## 36.12 Informed Consent

Informed consent is one of the chief ways that researchers can ensure 'respect for persons'. The decision whether to participate in the research should be based on adequate knowledge of the research in a format that is accessible and in sufficient detail to allow the decision to be informed. This decision should be voluntary without overwhelming incentives or fear of adverse consequences should they decline. Individuals should be competent to choose freely and, where possible, have the right to withdraw without penalty. Such informed, voluntary consent empowers participants and is key in most human research ethics codes.

While free, informed consent is a fundamental ethical principle; it is socially situated and may not be as simple in educational research as it may appear. In educational research the researcher may also be a teacher and/or practitioner; the relationship between them and their participants can be complex, each potentially having multiple identities with multiple responsibilities. Participants may perceive incentives or penalties that do not exist, even with full, clear information, and this may influence both participation and data.

There may be further complexity associated with particular methods. As previously mentioned, consent can be problematic online where identity can be uncertain. There can also be ambiguity in the distinction between private and public in the online space making consent less clear when, for example, using data from blogs or social networking. Informed consent can also be challenging in ethnographic educational research. Typically this involves observation, recording and interpretation of 'normal' behaviour in social context. Informed consent in advance in such circumstances may alter behaviour and invalidate data. Even where this is not an issue, it can be difficult to gain informed consent when it is often not possible to know in advance which aspects of language or behaviour will prove significant and become 'data'.

Given the complexity of educational research, particularly with ethnographic and action research methods, it may be appropriate to limit disclosure or take retrospective consent and allow withdrawal where, for example, fully informed consent may invalidate data or where the process of consenting may limit educational benefit (perhaps simply by taking time away from a valuable educational resource or opportunity). There is also a need for provision for appropriate implied consent, for example, by returning a voluntary survey. In all circumstances the process should be clearly explained and justified in ethics applications.

## 36.13 Power and Positionality

Educational research is almost always characterised by a status-power differential. Even if the research does not cross any obvious hierarchy, the roles of researcher and subject set up a power differential. While it could be argued that the subject holds the power in an interview as they choose what to say, the researcher exerts the ultimate control in interpreting and disseminating the data.

Researching with extreme power differentials such as when using the vulnerable, children or patients as subjects can be fraught with ethical concerns and usually necessitates a full review process. But in all cases where the balance of power lies with the researcher, it is particularly important to ensure participation is truly voluntary with no real or perceived coercion or obligation, perhaps using a neutral third party for recruitment. However the issues do not end with recruitment; power imbalance can influence data collection with participants being eager to please and win favour or being reluctant to criticise for fear of reprisal.

There are also potential ethical implications of a power gradient in the other direction. There can be risks to the researcher if they appear critical or take an opposing stance to senior figures. Power imbalances in this direction can also inhibit recruitment and influence data as a relatively junior researcher may be inhibited from probing a more senior subject's response or may lack the context to interpret the data.

A power imbalance in either direction can inhibit the process of gaining trust and establishing rapport with subjects, and this can limit data collection in interview situations. Researching one's own peer group may also raise ethical issues as it can make it difficult to establish the appropriate roles of researcher and subject and lead to assumptions when providing and interpreting data.

Power is not just a function of seniority; there are issues of relative power and positionality associated with age, gender, class, ethnicity, role, etc.; and these may interact to produce complex relationships. The key in terms of ethics is to acknowledge these issues and be clear how recruitment, data collection and interpretation are managed to mitigate their influence and how trust and rapport are established to facilitate quality data collection.

> **Vignette 2**
> Consider once again Julie, a surgical trainee doing a part-time Master's in education. She is contemplating the methods of her project for her ethics form. She wonders whether to exclude colleagues she works with, although she thinks they may be easier to recruit to the study. To make things easier for participants and maximise recruitment, she plans to conduct her interviews anywhere at their convenience. As all her potential participants will be more senior than her, she does not think she has any power relationships to worry about.
>
> **Consider:**
> *How might you advise her regarding:*
> *Who she recruits to her research?*
> *Where she conducts her interviews?*
> *Possible power relationships with more senior participants?*

## 36.14 Data Analysis and Dissemination

One's ethical obligations do not end with successful ethical review prior to research. Researchers have an ethical obligation to honestly obtain, manage, analyse and disseminate their data. Many national educational research associations, including those of Australia (AARE) and the UK (BERA), offer guidance on ethical educational data management. This is also covered in more detail in well-known educational research textbooks and in Brooks et al.'s excellent book on ethics and educational research [12].

In essence, the advice is for good research practice; researchers should not falsify data and be careful and transparent, paying attention to the limitations of methods and data. While intentional misrepresentation may be rare, research and ethical integrity demands consideration. While a researcher is required to analyse, interpret and present data, care has to be taken not to 'trim' data excluding 'outliers' that do not seem to 'fit' the hypothesis or exaggerate by selectively reporting those that do. Often this is considered less problematic in quantitative approaches where data and statistics 'speak for themselves'. However, reductivist graphical and statistical representation can be manipulated to fit a hypothesis or argument. The choice of analysis and representation can significantly colour an argument. Consider a study on a group of surgeons, a minority of whom are very experienced, reporting the mean number of years' experience will give a different impression than reporting the median or mode, and imply the whole group is more experienced than it is. Qualitative research has distinctive ethical demands in interpreting and presenting data. Even a modest interview-based study may produce many hundreds of pages of transcript. This cannot simply be described or graphically summarised; an appropriate analysis framework should be employed, and great care taken when choosing and framing quotes to represent the data. While picking an extreme but notable quote and claiming it is representative of all the data would be dishonest and unethical, using the same quote but explaining it illustrates the 'extreme' of views expressed in eight of ten interviews would be ethically acceptable, and better research.

## 36.15 Confidentiality

Protecting research participants' anonymity is a fundamental ethical principle and vital to show 'respect for persons'. However there can be tensions between this and data analysis, interpretation and dissemination. Confidentiality both protects the identity of participants and helps ensure full and honest data collection, but it requires attention throughout the research. The process for collecting, storing, interpreting and disseminating data while maintaining confidentiality has to be considered and communicated to participants. While collecting anonymous data from an online survey is relatively easy, interpretation can be limited by the difficulty in contextualising the information. In contrast, in an interview the context can be explored, but anonymity is more difficult. Whereas transcripts can be anonymised, this is often impossible with the raw recorded data. While all data should be treated with respect and stored securely, special care must be taken with data where individuals are identifiable. Keys to anonymisation should be kept secure, separate from the raw data which should be destroyed as soon as it has been transcribed (although all data may have to be securely stored until after assessment for student projects). It is technically harder to anonymise video or pictorial data, and care must be taken using published text where the original source and therefore identity can be determined even from redacted text using simple online search engines.

There is often a tension between retaining appropriate contextual detail to aid data interpretation and anonymisation. Pseudonyms can be used to retain say gender and ethnicity and give required context, and specific data can be replaced with carefully generalised information. For example, a hospital name replaced by just enough pertinent information, say, 'a large, teaching hospital'. However, care must be taken as it may be possible to deduce identity. Removing all clues to identity distorts data and can make it difficult for readers to contextualise and therefore interpret quotes and information. The quality and depth of reported data and the ease with which it may be interpreted have to be balanced with the risk to participants' identity, and this justified and explained to potential participants and in any ethics application.

Usually, the concern is protecting the identity of participants, but researchers also have to consider that participants may want to be identifiable. For example, a hospital may want to be associated with a study highlighting innovative practice or a company identifiable in a study about teaching using their product. This may be appropriate, but such identification may risk the research being regarded as partisan. While it is a researcher's obligation to report findings accurately, in qualitative research there may be more than one interpretation or 'voice' to report. Trying to report all possibilities can confuse and weaken the case, but selection limits the truth and requires clear positioning. Even with this care, honestly presented data may be interpreted differently by different readers.

> **Vignette 3**
> As part of her research, Julie is observing how trainees learn from small 'mistakes' and feedback in the operating theatre. She overheard a 'great comment' the head of department said under her breath in a surgery ... it would make a great section title in her thesis with a little editing to make it slightly less insulting.
>
> **Consider:**
> *How might Julie consent participants for this observational study?*
> *Is there an argument for less than fully informed consent?*
> *Are there any ethical issues surrounding the use of the overheard comment?*
> *Does it make a difference if the comment is quoted in a publication?*
> *Should the comment be attributed to the individual?*
> *Given the seniority of the person involved they may be identifiable even using a pseudonym – how could this be managed?*

Almost always, participants will have the right to withdraw from research without risk or prejudice, but it is not always easy to withdraw their data. While some data are relatively easily associated with an individual and may therefore be removed, this may not be the case after anonymisation. Even when data can be removed or excluded from quotation, it can be harder to exclude them from interpretation. One cannot 'un-hear' an interview or 'un-think' the thoughts it generated, and this inevitably influences interpretation. Given this, care must be taken when describing the process of withdrawal to participants.

While confidentiality is a core tenet of ethics, there may on occasion be a reason to break this. If during an interview a subject revealed illegal or unprofessional practice, or you felt there was a significant risk to the subject or others, there may be a legal and/or moral duty to break confidentiality. Where possible this should be done with the subject's consent and with appropriate support, but failing this, if the circumstances dictate, identity may be disclosed without consent. This should always be done in as professional and controlled a manner as possible. While such situations are rare, it is important to establish the process you would follow should the situation arise.

## 36.16 Education and Ethics

Given that virtue ethics recognises that the capacity to act in an ethical manner depends on education and perception, there is a moral imperative for ethics reviewers and researchers to learn from the review process and promote good practice. The review process should not only act as a gatekeeper for appropriate ethical behaviour but also promote virtuous ethical practice. It should not be seen as a bureaucratic barrier to be negotiated with minimal effort and then forgotten about. A good ethics review process improves research quality and impact, given careful consideration of ethical issues, and is invariably aligned with good research. Ethical research does not end with successful ethical approval but is ongoing iterative consideration of methods, data and the disseminated message that results.

## 36.17 Conclusion

Educational ethics is not a process barrier to research, but a framework for continual consideration of process to maximise benefit and minimise harm. Linking this principle of beneficence with respect for persons through appropriately informed consent, free participation and careful management of both privacy and data in a compassionate and honest way enables not only ethical practice but high-quality research. Researchers, educators and those who contribute to and manage local ethical review processes share in this ethical obligation.

> **Reflection on the Vignettes**
> While all research issues are to some extent governed by similar ethical principles and often require similar ethical review processes, there is seldom a universal 'right answer'. Issues have to be considered in context to optimise the cost benefit equation that underpins ethical review and ethical research behaviour.
> If we consider Julie the surgical trainee doing her Master's in education. Her research project is interesting, but interviewing colleagues from her specialty who have been through a disciplinary process frames the work in a challenging way. Given this relatively 'high stakes' and negative focus, recruiting within her disciplinary area raises issues about power and the sensitivity of the research. This is not to say it is inappropriate or unethical, but it is a challenging study for a relatively inexperienced educational researcher and would likely face serious ethical scrutiny. Simply reframing the work and interviewing successful surgeons from a different area about how they feel they have learnt from their mistakes retain much of the research but mitigates many of the more challenging issues. Given the time a challenging full ethics review may take, this may be wise for a student project with a tight deadline.
> By reframing the research in this more positive way, it may be more appropriate to recruit people she is more closely connected with in terms of the risk of sensitive issues, and closeness in context can give empathy and rapport and aid interpretation as well as make recruitment easier. However, the power relationships and positioning may be challenging for a novice researcher to

(continued)

negotiate, and this can influence data collection and interpretation and therefore limit value. Choosing participants who are able to reflect and answer her questions, with enough common context to provide rapport and contextual awareness, while at the same time maintaining enough separation to encourage honesty and freedom in participation, is the ideal. This can be hard to achieve, but it is important that this tension is acknowledged and managed. The location of the research is easier to consider; interviews should be conducted in a mutually convenient appropriately private space. She should also be aware that the exact location may impact on the need for additional gatekeeping processes to obtain management approval and access.

An observational component of the study perhaps triangulating views collected at interview with observable practice would add validity and may be possible given that Julie is a surgeon and comfortable in the environment. Such a study would require consent, but perhaps the information provided would need to be managed so as to not unduley influence behaviour and risk invalidating data; this would need to be explained and justified in an ethics application. The overheard comment raises several issues, how public was it and is it available as data, how could you clarify this. Should it be used to inform the analysis and/or be quoted and ascribed particularly given the circumstances are such that the person may be identifiable? One approach may be to include the quote in a transcript and check with the individual concerned whether she is happy with the quote being used. She may be happy to be quoted and not worried about anonymity, although that doesn't mean the data shouldn't be handled sensitively. The compromise is to try and retain the veracity of the data and the integrity of the narrative and interpretation to protect the identity of all concerned.

There is no right answer, just an obligation for careful and ongoing consideration balancing fidelity, justice and beneficence.

# References

1. Stewart, N. (2009). *Ethics*. Polity.
2. Churchill, L. R. (1999). Are we professionals? A critical look at the social role of bioethicists. *Daedalus, 128*, 253–274 259.
3. Robinson, R., & Foucault, M. Ethics. In *The internet encyclopedia of philosophy*. ISSN 2161-0002. http://www.iep.utm.edu/. Accessed 20 Jan 2017.
4. DHEW (Department of Health Education & Welfare), The Belmont Report. (1979). Available at: https://www.hhs.gov/ohrp/regulations-and-policy/belmont-report/index.html. Accessed 20 Jan 2017.
5. Bosk, C., & De Vries, R. (2004). Bureaucracies of mass deception: Institutional review boards and the ethics of ethnographic research. *Annals AAPSS, 595*, 249–263.
6. Bresler, L. (1996). Towards the creation of a new ethical code in qualitative research. *Bulletin of the Council for Research in Music Education, 1*, 17–29.

7. Ten Cate, O. (2009). Why the ethics of medical education research differs from that of medical research. *Medical Education, 43*(7), 608–610.
8. Jamrozik, K. (2004). Research ethics paperwork: What is the plot we seem to have lost? *BMJ, 329*, 286–287.
9. Resnik, D. (2011). What is ethics in research & why is it important. In *The national*. Available at: https://www.niehs.nih.gov/research/resources/bioethics/whatis/index.cfm?links=false. Accessed 20 Jan 2017.
10. Goldacre, B. (2013). *Building evidence into education*. Department for Education.
11. Ellis, C. (2011). Communicating qualitative research designs to research ethics review boards. *The Qualitative Report, 16*(3), 881–891.
12. Brooks, R., Te Riele, K., & Maguire, M. (2014). *Ethics and education research*. London: Sage.
13. Coupal, L. (2005). Practitioner-research and the regulation of research ethics: The challenge of individual, organizational, and social interests. *Qualitative Sozialforschung/Forum: Qualitative Social Research, 6*(1).
14. Walther, J. (2002). Research ethics in internet-enabled research: Human subjects issues and methodological myopia. *Ethics and Information Technology, 4*, 205–216.

# Chapter 37
# Remaining "Grounded" in a Laparoscopic Community of Practice: The Qualitative Paradigm

Rory Kokelaar

**Overview** Without doubt, conducting qualitative surgical educational research has been the most challenging but also the most rewarding part of my professional development. In this chapter I share my experiences of a research project exploring surgical trainees' learning in a laparoscopic community of practice [1]. My intention is to make explicit some of the challenges I experienced from my perspective as a surgical trainee studying surgical education and to offer guidance on key elements of a qualitative research project.

Without doubt, conducting qualitative surgical educational research has been the most challenging but also the most rewarding part of my professional development. In this chapter I share my experiences of a research project exploring surgical trainees' learning in a laparoscopic community of practice [1]. My intention is to make explicit some of the challenges I experienced from my perspective as a surgical trainee studying surgical education and to offer guidance on key elements of a qualitative research project.

Most doctors, like myself, have a background in a quantitative research paradigm; we want to know the $p$ value and the standard error; we look to meta-analysis and randomisation. The language of quantitative research is where we feel comfortable; it provides the tools we use to make judgements about the quality of research and clinical guidance and ultimately influences how we practise clinically. This paradigm, however powerful in determining effects over populations and between different interventions, is largely blind to the nuance of human interaction, the complexities of affective learning, and the depths of personal emotions. To understand how green newly qualified doctors develop into mature and resilient clinicians who embody the profession that they represent requires us to delve into the murky world of the qualitative.

R. Kokelaar (✉)
Swansea University, Swansea, Wales

A qualitative research paradigm, as traditionally applied in social sciences, is a relatively novel concept to most clinicians but underpins the discourse of surgical education. Examining surgical education through a qualitative lens is challenging and rewarding and may provide insights that are both revealing and reflective. A commonly employed and adaptable methodology is *Grounded Theory* [2], where theory is formed from the data as an emergent process towards the end of the research, rather than at the outset as a hypothesis to be tested. Starting with an open mind will increase the chances of discovering something novel, but the sense of stepping into the darkness not quite knowing what you should be looking for is challenging. I share three key guiding points: the research question and reflexivity provides direction, reference to existing theory assists in further framing your question and provides scaffolding to develop your enquiry, and appropriate methodology will ensure that your findings and later theory development are robust and meaningful.

My research sought to illuminate processes that influenced learning of laparoscopic surgical skills in the operating theatre. My starting point was that an interplay of factors, as yet unspecified but probably based upon the people and equipment in the operating theatre, influence the learning and professional development of surgical trainees in this working environment. Unlike quantitative research, which begins with the null hypothesis (theory) to be tested and variables to be measured, qualitative research often begins solely with a question based on personal experiences or ideas. Formulating a sound research question and reflexivity provides the basis by which you interpret and judge your work (see Box 37.1). In Grounded Theory the question should be framed in an open manner; how does this occur? What factors are at play? Who is important in this process? By deliberately keeping the research question based in open enquiry, you will ensure that you do not guide your research into a foregone conclusion; if you go looking for apples, you will likely find them. This does not however mean that your question should be vague or lack definition; you should provide thorough context, set limits of enquiry (such as the environment or groups of individuals), and reference your research to a timeframe. Try to be specific, but open minded. For example:

*What conceptions do junior surgical trainees have of the influence of laparoscopic surgery on their training? What are the effects of learning in the laparoscopic community of practice on professional identity formation?* [1]

In this example, which was the research question from my own dissertation, I constructed questions that were at the same time open-ended ("what conceptions"; "what ... effects") but also specific ("junior surgical trainees"; "laparoscopic community of practice").

The flip side to your research question is your reflexivity. Here you should set out your personal conceptions about the research question to provide personal context as the researcher, so that the research process and theory formation can be interpreted considering your conceptions. Do not be afraid or apologetic of your own opinions and theorems; they are valid even if the eventual data points in a different direction; it is important only that you acknowledge them and keep an open mind.

## Box 37.1 Elements and Principles Associated with Qualitative Research

| Element | Principle |
|---|---|
| Research question and reflexivity | Remain open minded |
| | Be as specific as possible without limiting your enquiry |
| | Do not be afraid to voice your own conceptions and feelings |
| | Avoid polemics and try to see the bigger picture |
| Theoretical framework | Use existing theory as scaffolding for enquiry and as a means of providing the language of a common discourse |
| | Do not allow existing theory to straightjacket your thinking |
| Methodology and methods | Consider your research question and which methods will help illuminate the field |
| | Be realistic about what you can achieve given your resources |
| | Employ your methods rigorously and transparently |

One way to imagine this element is as a documented rhetorical conversation; explore your own conceptions, how it makes you feel, how has it has materially affected you, and how this fits into the wider perspective. Do however try to avoid a polemic! Part of gaining the wider perspective is thinking about the research question as a researcher, rather than a participant in the system; you have to regain "objectivity" in order to unpack the concepts in an "unbiased" way. You may at this point also wish to include reference to existing theories you are familiar with and draw parallels with your own conceptions, and this in its self can help form the research question and provide a framework for enquiry.

Interpreting and applying existing theory to your research question is helpful in several ways. The most obvious benefit is that it provides initial guidance as to what you may discover for yourself and a common language by which to describe it. This will of course facilitate conducting your research by providing a structure and discourse in which to frame your enquiry, but be mindful also that it will also therefore shape your findings and conclusions. Correlation of your developing theory with existing theory may help to corroborate your work, but will simultaneously lay it open to the same criticisms of the theory it has been aligned with. From a Grounded Theory perspective, it is also difficult to produce a truly emergent and novel theory without having some prior knowledge of what others have already theorised, and thus a pragmatic post-positivist position is usually adopted. I used the theoretical notion of communities of practice [3, 4] to help frame my research question and provide some initial scaffolding to my enquiry. This approach was helpful in initiating my Grounded Theory research, but I was mindful to acknowledge the role this particular theory had on my research and in my later theory formation.

Considering several theories at an early stage may help to broaden the remit of your investigation, but may also contribute to confusion in the interpretation of your findings. This, in and of itself, can be constructive; emergent theory can be developed from a patchwork of existing principles, especially in complex environments where the factors influencing learning interact in a rich and miscible manner, but be mindful that theories ultimately rely on unified principles rather than endless parallel possibilities. Addressing and reconciling complexity in theoretical frameworks is in this way difficult; it is easy to find the exception that disproves the rule within a system and hence undermines the theory. This can be frustrating as a budding theorist, and as medical scientists, it is perhaps helpful to think of theory as guidance rather than a strict algorithm; it is there to develop our thinking in a particular direction based upon the commonality of past experiences examined by sound methodology; whilst acknowledging that inevitably, there will be exceptions and partial truths. This is the ontology of post-positivism.

Good methodology in qualitative research is also exceptionally important, although the methods are usually novel to most clinicians. To successfully complete qualitative surgical education research, it is important to consider what format of findings would best suit your research question and then to select from the plethora of methods available (which your supervisors and a good textbook will assist with). Many researchers in surgical education will however inevitably employ Grounded Theory, as I did, and thus gathering data that will aid the formation of a theory, rather than test one, is the most important consideration. Whichever method you choose, it is always important to keep in mind how best to answer your research question and then to execute the chosen methods rigorously and transparently, as it will underpin the theory that you will develop and espouse. Theory formation is therefore emergent and grounded in the research question, reflexivity, and sound methodology.

My research question asked how junior surgeons learn in the operating theatre. To begin to understand the fundamental relationships and interactions that may govern this process, and ultimately to develop theory, I needed a method of data collection that would provide a free hand to my participants and offer an opportunity for deep insight. For these reasons I chose to conduct face-to-face individual interviews, each of approximately an hour, with junior surgical trainees. This method produced very rich data and some profound reflections, which in turn facilitated theory formation. It took a considerable amount of time and effort in recruitment, data collection, and transcription. Although I might have employed another method, such as a questionnaire, the data it would produce and depth of analysis would have been greatly reduced. As well as technical considerations, it is also important to consider the ethics of your methods, for instance, I had to consider the implications of interviewing peers and how they might disclose sensitive working relationships (see Chap. 36).

The final and unifying process in performing Grounded Theory qualitative research in the domain of surgical education is theory formation. At this stage of the research process, you should have already laid solid foundations with your research question and reflexivity, acknowledged existing theories and executed rigorous methods in data collection, and thus theory formation should be almost inevitable. This is the essence of the emergent process; theory formation is an almost unavoidable result of good research and should feel to some degree natural and easy; never forced. It is always important however to relate back to your starting points and conceptions in interpreting your findings and forming theory and to be explicit about how these are related. By following a qualitative research process, I hope that your work will help illuminate the domain of surgical education and that you and others can view this complex world in a new light.

# References

1. Kokelaar, R. F. (2016). *Learning and identity formation in the laparoscopic community of practice – the conceptions of junior surgical trainees*. Masters thesis [MEd], C. Imperial, Editor. London.
2. Glaser, B. G., & Strauss, A. L. (1967). *The discovery of grounded theory: Strategies for qualitative research*. New Brunswick: Aldine Transaction.
3. Lave, J., & Wenger, E. (1991). *Situated learning: Legitimate peripheral participation*. Cambridge: Cambridge University Press.
4. Wenger, E. (1998). *Communities of practice: Learning, meaning, and identity*. Cambridge: Cambridge University Press.

# Chapter 38
# The Nature of Nurture in Surgery: A Drama in Four Acts (So Far)

**David Alderson**

**Overview** In 2010 I undertook research for a Master's of Education in Surgical Education at Imperial College London. In this chapter I have endeavoured to give a flavour of the approaches I have tried in sharing the research findings—a continuing journey to promote resonance and reverberation for a variety of audiences. My research thesis essayed novel modes of presentation, drawing on the medical humanities for inspiration; it was written using the conventions of a theatre script throughout and included word pictures, visual models and an allegory. Subsequently, I have transformed the work into an actual stage play ('True Cut') in order to reach wider audiences.

> *A painter takes the sun and makes it into a yellow spot*
>
> *An artist takes a yellow spot and makes it into a sun.* (Picasso [1])

In 2010 I undertook research for a Master's of Education in Surgical Education at Imperial College London.

In this chapter I have endeavoured to give a flavour of the approaches I have tried in sharing the research findings—a continuing journey to promote resonance and reverberation for a variety of audiences.

My research thesis essayed novel modes of presentation, drawing on the medical humanities for inspiration; it was written using the conventions of a theatre script throughout [2]. Subsequently, I have transformed the work into an actual stage play ('True Cut') in order to reach wider audiences. In the following sections, I have used short quotes from each of the 'Acts' of the thesis and from my subsequent work with True Cut to illustrate some of the approaches used.

---

D. Alderson (✉)
Torbay & South Devon NHS Foundation Trust, Torquay, UK
e-mail: david.alderson@nhs.net

© Springer Nature Singapore Pte Ltd. 2019
D. Nestel et al. (eds.), *Advancing Surgical Education*, Innovation and Change in Professional Education 17, https://doi.org/10.1007/978-981-13-3128-2_38

## 38.1 Prologue

*Development of expertise in surgery has always relied on extensive practice in the operating theatre, but opportunities for trainees have dramatically reduced in recent years. There is a need to examine the factors that lead to effective learning in this environment.*

This is a story about how people learn in theatre: learn to operate, learn judgement and learn how (and whether) to become surgeons. The wish to tell the story arose from my desire as a consultant ENT surgeon to teach better, to learn more and to help others to do the same.

## 38.2 Stagecraft

*A phenomenological approach was used to explore the lived experiences of trainee and consultant surgeons, as well as other members of the theatre team. Analysis, then synthesis of the data from semi-structured interviews allowed a richly textured description of the circumstances that are perceived as important for learning.*

Inquiry in this tradition focuses on the lived experiences of individuals—and on how they interpret these events. The researcher travels this world in search of the shared essence of individual meaning.

My starting point was the applicability of the concept of 'deliberate practice' to learning in the operating theatre. I was particularly interested in the role of the surgeon educator in nourishing, supporting and fostering the surgical learner according to their needs, using 'nurture' as a 'sensitising concept' to guide my exploration.

Some themes arose from my initial review of the literature; others emerged during the research; all became richer and more detailed through constant interplay between iterative review of transcripts, reading of the literature, discussion with colleagues and participants and reflection on developing images.

## 38.3 Act I: Pictures at an Exhibition

*Ten overarching themes are surveyed in order to illustrate the factors which enable the development of surgical expertise: repetitive practice, goal clarity, feedback, challenge, motivation, mindset, relationship, community, climate and context. 'Deliberate practice' thus appears to be a relevant but not entirely sufficient model.*

> Sounds and ideas float in the air
>
> and my scribbling can hardly keep pace with them (Mussorgsky [3])

In Act I, I presented a series of tableaux—word pictures showing different aspects of the emerging story. In accounts of qualitative research, it is customary for short verbatim extracts to be included—the participants' words indented—often in a smaller font than the main text. The message is clear: the words of the author are to be read on a higher level, with more authority and worth. Instead, I chose to join

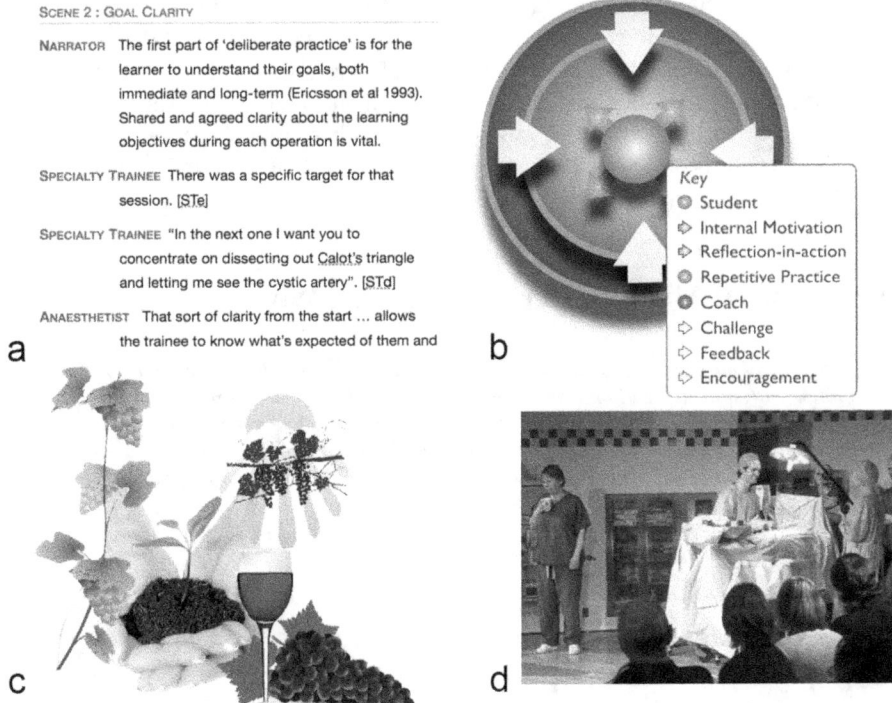

Fig. 38.1 Complementary modes of presentation to promote engagement with qualitative research. (**a**) Word pictures (**b**) conceptual models (**c**) extended metaphor (**d**) storytelling

the cast. As narrator I stood to one side of the stage, guiding the audience but addressing them on equal terms with the actors—who unfolded the story themselves (Fig. 38.1a).

## 38.4 Act II: Music of the Spheres

*Integrating these themes with the expertise literature and educational theory, a 'cosmological model' is presented, as a constructivist synthesis of six perspectives on learning: transmission, developmental, apprenticeship, social reform, nurturing and clinical.*

> The heavenly motions...
> 
> are nothing but a continuous song
> 
> for several voices,
> 
> perceived not by the ear
> 
> but by the intellect,
> 
> a figured music which sets landmarks
> 
> in the immeasurable flow of time (Kepler [4])

Act I provided rich insights into the factors needed for development of expertise in the operating theatre. However, the plot was fragmented and lacked coherence. In order to pull these varied strands together, Act II explored an abstract, conceptual model of surgical learning, moving from individual pictures to a more universal point of view. I presented a series of concentric sphere models, drawing together Kepler's 'cosmic bowl' with Pratt's 'Perspectives on Teaching and Learning' [5] (Fig 38.1b).

## 38.5 Act III: The Vine, the Fruit and the Wine

> *A 'viticultural allegory' is drawn, as an extended metaphor, in order to present a coherent overview with both educational 'meaning' and surgical 'sense'. Surgeon educators use 'professional artistry' to recognise and balance the constructive tensions between divergent ideals: challenge and motivation; experiential learning and performance bandwidth; training and service; supervision and safety; personal and professional needs of the trainee.*

> *Those whose pursuit of knowledge*
> 
> *takes them to the summit of the world,*
> 
> *Whose intellect penetrates the depths of the universe,*
> 
> *To them the sky shall be an upturned goblet*
> 
> *From which, their heads thrown back,*
> 
> *they shall drink to intoxication* (Omar Khyyam [6])

While the abstract models of Act II had utility in synthesising the individual stories with educational theory, they did not resonate with the majority of surgeon educators and surgical learners.

Metaphors provide powerful alternative routes to explore the world, linking seemingly disparate notions to enable new insights. By invoking a shared understanding and applying this in a novel context, they can communicate a concept's essence and suggest further areas for fruitful study. They can explain and engage in a way that simple descriptions and analytical models cannot.

In Act III, I used an extended metaphor, or allegory, to draw out and draw together the sub-plots of this story—exploring their application in the real world of surgery. I touched on the nurture of the vine, the importance of 'terroir' and the art of the vintner in creating fine wine (Fig38.1c).

## 38.6 Act IV: True Cut

> *Surprising and enlightening…a responsible and very 'grown up' meeting with the real people we put our trust in* [7]

> *My father died due to medical error…*
> 
> *the play helped me put what happened*
> 
> *into a perspective* (Audience member)

A recurring theme, which emerged despite rather than because of my initial aim, was the universal experience of making and living with mistakes—and the profound effects these had on clinicians. Within the profession this is often seen as 'just something to get used to'; while in the media mistakes are portrayed as indicators of unskilled, often uncaring doctors—who deserve to be ostracised.

I felt that there was an acute need for more nuanced considerations of the true complexity of surgical practice. I embarked on writing a stage play, able to open up dialogue with clinical, educational and lay audiences. I wanted to use the interviewees' own words where possible—as verbatim theatre—making the scenes believable for professionals, while opening this area to general audiences, engaged as much by a fictional drama as by the subject matter.

An area of weakness in early drafts was the lack of a patient perspective. I was fortunate enough to receive permission to integrate the words of Leilani Schweitzer into the play; her son died following medical error, and she has talked movingly about how this happened, its impact on her and on the staff involved [8].

The script has developed through dramaturgy, workshops, readings and productions. It has shown an ability to engage diverse groups in animated discussion about the place of error in surgical practice, the tensions between educational and patient safety perspectives and the potential boundaries to candour and compassion.

Healthcare professionals strongly identify with the situations presented, while general audiences are also stimulated to vigorous discussion. The script has had favourable responses from professional theatres. I am currently exploring ways to take the play to wider audiences, including medical schools, science festivals and radio drama (Fig. 38.1d). In recent months, I have worked with a professional creative team and Imperial College colleagues to organise a series of public performances of True Cut (https://youtu.be/eJJqUF2opBk).

## 38.7 Epilogue

Quantitative research portrays the world as small dots of black and white certainty; with sufficient granularity, a 'halftone' image can be created, and we perceive a continuous greyscale. However, qualitative researchers can paint on a broader canvas, using a rich palette of colours and textures (Fig. 38.2). Good qualitative research remains true to the original experience, but moves beyond personal impressions and technical analysis, to exploration of meaning.

This research has continued to lead me into new and unexpected areas. Starting with expert performance, and continuing to focus on 'nurture', I have become drawn into the very 'nature' of what makes and sustains a surgeon.

In naturalistic research many meanings are possible, and 'reality' lies in the interstices between the 'actors', the 'playwright' and the 'audience'. I have presented my thoughts, experiences and conclusions alongside the words of the 'cast'—mixing theory, abstract representation, metaphor and story with verbatim

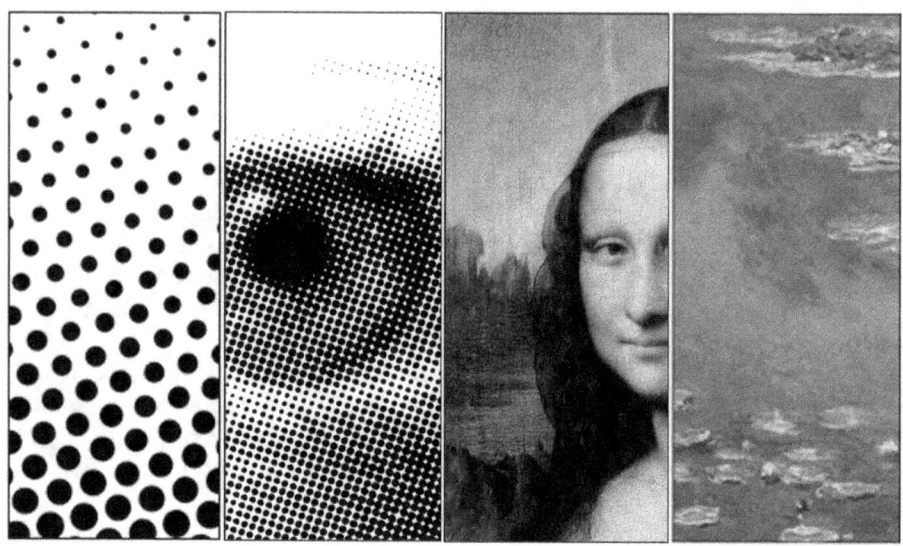

**Fig. 38.2** Comparing the realities portrayed by quantitative and qualitative studies

quotation. Each modality contains the potential to inform and inspire, but all rely on empathic engagement to bring the stories to life:

*Think when we talk of horses, that you see them*

*Printing their proud hoofs i' the receiving earth;*

*For 'tis your thoughts that now must deck our kings,*

*Carry them here and there; jumping o'er times,*

*Turning the accomplishment of many years*

*Into an hour-glass: for the which supply,*

*Admit me Chorus to this history;*

*Who prologue-like your humble patience pray,*

*Gently to hear, kindly to judge, our play.* (Shakespeare [9])

# References

1. Eisner, E. W. (1991). *The enlightened eye* (p. 9). Upper Saddle River: Prentice Hall.
2. Alderson, D. J. (2010). *The nature of nurture in surgery*. Thesis for Master's in Education in Surgical Education. Imperial College London.
3. Calvocoressi, M. (1956). *Modest Mussorgsky* (p. 182). London: Rockliff.
4. Banville, J. (2001). *The revolutions trilogy* (p. 488). London: Picador.
5. Pratt, D. (1998). *Five perspectives on teaching*. Melbourne: Krieger.
6. Khyyam, O. (1889). *The Rubaiyat of Omar Khayyam* (5th ed., E. Fitzgerald, Trans.).
7. Bristol Old Vic Theatre. 'True Cut' review. Personal communication 2015.
8. TED talk video https://www.youtube.com/watch?v=qmaY9DEzBzI Accessed 20 Nov 2018.
9. Shakespeare, W. (1998). *Henry V*. New York: Oxford University Press.

# Chapter 39
# Approaching Surgery Simulation Education from a Patient-Centered Pathway

**Kiyoyuki Miyasaka**

**Overview** Surgical simulation training has tended to focus on individual technical skills for procedures. While the acquisition of individual technical skills is desirable and should be encouraged, competence in clinical practice requires the application of multiple technical and nontechnical skills in their appropriate context as part of a continuous patient-centered pathway of care. To provide competency-based simulation education in a realistic clinical context, we implemented a pathway of preoperative, intraoperative, and postoperative simulation encounters for general surgery residents.

## 39.1 Rationale

Surgical simulation training has tended to focus on individual technical skills for procedures. While the acquisition of individual technical skills is desirable and should be encouraged, competence in clinical practice requires the application of multiple technical and nontechnical skills in their appropriate context as part of a continuous patient-centered pathway of care. To provide competency-based simulation education in a realistic clinical context, we implemented a pathway of preoperative, intraoperative, and postoperative simulation encounters for general surgery residents.

## 39.2 Method

We developed simulation pathways – sequences of immersive high-fidelity simulated encounters in the preoperative, intraoperative, and postoperative setting – that represent the continuum of care for patients presenting with selected common surgical disease states. Repeating the same simulation care pathway before and after a

K. Miyasaka (✉)
Simulation Center, St. Luke's International University, Tokyo, Japan

training intervention provided a mechanism for standardized evaluation of clinical competence in a realistic yet controlled context, while also allowing us to demonstrate the effectiveness of the educational curriculum. These simulation pathways were implemented as part of an integrated simulation-based training curriculum for 1st-year general surgery residents.

Three-day training modules were devised around pathways for 4 surgical divisions (acute care, biliary, colorectal, and foregut) and delivered to a class of 18 1st-year residents. Repeating each module with small groups allowed all residents to complete the curriculum without undue disruption to clinical services. Analysis of evaluations pre- to post-training showed significant positive impacts of training on faculty assessment of resident clinical performance.

This work was conducted within the residency program in general surgery at the Hospital of the University of Pennsylvania. The Institutional Review Board confirmed the protocol to be eligible for exemption from review, as human subjects research occurs within an established educational setting. Furthermore, written consent was sought from all participating residents regarding the collection of data related to their simulated clinical performances for the purpose of research and publication, with the understanding that their consent or refusal, as well as any data collected, would not have any impact on the provided educational content or their standing as a resident in the program.

We utilized the Penn Medicine Clinical Simulation Center, which contains simulated operating rooms, inpatient ward, and outpatient clinic environments, as well as classrooms and skills laboratories within a 22,000 ft$^2$ space [1]. Services of the Perelman School of Medicine Standardized Patient Program were retained to cast and train actors and actresses to fill the patient as well as confederate roles in the simulations.

## 39.2.1 The Simulation Pathway

The simulation pathway consists of sequential encounters that represent key points in the continuum of care for a specific patient. For most surgical disease processes, the continuum of care can be segmented into the three phases of the perioperative period: preoperative, intraoperative, and postoperative (Fig. 39.1).

### 39.2.1.1 Preoperative Encounter

The simulation pathway begins in the outpatient clinic with a SP presenting with a surgical problem. This "preop" encounter is much like a traditional objective structured clinical examination (OSCE), with the resident performing a medical interview including a history and physical exam, with additional focus on preoperative evaluations and consent for surgery as appropriate. Up to 15 min were assigned to this encounter in order to allow completion of the entire sequence in a reasonable timeframe.

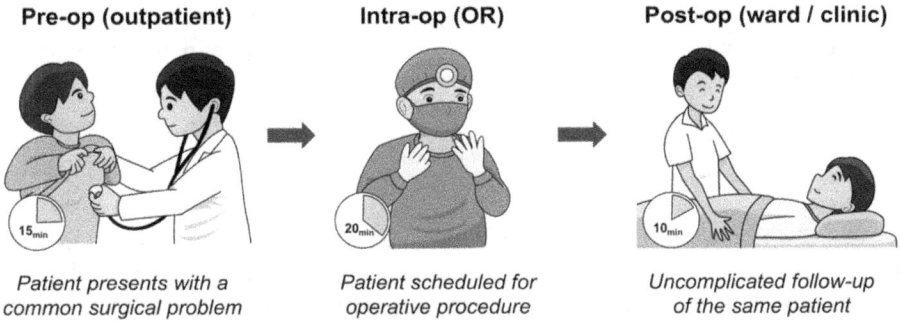

**Fig. 39.1** Phases of the simulation pathway

### 39.2.1.2 Intraoperative Encounter

Following the outpatient encounter, the resident proceeds to an operating room to perform a surgical intervention on the patient they just saw in the preop encounter. The fully immersive "intraop" simulation is set up with a procedure-specific animal tissue or synthetic model, as well as confederates like an assistant and anesthesia providers as appropriate for the operative context and interaction. The resident is given up to 20 min to proceed with the assigned operative task.

### 39.2.1.3 Postoperative Encounter

The same SP reprises their role for the final "postop" encounter in a simulated ward or clinic setting. The resident assesses and explains the patient's postoperative course and provides instructions and counseling as appropriate. The postoperative encounter may be completed within a 10-min window.

### 39.2.1.4 Evaluation of Resident Performance

During each encounter, residents are observed and evaluated by attending faculty in a separate room watching via live video. The use of an electronic audiovisual system allows for simultaneous live monitoring as well as recording and playback of simulated encounters for this purpose. Both faculty and the SP also provide feedback to each resident at the conclusion of the pathway.

While a variety of measurement tools exist for the evaluation of clinical performance, validity evidence remains limited [2]. For each phase of the pathway, we selected rating scales strongly suggested as the best available for use by the American Board of Surgery (ABS). Multiple assessments using these tools are required by the ABS for residents completing surgery residency programs in the 2012–2013 academic year or thereafter, with the requirement increasing to six assessments each from the 2015 to 2016 academic year [3]. Other specialties such as anesthesia, internal medicine, and family medicine also have similar requirements with more expected to follow suit [4].

## CAMEO

The Clinical Assessment and Management Exam – Outpatient (CAMEO) is designed to evaluate surgery residents' ability to assess and manage a patient in an initial outpatient clinic encounter [5]. The assessment is based on five criteria (test ordering and understanding, diagnostic acumen, history taking, physical examination, and communication skills) in addition to overall performance, each scored on a 5-point Likert scale. During the pathway simulations, attending faculty observe the residents' simulated outpatient encounter on video and perform a live rating of their performance. Immediately following the encounter, each resident evaluates their own performance using the same criteria.

## OPRS

The Operative Performance Rating System (OPRS) is used to rate the intraoperative technical skills of a surgeon [6, 7]. The assessment consists of four general criteria (instrument handling, respect for tissue, time and motion, operation flow), several additional procedure-specific criteria as available, as well as an indication of overall performance. Again, each criterion is rated on a 5-point Likert scale. Attending faculty observe the residents' simulated operative encounter on video and rate their performance. Each resident also evaluates their own performance immediately following the encounter.

## Mini-CEX

The Mini Clinical Evaluation Exercise (Mini-CEX) is a tool for assessment of trainees in any medical setting [8]. It is the most studied tool and is associated with the strongest available validity evidence [2]. The Mini-CEX assessment consists of six criteria (medical interviewing skills, physical examination skills, humanistic qualities/professionalism, clinical judgment, counseling skills, organization/efficiency) in addition to overall clinical competence. Each criterion is scored on a 9-point scale, grouped into three performance categories (1–3 for unsatisfactory, 4–6 for satisfactory, and 7–9 for superior). Like the previous encounters, each resident evaluates their own performance immediately following the postoperative encounter.

### 39.2.1.5 Results

Simulation pathways were developed for four surgical divisions (acute care, biliary, colorectal, and foregut), each serving as the cornerstone of a 3-day multimodal educational module. Each training module consisted of a series of didactic, hands-on, and peer-engaged simulation sessions [9, 10]. Data was collected over the course of the 2013–2014 academic year for a class of 18 residents taking part in 4 training modules, each with paired performance assessments pre- (day 1) and post-training (day 3) conducted using repeated pathway simulations. Wilcoxon signed-rank tests for paired nonparametric measurements showed significant improvements in faculty assessment of resident performance for the majority of simulated encounters and significant improvement across all encounters and modules for resident self-assessments.

## 39.3 Key Messages

By using simulation to recreate a pathway of surgical patient care, training and assessment of clinical competence were achieved in a time-efficient manner. Repeating the pathway simulation enabled evaluation of the educational intervention in addition to residents' level of achievement. Simulation program leadership and staff were the key to implementation, providing structure and oversight to participating faculty and residents.

Just as clinical pathways provide structure to the delivery of clinical care, simulation pathways served to focus educational efforts to be delivered in a time-efficient manner. Repeating these simulations provided a mechanism for standardized pre- and post-training evaluation of clinical competence in a realistic context and may have further applications to assess the benefits and translation of training to the clinical setting to show return on investment [11].

The concept is versatile and can be applied to any patient narrative with an introduction, development, turn(s), and conclusion. It can thus provide a practical framework to address competency-based training and integration of simulation for varying levels of providers, other clinical disciplines, as well as interprofessional teams. Institutional support was key, and we emphasize the role of a dedicated simulation program with adequate leadership, resources, and support personnel required to provide the structure and oversight to ensure coordination of training as well as research output.

Education research has many parallels with a clinical study. A clinical study is not simply an academic exercise, but a significant administrative and logistical undertaking. The same can be said for education research. While use of simulation center and standardized patient resources were essential, many other factors were necessary to execute this work. We were fortunate to have an existing allocation of PGY1 resident time for simulation, so that coordination of resident schedules to participate occurred as part of the residency program. An existing mechanism to compensate faculty for time committed to simulation education was also essential. Just as one cannot conduct a quality clinical study without any support infrastructure, conducting education research requires a lot of groundwork to be done in advance.

A personal challenge was finding ways to improve the educational experience (as an educator) without altering the parameters of the research intervention (as a responsible researcher). Clinicians conducting clinical studies may find it difficult to defer a treatment decision to a fixed protocol rather than their own judgment. However, this level of rigor is necessary to ensure a uniform intervention to produce meaningful research output, which ultimately benefits learners and patients.

# References

1. Williams, N. N., Mittal, M. K., Dumon, K. R., Matika, G., Pray, L. A., Resnick, A. S., & Morris, J. B. (2011). Penn medicine clinical simulation center. *Journal of Surgical Education, 68*(1), 83–86.
2. Kogan, J. R., Holmboe, E. S., & Hauer, K. E. (2009). Tools for direct observation and assessment of clinical skills of medical trainees: A systematic review. *JAMA, 302*(12), 1316–1326.
3. American Board of Surgery: General Surgery Performance Assessments. http://www.absurgery.org/default.jsp?certgsqe_resassess. Accessed 5 Aug 2016.
4. Levine, A. I., Schwartz, A. D., Bryson, E. O., & DeMaria, S. (2012). Role of simulation in US physician licensure and certification. *Mount Sinai Journal of Medicine, 79*, 140–153.
5. Wilson, A. B., Choi, J. N., Torbeck, L. J., Mellinger, J. D., Dunnington, G. L., & Williams, R. G. (2014). Clinical Assessment and Management Examination-Outpatient (CAMEO): Its validity and use in a surgical milestones paradigm. *Journal of Surgical Education*. pii: S1931-7204.
6. Williams, R. G., Sanfey, H., Chen, X. P., & Dunnington, G. L. (2012). A controlled study to determine measurement conditions necessary for a reliable and valid operative performance assessment: A controlled prospective observational study. *Annals of Surgery, 256*(1), 177–187.
7. Larson, J. L., Williams, R. G., Ketchum, J., Boehler, M. L., & Dunnington, G. L. (2005). Feasibility, reliability and validity of an operative performance rating system for evaluating surgery residents. *Surgery, 138*(4), 640–647.
8. American Board of Internal Medicine, Assessment Tools. http://www.abim.org/program-directors-administrators/assessment-tools/mini-cex.aspx
9. Buchholz, J., Miyasaka, K. W., Vollmer, C., LaMarra, D., & Aggarwal, R. (2015). Design, development and implementation of a surgical simulation pathway curriculum for biliary disease. *Surgical Endoscopy, 29*(1), 68–76.
10. Miyasaka, K. W., Buchholz, J., LaMarra, D., Karakousis, G. C., & Aggarwal, R. (2015). Development and implementation of a clinical pathway approach to simulation-based training for foregut surgery. *Journal of Surgical Education, 72*(4), 625–635.
11. Griswold, S., Ponnuru, S., Nishisaki, A., Szyld, D., Davenport, M., Deutsch, E. S., & Nadkarni, V. (2012). The emerging role of simulation education to achieve patient safety: Translating deliberate practice and debriefing to save lives. *Pediatric Clinics of North America, 59*(6), 1329–1340.

# Part V
# Future Directions in Surgical Education

**Debra Nestel, Kirsten Dalrymple, and John T. Paige**

Finally, in this part we move from past and contemporary practices with a view to looking to 2030. Rashid and McCammon imagine surgical education considering curriculum structures and educational methods at medical school and in surgical training (Chap. 40). The structures and methods described by the authors all appear in the chapters of this book. However, it is unlikely that there is any single institution that incorporates all these ideas and practices. Finally, we close the book with considerations of the role of surgical educators. Nestel et al. consider a new lexicon and offer perspectives of current content as viewed from 2030 (Chap. 41). The authors share two excerpts of diaries from a working week and a letter from a surgeon graduate! Although technology plays a critical role in shaping practices as surgical educators and surgeon educators, interpersonal relationships remain at the heart of our practice whether with patients, their families, and our colleagues.

D. Nestel
Faculty of Medicine, Nursing & Health Sciences, Monash Institute for Health and Clinical Education, Monash University, Clayton, VIC, Australia

Faculty of Medicine Dentistry & Health Sciences, Department of Surgery, Melbourne Medical School, University of Melbourne, Parkville, Australia
e-mail: dnestel@unimelb.edu.au; debra.nestel@monash.edu

K. Dalrymple
Faculty of Medicine, Imperial College London, London, UK

J. T. Paige
Department of Surgery, Louisiana State University School of Medicine, New Orleans, LA, USA
e-mail: jpaige@lsuhsc.edu

# Chapter 40
# Surgical Education in the Future

**Prem Rashid and Kurt McCammon**

**Overview** This chapter explores an ideal surgical programme for the future. Previous chapters have primed us for what we know we can achieve. Here, we amalgamate the many solutions to the challenges we currently face. We gaze into our crystal ball looking to the year 2030. In doing so, there will be focal aspects of surgical education where changes in the way we consider, teach and evaluate what we do has conceptually evolved. Using some focal points below, we can consider the way surgical education and training programmes will eventually look and feel.

## 40.1 Introduction

We were asked to consider the future of surgical education with 2030 in mind. We write from our perspectives as academic surgeons who have a strong interest in surgical education and its progressive development. We imagined we were in 2030 and looking back on the development of surgical education and training. We explore key points – training time and scope, mentoring, simulation, robotics, e-learning, social media, communication, work-based assessment, mental health, bullying and harassment and gender and race inequality.

---

P. Rashid (✉)
Department of Urology, Port Macquarie Base Hospital, Rural Clinical School,
The University of New South Wales, Port Macquarie, Australia
e-mail: premrashid@me.com

K. McCammon
Department of Urology, Eastern Virginia Medical School, Norfolk, VA, USA
e-mail: MccammKA@EVMS.EDU

© Springer Nature Singapore Pte Ltd. 2019
D. Nestel et al. (eds.), *Advancing Surgical Education*, Innovation and Change in Professional Education 17, https://doi.org/10.1007/978-981-13-3128-2_40

## 40.2    2030 and Looking Back

We've much to reflect on… The process started with how medical students were educated and inspired because of their clinical attachment. Each speciality fostered and created a clinically sound interesting programme for students. This included formal surgical teacher programmes so that clinical educationalists drove the process. Junior doctors gained access to terms where useful clinical skills can be acquired. Part of that involved access to teaching and skills development. Along with that are defined preselection criteria for surgical training with the facility to achieve the required skill base. Selection into programmes became fair, transparent and objective. Curricula were clearly defined and resourced to deliver what was expected. This encompassed an enriching environment for safe learning and the tools to ensure that theoretical and practical knowledge were developed at the expected rate. Engaging with technology in a useful and efficient manner was essential. Assessments were both formative and summative with validated whole activity tools and constructive feedback. It has been challenging for any programme to achieve all the ticks, but striving to do has fostered an ethic of constant improvement.

Elements of graded responsibility in surgical training, based on the original master-apprentice model, have been preserved in some form as a way to sequentially acquire complex skills. To be acceptable to jurisdictions, professional training institutions and surgical trainers and trainees, change has had to be gradual and with purpose.

Surgical education focusses on learning opportunities, safe working environments as well as adherence to set staged and achievable curricula. Efficient systems offer high-quality surgical education within a shorter working week and timeframe.

Re-engagement with medical schools ensured that undergraduate curricula received a reinvigorated surgical emphasis to offset the dilution in the years preceding 2018. This involved partnered integration of postgraduate programmes by providing stepwise 'primers' into the undergraduate curriculum. Formal curricula have been developed in partnership with undergraduate educators using the changes in technology. Graded simulation and surgical education has been progressively formalised with the goal of better preparation of trainees for clinical operative exposure [1]. *Opt-in* formal structured programmes via online delivery for junior residents or even medical students who aspire to a surgical career path are now offered. Much of this has been integrated into procedural skill sets to help junior doctors keep their options open building on the primers from their undergraduate degree [2].

Surgical societies in conjunction with postgraduate training colleges have developed collaborative models to offer additional technical and nontechnical skills development programmes to help those who desire additional learning. Flexible mode, easy access and timing remain the key.

**Table 40.1** The ten FMEC recommendations for MD education [3]

| |
|---|
| 1. Address individual and community needs |
| 2. Enhance admissions processes |
| 3. Build on the scientific basis of medicine |
| 4. Promote prevention and public health |
| 5. Address the hidden curriculum |
| 6. Diversify learning contexts |
| 7. Value generalism |
| 8. Advance inter- and intra-professional practice |
| 9. Adopt a competency-based and flexible approach |
| 10. Foster medical leadership |

## 40.3 Training Time and Scope

Surgical training programmes have developed a two-stage qualification where the primary training of 3–4 years offers a core set of skills for general specialty practice and a second stage of 2–3 years for higher level subspecialised 'fit-for-purpose' qualification. This has added flexibility in some branches of surgery and will likely extend into other areas as jurisdictions formalise scope of practice.

The Future of Medical Education in Canada Postgraduate (FMEC PG) Project culminated in ten recommendations for change (Table 40.1) [3]. Many of the recommendations have been applied to other jurisdictions and serve as a template for institutions looking to address programme deficiencies.

One of the major changes in earlier decades was the focus on graduates' readiness for general practice by medical schools. This was understandable as most graduates entered a career in general practice. The challenge with this concept was that there had been a de-emphasis on the needs of those students who aspired to a surgical career path. Parallel electives in surgical sciences and skill development began to be offered to those who choose a procedural path and this was further integrated into non-surgical procedural medical careers as well [2]. This not only allowed for development of skill but also generated and consolidated interest in a procedural career path.

## 40.4 Mentoring

Surgical mentoring became multifaceted and formalised [4]. This was achieved by the increased use of technology, 24/7 access and tele-mentoring. Surgical trainees now use multiple sources of mentoring with each offering different expertise. This 'mosaic mentoring' also fits the needs of trainees (Fig. 40.1) [5, 6]. Mentors can

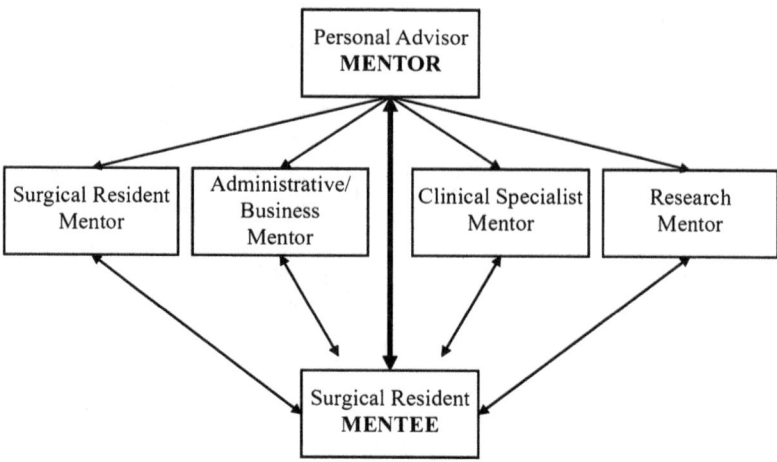

**Fig. 40.1** Mosaic mentoring [7]

provide multifaceted nontechnical guidance or coaching to help manage interpersonal issues and work-life balance – an area most surgeons continue to struggle with. Despite simulation technology, ongoing mentor support remains vital in the global education process.

## 40.5 Simulation

Simulation has developed into a viable adjunct to the apprenticeship model. Exciting possibilities with detailed 3D imaging and printing as a teaching tool continue to evolve [8].

Collaborative resourcing between various institutions help with cost structures. Adjunctive simulation is now delivered starting with basic aspects and leading to a full immersive scenario to bring together all the technical and nontechnical skills [9].

Trainers and trainees intuitively recognise and accept that the use of simulation is worthwhile. Virtual reality simulation assists in 'whole activity' simulation encompassing technical and nontechnical skills with good face validity and the ability of repeat tasking.

Models for investment in simulators have been developed with better access for trainees, needs analysis and validity research along the way to offer standardised definitions and valid methods of measurement (Fig. 40.2) [10]. Trainers routinely apportion time and resources as well as ensuring that their own train-the-trainer needs are met.

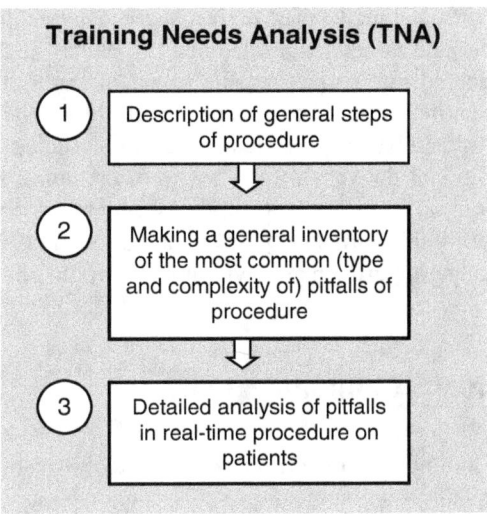

**Fig. 40.2** Training needs analysis [10]

## 40.6 Robotics

Robotic surgery, single port and natural orifice minimally invasive surgery continue to evolve with innovative clinical applications in time. With introduction of new technology comes the learning curve that qualified surgeons need to acknowledge. Simulation and parallel console programmes have been able to provide the early modular structured learning required [11]. More conventional procedures be they open, endoscopic or laparoscopic have been modularised for stages in training.

## 40.7 E-Learning

E-learning has increasingly become an acceptable and efficient way to educate with access to technology and progressive online tools [12]. Online education tools being progressively introduced are promoted and complement traditional methods. E-learning modules with smart device access are used to rapidly introduce and progress key concepts in the learning continuum making face-to-face interactions more worthwhile and efficient.

## 40.8 Social Media

Technology helps positively address power imbalances in traditional hierarchical structures. Smart devices and wearable technology continue to be dual-edged swords in being enormously helpful and adding to efficiency but equally can be distracting and a source of abuse (e.g. during examinations).

Social media (SoMe) has become a valid method of exchanging legitimate clinical and educational content [13]. Much of this continues to grow at an unprecedented rate surpassing the speed of traditional models [14]. The SoMe platform continues to prove to be powerful, influential and efficient, transcending many traditional barriers. SoMe now delivers efficient piecemeal updates to supplement traditional delivery of education. Short quizzes, highlighting key research findings, journal club, meeting updates and rapid communication all lend themselves to SoMe platforms [15]. SoMe and online networking in general will remain an ever-changing growth area with novel ways to educate and engage between peers.

## 40.9 Communication

Communication errors continue to be responsible for adverse outcomes. High-quality communication skills cannot be assumed for any individual as failure to engage the team can affect the complexity of surgical processes. Communication failures can occur for a number of reasons [16]:

- Error of judgement
- Carelessness
- Inadequate hand over
- Unclear responsibilities
- Failure to convey critical information
- Knowledge gaps
- Fear of loss of autonomy

Focussing on communication from a situational and cognitive perspective has tangible benefits for the surgical staff and patient care. Reflective writing and discussion forums are used to bolster insight and empathy. We have left behind the original methods of allowing junior surgical trainees the 'opportunity' of 'learning from their mistakes' while engaging in unfamiliar clinical situations that could lead to patient harm.

Interpersonal communication skills remain a vital core competency. Correct situational awareness, assessment and handling are key components in complex environments like the operating room. Multiple points of source information and recording make this type of learning feasible and, most importantly, valuable. Updating in real time via smart devices continues to be key in making the process seamless.

Nontechnical skill and communication tools have been used to improve skills of surgical trainees including specific feedback [17]. Much of this is assessed and corrected via interpersonal observation and counselling and via instructional video capture, team scoring and analysis.

## 40.10 Workplace-Based Assessments (WBAs)

Ongoing evaluation of the types and effectiveness of the different WBAs has led to their increasing usefulness within each programme [18]. Trainer upskilling in the use of assessment processes remains essential. This is accomplished in real time, formalised and credentialed to ensure trainers meet their obligations as well.

Whole activity competency from the first consult to discharge and aftercare is what the practice of surgery requires and is now achievable. Entrustable professional activities (EPAs) remain an ideal tool for assessing discrete milestones and competencies [19]. Improvement in these types of tools continues to be developed and evaluated on an ongoing basis for quality and supplemented where required.

## 40.11 Mental Health, Bullying and Harassment

Mental stress is a significant issue for all doctors. It can emerge in a variety of forms including underperformance, mood swings, increased tendency to depression, substance abuse and suicide. Stress management training and appreciation has become an integral part of the ethic of surgery and surgical education.

There was enough evidence to suggest that bullying and harassment needed to be addressed and workplace environments free of intimidation. Mechanisms are in place with most workplace environments instituting policy about the issue. The culture of bullying and harassment was once pervasive in the surgical environment. Change started when the President of the Royal Australasian College of Surgeons issued an unreserved apology and promised to begin a process of rectifying this long standing issue [20].

Addressing these issues was much more than just instituting policy. There needed to be open acknowledgement and a mechanism to address poor behaviour in a manner that fostered permanent change for the better. It helped enormously when this came from the leadership of all organisations involved in healthcare and education instituting with a 'mindset' change [21].

## 40.12 Gender and Race Inequality

Race and gender inequality issues continue to exist but discrimination has become less pervasive in surgery. Inequality in remuneration and workplace discrimination have been progressively addressed by the surgical leadership in all jurisdictions [22]. Focus on flexibility of training with jurisdictions and training colleges was acknowledged and with that came progressive moves to help address race and gender inequalities.

## 40.13 Conclusion from 2019

Surgeons at all levels should inspire their teams and push to empower the system to reconstruct surgical training and education into the new age. It takes leadership, vision and access to the decision-makers that will allow for progressive change. Resource allocation, tailored solutions and technology continue to be pivotal to improving surgical education into the future. Patient safety, cost and time limitations will be key issues curtailing some of the ideal models. Faculty development will be essential in tandem. Seamless cooperation between undergraduate and postgraduate training bodies should offer the benefits that come with cohesive synergy. Additionally, engaging medical students with a positive experience during a surgical term continues to be an important part of the first step of recruitment into surgery as a career. All this could lead to supportive frameworks for surgical training as outlined in the following diary extract (Box 40.1).

> **Box 40.1: Excerpt from the Diary of a Surgical Graduate in 2030**
> *It's just 8 years since I completed medical school at my local university. I was fortunate to get the grades to enter a progressive school where we were exposed to many branches of medicine – not just on our largely screen-based resources but in real clinical settings. In my second last year, I had a placement in a urology unit where I could see the breadth within the specialty. We were offered mosaic mentoring. This allowed me to access several mentors who could guide me as the challenges of life presented themselves – not all work related. The surgical trainees I worked with were clearly well supervised and seemed happy in their career choice. One of the consultants took the time to take an interest in who I was as a person and listened to my reasons for doing medicine. I was encouraged to consider writing a review paper which not only allowed me to focus on how to write for scientific publication but the resultant paper was published. My new mentor was supportive and helpful in getting the project to completion despite my cursory first draft.*
>
> *I continued along my path to complete my medical degree but an interest in surgery had developed. I could attend optional basic skills workshops and simulation labs to acquire an understanding of the skills I would need. The virtual reality platforms were conducive to learning, correcting as I went along. Many of the skills included nontechnical aspects of clinical practice which I had not associated with being a surgeon. Collaborative team practice using smart device technology made learning on the run very easy. My mentor continued to guide me through my early postgraduate years as I undertook clinical projects and slowly built up skills and experience a range of clinical terms in surgery.*

(continued)

**Box 40.1** (continued)

> The selection process for advanced training was transparent and achievable. I was not successful at my first attempt but with encouragement, I found the will to continue trying to improve my CV and skill base. I was successful on the second attempt but did find the early years challenging. I also experienced a personal crisis and needed time to resolve a family matter. Fortunately, I was supported to take a year off during my training to care for my sick child. It was a time when I experienced significant self-doubt about the path I had chosen. All through this period my mentor seemed to be there when I needed her. I could continue to attend teaching sessions and simulation skills labs. The programme was run by amazing teachers who knew how to extract from me what I didn't know I had and progress my rate of growth as a surgeon. Real-time assessment online portals allowed me to evaluate areas where I was doing well and aspects that needed attention. It made me realise that I was doing what I wanted to do.
>
> My final exams were a challenge and I failed the first time but again when self-doubt crept in, I found amazingly supportive peers and seniors. I have now completed my training and have two lovely children. My mentor offered me a position as an associate in her practice and continues to appreciate my responsibilities outside of work. I have been fortunate to have found my place thanks to the people who knew how to bring out the best in me. My experience has helped me better see the needs of the medical students and juniors I work with. Hopefully I will be able to offer to them what was offered to me.

Finally, surgical education and training programmes must establish a mindset that embraces change, finding ways to better tap into progressive thinking and monitoring quality in a meaningful way to foster improvement.

# References

1. Pearce, I. (2016). *BAUS Nedical students' section*. Available from: http://www.baus.org.uk/professionals/sections/medical_students.aspx.
2. RACS. (2014). *JDocs framework*. Available from http://www.surgeons.org/news/junior-doctors-competency-framework/. 1 Jan 2015.
3. AFMC. *The future of medical education in Canada (FMEC): A collective vision for MD Education*. Available from https://www.afmc.ca/future-of-medical-education-in-canada/medical-doctor-project/. 29 Apr 2016.
4. Rashid, P., Narra, M., & Woo, H. (2015). Mentoring in surgical training. *ANZ Journal of Surgery, 85*(4), 225–229.

5. Singletary, S. E. (2005). Mentoring surgeons for the 21st century. *Annals of Surgical Oncology, 12*(11), 848–860.
6. Morahan, P. S., & Richman, R. C. (2001). Career obstacles for women in medicine. *Medical Education, 35*(2), 97–98.
7. Rombeau, J., Goldberg, A., & Loveland-Jones, C. (2010). Ch 9 – Future directions. In *Surgical mentoring – Building tomorrow's leaders* (pp. 145–164). New York: Springer.
8. Zheng, Y. X., et al. (2016). 3D printout models vs. 3D-rendered images: Which is better for preoperative planning? *Journal of Surgical Education, 73*(3), 518–523.
9. Grantcharov, T. P., & Reznick, R. K. (2009). Training tomorrow's surgeons: What are we looking for and how can we achieve it? *ANZ Journal of Surgery, 79*(3), 104–107.
10. Schout, B. M., et al. (2010). Validation and implementation of surgical simulators: A critical review of present, past, and future. *Surgical Endoscopy, 24*(3), 536–546.
11. Pietrabissa, A., et al. (2013). Robotic surgery: Current controversies and future expectations. *Cirugía Española, 91*(2), 67–71.
12. Jayakumar, N., et al. (2015). E-learning in surgical education: A systematic review. *Journal of Surgical Education, 72*(6), 1145–1157.
13. Chung, A., & Woo, H. (2016). Twitter in urology and other surgical specialties at global conferences. *ANZ Journal of Surgery, 86*(4), 224–227.
14. Branford, O. A., et al. (2016). #PlasticSurgery. *Plastic and Reconstructive Surgery, 138*(6), 1354–1365.
15. Thangasamy, I. A., et al. (2014). International urology journal club via twitter: 12-month experience. *European Urology, 66*(1), 112–117.
16. Graafland, M., et al. (2015). Training situational awareness to reduce surgical errors in the operating room. *The British Journal of Surgery, 102*(1), 16–23.
17. Nestel, D., et al. (2010). Evaluation of a clinical communication programme for perioperative and surgical care practitioners. *Quality & Safety in Health Care, 19*(5), e1.
18. Shalhoub, J., et al. (2015). A descriptive analysis of the use of workplace-based assessments in UK surgical training. *Journal of Surgical Education, 72*(5), 786–794.
19. ten Cate, O. (2005). Entrustability of professional activities and competency-based training. *Medical Education, 39*(12), 1176–1177.
20. RACS. (2016). *About respect*. Available from http://www.surgeons.org/about-respect/. 30 Apr 2016.
21. RACS. (2017). *Operating with respect: E-learning module*. Available from: http://www.surgeons.org/news/operating-with-respect-%E2%80%93-e-learning-module-launched/. 05 June 2017.
22. Frohman, H. A., et al. (2015). The nonwhite woman surgeon: A rare species. *Journal of Surgical Education, 72*(6), 1266–1271.

# Chapter 41
# Finally, the Future of Surgical Educators

**Debra Nestel, John T. Paige, and Kirsten Dalrymple**

**Overview** Having reviewed each chapter in this book, thinking about the future of surgical education is a truly exciting prospect. Across the four parts, authors have made offerings on various topics from the past and the present. In this final part, the previous chapter considered the state of surgical education in 2030 while here we shift our focus to the role of the surgical educator in the same year. First, we consider about whom we are writing; second, we reflect on the contents of the book as a guide to the surgical educators' practices; and third, we offer pages from our 2030 diaries before concluding.

## 41.1 What's in a Name in 2030?

So, here we are in 2030 and debate on the proper moniker with which to describe the overarching role of the dedicated individuals who teach and mentor surgeons and surgical trainees has settled with "surgical educator." This label encompasses surgeons and other experts who may function as educators for surgeons – psychologists, sociologists, engineers, behavioural scientists, economists and, of course, surgeons themselves who also choose on occasion the more defined descriptor of "surgeon educator". Although these surgical educators still employ the term

---

D. Nestel (✉)
Faculty of Medicine, Nursing & Health Sciences, Monash Institute for Health and Clinical Education, Monash University, Clayton, VIC, Australia

Faculty of Medicine Dentistry & Health Sciences, Department of Surgery, Melbourne Medical School, University of Melbourne, Parkville, Australia
e-mail: dnestel@unimelb.edu.au; debra.nestel@monash.edu

J. T. Paige
Department of Surgery, Louisiana State University School of Medicine, New Orleans, LA, USA
e-mail: jpaige@lsuhsc.edu

K. Dalrymple
Faculty of Medicine, Imperial College London, London, UK
e-mail: k.dalrymple@imperial.ac.uk

"training", they now use it to refer to specific acts of practice or rehearsal to develop a component of surgical practice, much like an athlete "trains" for a match, rather than to describe the entire educational experience of those learning the craft of surgery. Athletes would be unlikely to refer to their performance in a match as "training". Well, same for surgery.

In 2026, after weeks of professed outrage in social media outlets that surgical trainees should not be "training" on real patients, the surgical education community was forced to think hard about the language used to describe progression from medical student to surgeon. This controversy was triggered by publicly released audio recordings of surgeons and trainees talking about patients as *training fodder*. These stories were more nuanced than portrayed, but the media coverage was intense and decisive. The verdict from the general public who would comprise the future and current patient population was clear; "training" on people was unacceptable. Again, because of a small number of individuals, the surgical community was forced to reflect on its behaviour and to rethink its language.

Almost overnight, the terms "surgical trainee" and "surgical resident" were dropped from the lexicon, replaced by the expression "associate surgeon". Today, these associate surgeons are still under the supervision of senior consultant or attending surgeons, but such supervision is no longer framed as "training". Instead, "training" is now only used to refer to elements of surgical practice that take place using simulation – in situ, peri-situ or ex cura settings. The term ex cura, which originally referred to simulation-based activities occurring in specialised simulation centres away from care environments, has now expanded to include cost-effective practice on home-based simulators. "Surgical trainers" today, therefore, only work in these simulated settings, and their focus is typically on supporting the development of specific, often psychomotor skills.

The "surgical coach" (and yes, surgeon coach) has now transformed into a specialist role working mainly with experienced surgeons to achieve excellence. Even small nuanced changes may be achieved as a consequence of observation and conversation by coaches with surgeons. It is commonplace for consultant and attending surgeons to intermittently have a coach in operating theatres, wards and outpatient departments. The surgical coach role is prestigious and sometimes performed by a discipline outside of surgery – someone whose focus is on a targeted element of practice (e.g. verbal communication). And of course, there are still mentors who may or may not have the "surgical" or "surgeon" prefix. As they did in 2018, these individuals may not be in the same workplace but forge a long-term relationship with a surgical aspirant or surgeon.

We are also starting to see the new interprofessional surgical practitioners too. These individuals complete interprofessional curricula equipping them to work in various roles in the operating theatre, pre- and post-operatively. The roles are proving especially valuable, given their flexibility and its practitioners' abilities to work effectively in diverse activities. Some of these individuals have even entered programmes to become surgeons, while others are specialising in specific tasks within theatre. The scope of practice of traditional professions has shifted and new roles formed. Surgical educators have played an important role in shaping these developments.

## 41.2 Reflecting on the Contents of This Book in 2030

From Part I in the *Foundations of Surgical Education*, we see many changes and most of them advances. While acknowledging variations across the world in 2018, in 2030 we have witnessed shifts from the single dominant national regulatory body to alternate forms. This decentralisation has been reflected in the shift away from super specialisation seen in 2018 towards developing surgeons possessing a broader range of surgical skills in order to be able to practice in a variety of healthcare settings (i.e. rural, austere, urban environments). Knowing a wide range of fundamental procedures within and across specialties is once again in vogue.

Regulatory practices have extended to those in educator roles through professional bodies and academies. Different levels of membership acknowledge developmental stages of surgical educators. Academicians hold high status in the surgical, health professions and health service communities. Academies offer exciting professional development opportunities drawing on expertise from outside the profession as much as from within. Universities host postgraduate courses in surgical education that are mandatory for individuals in surgical education leadership roles. These courses are offered in a variety of ways, often blended forms including virtual communities with synchronous and asynchronous interactions for students and faculty. Acknowledging the importance of context and community for learning, students also meet in person to share their knowledge and practice of surgical education in structured learning activities, and faculty support their learning in health service settings. Awarding institutions have sufficient flexibility to facilitate students selecting subjects across diverse programmes, some crossing national boundaries. The surgical education community has developed the language, knowledge and influence to sway health policy in ways that show responsiveness to societal concerns but also to the community's members need to develop and thrive as professionals.

In crafting Part II – *Theories Informing Surgical Education* in 2030 – we have a similar range of theories with which we can examine learning. Our understanding of cognitive neuroscience has advanced and helps us to better manage the exponential growth of medical knowledge. These theories help surgical educators to provide learners with skills to sift through the vast amount of information that is instantly available. Theories that help us improve understanding of how technology supports learning to distributed groups is privileged as screen-based learning continues to emerge as a key source of knowledge. Of course, we continue to seek to understand how expertise develops in the quest for excellence. Deliberate practice and mastery learning are embedded in all skills-based activities. The complex role of emotion in the process of learning, development and being a surgeon has become well ingrained into our thinking and educational practice.

Social learning theories remain of interest as formal and informal learning groups continue to support individuals at all stages of their careers. We have shifted focus to socio-material theories and other theories that offer insight to learning in complex environments. Other work-integrated learning theories are also valued. We continue to advance our understanding of how individuals develop and manage their multiple identities across surgical careers. We also have theories that address issues of team identity, as yet in 2018 an understudied but emerging topic of interest. We do not have a grand theory of surgical education but theories of the middle ground that are advancing surgical practice.

Surgical education's complexity has been fully recognised by the community and its practitioners better equipped to respond to this. An understanding of the full range of disciplinary thinking and practices the field of education has to offer is now seen as a way to make sense of surgical educational problems. When seen as conceptual frameworks to guide our educational practice and research, ideas about clinical judgement may well be seen through Aristotle's philosophical writings on phronesis as they are through psychology's findings on cognitive biases and metacognitive function. By 2030, ways to integrate disparate types of knowledge drawn from theory and beyond have been born, freeing up our ability to investigate and offer educational approaches that bring together the art and science of surgical education and surgical practice.

From Part III – *The Practice of Surgical Education* – we see many advances.

Recruitment and selection approaches have been successful in widening participation of diverse communities in surgical practice.

The use of artificial intelligence, augmented reality and robotics has enabled changes in surgical practice and therefore the ways in which surgical education occurs. These developments in technology enable surgeons and educators to *step back* from the operative site with advanced technologies performing a range of operative skills.

Improved visualisation and imaging devices have enhanced teaching and learning at the operative site. This enables operative skills that have been learned and assessed in objectives-driven, simulation-based curricula to be safely implemented under supervision in real clinical settings. All curricula are based on sound educational principles aligned with deliberate practice and new theories related to enhanced cognitive imprinting[!] There are very few procedures or techniques that cannot be learned in this stepwise simulation-based fashion followed by refinement in the actual operating theatre. Patient-specific rehearsal of procedures using simulation is commonplace for less experienced surgeons. Verbal and non-verbal communication strategies to support teaching and learning at the operative site have evolved. Screen-based supervision of surgical techniques and team-based interactions has even become a specialist educational practice.

Curricula are highly sophisticated. Patients are now routinely involved in their development. In fact, surgical educators work closely with "patients" as co-faculty in all facets of curriculum design from recruitment and selection, technical and team-based competency learning and assessment. Simulation-based activities are designed to provide full immersion in clinical experiences. Technology allows for robust curricula ensuring all surgeons across the educational continuum receive standardised materials, while surgical educators add resources and activities to address local conditions as required. For learning methods, screen-based learning forms the basis of many learning activities. Surgical educators have adapted smoothly to their incorporation in curricula and have combined them with more advanced technologies such as three-dimensional (3D) immersive environments and the now pervasive 3D printing.

Technology facilitates the delivery of surgical services in rural locations. Surgical educators support learning needs associated with these technology-based changes in surgical practice. Technology-enabled "remote" supervision of associate surgeons in rural locations is a specialist surgeon educator practice.

The process by which learners in surgical education advance has completely transitioned from the time-based apprenticeship model still practised in 2018 to truly learner-centred, competency-based progression. Associate surgeons advance at their own pace and with individualised curricula and experiences. Learning activities are sufficiently flexible to accommodate this individuality. Thus, the traditional start and end time for surgical training that centred on the academic year has transformed into a continuous cycle of learners entering programmes as individuals within them complete their educational experience and graduate, opening up spaces. In this setting, proper programme evaluation is paramount, and curricula are constantly evaluated for outcome data and refined as needed.

To date, the results are encouraging, with evaluations consistently demonstrating that we are producing technically competent, emotionally intelligent and well-rounded surgeons able to cope with stress; recognise and successfully treat rare, life-threatening events; and "connect" with patients under their care. Reflective practice is now a daily part of the surgical work with all level of surgeons debriefing after procedures and events with specialised surgical educators/coaches and within their interprofessional teams in order to refine continually knowledge, skills and attitudes to enhance patient care.

Another routine part of the surgical learning environment is the incorporation of assessments into everyday practice. In the first instance, surgical educators like ourselves can now assess their educational practice more frequently and less obtrusively by recording our educational interactions with *smarterphones* [2030 version of mobile technology], reviewing segments and making global judgements of our performance using evidence-based rating forms for the particular educational practice. These forms are used to start conversations about the quality of our work with others and not to tick boxes. Such data is cumulative and creates longitudinal pictures of our progress.

Secondly, as surgical educators, we work with surgeon colleagues who are continually making judgements on the surgical practices of surgeons, consultants and attendings. Surgeon profiles are built from thousands of measurements providing comprehensive progress reports. Entrustable professional activities have shifted to reflect new roles and scope within the practice of surgery. Evidence-based assessments occur as part of a surgeon's practice with the data collected electronically. Other objective-based performance data are collected from surgical instrumentation and wearable technologies. The cumulative feedback from these observer-based and objective-based measurements offer meaningful insights related to the strengths and weaknesses, referred to as "development foci", of individual practitioners. Patients also participate in these judgements. In addition to this individual feedback, surgeons are also evaluated on their team-based competencies.

Although teams are routinely debriefed at the end of the work sessions (e.g. multidisciplinary team meetings, ward rounds, operating theatre lists, etc.), data is now gathered from multiple sources – objective measurements related to biometric badges, movement, eye tracking and physiologic/thermal variations as well as human-derived assessments using quick, easy-to-use tools within the clinical sphere. As with aviation, "black boxes" are ubiquitous, recording procedures from multiple vantage points.

Critical junctions of the operation are now characterised by periods of only necessary communication and action, much like aviation's "sterile flight deck", referred to as operating theatre "showtime". During such periods, the black box is most active in recording pertinent information. Such monitoring only came about after tort reform in which the recordings could not be used in litigation if the surgeon reported an adverse event or near miss to the monitoring body tracking them, the Federal Aviation Administration in the United States. As a result, the data from these black boxes are combined with the other measurements of performance, linked with patient outcomes, and used to help surgical educators establish effective, steam-lined surgical practices through personalised curricula targeting identified areas for development.

This data is a key resource for surgical educators as they support associate surgeons. Surgical educators have undertaken specialist programmes to help them meaningfully use this data to support learning.

Interprofessional education is well established, and the competencies of interprofessional collaborative practice are as well-known as the CanMEDS competencies in 2018. Learning in and about surgical teams is as fundamental as learning basic wound closure skills. In fact, health professional education has been reformatted to be interprofessional in character from Day 1. In this manner, students from all the professions taking care of patients are truly learning with, from and about each other as they prepare for clinical practice. In the field of surgery, the above-mentioned interprofessional surgical practitioners play a critical role in helping surgical educators develop effective curricula.

On the information technology front, surgical educators can now work closely with education managers who can bring to bear the ever-increasing computing power and sophisticated software to prospectively identify and resolve logistical issues early. In this manner, bottlenecks are avoided and individualised learning proceeds with minimal delays or conflicts.

Beyond the exciting advances made through systems improvements, technology and enhanced performance metrics, surgical education has also incorporated approaches from the humanities ensuring that our work holds the wellbeing of all people central to our practice, including healthcare professionals themselves.

From Part IV, *Research* in surgical education now involves an established community of surgical educators, many of whom hold relevant doctoral degrees. Through needs assessments, surgical education priorities have been established at local, national and global levels and are revisited regularly. This development has already resulted in advances in the practice of surgical education as we better understand how learning occurs in complex environments. Such assessments now include patients who have voices in all our research questions. Every major surgical society, irrespective of speciality, now has educational research sessions as part of Annual Meeting programmes. To forego such sessions now risks falling behind in the dynamic world of training and education. Such a trend reached a tipping point with the refinement and development of unobtrusive, objective-based technologies for measuring surgical and team performance in the operating room. These audio-visual and sensory capture data provided a more solid link between educational interventions and performance. Finally, progress towards linking surgical education practices with patient outcomes continues apace.

## 41.3 March 2030 Diaries and a Letter to a Surgeon Educator

Finally, we share notes on our diaries as we anticipate our work practices in 2030 (Boxes 41.1, 41.2 and 41.3).

---

**Box 41.1: March 2030 – Professor Debra Nestel: Notes on My Forthcoming Week**

I'm looking forward to my week. So much to do. Some things don't change. On Monday and Thursday mornings, I'm on to that monthly cycle when I shadow two surgical consultants across their work. We check in first thing to see how their educational practice has shifted since we met last month. We discuss what they'd like to work on, why and how and then off we go. Can be anywhere in the hospital. Usually starts super early before ward rounds and then off to theatre. At the end of these coaching sessions, we revisit their goals and think about strategies to strengthen their practices and develop areas that might need work. I've worked with them for years now. It's so exciting to see their expertise in action. Both were graduates of the Master of Surgical Education programme at my University and it's really impressive to see how they have responded to these surgical coaching sessions.

On Monday afternoon, I've a planning meeting for the international surgical education conference – it used to be biannual but now annually as the global community of surgical educators has grown. This year we've had interest from the anaesthetic and operating room nurses' professional communities so it looks like the next conference will be truly interprofessional. It's taken awhile but really exciting to have this interprofessional focus on teaching and learning in the operating theatre at the next conference.

Tuesday, I've got the Graduate Programs in Surgical Education subjects on "Managing the Underperforming Surgeon (MUS)" and "Teaching Professionalism in Surgery (TPS)". On the one hand, the subjects have not changed very much since we first started them in 2010 but in other ways they've changed a lot. Selection processes seem to be addressing some of the underperformance issues that we faced early on. In the subject MUS, students identify underperformance issues from their practices. Now we have issues associated with the flexible programs (they are a bit too flexible such that surgeons are not getting sufficient experience) and all the data we now capture identifies underperformance. Often it is "not enough" performance that is at

(continued)

**Box 41.1** (continued)

issue and needs to be addressed. We don't have so many mental health issues as we did when we first started. That's really impressive. The initiatives taken by the Royal Australasian College of Surgeons on operating with respect have led to some really positive cultural changes in the work environment. It's interesting to me that the students on the Graduate Programs in Surgical Education are now mainly new consultant surgeons. These days about one-third of them go on to doctoral studies in surgical education.

Wednesday is PhD supervision day. It starts with "doctoral club" – a virtual community that meets monthly – small groups of students and although it is student-led, this month I've been invited to talk with them about the human research ethics issues for visual methodologies projects set in theatre. I then meet with students individually across the day for PhD supervision.

The rest of the week is taken up with meetings – curriculum committees, patient safety advisory, simulation. The Professor of Surgery and Professors of Surgical Education meet monthly to make sure we are informed of each other's activities.

Thursday night we're celebrating 20 years of the Academy of Surgical Educators. It will be fun to catch up with colleagues and celebrate those who have contributed so much for so long.

I no longer officially work Fridays (or Saturdays and Sundays), but old habits die hard, and I expect I'll be reviewing another manuscript submitted to the open access journal on surgical education.

Hmmm – a note has just popped up on my calendar stating that Nestel et al. (Eds.) need a third edition. Time to handover that one to some new editors. I'll enjoy looking at that Chap. 41.

**Box 41.2: March 2030 John Paige: Notes on My Forthcoming Week**
Let's see what is on the docket for this upcoming week. Looks jam packed as usual; just as I like it! I have the usual practice items: clinic all day Tuesday and operating room time Monday and Wednesday morning and all Friday. They look like typical general surgical cases, computer-aided cholecystectomies and hernias. On Friday, however, I have that complex retroperitoneal mass excision. I'm glad I get to do the rehearsal procedure Thursday afternoon using the 3D printed model that I ordered to determine the most efficient approach. I can then have the associate surgeon go through it with me and make sure we are on the same page regarding steps. I can also make sure that we go over those areas for development that were identified during the

(continued)

**Box 41.2** (continued)

associate surgeon's simulation-based training to ensure a quick, safe surgery. We will debrief after both the rehearsal and the actual procedure to help the associate surgeon identify the "take home" from each on which to work. I am glad that such debriefing is now considered a step in every procedure; it ensures that it is now done and gives the necessary time to do it, without harming efficiency in the theatre thanks to its structured, standardised protocol. The same is true for the team debriefs. They sure have helped identify systems-based issues and with efficiency and safety. The quick teamwork assessment tool that everyone completes and compares makes it work. I have my monthly assessments this week as well so Wednesday OR will be filled with "showtime" moments with black box recordings of activities that will go to the surgical coach and educators to evaluate. The surgical associate assessments will be Friday after the sarcoma excision. Team assessment is Monday morning. It seems such evaluations never stop! Fortunately, they are now used to develop individualised learning plans to improve practice and not for punitive measures!

Monday afternoon we have the new applicants coming in for surgical associate positions. We will run them through the multiple mini interviews to get help us identify those individuals who will best fit our programme. Since these simulation-based activities have become universal, attrition has plummeted and we have far fewer people encountering mental health issues. I'm sure the associate surgeons' monthly meetings with educational psychologists have helped as well. Although these interviews are continuous, we only do a few at a time, making it more doable. Wait! Monday morning I'm meeting with Debra, my surgical coach! Perfect timing. I wanted to go over some fine points in my practice, and she will be able help organise a learning programme for me. I'm still amazed we can chat real time Monday evening her time and early morning mine.

Tuesday afternoon after clinic is the Professional Development Committee (PDC) meeting to go over target items for improving learning efficiency of practicing surgeons as they perform their individualised training programs to acquire new procedural skills. With the ever-shortening doubling time of medical knowledge, it is hard to keep up and surgical educators are now more valuable than ever. After the PDC is the Credentialing Committee meeting. I am sure, we will need to advise on learning plans developed by surgical coaches for helping surgeons who want to expand their practice.

Wednesday afternoon, I have my medical education research activities within the Center for Human Factors in Healthcare. I'm so happy we have our PhD in Behavioral Psychology as the Director. She is essential to helping with

(continued)

**Box 41.2** (continued)

obtaining grants and making sure everything is running and progressing according to plans. I am sure we will have a near-miss simulation scenario to run through in order to identify systems-based issues or to test potential solutions to them. Also, we will be running more simulation-based scenarios as part of our Objective Measures in Teamwork Project. This long-running federally funded project has uncovered some truly amazing measures of highly reliable teamwork. After all that, I will need to work on manuscripts, chapters and my upcoming presentation at Australasian Simulation Congress. Too bad, I cannot go in person this year, but the Internet-based stream allows me to participate in at least some of it.

Thursday is Morbidity and Mortality (M&M) Conference followed by Grand Rounds in the morning. These standbys harken in a way back to the Halstedian days of training. They do have some significant changes though. In addition to surgical complications, M&M now have system complications presented, and the use of three-dimensional holographic images of conditions and situation combined with the black box recordings add to its value. Grand Rounds invariably involve some immersive rehearsal or practice to emphasise a topic's point. Much more interactive too with the response systems and real-time tweets. After these conferences, the surgeon associates will go do their individualised simulation-based learning plans with faculty helping to coach. Thursday afternoon is rehearsal time. This week is the 3D printed sarcoma excision. Next week is team rehearsal.

This weekend I'm covering for the group, but it will give me time to work on the curricula we are developing for the incoming associate surgeons based on the programme evaluation results from the graduating ones.

Hmmm – a note has just popped up on my calendar stating that Nestel et al. (Eds.) need a third edition. I wonder what we'll be discussing come the fifth one.

**Box 41.3: March 2030: A Letter to Dr. Paige from an Associate Surgeon**
John

It's Jamie, your favourite associate surgeon, dropping a line to let you know that I just successfully completed my final required Professional Care Performance Unit (PCPU) over at the holo-suite; I am done! It's hard to believe that I have completed my childhood dream of becoming an attending surgeon. I have taken your advice to reflect on the journey and am writing to key individuals who helped me along the way notes of appreciation (as you

(continued)

**Box 41.3** (continued)

say, doing one of these a day has been demonstrated to increase one's happiness and improves performance). I decided that you should receive my first letter, since your mentorship has been indispensable in helping me get through my associate surgeon years.

I remember how overwhelmed I felt when I first became an associate surgeon to see all the PCPUs that had to be satisfied and the criteria for each that had to be met! Each PCPU had its knowledge component that had to be mastered, its skill components with its simulation-based training and then its immersive experience in 3D that had to be passed before being allowed to use the robots to cut on a patient. Each step of the way, this or that criterion had to be reached to go to the next step. Then there were the Touchstones that had to be reached at certain points along the way. I thought I would never make it! Your advice regarding approaching each PCPU one at a time, satisfying the Touchstones along the way and going at the pace that worked for me was a really calming influence. I am still amazed at how fine the assessment devices have become: tensiometers, eye trackers, motion analysis, biometric badges and pattern evaluation software now so advanced that the devices are unobtrusive and almost unnoticeable when applied. I still go back and print up 3D models for practice based on the particular patient anatomy and case I am doing. I learned that from you and the other attending surgeons who go through the simulations and training to learn new procedures and practice on 3D models for difficult cases. I know I will be ready for the annual return to the immersive 3D environment for the required touch-ups and refinements needed based on my performance as an attending surgeon.

I want to especially thank you for your teaching in the operating room. I will miss those pre-briefs, the structured interoperative teaching and our debriefings afterwards. Most of all, however, I will miss those wonderful "take home" points that each debriefing ended on. They really helped to direct and focus my learning and practice. Thank you.

As I said, you are only the first of a series of people I am going to reach out to. Since it was your idea, I will give you the run down. Tomorrow, I am going to contact my Sociology Professor from my College days. I remember thinking that the required "minor" in soft science/liberal arts topics (psychology, sociology, history, philosophy) for pre-preparation was a waste of time. Hard sciences like biology and chemistry were only needed! I now appreciate how this requisite really helps with empathy and emotional intelligence development, something really needed in surgery. Those mini multiple interviews before boot camp work (BCW) showed that this was lacking before the minor requirement came into being.

(continued)

**Box 41.3** (continued)

The next day, I am going to reach out to my good friend from my first year learning team from my pre-licensure training (PLT) days at the Health Sciences Centre. I think he is a respiratory therapist (RT) now. We met Day 1. I remember our learning team, like all others at the Health Sciences Centre, was a mélange of interprofessional pre-licensure students. We had my RT buddy, a dental student, an occupational therapy student and an undergraduate nursing student. We did everything together that first year. I still can't believe how seamlessly fused the curricula are at the pre-licensure level now. Sure, we did break out into our track teams after the first year to focus on more in depth/specialty specific topics. We all came together as interprofessional teams on the wards, however, and everyone had the simulation-based training before the wards to hit the PCPUs of PLT: teamwork, history taking, physical exam, technical skills and emotional intelligence. That last year on clinical rotations was intensive, especially the BCW everyone did the last half.

That brings me to the next person, the head of the BCW selection process. I remember all those simulation scenarios to go through: the immersive simulations in virtual 3D that may or may not have been in a clinical setting, the skills teaching with faculty in which they really assessed your ability to learn, the high-fidelity mannequin and tabletop sessions assessing teamwork and clinical knowledge, give a 2-min presentation challenge in which one had to demonstrate their ability to quickly locate and assimilate evidence-based information, the standardised patient interactions, etc. They really knew how to select the best candidates for each programme this way, and I wanted to thank him for getting me into the BCW and then pairing me up as an associate surgeon at this program.

I am really looking forward to working with you as new faculty here to teach the up and coming associate surgeons. I still can't believe I succeeded in getting the position! Thank you for your help with that as well!

I appreciate all the hard work and dedication you put into teaching; it was my motivation to do the same!

Sincerely,
Jamie

## 41.4 Closing in 2018

Surgical practice and surgical education are intricately interwoven. A change in one profoundly impacts the other. At times, surgical education will lead to shifts in surgical practice and vice versa – always meeting societal needs as the endpoint. Sometimes surgical education work can feel very distant to that endpoint but by supporting the development of surgeons who work directly with patients and their relatives, the value of the work must not be underestimated. Whatever facet of education, the surgical educator has a tremendous responsibility. This chapter has offered a glimpse into how competency-based curricula, simulated-based practice and work-integrated learning will develop by 2030. However, the human interactions with patients and their families will remain a rich source of learning, together with relationships with colleagues. These personal interactions will likely continue as the most compelling source of learning. It has been exciting to work with our colleagues who have contributed to this book. We value their breadth of experience and willingness to share it within this volume. We hope you have enjoyed this collection.

# Index

**A**
Academia, 33, 36, 37, 41, 42
Academy of Master Surgeons, 2
Academy of medical Educators (AoME), 25, 139
Academy of Surgical Educators, 2, 26, 349, 358, 476
Acquisition, 5, 14, 24, 36, 71, 74, 82, 106, 107, 112, 130, 150–152, 155, 183, 184, 188–191, 242, 248, 250, 270, 276, 316–318, 330, 331, 351, 365, 451
Activity theory, 56, 105–112
Actor-network theory (ANT), 107, 108, 112
Acts, 136, 425, 445–450, 470
Alder hay Children's Hosp, 12
Analysis, 14, 35, 36, 38, 55, 70, 83, 85, 106, 116, 137, 159, 168, 172, 198, 240, 261, 294, 330, 339, 342, 344, 346, 347, 355–358, 360, 364, 373, 379, 383, 384, 386, 393–395, 397–398, 400, 401, 407–410, 412–415, 417, 418, 433–434, 437, 442, 446, 449, 452, 453, 462, 464, 479
Anticipatory socialisation, 128
Apprenticeship, 2, 7, 10, 11, 46, 95, 96, 106, 136, 213, 229, 230, 234, 236, 271, 330, 353, 356–357, 364, 367, 408, 410, 447, 462, 473
Aptitude testin, 163, 168
Artefacts, 107–110, 112
Assessment, 8, 11, 18, 46, 61, 70, 91, 96, 107, 116, 129, 134, 146, 163, 174, 185, 199, 209, 221–226, 230, 241, 257, 270, 293, 305, 315, 330, 344, 364, 379, 389, 427, 452, 459, 472

Association of Surgeons in Training (ASiT), 135
Attitudes, 22, 23, 26, 35–37, 41, 57, 135, 136, 138, 139, 153, 159, 164, 175, 205, 230, 273, 283, 291, 292, 295, 297, 298, 320, 330, 390, 399, 473
Audiences, 63, 64, 117, 178, 263, 265, 266, 340, 344, 359, 374, 445, 447–449
Augmented reality, 472

**B**
'Becoming', 9, 56, 80, 83, 92, 102, 103, 123–130, 133–139, 175, 205, 232, 234, 294, 306, 307, 335, 357, 370, 374, 478
Behaviour, 19–22, 25, 39, 40, 80, 81, 87, 103, 109, 116, 118–121, 126–128, 138, 160, 165, 167, 175–177, 179, 211–213, 231, 304, 306, 313, 315–317, 320–324, 335, 343, 357, 359, 393, 399, 400, 407, 415, 416, 418, 424, 426, 431, 436, 437, 465, 470
Behaviourism, 59, 61
'Being', 2, 11, 15, 18–20, 22–24, 27–29, 37, 39, 42, 47, 50, 53, 59, 61, 63, 65, 69, 70, 72, 73, 75, 81–83, 85, 86, 90, 91, 96, 97, 106, 107, 109, 110, 115–120, 123–130, 134–139, 143, 153, 154, 160–162, 165, 175, 179, 185, 188–191, 194, 197, 198, 203, 206, 212, 214, 224, 233–237, 239, 242, 245, 256, 261, 263, 285, 286, 305, 306, 308, 318, 322, 332, 333, 344, 345, 347, 350, 354, 356–361, 364, 371, 379, 385, 386, 390, 394, 406, 408, 411–413, 416, 417, 425, 426, 431, 432, 434, 463, 471

Beneficence, 12, 371, 425, 427, 436, 437
Best evidence Medical Education (BEME), 137
BID, 142, 174, 179, 186, 191–195
Biomedical, 3, 5, 14, 21, 135, 199, 201, 291, 347, 348, 350, 356, 361, 365, 367, 371, 397, 406, 420, 427
Bleakley, A., 108, 419
Boundary object, 109
Briefings, 174, 179, 186–187, 194, 195, 290, 334
Bullying and harassment, 19, 459, 465

## C
Career information, 160
Case study, 103, 108–111, 124–126, 128, 407, 419
Certification, 8, 47, 51–52, 143, 222, 225, 235–237, 239, 240, 243, 244, 246, 249, 250
Checklists, 209, 283, 290–292, 298, 329, 334, 390, 391, 396, 398, 419
Chunking, 60, 71
Clinical
  competence committee, 116, 339, 452, 454, 455
  tasks, 230, 231, 233, 234, 237
Cognitive, 19, 23, 37, 55, 57–66, 71, 87–90, 106, 110–112, 154, 165, 172, 183, 184, 186, 189–191, 225, 281, 297, 331, 332, 334, 355, 357, 360, 408, 410, 416, 464, 471, 472
  load, 58, 63–64, 191
  neuroscience, 57–66, 471
Coherence, 406, 408, 411, 420, 448
Colleges, 8, 20–22, 24, 28, 29, 45–53, 176, 236, 243, 460, 465
Communication, 19–21, 23, 25, 37, 96, 99, 126, 129, 130, 152, 176, 178, 179, 200–203, 214–219, 223, 240, 242, 245–247, 250, 273, 274, 284, 285, 290–293, 296, 315–317, 329, 331–333, 357, 401, 419, 454, 459, 464, 470, 472, 474
Communities of practice, 3, 40, 55, 56, 95–103, 107, 125–126, 137, 138, 355, 358, 382, 415, 441
Community, 2–4, 7, 11, 13, 14, 20, 27–29, 34, 73, 82, 95–102, 106, 107, 119, 125–129, 134, 138, 139, 142, 151, 166, 173, 204, 205, 236, 303, 340, 342, 348, 349, 353, 358, 390, 415, 419, 439–443, 446, 461, 470–472, 474–476
Community of practice, 20, 95–103, 134, 139, 173, 340, 353, 358, 419, 439–443
Competence, 19, 22, 29, 34, 71, 72, 97, 116, 142, 158, 163, 226, 231, 233, 242, 244, 313, 315, 321, 339, 347, 350, 451, 452, 454, 455
Competency-based assessment, 129
Competency-based education, 2, 188
Complexity, 36, 39, 56, 62, 70, 85, 90, 91, 106, 124, 126, 137, 144, 158, 174, 187, 281, 283, 289, 330, 331, 334, 345, 381, 407, 414, 419, 428, 430–432, 442, 449, 472
Conceptual framework, 143, 164, 190, 258, 346, 350, 411, 472
Confidentiality, 308, 330, 434–435
Connections, 108, 109, 260, 366
Consensus statement, 158–159, 167
Consent, 12, 199, 202, 266, 308, 371, 372, 431–432, 435, 437, 452
Constructivist, 116, 135, 137, 138, 213, 344, 345, 406, 408, 411, 415, 447
Contemporary challenges, 9
Continuing professional development, 20, 21, 240–243, 246, 295
Cosmological model, 447
Creating a Research Space (CARS), 368, 374
Curriculum design, 91, 130, 141, 150, 257, 472

## D
Data, 15, 70, 103, 134, 154, 160, 223, 242, 256, 273, 313, 331, 342, 355, 366, 378, 389, 406, 430, 440, 446, 452, 473
Dave taxonomy, 184–186, 189, 190, 194
Davydov, V.V., 110
Debriefing, 5, 142, 174, 175, 179, 186, 188, 193–195, 274, 294, 296, 297, 332, 333, 473, 477, 479
Deliberate practice, 20, 55, 70, 75, 152, 184, 186, 190, 191, 248, 262, 330, 446, 471, 472
Deontology, 425, 426
Design frameworks, 142, 391
Dialogue, 24, 27, 28, 39, 81, 130, 142, 217, 218, 237, 265, 344, 356, 358, 430, 449
Disciplinary power, 118, 119
Discourse, 14, 90, 116–121, 123, 142, 183, 218, 240, 246, 305, 440, 441

Index

Documentation, 98, 166, 226, 315, 359, 395, 428
Domain, 63, 70–72, 74, 75, 95, 97, 98, 124, 150, 154, 159, 162, 168, 177, 184, 188, 223, 332, 347, 349, 354, 411, 442, 443
Domains of surgical performance, 155
Double stimulation, 109, 110

**E**
Educational
  alliance, 210, 213, 218
  change, 12, 134
  strategies, 65, 136, 151, 177
Educationalist, 14, 15, 62, 139, 353–355, 359, 460
E-learning, 23, 91, 92, 210, 459, 463
Emotional intelligence (EI), 164, 479, 480
Entrustment, 237
Epistemological shift, 80, 83
Epistemology, 307, 342, 343, 356, 367
Ethics, 5, 115, 199, 244, 265, 266, 340, 359, 371, 373, 423–437, 442, 476
Evaluation, 2, 24, 110, 141, 146, 149–151, 154–155, 166, 217, 221, 223, 225, 232, 237, 248, 256–266, 272, 276, 281, 294, 307, 319–321, 324, 341, 342, 344, 347, 364, 389–402, 427, 452–455, 465, 473, 477–479
Evidence-based medicine, 332, 378
Expansive learning, 109, 110, 112
Expertise, 2, 4, 12–15, 19, 21, 47, 48, 55, 69–75, 83, 128, 133–135, 137, 139, 152, 164, 188, 194, 199, 201, 249, 274, 280, 283, 294, 306, 342, 379, 382–384, 398, 414, 415, 446–448, 461, 471, 475

**F**
Faculty development, 5, 24, 137, 149, 195, 235, 250, 251, 276, 347, 466
Faculty of Surgical Trainers, 2, 349
Feedback, 20, 23, 24, 38, 41, 55, 61, 71, 74, 81, 89, 103, 134, 138, 142, 143, 149, 151, 152, 154, 166, 172, 174–176, 188–190, 192, 193, 195, 205, 209–219, 221, 222, 224, 230, 233, 235, 237, 241, 244, 245, 247, 248, 257, 262, 272–274, 294, 318, 320, 322, 331, 379, 410, 430, 435, 446, 453, 460, 464, 473
"FINER," 368
Flexner Minimally invasive surgery, 10

Formative, 49, 66, 136, 154, 210, 218, 221, 222, 224, 233, 234, 257, 262, 263, 330, 390, 391, 460
  evaluation, 257
Foucault, 115–119, 121, 124, 426
Framework, 2, 10, 19, 21, 52, 55, 58, 69, 72, 79–92, 96, 102, 103, 125, 139, 142, 143, 164, 185, 186, 190, 198, 218, 222–224, 233, 237, 242, 244, 246, 258, 260, 293, 298, 308, 318, 332, 334, 342, 344, 345, 350, 357, 372, 374, 391, 406, 408, 411, 424, 427, 433, 436, 441, 442, 455, 456, 472
Fundamentals of laparoscopic surgery, 225, 271

**G**
General Medical Council (GMC), 36, 45, 46, 137, 245
Global revalidation, 242–246
Governance, 8, 21, 45–53, 329
Graduate programs in education, 3, 4, 26, 475, 476
Grounded theory, 343, 356, 414–419, 440–442

**H**
Halftone, 449
Harold Shipman, 12
Hidden curriculum, 20, 21, 89, 119, 137, 151, 153, 161, 179, 284, 347, 461
High reliability, 283, 284, 293, 328, 398
Human factors (HF), 5, 19–21, 143, 144, 259, 280–284, 290, 328, 477
Human research ethics, 340, 371, 427, 431, 476

**I**
Identity, 2, 11, 14, 15, 39, 56, 80–83, 88, 92, 97, 99, 102, 103, 109, 118, 119, 124–129, 133, 134, 136–138, 153, 179, 205, 206, 233, 304, 356, 374, 420, 431, 434, 435, 437, 440, 472
  formation, 125, 127–129, 138, 440
Impact evaluation, 263, 390–402
Individual interviews, 84, 371, 442
Informal learning, 105, 471
Information processing, 58–62, 66, 281
Innovation, 4, 7, 10, 12, 15, 29, 42, 80, 269, 276, 279, 339, 341, 357, 411, 414, 419

Intercollegiate Surgical Curriculum
    Project, 14, 85
Interpretivist, 138
Inter-professional education (IPE), 5, 143,
    197, 289, 293, 297, 474
Interprofessionalism, 126–127
Interprofessional surgical practitioner, 470,
    474
Interrupted time series, 396, 398
Interviews, 81, 84, 85, 87, 138, 159, 164–166,
    315, 343, 356, 360, 371, 373, 407, 408,
    411–413, 416–418, 433, 434, 437, 442,
    446, 477, 479

**J**
Journals, 3, 98, 161, 339, 346, 349, 365, 429
Justice, 40, 371, 425, 427, 437

**K**
Keyhole surgery, 12–15
Kirkpatrick, 138, 262, 263, 297
Knot working, 109, 112
Knowledge synthesis, 332

**L**
Language, 4, 33, 55, 62, 71, 80, 87, 99–101,
    136, 138, 162, 191, 203, 265, 285,
    305–309, 321, 359, 364, 365, 385, 409,
    413, 431, 439, 441, 470, 471
Laparoscopic community of practice, 439–443
Latour, B., 107, 108
Lave, J., 95, 97, 107, 408, 415
Leadership, 5, 7, 8, 19, 20, 25, 26, 33–42, 51,
    147–149, 152, 255, 274, 292, 294, 319,
    331–333, 419, 455, 461, 465, 466, 471
Learner-centred, 18, 22, 74, 91, 137, 210,
    215–217, 219, 473
Learning, 3, 9, 18, 37, 56, 70, 81, 95, 105,
    118, 134, 147, 158, 171–179, 186,
    197–206, 210, 221, 233, 241, 256, 269,
    290, 305, 317, 330, 342, 354, 365, 379,
    393, 405–420, 428, 439, 446, 460, 470
    curve, 74, 90, 99, 138, 147, 179, 270–272,
        276, 330, 463
Legitimacy, 36, 99, 125, 126, 128, 129
Legitimate peripheral participation (LPP), 98,
    100, 102, 103
Leont'ev, A.N., 106

Levels of evidence, 355
Liminal states, 82
Literature review, 293, 317, 339, 355, 367,
    373, 374, 377, 378, 380, 382, 383, 387,
    416
Lived experience, 446
Living curriculum, 97
Logic Model, 258–260
Longitudinal development, 138
Long term memory, 60, 62, 63, 65

**M**
Macro, 2, 7, 18, 21, 24, 210, 262
Maintenance of certification (MOC), 240, 243,
    249, 250
Mastery learning, 55, 58, 59, 64–66, 330, 471
Meaning frames, 90
Measurement, 2, 134, 139, 164, 260, 262, 296,
    297, 334–335, 339, 347, 390, 391, 394,
    396–402, 453, 455, 462, 473, 474
Medical education, 11, 18–20, 24, 26, 52, 74,
    82, 115, 119, 142, 148, 150, 167, 188,
    197, 198, 202, 206, 210, 212, 213, 215,
    224, 236, 321, 346–348, 367, 374, 377,
    397, 414, 461, 477
Mental health, 39, 319, 459, 465, 476, 477
Mentor(ing), 26, 53, 91, 148, 212, 271, 318,
    365, 366, 459, 461–462, 466, 467, 469
Meso, 7, 18, 21, 24
Meta-ethnography, 380, 383, 386
Metaphor, 106, 204, 367, 447–449
Methodology, 5, 50, 159, 294, 342, 343, 349,
    356, 365, 367, 370–374, 378–384, 386,
    393, 394, 402, 406, 407, 409, 411,
    414–416, 418, 440–442
Micro, 2, 12, 18, 21, 24, 210
M&M rounds, 117–121
Modelling, 20, 138, 167, 179, 306
Moral education, 35
Motor skills, 13, 172, 175, 324
Multi-disciplinary learning, 139

**N**
National Health Service (NHS), 10, 46, 47,
    198, 245, 428
'Newcomers', 83, 98–100, 103, 107
Nobility of purpose, 36, 42
Non-technical competencies, 19–21, 23, 24,
    130, 357

Index 487

Non-technical skills, 7, 13, 20–21, 25, 26, 73, 202, 270, 273–275, 293, 316, 324, 328, 331–333, 357, 398, 451, 460, 462

**O**

'Old timers', 98, 99, 103
Ontological shift, 80, 83, 89, 91
Ontology(ies), 112, 307, 309, 342, 343, 356, 367, 442
Operation, 61, 89, 107, 110, 111, 117, 136, 172, 174, 175, 177, 178, 186, 205, 234–237, 249, 257, 273, 274, 276, 281, 283, 407–410, 413, 416, 417, 454, 474
Opportunistic learning, 96
Outcome measurements, 134, 297, 334, 335, 347, 391, 397–399, 401, 402

**P**

Paradigm(s), 5, 13, 116, 135–136, 151, 152, 270, 276, 339–346, 348–350, 353–357, 363–367, 370–371, 374, 383, 409, 412, 417, 418, 420, 429, 439–443
Participation, 29, 35, 96–100, 102, 103, 106, 107, 112, 125, 138, 162, 173, 177, 187, 198, 218, 242, 245, 249, 258, 259, 275, 291, 296, 343, 345, 349, 371, 413, 430–432, 436, 437, 472
Pastoral power, 119, 120
Patient involvement, 197–200, 204, 206
Patient voice, 198
Performance, 10, 18, 23, 37, 55, 61, 70, 89, 96, 108, 116, 134, 149, 158, 174, 184, 209, 222, 229, 240, 256, 270, 283, 290, 304, 315, 330, 348, 394, 416, 448, 452, 470
Personality assessment, 157, 163, 164
Personal statements, 162–166
Person specification, 157, 159, 160, 167, 168
Phronesis, 304, 306, 309, 472
Positivist paradigm, 116, 344, 363–366, 374
Power and positionality, 423, 432–433
Practice, 1, 10, 18, 34, 47, 58, 70, 79, 80, 95–103, 105, 115, 116, 123, 134, 145, 158, 172, 183, 197–206, 209, 222, 230, 239–251, 258, 269, 279, 290, 303–310, 313, 329, 341, 353, 364, 382, 389, 405, 423, 439–443, 446, 451, 461, 469
Practice-based learning and improvement (PBLI), 242
Pre-/post-test design, 396

Primacy, 53, 61
Procedural skill, 57, 65, 242, 270, 401, 460, 477
Professional
 activities, 142, 229–237, 473
 identities, 56, 102, 119, 123–126, 130, 133, 134, 136, 138, 153, 179, 304, 440
Professionalism, 9, 15, 19, 20, 24, 29, 96, 99, 116, 125, 143, 152, 165, 177, 206, 213, 240, 242, 245, 247, 303–310, 315, 319, 322, 323, 454
Professionalization, 363
Program evaluation, 145, 146, 154, 155, 255–266, 364, 389–391, 394, 395, 397
Psychomotor skills, 18, 65, 142, 163, 183–195, 470

**Q**

Qualitative, 5, 14, 83, 136, 138, 139, 172, 198, 209, 226, 340, 342–348, 356–360, 363–367, 370–371, 377–387, 405–420, 428–430, 433, 434, 439–450
Qualitative surgical education research, 442
Quality, 2, 18, 37, 45, 69, 141, 143, 147, 166, 173, 185, 200, 217, 229, 240, 256, 269, 279, 297, 319, 328, 347, 356, 379, 390, 405, 428, 439, 456, 465, 473
Quantitative measurements, 226, 339, 389–402
Quasi-experimental design, 395, 396

**R**

Rapport, 81, 138, 432, 436, 437
Realist review, 380, 381, 383, 386
Recency, 61
Recruitment, 42, 51, 141, 150, 157, 158, 160, 167, 258, 317, 371–373, 409, 429, 430, 432, 433, 436, 442, 466, 472
Reflection, 3, 4, 21, 87, 88, 110, 121, 127, 128, 130, 136–138, 142–144, 175, 186, 307, 309, 364, 366, 367, 410, 436, 442, 446
Reflection-in-action, 136
Reflexivity, 370, 408, 415, 418, 440–442
Regulation, 118, 135, 243, 250, 284, 305, 319
Reliability, 150, 159, 162, 165–167, 211, 224, 283, 284, 289, 293, 328, 332, 339, 345, 380, 398, 399, 431
Remediation, 20, 24, 154, 313, 315, 321–324

Research
  design/standards, 341, 356, 360, 364, 370, 406, 408, 429–430
  integrity, 371
  methods, 256, 346, 356, 358, 365, 371–372, 374, 389, 394, 408, 428, 430, 432
  paradigm, 5, 341–346, 350, 353, 355–356, 363, 371, 374, 412, 420, 439, 440
  questions, 341, 343, 344, 346, 358, 365–368, 370, 372, 377–380, 382, 383, 387, 406, 407, 409, 411, 414, 415, 428–430, 440–442, 474
  Spider, 364, 365
Researcher, 3, 41, 42, 139, 172, 221, 274, 284, 341–346, 348–350, 357, 358, 360, 363–366, 370–372, 374, 384, 387, 392, 405–409, 412–418, 420, 423, 424, 426, 428–436, 440–442, 446, 449, 456
Resources, 19, 23, 27, 28, 41, 42, 47, 50, 63, 64, 88, 92, 96, 98, 141, 146–152, 155, 165, 191, 195, 246, 248, 255–258, 260, 261, 264, 266, 293, 294, 323, 324, 333, 349, 370, 382, 393, 394, 416–418, 426, 432, 441, 455, 462, 466, 472, 474
Respect for persons, 423, 427, 431, 434, 436
Revalidation, 21, 24, 143, 239–251
Robotics, 15, 459, 463, 472

S
Safety, 5, 13, 19–21, 23, 24, 29, 34, 47, 108, 117, 144, 147, 151, 154, 186, 188, 191, 194, 198, 204, 205, 232, 236, 240, 244, 245, 270, 271, 273, 274, 283, 284, 290, 293, 296–298, 318–320, 322, 327–335, 371, 390, 391, 396, 407, 410, 411, 414, 419, 430, 448, 449, 466, 476, 477
Sampling, 380, 394, 397, 400, 409, 415–418
SBT, *see* Simulation-based training
Schema, 57, 58, 63, 64, 66, 223
Scholarship, 6, 22, 26, 29, 35, 138, 339, 364
Scientific surgery, 10
Selection methods, 157–161, 168
Self-awareness, 39, 137, 332
Self-regulated learning, 188
Sensitising concept, 446
Sfard, A., 106
'Silver Scalpel', 135
Simulation, 4–6, 12–15, 21, 23, 24, 55, 65, 69, 72–75, 91, 92, 96, 101, 105, 115, 143, 144, 147, 151, 152, 154, 183, 184, 186, 190, 200, 201, 203, 210, 211, 216, 225, 236, 241, 245, 247, 250, 256, 269–277, 279, 289, 291–298, 322, 324, 327–335, 339, 340, 347, 357, 381, 401, 419, 451–456, 459, 460, 462–463, 466, 467, 470, 472, 476–480
Simulation-based training (SBT), 10, 74, 270, 273, 276, 290, 291, 293–298, 330, 452, 477, 479, 480
Simulation care pathways, 275–277, 451
Situated, 98, 99, 106, 134, 172, 345, 424, 431
Situated learning, 97–99, 105, 107, 108, 408
Socialisation, 20, 89, 124, 127, 128, 138
Social media, 459, 463–464, 470
Social obligation, 27–29
Social science, 4, 14, 19, 133–135, 139, 347, 363, 368, 370–371, 384, 389, 427, 440
Social system, 109
Socio-cultural, 419
Socio-cultural learning theory, 95, 102
Socio-material, 471
Specialities, 85, 105, 109, 110, 159, 230, 313, 460, 474
Stakeholder, 49, 73, 141, 150, 219, 223–225, 241, 250, 257–260, 262–266, 344, 350, 370–372, 374, 391, 393, 395, 398, 425
Standards, 2, 10, 13, 18, 21, 22, 24, 25, 27, 29, 37–38, 47, 49–53, 66, 127, 143, 166, 185, 188, 190, 191, 193–195, 201, 202, 213, 215, 216, 223, 225, 234, 239, 241–243, 245–248, 250, 257, 266, 274, 275, 306, 315, 319, 320, 323, 379, 381, 386, 394, 397, 399, 406, 439
Strategy, 24, 27, 29, 35, 37, 65, 66, 89, 92, 136, 142–144, 151, 153, 172–175, 177, 178, 184, 185, 190, 193–195, 209, 211–218, 221–224, 226, 239, 242, 243, 247, 248, 264, 269, 284, 290, 293, 313, 329, 331, 332, 334, 342, 356, 357, 360, 365, 366, 380, 385, 411, 472, 475
Summative, 49, 50, 142, 154, 210, 221–226, 229, 230, 235, 263, 330, 390, 460
Summative evaluation, 257
Supervision, 10, 23, 24, 27, 47, 99, 101, 143, 147, 151, 153, 174, 183, 186, 211, 229, 230, 232, 233, 236, 237, 249, 306, 307, 318, 321, 381, 448, 470, 472, 473, 476
Supervisor, 5, 25, 26, 65, 137, 143, 166, 209–215, 218, 229, 235, 237, 307–309, 316, 318, 320, 321, 364–366, 378, 379, 381, 382, 393, 442

Surgeon coach, 470
Surgeon educator, 2, 15, 24, 96, 102, 133–139, 149, 167, 175, 177, 179, 304, 446, 448, 457, 469, 473, 475–480
Surgery, 2, 9, 18, 35, 46, 69, 79–92, 96, 105, 117, 124, 133, 145, 157, 171, 183, 198, 212, 222, 229, 243, 256, 269, 279, 289, 303, 314, 328, 347, 354, 371, 378, 406, 435, 440, 445–456, 461, 470
Surgical coach, 470, 475, 477
Surgical community, 14, 29, 40, 73, 97–103, 126, 128, 142, 151, 470
Surgical consultants, 73, 475
Surgical education, 1, 4, 15, 18, 28, 42, 57, 206, 229, 237, 335, 339, 341, 350, 460, 472
Surgical education research, 3, 55, 56, 172, 179, 339–351, 353–361, 363–374, 402, 408, 423–437, 442
Surgical educator, 2, 3, 7, 9, 24–26, 49, 55–58, 65, 66, 80, 92, 100–102, 121, 130, 137–139, 143, 144, 150–152, 171–173, 213, 216, 235, 258, 279, 280, 289, 290, 293, 294, 298, 339, 342, 349, 350, 358, 363, 367, 371, 374, 396, 401, 407, 420, 457, 469–481
Surgical firm(s), 10, 233
Surgical identity, 11, 14, 15, 123–130, 133–139
Surgical knowledge, 4, 95, 98, 99, 101, 242, 247, 248, 371
Surgical procedure, 49, 96, 107, 109, 110, 118, 120, 183, 215, 270, 280, 322
Surgical program evaluation, 261
Surgical team(s), 12, 101, 106, 143, 174, 178–179, 205, 206, 233, 274, 279–286, 289–298, 332, 368, 392, 396, 474
Surgical trainees, 20, 22, 23, 26, 42, 51, 52, 55, 80, 84, 85, 92, 95–97, 99, 101, 103, 119, 121, 125, 126, 147, 152, 157, 162, 163, 166, 167, 177, 198, 211, 218, 225, 229, 231, 233, 234, 273, 313, 314, 316, 317, 347, 366, 394, 398, 439, 440, 442, 461, 464, 466, 469, 470
Surgical trainer, 2, 95, 134, 349, 460, 470
Surgical training, 4, 7, 8, 11, 12, 17, 19–24, 26–29, 45–53, 65, 69, 72–75, 79, 83–88, 95–103, 106, 115, 116, 118, 119, 121, 129, 135, 136, 138, 141, 145, 146, 150, 153, 160, 161, 163, 164, 167, 186, 189, 206, 210–211, 225, 226, 230–237, 271, 272, 276, 277, 317–319, 349, 356, 374, 390, 391, 397, 419, 457, 460, 461, 466, 473

Systematic review(s), 225, 293, 330, 339, 346, 355, 378, 379, 381, 383, 384, 386, 387
Systems approach, 273

**T**
Tactics, 35, 37
Teaching, 3–5, 15, 17, 18, 20–27, 41, 61, 65, 75, 81, 91, 101, 116, 118, 135–138, 141–143, 147–150, 152–155, 158, 171–179, 185–188, 194, 195, 200, 202, 203, 215–217, 246, 256, 260, 264, 269, 276, 279, 280, 290, 293, 297, 304–310, 322, 328, 330, 333, 347, 354, 357, 371, 381, 407–410, 412, 420, 434, 448, 460, 462, 467, 472, 475, 479, 480
Team training, 5, 143, 152. 279, 289, 291–296, 298, 328, 333–335
Teamwork, 21, 23–25, 96, 99, 139, 245, 247, 250, 273, 279, 280, 284–286, 289, 290, 292, 293, 295, 297, 298, 329, 332, 333, 401, 477, 478, 480
Technical skills, 13, 14, 19, 34, 49, 85, 86, 96, 145, 151, 152, 163, 202, 211, 225, 230, 232, 239, 247, 270, 271, 273, 274, 276, 279, 280, 297, 315, 316, 318, 322, 328, 330–331, 335, 451, 454, 462, 480
Technology, 12, 74, 105, 110, 145, 186, 211, 244, 257, 276, 280, 281, 296, 330, 406, 431, 457, 460–463, 466, 471–474
Temple report, 136
Theatre, 11, 13, 15, 74, 83, 88–89, 98–101, 105, 106, 110, 112, 141, 142, 171–179, 205, 206, 210, 215, 230, 236, 304, 309, 322, 331, 332, 334, 335, 354, 406, 407, 410, 412, 414, 418, 435, 440, 442, 446, 448, 449, 470, 472–477
Theatre script, 445
Theoretical framework, 102, 125, 190, 346, 406, 441, 442
Theory, 1, 35, 55, 57, 70, 79, 95, 105–112, 137, 172, 218, 232, 259, 279–286, 296, 307, 341, 354, 383, 393, 408, 424, 440, 447, 472
Thesis, 435, 445
Threshold capability
theory, 89
Threshold concepts, 55, 79–92, 172, 353, 355–358
Time for Training
Report, 136
Time management, 165, 353, 354, 360, 361

Training, 2, 10, 17, 33, 45, 65, 69, 79, 95–103, 106, 115, 125, 134, 145, 157–168, 177, 186, 198, 210, 221, 229, 239, 256, 270, 279, 289, 313, 327, 349, 354, 363, 378, 389, 410, 429, 440, 448, 451, 459, 469
Training-the-trainer, 26, 138
Transformative, 7, 12, 33, 34, 36, 80–83, 90, 91, 138, 139, 345
Transitions, 39, 79–92, 106, 121, 148, 222, 232, 233, 235, 246, 272, 370, 374
Trends, 280, 305, 342, 346–347, 474
Troublesome knowledge, 79–92
Trust, 2, 12, 15, 53, 109, 194, 209, 210, 212, 239, 245, 432, 448

**U**

Uncertainty, 13, 15, 42, 83, 85, 88–92, 410–414, 416, 420
Underperformance, 144, 313–324, 465, 475
Unprofessional, 127, 128, 320, 322, 324, 435
Urgency, 19, 37, 42, 230, 354
Utilitarianism, 424–426

**V**

Validity, 88, 150, 159, 162, 164–167, 223, 224, 231, 234, 294, 297, 339, 345, 347, 374, 386, 396, 398–401, 406, 409, 430, 437, 453, 454, 462
Values, 4, 5, 15, 23, 35–37, 39, 41, 96, 99, 101, 112, 116, 118, 119, 121, 125, 127–129, 137, 138, 142, 150, 153, 159, 206, 214, 283, 305–307, 345, 379, 380, 382, 406–410, 416, 418, 420, 424

Verification and Validation Model, 248, 394, 399, 401, 402
Virtual reality, 6, 74, 271, 275, 330, 394, 462, 466
Virtue ethics, 425–426, 435
Virtues, 303–310, 426
Vision, 13, 35–37, 124, 127, 466
Vygotsky, L., 106, 109, 110

**W**

Wenger, E., 95, 97, 98, 103, 107, 125, 138, 355, 408, 415
Wickham, J., 12, 13
Work-based assessment, 23, 210, 232–235, 459
Workforce planning, 27, 51
Working hours, 22, 105, 136, 319
Working memory, 58, 60–63, 65
Workplace, 22, 24, 49, 55, 56, 95, 96, 99, 100, 102, 105–112, 134, 136, 142, 154, 162, 164, 167, 168, 209–215, 229, 233, 234, 241, 247, 281, 283, 317, 364, 419, 465, 470
Worldviews, 56, 125, 199, 342
World War II, 10, 280, 281

**Y**

Yrjo Engeström, 106

**Z**

Zone of proximal development, 41, 110, 194

GPSR Compliance

The European Union's (EU) General Product Safety Regulation (GPSR) is a set of rules that requires consumer products to be safe and our obligations to ensure this.

If you have any concerns about our products, you can contact us on

ProductSafety@springernature.com

In case Publisher is established outside the EU, the EU authorized representative is:

Springer Nature Customer Service Center GmbH
Europaplatz 3
69115 Heidelberg, Germany

www.ingramcontent.com/pod-product-compliance
Lightning Source LLC
LaVergne TN
LVHW020349080526
838201LV00123B/155